Forensic Medicine, Toxicology and Medical Jurisprudence

Second Edition

W0225633

Forensic Medicine, Toxicology and Medical Jurisprudence
Second Edition

ISBN: 978-93-88178-87-7

Second Edition: 2019

First Edition: 2004

Reprint: 2008

Published by Satish Kumar Jain and Produced by Varun Jain for

CBS Publishers & Distributors Pvt Ltd
4819/XI Prahlad Street, 24 Ansari Road, Daryaganj, New Delhi 110 002, India.
Ph: 23289259, 23266861, 23266867   Fax: 011-23243014   Website: www.cbspd.com
e-mail: delhi@cbspd.com; cbspubs@airtelmail.in.
Corporate Office: 204 FIE, Industrial Area, Patparganj, Delhi 110 092
Ph: 4934 4934   Fax: 4934 4935   e-mail: publishing@cbspd.com; publicity@cbspd.com

Branches

- **Bengaluru:** Seema House 2975, 17th Cross, K.R. Road,
  Banasankari 2nd Stage, Bengaluru 560 070, Karnataka
  Ph: +91-80-26771678/79   Fax: +91-80-26771680   e-mail: bangalore@cbspd.com
- **Chennai:** 7, Subbaraya Street, Shenoy Nagar, Chennai 600 030, Tamil Nadu
  Ph: +91-44-26680620, 26681266   Fax: +91-44-42032115   e-mail: chennai@cbspd.com
- **Kochi:** 42/1325, 1326, Power House Road, Opp. KSEB Power House
  Ernakulam 682 018, Kochi, Kerala
  Ph: +91-484-4059061-65   Fax: +91-484-4059065   e-mail: kochi@cbspd.com
- **Kolkata:** 6/B, Ground Floor, Rameswar Shaw Road, Kolkata-700 014, West Bengal
  Ph: +91-33-22891126, 22891127, 22891128   e-mail: kolkata@cbspd.com
- **Mumbai:** 83-C, Dr E Moses Road, Worli, Mumbai-400018, Maharashtra
  Ph: +91-22-24902340/41   Fax: +91-22-24902342   e-mail: mumbai@cbspd.com

Representatives

• **Bhopal**	0-8319310552	• **Bhubaneswar** 0-9911037372	• **Hyderabad** 0-9885175004	• **Jharkhand**	0-9811541605
• **Nagpur**	0-9021734563	• **Patna** 0-9334159340	• **Pune** 0-9623451994	• **Uttarakhand**	0-9716462459
• **Dhaka (Bangladesh)**	01912-003485				

Printed at Goyal Offset Printers, GT Karnal Road, Industrial Area, Delhi, India

Forensic Medicine, Toxicology and Medical Jurisprudence

Second Edition

BV Subrahmanyam MD, DCrL, AAFS, FIAFM, FICFMT, DYo

Medicolegal Consultant
former Professor and Head
Department of Forensic Medicine and Toxicology
Narayana Medical College, Nellore
Chairman, Paraclinical Studies, Faculty of Medicine
Head, PG Centre and Department of Forensic Medicine
South Gujarat University and Government Medical College, Surat
Dean, Medical College, Bhavnagar
Medical Superintendent, Govt. Medical College and New Civil Hospital, Surat
Professor and Head, Department of Forensic Medicine, Medical College, Baroda
Professor and Head, Department of Forensic Medicine, MP Shah Medical College, Jamnagar
Professor and Head, Department of Forensic Medicine, Regional Institute of Medical Sciences, Imphal
Reader, Institute of Medical Sciences, Banaras Hindu University, Varanasi
Assistant Professor, Institute of Medical Sciences, Osmania Medical College, Hyderabad
Faculty Member, Sri Venkateswara Medical College, Tirupati

SV Phanindra MD

Professor and Head
Department of Forensic Medicine and Toxicology
Narayana Medical College
Nellore

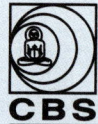

CBS

CBS Publishers & Distributors Pvt Ltd

New Delhi • Bengaluru • Chennai • Kochi • Kolkata • Mumbai
Bhopal • Bhubaneswar • Hyderabad • Jharkhand • Nagpur • Patna • Pune
Uttarakhand • Dhaka (Bangladesh)

_to_

---

my Forensic Medicine
teachers, students and life-partner
Dr Saraswathamma for
her devotion, patience and
perseverance

Contributors

Amit Agrawal
Professor and Head
Department of Neurosurgery
Narayana Medical College, Nellore

G Veera Nagi Reddy
Professor
Department of Forensic Medicine
Principal, Narayana Medical College, Nellore

I Mohan Prasad
Associate Professor
Department of Forensic Medicine
Narayana Medical College, Nellore

Krishna Dutt Chavaili
Professor and Head
Department of Forensic Medicine
All India Institute of Medical Sciences
Raipur

P Suresh
Assistant Professor
ACSR Medical College
Nellore

Swapnil Agarwal
Professor
PS Medical College
Karamsad, Gujarat

Vishnu Vardhan Reddy V
Research Associate
Narayana Medical College and Hospital
Nellore

Z Sasikanth
Associate Professor
Department of Forensic Medicine
Rajiv Gandi Institute of Medical Sciences
Kadapa

Foreword

Dr BV Subrahmanyam is known to me for the last 50 years as a teacher, academician and as an administrator in various places like Hyderabad (Osmania), Manipur (RIMS), BHU, Varanasi, Jamnagar, Baroda, Bhavnagar, Surat and Nellore. He is well known in the field of Forensic Medicine and I am happy to write the Foreword to *Forensic Medicine, Toxicology and Medical Jurisprudence, second edition*. I am sure this book will continue to be popular among the medical students, doctors, lawyers, judiciary and the investigating officers.

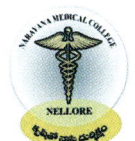

Dr G Veera Nagi Reddy MD
Principal
Narayana Medical College
Chinthareddypalem, Nellore, AP, India

Preface to the Second Edition

It is my pleasure to present the second edition of *Forensic Medicine, Toxicology and Medical Jurisprudence*.

This book is student-friendly and updated according to the latest academic curriculum and examination pattern. Efforts are made by the author, co-author and all other contributors to keep the book in simple language instead of the difficult and daunting task of the subject with legal and highly technical vocabulary in this edition. Advantages and disadvantages of DNA profiling, criminal responsibility in relation to section of IPC, lividity positions, sudden deaths, autopsy and dissection, embalming disadvantages, avulsion injury of face, hinge fractures of skull, microwave burns, rape trauma syndrome, deaths during sexual activity, sex-related deaths, POCSO Act, new offence after the changes in IPC and CrPC like voyeurism, stacking and acid attacks, all definitions connected with assisted reproduction. Cryopreservation, hair dye poisoning, paraquat poisoning, and surrogacy are newly added. Besides these, many new tables, colour photographs, additional MCQs, new case studies, revision MCQs test, etc. are also added. All efforts are made to bring forward simple, lucid and succinct study material, catering to the needs of medical students, doctors, lawyers, judiciary and the investigating agencies.

My sincere thanks to my colleagues and friends for their valuable help and suggestions in the preparation of this book at various stages.

Trust! This book will be of great help to the concerned people.

BV Subrahmanyam

Preface to the First Edition

I feel pleasure in presenting the book *Forensic Medicine, Toxicology and Medical Jurisprudence*.

The book is student-friendly, and is written according to the new academic curriculum and examination pattern.

I hope that this book will benefit the government and private medical practitioners, the students of MBBS, homoeopathy and other disciplines, who want to strengthen their fundamentals on *Forensic Medicine, Toxicology and Medical Jurisprudence*. Moreover, it will also help lawyers while preparing their medicolegal cases and the police officers involved in the investigation of crime.

My sincere thanks to my colleagues and friends for their valuable help and suggestions in the preparation of this book at various stages.

Trust! This book will be of great help to the concerned people.

BV Subrahmanyam

Acknowledgements

I am grateful to the Municipal Administration Minister Dr P Narayana Garu and Founder Chairman of Narayana Medical Institutions. Thanks are due to all my friends and well wishers who encouraged me in this venture. My special thanks are due to Dr G Veera Nagi Reddy who wrote Foreword for this edition, Dr I Mohan Prasad, Dr Maniganda Raj, Dr S Ganesh Kumar, Dr Niranjan Kumar G, Dr Aswani Kishore and other staff members who helped me in many ways in completing this work.

Thanks are due to CBS Publishers and Distributors, Mr YN Arjuna and other members of the dynamic team who stopped this book.

Thanks are due to many students and teachers who gave me feedback and asked me to continue the book in the same style.

My sincere thanks to Mrs A Karuna for the help in the preparation of the text material.

I fail in my duty if I do not thank my wife Dr Saraswathamma who was behind my academic pursuits.

BV Subrahmanyam

Contents

SECTION I: Forensic Medicine

SECTION II: Forensic Toxicology

SECTION III: Medical Jurisprudence

Section I

Forensic Medicine

CHAPTER 1

Forensic Medicine

INTRODUCTION

"Forensic Medicine is the knowledge of all the branches of Medical Sciences applied in the Court of Law of the purpose of Administration of Justice". It deals with personal injury, murder and legal proceedings.

The term 'Forensic' is derived from the ancient Roman practice for settlement of disputes in 'Forum' (debating place in ancient Rome). It was done by 'Panchayat' where a group of 'five' village elders were authorized to settle the disputes.

The knowledge of forensic medicine is becoming necessary for the doctors doing their own practice or those in government services, private service, trust service or any other service for that matter, because during the medical practice, doctors come across cases which at a later date may require their presence in a Court of Law, to give evidence about the relevant facts-in-issue before the presiding officers.

Injury cases, medical certificates, disability certificates, sexual offences, surgical procedures leading to complications, vehicular accidents presented before accidental claims tribunal, any case coming before consumer forum demanding compensation, are the common examples when the doctor has to attend the Court of Law.

MEDICOLEGAL CASE

Whenever a doctor examines a patient and feels that there is need to inform the matter to the police because later it may become a case of police investigation, e.g. bleeding injury on face, internal head injury, suspected case of poisoning, road traffic accident, stab injury, firearm injury, etc. then the doctor must inform the police in writing.

These cases are known as medicolegal cases and are also called emergency police report case (MLC/EPR). Whenever a police report is made for the first time about any such case and the police register, it becomes the First Information Report. At times doctor also informs about such cases to the police for the first time. The FIR starts the chain of evidence in any investigating process. The FIR should be lodged at the nearest police station.

CORPUS DELICTI

Corpus delicti means body of evidence or chain of evidence. In any legal case, the court requires the whole body of evidence to be produced before it and it should be completed from beginning to the end without any missing links in-between.

If there are missing links then the court does not accept the body of evidence as complete fact and consequently the case fails in the eyes of law.

Many times as doubts arise as to why a case of stabbing incident occurring at a busy road junction in broad daylight results in acquittal of the accused. This is because the corpus delicti is not proved beyond reasonable doubt leading to dismissal of the case.

Res judicata means that the case is already judged. Therefore, it will not be taken up and it will be dismissed.

THE ESSENTIAL INGREDIENTS OF A CRIME

- Intention
- Motive
- Preparation
- Attempt
- Execution

'B' loves the girl 'G' but 'G' is interested in another man 'M', so 'B' feels that if he can eliminate 'M', he can bag 'G'. Here, 'B' wants to eliminate 'M'; that is his intention. Why he wants to eliminate 'M'? Because he wants to bag 'G', that is his motive. So he makes the necessary preparations to kill 'M' and keeps on observing where he can be found alone. The last step is to buy a sharp knife from the market to complete the preparation. He finds 'M' and 'G' alone, but before the crime is committed he suddenly changes his mind and thinks that he can look for another woman 'W' instead of bothering for 'G' and he forgets about the whole preparation. In this process no crime is committed.

B finds the man (M) and the girl (G) in the bush. He takes out the knife, raises it and attacks 'M'. In another situation 'B' attacks 'M' with the knife, 'M' sustains injury to vital organ heart and dies. 'B' has successfully executed crime of killing 'M'. Here 'B' had completed the crime with all ingredients of offence, i.e. motive, intention, preparation, attempt and execution, so this killing becomes homicide and hence amounts to murder.

In the legal terminology, it becomes culpable homicide amounting to murder.

MENS REA (MENS—MIND: REA—CRIMINAL)

"The law presumes that no guilty act can be committed by a person who does not have a guilty mind".

In any crime, the person who suffers is called victim, the offender or the perpetrator of crime is known as accused, the place where crime is committed is known as scene of offence or the scene of crime. The weapon or the object used for the crime becomes an important link between the victim and the accused.

LOCARD'S PRINCIPLE OF EXCHANGE

One of the fundamental principles to be remembered is *Locard's Principle of Exchange* which states that—whenever two objects come in contact with each other, there is exchange of matter and in relation to the crime this exchanged matter from the victim may be found on accused, from the accused may be found on victim and from one or both of them on the weapon or is likely to be found at the place of occurrence or scene of crime. In a case where the doctor feels it necessary, he can ask the investigating officers to arrange for scene visit. The doctor has to examine the scene in a systematic fashion without leaving any area from careful observation. At the scene of crime the doctor should look for trace evidences linking the accused, the victim and the scene.

The investigation of crime is essentially the job of the police. Commonly the cases are investigated by subinspector of police. The traffic crimes are investigated by the traffic police.

In cases where the government feels, the investigations are handed over to special teams. The investigating officer incharge of a particular case is expected to complete the investigation within 90 days and file a charge sheet before the judicial magistrate. The cases are divided into *civil cases* and *criminal cases*.

Civil cases deal with matters of compensation as in accident claims. Cases connected with divorce, nullity of marriage, inheritance, disputed paternity are some other examples of civil cases.

Criminal cases deal with injuries to the human body or death of a human being or sexual offences like rape, etc. When the punishment awarded is below two years, the cases are designated as summon cases and where the punishment given is more than two years, the cases are called warrant cases.

In India, cases are brought before various types of Court of Law. The criminal courts are:
- Magistrate Court.
- Sessions Court.

- High Court.
- Supreme Court of India.

Magistrates are judicial magistrates and executive magistrates.

Executive magistrates perform the *inquest* or *inquiry* in cases of:
- Police firing
- Deaths in jail
- Deaths in police custody
- Dowry deaths
- Exhumations, etc.

At the sub-division level, the sub-divisional Magistrate and at the district level the District Magistrate or Collector also enquires as and when ordered.

In fact, every crime that is committed is brought to the knowledge of area magistrate by investigating police officer.

Executive magistrates do not have the power of trial and penalisation, i.e. giving punishment. In contrast, the judicial magistrates and the judges have the power of awarding sentences and fines.
- A second class judicial magistrate can award an imprisonment up to three years and fine of 3000 rupees.
- A first class judicial magistrate can award imprisonment up to five years and fine up to 10000 rupees. He is called Metropolitan Magistrate in Metropolitan cities.
- The chief judicial magistrate has the power of giving punishment for seven years and unlimited fine. He is called Chief Metropolitan Magistrate in Metros.
- The powers of magistrate are prescribed under Section 29 of CrPC.

The Session Courts are located at the district headquarters. The session judge can pass any punishment including the death sentence. However, the death sentence cannot be carried out unless it is confirmed by the High Court. Additional session judges have same powers as district session judges. An assistant session judge can give imprisonment up to ten years.

Accident cases are tried by accident claims tribunal headed by session judges. The High Court can pass any sentence authorized by law (Section 28 of CrPC).

The offences where a police officer can arrest a person without obtaining a warrant from a magistrate, are known as cognizable offences. The state takes the responsibility of recognizing the offences and proceeding with investigation in cases of cognizable offences.

In the case of non-cognizable offences, the responsibility lies with the victim in brining to the notice of the police or the magistrate about the offence. A person accused of any crime cannot be labeled as a criminal unless the crime is proved and he is convicted.

Any conviction is not implemented until it is confirmed. Any conviction in a lower court can be challenged in a higher court on an appeal with the permission from the convicting court.

Crimes commited by children below the age of 16 years are dealt by Chief Judicial Magistrate or by any other court empowered for that purpose, e.g. magistrates of juvenile courts.

INQUEST

Officers incharge of police stations are empowered to enquire and report regarding suspicious deaths, accidental deaths, suicides, death caused by animals, death caused due to machinery or murder case. The police officer goes to the place where dead body of person is lying. In the presence of two or more respectable persons of that area he will draw a report of the apparent cause of death. He will describe the wounds, fractures or bruises or any other mark of violence found on the body. He will also record in what manner or by what instruments, such marks have been inflicted. The report is signed by the witness and the police officer. It is forwarded to the Sub-divisional or District Magistrate.

However, when any person dies in police custody or the death is in jail or due to police firing or dowry case the nearest executive magistrate holds the inquest. He will also inform the relatives like parent, brother, sister, children and spouse to be present at that time.

In the United States of America, the inquest is authorized to be carried out by a medical examiner, in cases of deaths due to violence, accident or suicide, pregnancy related deaths, deaths due to poisoning, death connected with anaesthesia and operating procedures, unexpected and unexplained deaths, deaths of mentally ill persons, deaths in jail, police custody or police firing, etc. The medical examiner who is an expert in forensic medicine and pathology, is better equipped to do more scientific and objective enquiry. This system is practiced in Japan and Canada also. In UK and some other countries a coroner's system of inquest exists. The coroner holds a court of enquiry and pronounces verdict regarding cause and manner of death.

In India, death sentence is given in the rarest of the rare cases. It is executed by hanging until death. In rape cases of minor twelve years and below maximum sentence given in death sentence.

CHAPTER 2

Court Procedures

INTRODUCTION

Registered medical practitioners may be asked to attend Court of Law and depose evidence based on observations and inferences in relation to the patients examined or treated.

Ordinarily, the Court of Law understand that the medical doctor is very busy person helping the patients in distress. Even the Supreme Court of India has directed that the primary duty of the doctors is to attend the patient and therefore the Court of Law should not unnecessarily call them to give evidence if the matter can be managed without their presence.

The process of doctor's attendance to a court starts with examining the case or issuing a certificate. The court compels the attendance of a witness by issuing a subpoena (sub—under; poena—penalty).

A subpoena is issued by the presiding officer of the court in duplicate. It is on the witness. He has to take the original and sign on the duplicate and return it to the person delivering the summons. He is asked to be present on a stipulated date, at a fixed time and at a given place. If he fails to do so, he is liable to be punished for contempt of court. Non-compliance of summons leads to fine or imprisonment. When a person receives summons from civil court and criminal court on the same date, he should attend the criminal court and inform the civil court accordingly. If he receives summons from same category of courts, the higher court should be obeyed and lower court should be informed (civil/criminal). If the summon is from two sessions courts at the same time, for the same date, then the one received by him earlier, should be given priority with intimation to the other. Sometimes a person may be summoned to submit only a document. This is known as **subpoena duces tecum.**

After receiving the summons, the doctor shall collect the case reports and subject matter connected with the case. He shall prepare to give evidence by refreshing the knowledge of case and the recent developments about the subject from standard books, reference books and journals. After due to preparation on stipulated date and stipulated time, he will present himself before the court wearing proper dress. It is customary to wear a suit and tie.

The doctor should present his summons to the court clerk and inform him that he has arrived. He should also contact the lawyer of the party calling him. Generally, the doctor is summoned on behalf of public prosecutor. He can try to learn about the case as it is to be presented before the court because the doctor may not be aware of matter. This **pretrial conference** is helpful to the court.

The doctor shall greet the presiding officer of the court without fail. When he is called upon to enter into the witness box, he will take his position in witness box upright, is permitted to look into records and answer questions. His answers should be loud, clear, as much nontechnical in language as possible so that the judge and lawyers are able to understand well and appreciate his evidence. When he does not know the answer, he should say so.

The main examination is carried out by the lawyer of summoning party who generally asks the doctor to read his report and his opinion. The opposing counsel, i.e. the opposite party lawyer starts his cross-examination with a view to assess the credibility of his evidence. The doctor should answer within the limits of science. As he is an expert, hypothetical questions are put to him many times; he should answer them.

However, if his answer to that particular question is different, he has a right volunteer a statement without being asked by lawyer or the court. If he thinks that in the interest of justice, he should clarify the matter, he should do so. During the whole process of court evidence, the doctor should remain polite and keep up the dignity of himself and his profession. If irrelevant questions are put, judge can prevent such questions being answered. Cross-examination is a double-edged weapon in as much as it exposes the deficiencies of witness if there are any, at the same time an overzealous and overconfident cross-examination may harm his own case. When doctor is confident in his subject he can raise questions to steer the ambiguities of cross-examination.

Many intelligent defence lawyers show restraint in putting questions to medical experts. In fact, once the judge and lawyers understand the impartiality of doctor and his competence and expertise, they treat him with due regards and may even ask him about his opinion to be incorporated duly, ultimately in the judgement.

Re-examination and re-cross examination may be required sometimes. The presiding officer of the court may put questions at any time during procedure. The court questions help the judge to get clarification.

The prerequisite of any evidence in any court of law is to bind the witness to speak the truth, only the truth. Initially therefore, as soon as the witness enters the witness box, he is administered oath. The witness can take oath in name of God or Solemn affirmation depending on his faith.

After the evidence is over, the doctor may be asked to go through the evidence and make corrections with a pencil regarding spellings, etc.

The government doctors are given a court attendance certificate so that they can claim traveling expenses from the office. For private practitioners the court decides the quantum of fees to be paid to the doctors.

In civil cases, at the time of serving the summons, money to cover traveling expenses is paid to the doctor to conduct himself to civil court to give evidence. This is known as conduct money. If the doctor feels that money given is meagre he can inform the court and return the summons. However, the final decision regarding payment is made by the court.

In criminal cases, the doctor cannot demand particular amount of money. After taking oath to speak the truth, if it is found by the court that the doctor is speaking lies, for the deliberate utterance of lies, the witness is charged with perjury and he is punished for the same, if it is proved.

Perjury is liable for severe punishment even up to seven years of imprisonment. During the court examination, questions leading to answers or leading questions are not allowed during main examination. They are allowed during cross-examination. However, when witness is declared **hostile, leading questions** are permitted during examination of hostile witness by summoning lawyer himself.

A witness is declared hostile when he deliberately speaks against the interests of the party that has summoned him. Whenever some confidential matter in relation to the patient is asked, which the doctor has known during his doctor–patient relationship, as it is known as professional secret, the doctor can politely refuse to give the reply. However, if the court insists he has to answer, because the doctor does not enjoy any legal immunity to keep professional secrets to himself.

EVIDENCE

"Evidence means includes all statements which the court permits in relation to matter of facts and inquiry". The statement made before Court of Law by a witness, under oath is oral evidence.

When a document is produced in a case for the inspection of the court, it is called documentary evidence. Besides these, material objects are produced before inspection of court like weapon of assault, the blood stained clothes of victim and accused. These materials when approved by the court are treated as exhibits.

Types of Evidence

- Direct evidence and circumstantial evidence.
- Real and personal evidence.
- Original and unoriginal evidence.
  - Direct or positive evidence is evidence about the real point in controversy for example when a person says that he saw the accused, inflicting a blow on the victim, it becomes direct evidence.
  - Circumstantial evidence is one which relates to the fact in question for example when footprints are found on sand, one can find out whether they belonged to a bird, animal or man.

A direct evidence acts as a proof to establish that the accused person has committed the offence, whereas in case of circumstantial evidence, the circumstances which are established by evidence point out that the accused has committed the offence.

Hearsay evidence is different from circumstantial evidence. In hearsay evidence, the evidence is neither direct nor circumstantial. It is only secondary evidence. It is a third party knowledge. In other words a person says what others have said to him.

Medical Evidence

It is documentary evidence as well as oral evidence.

Documentary evidence comprises medical certificates, e.g. sickness, death certificate, medicolegal reports (postmortem reports, dying declaration). A medical certificate issued only by registered medical practitioners is accepted in a Court of Law. It is an offence to issue false certificate.

Medicolegal reports are reports prepared by doctor in compliance to a requisition received from magistrate or police officer. Injury certificate, postmortem report, rape examination reports, etc. are some of the examples.

DYING DECLARATION

It is a declaration made by a person who is deceased (died) regarding the cause of his condition or the circumstances which have resulted in his death.

It is verbal or written, recorded by a medical officer or magistrate. Ordinarily the doctor calls for the nearest authorized magistrate to come and record the dying declaration of any patient under his care who is about to die.

When the death is nearing fast and there is no time available to wait for magistrate, the medical officer has to do the recording of declaration. The mental status of the person about to die must be in a state of sound mind and capable of making a statement. Gestures are permitted if he is unable to talk. The dying declaration should be recorded in the language in which it is spoken.

After the recording of the declaration, it has to be signed by two witnesses. During the process of declaration, if the person becomes unconscious or dies leaving the statement incomplete, that fact should be mentioned and the declaration closed at that stage. **Dying declaration** is accepted as an important piece of evidence in the court of law. However, if the patient survives, it requires to be corroborated by oral evidence of the person. When the magistrate in the presence of accused records the deposition it is called dying deposition. Here opportunity is given to accused to cross-examine the victim, therefore it becomes a **bed side court.**

Exceptions to Oral Evidence

- Dying declaration.
- Expert opinions expressed in treatise.
- Evidence of a witness tendered in a previous judicial proceeding.
- Deposition of medical witness in lower court.
- Forensic science laboratory report. Parties inform the court to treat it as an exhibit.
  - Whenever the court so feels, the forensic science laboratory officer issuing the report can also be summoned to the court.
  - Oral evidence is superior to documentary evidence because it can subjected to cross-examination.

WITNESS

Witnesses are of two types:
1. Common witness.
2. Expert witness.

Common witness: A common witness is an ordinary witness who is capable of talking about the facts observed by him.

Expert witness: An expert witness on the other hand is a skilled person who is not only able to testify about the facts observed by him but also is capable of making inferences and giving opinions based on his technical/professional/scientific knowledge or experience in a concerned skill over a period of time making him competent enough to be designated as an expert by Court of Law. The medical witness is a common as well as expert witness at the same time. When he is testifying about the patients examination details, observed by him, he is a common witness and when he speaks about his diagnosis and other opinions like cause of death, manner of death, time since death, age of injuries and so on, he is acting as an expert witness.

CHAPTER 3

Identity (Biometric Profiling)

INTRODUCTION

By identity we mean establishment of individuality of the person.

- The question of identity may arise in the living as well as in the dead. In fact, from the womb to the tomb and even after, question arises about the identity of the person. In the hospital when two babies are changed in neonatal period.
- For admissions into schools.
- In the cases of disputed paternity.
- Insurance purposes.
- Joining of service.
- Drawing pension every month.
- Property inheritance.
- Cases of impersonation by people accused of crimes or substitution of persons stealthily to escape from custody or jail or hospital or psychiatric hospital or defence forces the biometric profile (Fig. 3.1) is taken for identification.

The question of identification of dead arises when unknown dead bodies are recovered from rivers, wells, roadside places, railway tracks, jungles, uninhabited places, etc. In cases of mass disasters like flood, famine, earthquake, cyclone, shipwreck, air crash, bombardment during wars, epidemics like plague, anthrax, food poisoning, mass diarrhoea, identification may or may not be possible. Living persons are sometimes identified by identification parade where the person known to the suspected person or criminal or accused are asked to identify the person while passing through parade of a mixed group of persons including the suspect also.

Biometric Profiling

The *certain features* for identification of biometric profiling (Fig. 3.1) are:
- Fingerprints
- Footprints
- Poroscopy
- DNA profile

Other features useful for identification are

1. Race
2. Sex
3. Age
4. Tattoo marks
5. Moles
6. Scars
7. Deformities
8. Photographs
9. Hair
10. Superimposition photography, video superimposition.
11. Teeth
12. Lip prints
13. Ear prints
14. Nose prints
15. Palate prints
16. Frontal sinuses
17. Signature
18. ECG (Dr Srinivas method).

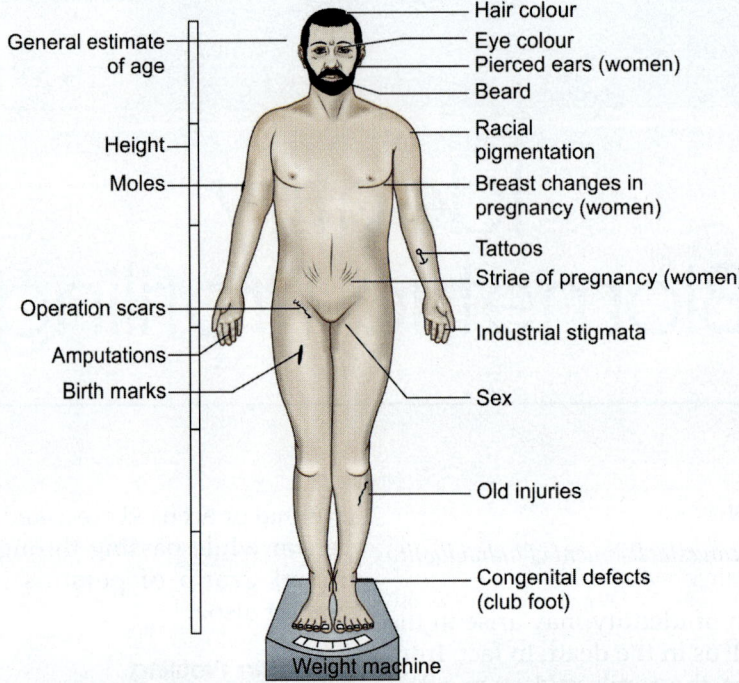

General estimate of age

Height

Moles

Operation scars

Amputations

Birth marks

Hair colour

Eye colour

Pierced ears (women)

Beard

Racial pigmentation

Breast changes in pregnancy (women)

Tattoos

Striae of pregnancy (women)

Industrial stigmata

Sex

Old injuries

Congenital defects (club foot)

Weight machine

Fig. 3.1: Biometric profiling: Features to be examined for identification

19. Namaste technique (Dr Subrahmanyam method).
20. Complexion and features.

When unknown bodies are recovered, they are labeled as A, B, C, D or 1, 2, 3, 4, etc. for the purpose of registration and identification of the body, also for investigation and legal purposes, until the real name, age, etc. of the person are obtained and the person is finally identified by name like, e.g. A is Chhagan, B is Magan, etc. Initial examination of outer features is very important in identification of a person (Fig. 3.2).

FEATURES FOR IDENTIFICATION

Fingerprints

In ancient Egypt, fingerprints were found on slabs of clay. Ts-in-she, a Chinese Emperor (B.C. 246–210) used fingerprints on the seals made of clay. On one side, king's thumb impression was taken and on the other, the name of the owner was written. In India, 'Panja', i.e. print of the palm and the fingers was used during the period of Mughals.

Sir William Herschel used fingerprints in official documents and contracts between 1858–1880. Dr. Henry Faulds was the first person to give the idea of tracing a criminal from marked impressions.

In 1880, he wrote an article on '*Journal Nature*' describing the science of fingerprint system. In 1892, Edward Henry, improved the system. *The first fingerprint bureau was established in Kolkata in 1897.*

Classification of Fingerprints (Fig. 3.3)

1. Loop 65%
2. Whorls 25%
3. Arch 6–7%
4. Composite 3–4%
5. Accidental 1–2%.

The Fingerprints Follow Quetelet's Rule

All nature made things have unlimited and infinite variation of forms.

According to Galton, the system of classification is based on the variations in the patterns of the ridges, which are grouped into arches, loops and whorls, i.e. ALW or Arch-Loop-Whorl system.

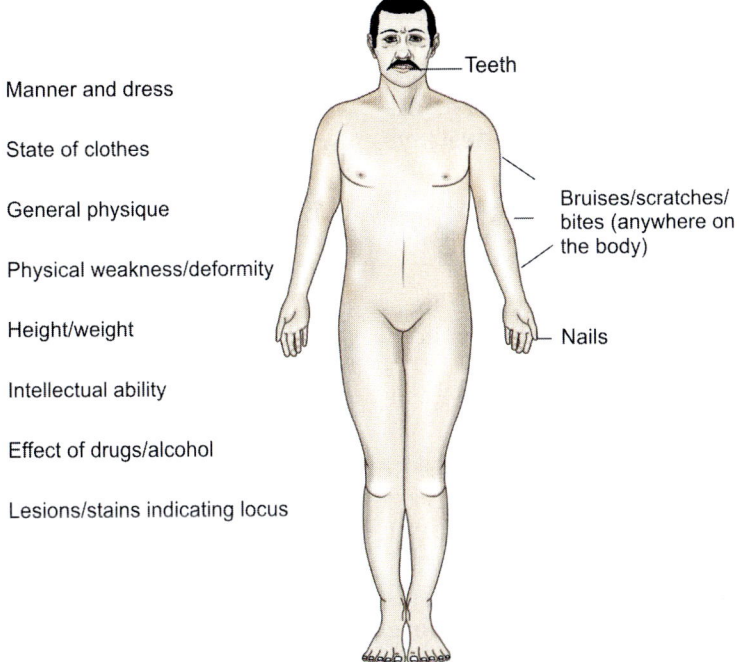

Fig. 3.2: Features for examination (outer apperance)

Manner and dress

State of clothes

General physique

Physical weakness/deformity

Height/weight

Intellectual ability

Effect of drugs/alcohol

Lesions/stains indicating locus

Teeth

Bruises/scratches/ bites (anywhere on the body)

Nails

Even the fingerprints of identical twins developed from same ovum are not the same.

This system is simple and infallible with an accuracy of 100%. When a suspected fingerprint is compared with known fingerprint, 16–20 points of similarity are accepted as proof of identity.

Recording of fingerprints is easy. The fingers must be thoroughly cleaned and dried. The fingerprint is taken with printers ink on unglazed white paper. There are two ways of taking fingerprint.

Plain fingerprint: A plain print is taken by simply pressing the inked finger on the paper and just lifting it.

Rolled fingerprint: The rolled print is taken by turning ridged surface of the inked finger from one side to the other. Rolled fingerprint is superior to plain one because a better study of ridge pattern can be made. When fingerprints are invisible or latent, then the latent fingerprints are made visible or patent by using suitable dusting powder, with a brush or sprayer and then taking photograph of the same.

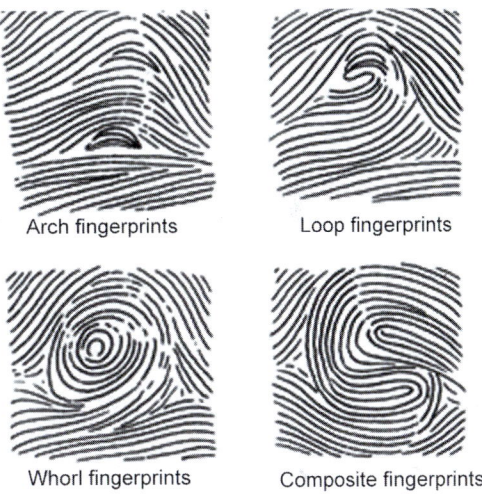

Arch fingerprints   Loop fingerprints

Whorl fingerprints   Composite fingerprints

Fig. 3.3: Fingerprint types

Fingerprints on the neck or on the body or clothes are made visible by X-ray techniques using radioopaque dusting powder (lead dust). Fingerprints on material like soap, wax are called plastic prints. They can be recorded by photography.

The dusting powder consists of grey and white powder. Grey powder contains chalk and mercury and white powder contains lead carbonate or French chalk. Iodine vapour, silver nitrate and osmium tetroxide are also used to bring out invisible fingerprints completely. Leprosy completely destroys fingerprint pattern.

Temporary changes may occur in celiac disease. The point of entry of electricity also destroys the fingerprints.

In the famous case of Ruxton the finger impressions of maid servant were recovered even after three years.

Footprints

Footprint is also called a **podogram.** The skin patterns of toes and heels are specific and permanent like the fingerprints. A footprint can also be taken similar like fingerprint.

A walking footprint is larger than a still footprint. Imprints left on soft and loose material like sand are smaller than the real size of foot. Footprints left at the scene of crime help in identification of accused. Deformities of the foot like flat foot, web foot, supernumerary toes can also be identified from footprints.

Poroscopy

Papillary ridges of fingers and palms have minute pores which are the opening of ducts of sweat glands. These pores are permanent and vary in size, shape, position and number in given length of the ridges for each individual.

Identification by utilizing the pores is called poroscopy and is called Locard's method of identification after the name of Edmund Locard who first introduced it. Poroscopy helps in positive identification like fingerprint.

DNA Profiling (Fig. 3.4)

The term DNA fingerprinting is wrongly used by many people because DNA profile has nothing to do with fingerprints. The DNA profile aims at the determination of sequence of bands on the DNA strand within chromosomes. The backbone of DNA (which consists of adenine, thymine, guanine, lysine, cystosine) strand is a sugar base component and a phosphate group. The DNA molecule is composed of two DNA strands coiled in double spiral (helix). In DNA typing,

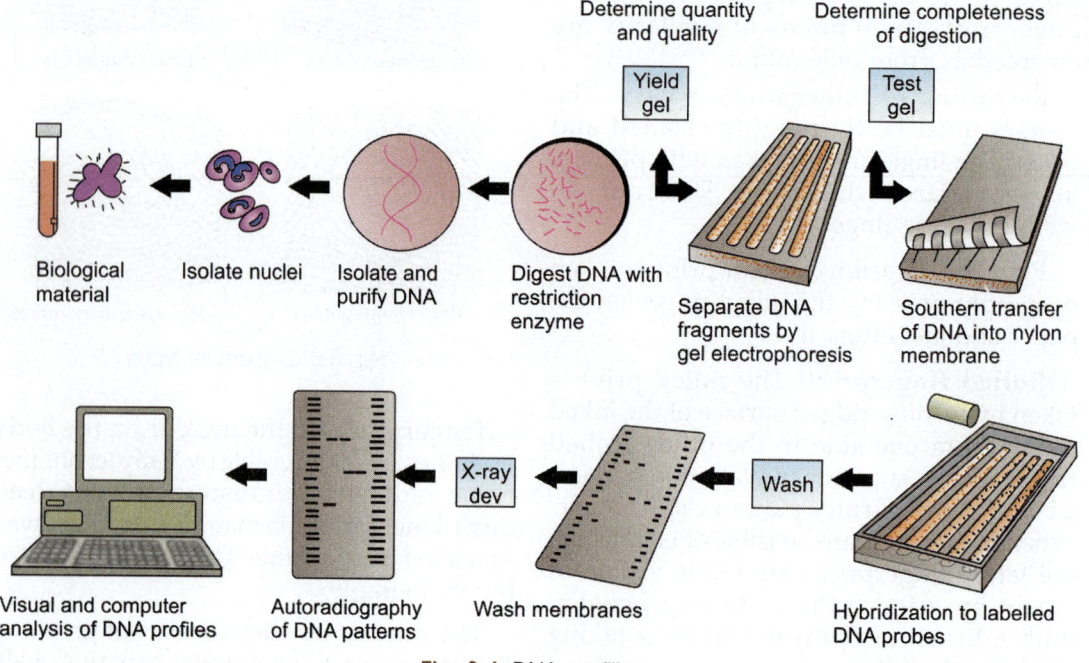

Biological material → Isolate nuclei → Isolate and purify DNA → Digest DNA with restriction enzyme → Separate DNA fragments by gel electrophoresis (Determine quantity and quality — Yield gel) → Southern transfer of DNA into nylon membrane (Determine completeness of digestion — Test gel)

Hybridization to labelled DNA probes → Wash → Wash membranes → X-ray dev → Autoradiography of DNA patterns → Visual and computer analysis of DNA profiles

Fig. 3.4: DNA profiling

samples like blood, semen, hair, buccal smear, mouth swab, vaginal swab are used.

Samples frozen at –20°C, yield good results, otherwise dried samples should be sent for analysis. Stains on clothes should be sent including nonstained areas for control purpose. The samples sent for analysis are subjected to DNA isolation, DNA quantitation, DNA digestion, DNA electrophoresis, DNA transfer, hybridization and autoradiography.

The whole procedure takes 10–15 days. The DNA from the samples is cut into fragments of sequence patterns using a specific enzyme, e.g. reverse transcriptase. The fragments are separated into bands by gel electrophoresis. Since Agarose gel is extremely fragile, this DNA fragment is transferred to a nylon membrane and fixed to the nylon membrane using heat or air drying.

In India, a multilocus probe isolated from a female banded krait is used for hybridization. Once the probe binds to the nylon membrane, it is invisible to the naked eye and is only visualized by autoradiography. First the excess probe is washed away then the membrane is raised against an X-ray film. It is exposed for 1–10 days and the X-ray film is developed. It shows the DNA bands. These bands are matched with the standard, genetic analysis and requires examination of 13 specific loci in human chromosome. Extraction of DNA sample takes 2 hours, so minimum laboratory time required is 10 hours approximately.

The accuracy of identification by DNA profile is said to be one in 30 billion to 300 billion.

In Bill Clinton's case regarding seminal stains on the dress of Monika Lewinsky, the stain was of Mr. Clinton's Monika Lewinsky, the stain was of Mr. Clinton's DNA. There was only one in 7.87 trillion chance that it was not of Mr. Clinton.

In India, in the case of Harivallabh Parikh, where a girl was aborted and the delivered foetus was subjected to DNA analysis, the suggestion made was that Parikh was the father of the child. The court did not agree to the opinion of laboratory on the ground that the data bank was inadequate, i.e. the test was not carried out to the expected level of accuracy.

The DNA profiling is useful in cases of rape, murder, identification of mutilated, dismembered or burnt bodies and in paternity disputes.

Advantages of DNA Profile

- It is the most conclusion test.
- It can be carried out with very small quantity of samples.
- Tissues buried under the soil preserve DNA better. DNA survives for many years in bones, teeth and hair.

Disadvantages of DNA Profile

- Very expensive, time consuming and interpretation of results require high level of skill and experience.
- DNA has a risk of destruction from humidity, smouldering fires and chemicals.
- It has a tendency to deteriorate easily from soft tissue and muscles. In cases where fingerprints are not available, DNA profiles can be utilized in forensic work for purpose of comparison. Samples obtained from combs, toothbrushes, or any personal articles can also be used.

OTHER FEATURES OF IDENTIFICATION

Hair

Except in very rare cases of agenesis of hair (congenital absence of hair), hair as a trace evidence in forensic investigation is very useful for identification purposes (Fig. 3.5).

The cuticular scale pattern (Fig. 3.6) on the surface of hair and the number of cuticles in a given length of hair are very helpful in individualization of hair.

Human hair differs from animals hair, because the medulla is very small in human hair. Some of the hairs are even non-medullated. Hair plucked with roots can help in sex determination because the cells in the root sheath of hair present Barr bodies.

The **lanugo hair** of newborn babies is light pigmented and thin. The hair which is coloured or dyed can be easily identified by

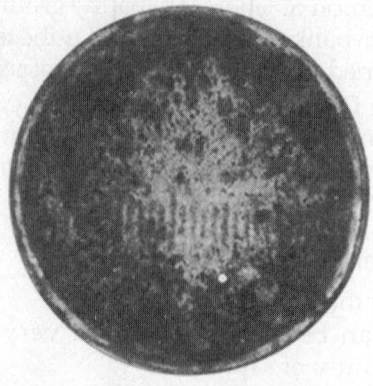

Fig. 3.5: Cross section of human hair with micrometre scale

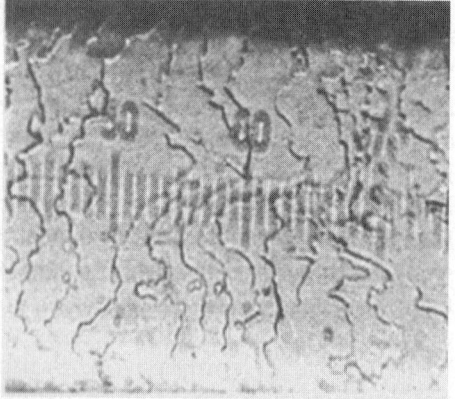

Fig. 3.6: Cuticular scale pattern (human hair)

examining under microscope as the dye forms a distinct layer on the surface of the hair.

The hair is present on various body parts and are termed eyelashes, sclap hair, axillary hair and pubic hair.

- Fraying or splitting is seen in scalp hair.
- Scalp hairs are oval or round.
- Moustache and eyelash hair are triangular. Injury to hair can be found out by examining under a simple magnifying glass. When the hair is exposed to burns/fire they become swollen, fragile, twisted, curly with carbon particle deposition. Further analysis is carried on by examining the cut end, if the cut end is clean—weapon is sharp, if the end is crushed—weapon is blunt, if bulb is distorted—it is forcible plucking. Certain poisons are deposited in hair, e.g. arsenic.

In cases of periodic consumption of poison, it can be detected by analysis the hair in bits.

Hair grows at a rate of 0.4 mm/day. Negroid hairs are very short and curly. Presence of hair as a trace evidence at the scene of crime, on the body of victim, accused and the weapon.

Hair does not grow after death. Due to dryness the skin shrinks after death, and so there is a wrong impression that hair has grown. The known sample hair and the hair from suspected victim, weapon or place are studied under comparator microscope. Neutron activation analysis (NAA) by exposing the specific hairs to neutrons in a nuclear reactor gives quantitative estimation of trace elements in the hair. This trace element pattern is unique for each individual. Identification by NAA of hair is accurate up to 90%.

Deformities

Deformities form an excellent means of identification (Fig. 3.7). They may be congenital or acquired, e.g. cleft palate, harelip, overriding teeth, supernumerary teeth, talipes, etc.

Scar

Scar is the result of repair process. It is a mass of fibrous tissue covered by simple epithelium. It does not have pigment, sweat glands, sebaceous glands and hair follicles.

A new or recent scar is somewhat red, soft and tender. This is formed in 10–14 days time.

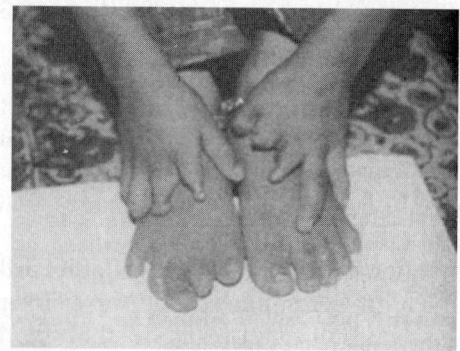

Fig. 3.7: Microdactyly and polydactyly in a 12-year-old girl

As the age advances, the scar loses vascularity, becomes smaller in size, denser, less sensitive and shines more.

Scars older than six months become white in colour, glistening, contracted and tough in consistency (Fig. 3.8). Sometimes excessive scar formation leads to keloids and these keloids may even turn malignant. From the examination of scar, it is possible to say about the nature of the wound, its size, the method of healing, the nature of the weapon, age of injury, etc.

- Liner scar suggests use of sharp weapon.
- Old surgical scars show satellite transverse scars of stitches.

An irregular scar suggests delayed and infected healing and healthy scar may heal faster in healthy adult persons. A circular depressed scar may be due to a bullet wound. An elliptical scar may be due to a stab wound. Thin tissue paper like scars on genitals may be due to syphilis. Multiple rounded scars around ribs may be due to herpes zoster.

Scars help in identification, in knowing the injury and nature of weapon. Rarely, criminals may try to remove scars by excision and skin grafting, to create problems in identification.

Moles

Moles are the birth marks. They are benign naevus. They may be located on any part of the body, ordinarily rounded, brown or black, raised or non-raised, with or without hairs.

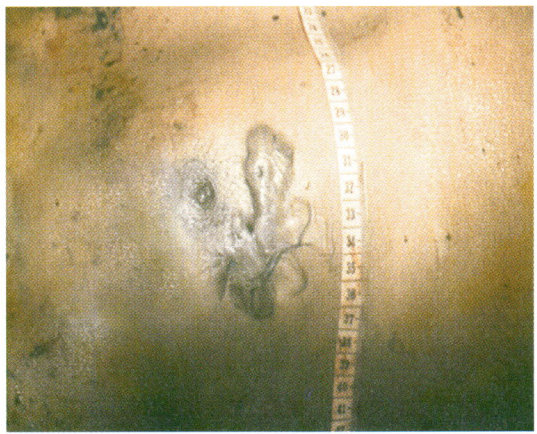

Fig. 3.8: Old scar

Moles rarely become active and then they show itching or increase in size, require excision and biopsy to rule out malignancy.

It is common practice to describe at least two moles as identification marks while issuing the certificates of medical and medicolegal examination. Those present on exposed parts of the body are commonly described in relation to body landmarks.

For specific purpose such as insurance, passport, vehicular license, etc. Moles are considered as important identification marks.

Moles are birthmarks and remain permanent unless intentionally removed. They are the most commonly used identification marks.

Photographs

It is very common practice to provide passport size photographs for purpose of identification for procuring hall tickets, train tickets under tatkal seva. For identity cards, passports and different applications recent passport size photographs are demanded. Photographs are also useful in cases of superimposition methods of identification.

Signatures and Handwriting

Signatures are supposed to be individualistic, written in any language. Signatures are taken for opening of bank accounts, deposition and withdrawl of money, on identification cards, in all applications and in all court matters like civil marriages, property transactions and so on.

Tattoo Marks (Figs 3.9 and 3.10)

The word tattoo is derived from Polynesian (*Ta*—to, *Tau*—mark). A tattoo mark is a design made on the skin by means of a needle dipped in a dye. The particles of insoluble pigments are introduced into the dermis, so tattoo marks remain more or less permanent.

- Carbon, Chinese ink and Indian ink produce black-coloured tattoos.
- Cinnabar and vermilion cause red tattoo.
- Chronic oxide causes green-coloured tattoo.
- Indigo, cobalt, Prussian blue and ultramarine blue cause blue-coloured tattoo.

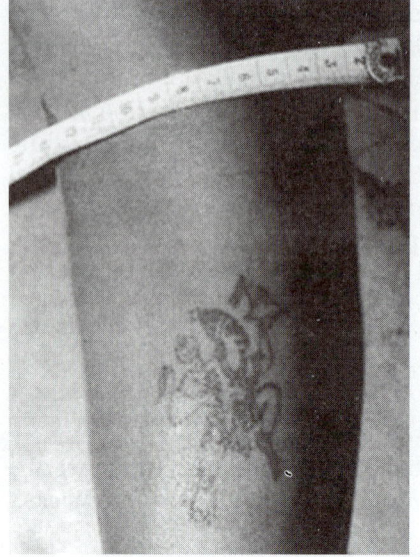
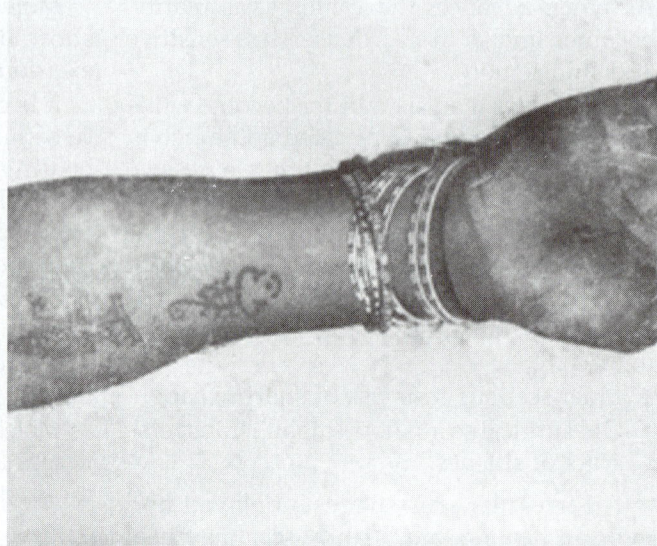

Fig. 3.9: Tattoo marks

• Tattoos may be found on any part of the body. All conceivable designs are found on tattoos such as figures of God, names of God, marks of particular tribe, marks of particular behaviour groups like homosexuals, drug addicts.

When tattoos are made with unstable substances like aniline dyes they may disappear in course of time. While describing a tattoo mark the site, size, shape, design, colour and meaning, if any is to be noted, e.g. Lord Krishna with flute, cross, birds, etc. Tattoo marks can be removed by surgery, carbon dioxide snow and exposure to laser beams. Only surgical removal with skin grafting can remove tattoo marks permanently, however, even in this case, if regional lymph node biopsy is taken, the pigments deposited in regional lymph nodes give the witness to prove that tattoos were excised from area of drainage.

Many times tattoo marks help in identification of person because people get their own names tattooed. Sometimes the name may belong to a friend or a lover. Religious belief and religious cult is obtained from tattoo marks like name of Sri Ram, Cross, Om, Swastik, Snake, etc. Psychology of the individual may be exposed like having tattoos of naked women or erotic tattoo marks. In fact, cases are known where people have not even left a single area of the body without a tattoo mark (Fig. 3.10). Tattoo marks on penis, thighs, chest, breast, buttocks, etc. area also seen. Tattoo marks can be erased by laser therapy also.

Complexion and Features

Europeans are white, Mongolians are yellow, Negroes are black in complexion. Indians being a mixed race do not subscribe to any particular complexion. Features like shape of the nose, shape of the ears, colour of iris, colour of hair are also considered in the identification process.

Many Indians are wheat complexioned, some of them are fair especially from the cold

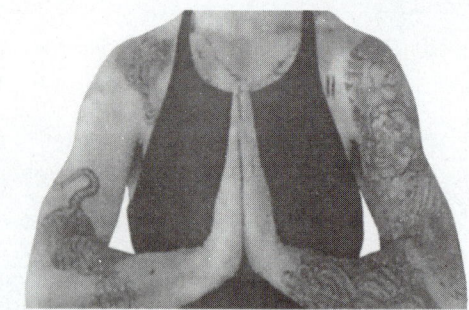

Fig. 3.10: Tattoo marks

climatic regions and mountainous areas. People from hot climatic zones like Gujarat, South India, Bengal are darker in complexion. Generally females confined to houses have better complexion compared to females working in fields.

Europeans have blue or grey eyes. Contact lenses, intraocular lenses, artificial eyes, leucoma (corneal scar) are helpful in identification.

Sex

The question of sex determination arises in relation to identification, marriage, employment, rape, participation in games, joining army services, inheritance, paternity, legitimacy, infertility, etc.

In human beings the two differentiated sexes are male and female. Up to a certain stage of development of the foetus, the sex differentiation is not possible.

By the time of delivery, the sex differentiation is complete and from the external genital examination, the sex is identified. However sometimes, sex determination becomes difficult due to developmental abnormalities in relation to genitals. In cases of chromosomal abnormalities, overlapping of sexual characters create difficulties in identification of sex.

Male or female characters and based on dominant features of sex in a given person. Sex parameters are anatomical, physiological, hormonal, endocrinological, chromosomal, gonadal, genetic, psychological and social. Genetic characters like sex chromatin determination in the hair bulbs, buccal mucosa, amniotic fluid, polymorphonuclear leucocytes, etc.

Anatomical sex is determined by physical examination of the body parts like the presence or absence of breast, vagina, penis, testes, hair on face, chest, etc.

Gonadal sex is determined by identification of testes and ovary.

Hormonal sex is determined by testicular and ovarian hormone determination.

The *chromosomal sex* is determined by chromosomal analysis of X an Y chromosomes.

By the general appearance, social behaviour and dress code, the social sex is determined.

Psychological sex depends upon the psychological feeling of an individual, mainly feeling of belonging to the same sex group.

Positive signs of sex identification are the presence of XY chromosomes and testes in case of males of XX chromosomes is further supported by the external genitalia of the corresponding sex. Persons showing ambivalence in sex are generally known as intersex or hermaphrodites.

When both, testes and ovaries are present in the same person, such person is a true hermaphrodite or double sex.

When a person has external female genitalia, but also has testes such person is called female pseudohermaphrodite.

It is of interest to note that the word hermaphrodite is derived from name of the child 'hermaphrodites', who was the child of 'hermis' and 'aphrodite' (story from Greek Mythology).

Common examples of intersex are

- Klinefelter's syndrome.
- Turner's syndrome.

In Klinefelter's syndrome, the chromosomal pattern is XXY. There is male type of differentiation of gonad (testes). There is hypogonadism associated with hypospadias, gynaecomastia, testicular dysgenesis. Male secondary characters are undeveloped. Azoospermia is seen.

In the case of *Turner's syndrome*, the chromosomal pattern is XO. Clinically the person is a woman of short stature with webbed neck, low posterior hairline, spina bifida, cubitus valgus, coarctation of aorta, renal defects like horseshoe kidney, endocrinal defects like diabetes and Cushing's syndrome. The nipples are pinpointed and there is history of primary amenorrhoea. The woman is unable to conceive.

Whenever confronted with a case of determination of true sex, a careful history, a thorough clinical examination, gonadal biopsy, Barr body and Davidson body study and chromosomal pattern by karyotyping must be done. Sometimes people conceal their sex as in the case of Dr. James Barry who lived up to the age of 80 years and even wrote a will that his body should not be subjected to autopsy. An autopsy was indeed done and 'he' was found to be 'she'.

Age

The question of age arises throughout life for various purposes such as in the determination of the age of the foetus, in relation to viability, in cases of infanticide, in cases of admission to schools, admission to professional colleges, in joining service, marriage and so on. A foetus is unable to survive apart from its mother unless it has completed 210 days of intrauterine life.

Legitimacy of a Child

Whether the child is born within legally viable wedlock or not is determined, based on whether the child is born within 280 days of divorce or death of the partner.

AGE AND MEDICOLEGAL IMPORTANCE

A child below the age of 6 years is not liable for any act including the acts which are against law, i.e. crimes. Above 6 years and below 7 years under the Railways Act the child can face punishment.

Regarding other Acts, till the completion of 7 years the child is considered to be incapable of having an intention of committing a crime. It is *Doli incapax* (*Doli*—infant, *incapax*—incapable of).

A child above the age of 7 years, but under the age of 12 years, is presumed by law to be mature enough to understand the nature and consequences of its actions, hence liable for punishment. However, whether the child has sufficient maturity of understanding or not, is required to be medically assessed.

A child up to the age of 12 years, cannot give consent for purpose of surgery or any other treatment for any medical problem, required to be carried out for the benefit of the child.

Any person above 12 years of age becomes legally responsible for his/her acts.

Up to the age of 16 years, the persons are tried in Juvenile Courts presided over by lady magistrates. A girl below 18 years and a boy below 21 years cannot engage in a legally valid marriage. A girl above the age of 16 years

Section of IPC	Criminal responsibility
82	A child under the age of seven is incapable of committing an offence. This is so because action alone does not amount to guilt unless it is accompanied by a guilty mind. And a child of that tender age cannot have a guilty mind or criminal intention with which the act is done. This presumption. However, is only confined to offences under the IPC but not to other Acts, e.g. the Railway Act.
83	A child above seven and under twelve years of age is presumed to be capable of committing an offence it, he has obtained sufficient maturity to understand and judge the nature and consequences of his conduct on that occasion. The law presumes such maturity in a child of that age unless the contrary is proved by the defence
89	A child under 12 years of age cannot give valid consent to suffer any harm which can occur from an act done in good faith and for its benefit, e.g. a consent for an operation. Only a guardian can give such consent
87	A person under 18 years of age cannot give valid consent, whether express or implied, to suffer any harm which may result from an Act no intended or not known to cause death or grievous hurt, e.g. consent for a wrestling contest
84	Nothing is an offence which is done by a person who at the time of doing it, by reason of unsoundness of mind, is incapable of knowing the nature of act (i.e. it is wrong or contrary to law)
85, 86	Drunkenness and criminal responsibility

can give a legally valid consent for sexual intercourse.

A child below the age of 10 years taken away from parent/guardian is said to have been kidnapped for purpose of removing valuables (ornaments or costly belongings) from the body of the person. For the purpose of offence of kidnapping a minor from lawful guardianship, the age of girl should be below 18 years and of a boy below 16 years. For transporting a girl from one country to other the age limit is 21 years for purpose of illicit intercourse. So, if a girl below 21 years of age is transported, it becomes an offence. Sexual intercourse with a girl below 18 years of age without consent is considered as rape.

Oath is administered in a Court of Law for giving evidence. However, for a child up to age of 12 years, there is an exception from administering oath. For the purpose of employment, a child below the age of 14 years cannot be employed under the Factories Act, 1948. To take up a government job, a person must have completed 18 years of age.

The age of recruitment is variable and is prescribed from time to time by the employer. Similarly, the age of retirement is also variable. Supreme Court judges do not retire up to 65 years of age. To contest for the post of a member of a parliament, the person must be above 35 years of age. State government employees retire at age of 58 years. However in Kerala, they retire by 55 years and in central government set up they retire by 60 years. In the university setup, the teachers retire by 62 years. Teaching doctors can work up to the age of 70 years according to medical council of India regulations. For central retirement age is 65 years. There is no age of retirement prescribed for a politician in India.

Estimation of Age

It is carried out reasonably accurately up to 25 years of age. Beyond that age it becomes increasingly inaccurate. Consent of the person for examination has to be taken. Consent is not required, if the person being examined is accused under arrest brought for the purpose by the police.

For the purpose of age estimation, general history of the patient regarding sexual development, menstrual history, followed by general growth like height, weight development of genitalia are noted. Then the dental formation examination in relation to number and nature is carried out. A radiological examination is done of the important and required centres of ossification depending upon suspected age. Opinion, regarding age is given by general, dental and radiological examinations.

The final opinion is given as: About 18 years, about 20 years. A range like 19–21 years, may also be kept in brackets for purposes of clarity.

Data for age estimation: Hairs begin to grow first on pubic and then on axilla regions. In girls pubic hair appear one year earlier than the boys at the age of thirteen years. Axillary hairs grow later around 14 years of age.

In the beginning when it first appears the hairs are lighter in colour, thinner and become dark and thicker within two years. In boys hair grow on chin followed by upper lips around 16–18 years. Greying of hair occurs from 40 years onwards starting near the temples then the sclap, beard and moustache, chest, axilla, pubic and body hairs. Generally scalp hairs become thinner in males as age advances and axillary hairs in females.

The breasts develop in girls between 10–14 years. It develops in 4 stages starting from 10 to 14 years. In the first stage, a small elevated enlargement of breast and nipple together occurs. In the second stage, enlargement of breast and areola occurs but the contours are not separated. In the third stage, there is projection of nipple and areola over the level of breast. In the fourth stage or adult stage only the nipple projects out and the areola merges with general contour of the breast. Beginning with small growth, each breast continues to grow gradually in size till it becomes elastic and hemispherical. Menarche sets in the girls around the age of 12 years. The voice in the boys becomes hoarse between 16 and 18 years. After 40 years, a whitish ring appears in the periphery of cornea due to degenerative changes. *Arcus senilis* is rarely complete before the age of 60 years. Increase of LDL affects the formation of arcus. When it occurs in young adults due to hyperlipidaemia, it is called *arcus juvenilis*. Wrinkles appear on the face around 50 years. Cataracts occur around 60 years (it may occur earlier also).

Height and weight are not very reliable means of age estimation. The areas which are radiographed for age estimation, are:

- Wrist in children.
- Elbow region, knee region in adults, skull in old people.
- Pelvis in all age groups.

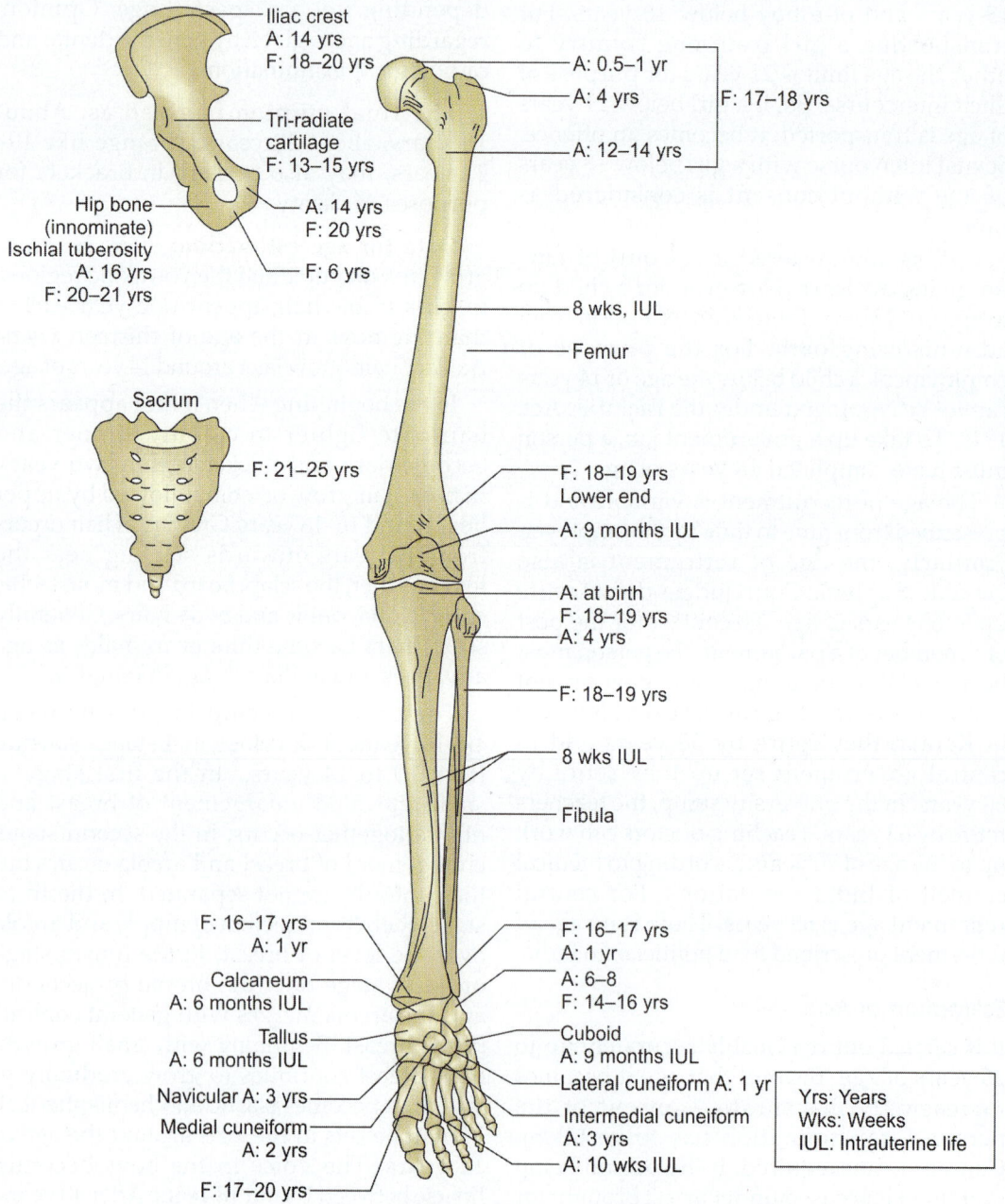

Fig. 3.11: Appearance and fusion of centres of ossification

The extent of ossification of bones varies depending upon diet, hereditary and geographic factors. The posterior fontanelle closes just after birth. The anterior fontanelle closes between 11 and 12 years. Pisiform ossifies at 10 years. Between 14 and 16 years, upper end of fibula unites with the shaft. The upper end of tibia unites with shaft between 14 and 17 years (Figs 3.11 and 3.12).

Between 14 and 18 years, crest of ilium unites with rest of the body. In South Indians and in other parts of India, it may be delayed up to 21 years. The olecranon unites with shaft of ulna by 16 years. The head of the radius, the lower end of humerus unites with the shaft between 15 and 17 years. Between 18 and 20 years, head of femur unites with the shaft. As general criteria, we can say about 15 years for the wrist, about 16 years for the elbow, about 18 years for knee joint and about 18 years for ankle joint +/– 6 months.

The four pieces of sternal body unite with one another between 14 and 25 years from below upwards (Fig. 3.13). The *xiphoid* unites with the body around 40 years, the *manubrium* with the body around 60 years. The sutures

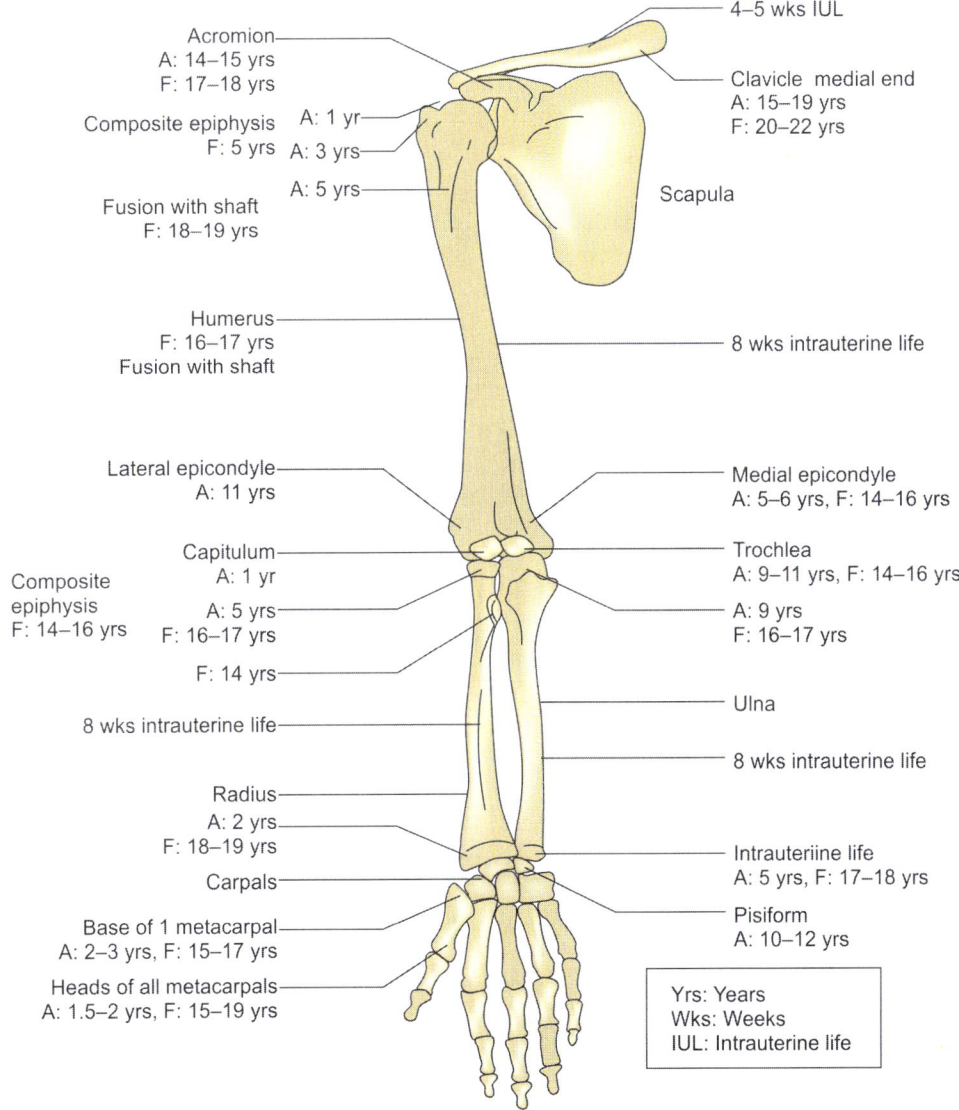

Fig. 3.12: Appearance and fusion of centres of ossification

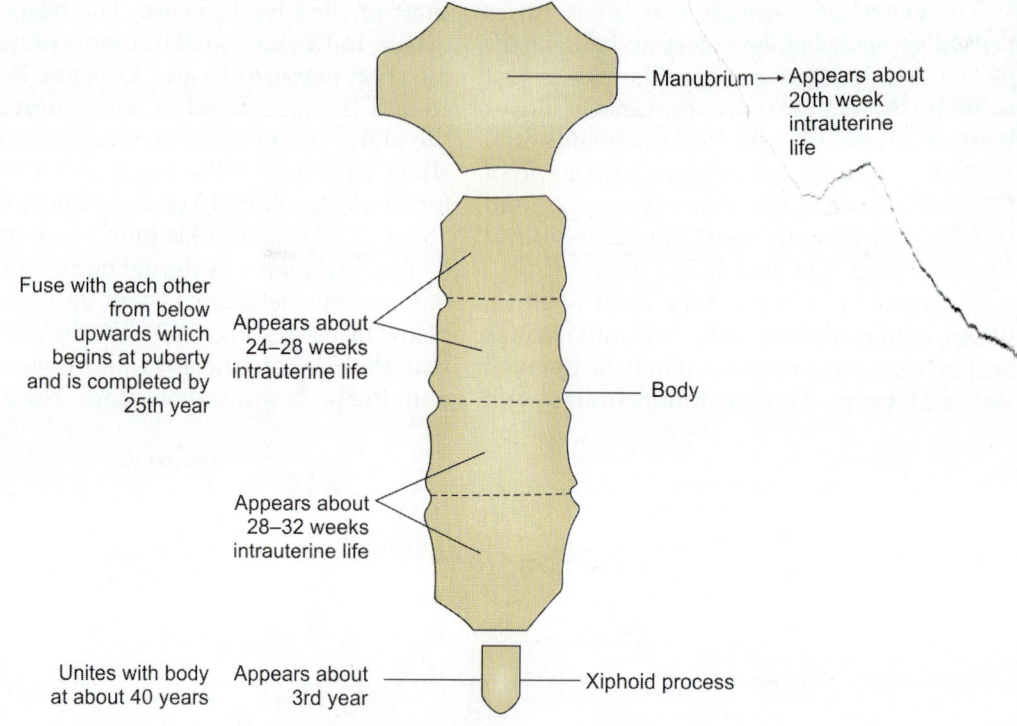

Manubrium → Appears about 20th week intrauterine life

Fuse with each other from below upwards which begins at puberty and is completed by 25th year

Appears about 24–28 weeks intrauterine life

Body

Appears about 28–32 weeks intrauterine life

Unites with body at about 40 years

Appears about 3rd year

Xiphoid process

Fig. 3.13: Ossification of the sternum

of the vault of the skull get obliterated first in endocranial aspect later in ectocranial aspect. The *basiocciput* unites with *basisphenoid* around 21 years.

Lipping of the bones starts after 40 years in lumbar vertebrae (Figs 3.14 and 3.15), knee joints, etc. The greater *cornu of hyoid bone* unites with the body after 40 years and below 60 years. Other neck cartilages and rib cartilages ossify in old age (Fig. 3.16). As the person grows older, the height of a person is said to go down 0.6 cm each year after

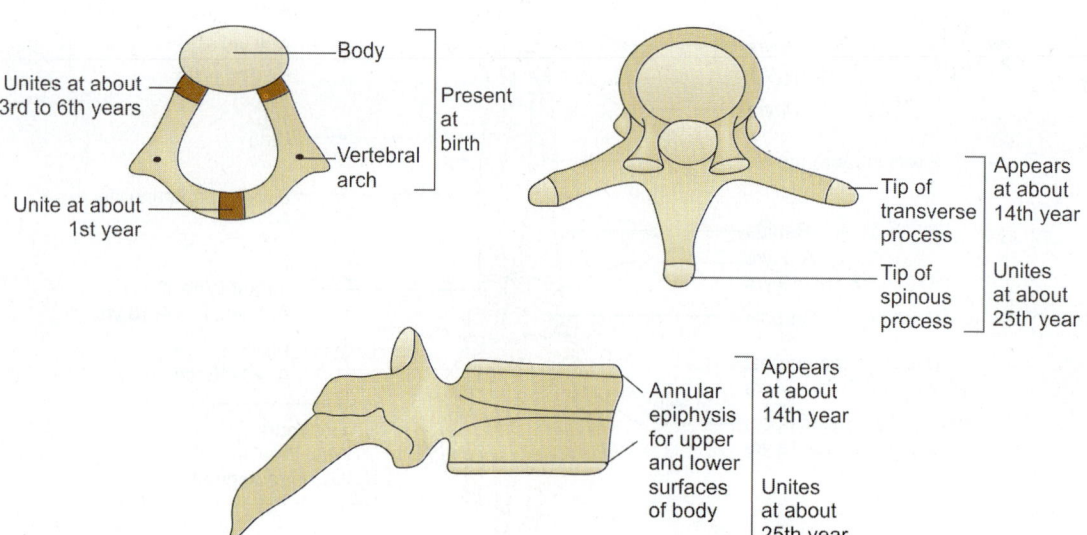

Unites at about 3rd to 6th years

Body

Present at birth

Vertebral arch

Unite at about 1st year

Tip of transverse process

Appears at about 14th year

Tip of spinous process

Unites at about 25th year

Annular epiphysis for upper and lower surfaces of body

Appears at about 14th year

Unites at about 25th year

Fig. 3.14: Vertebral ossification

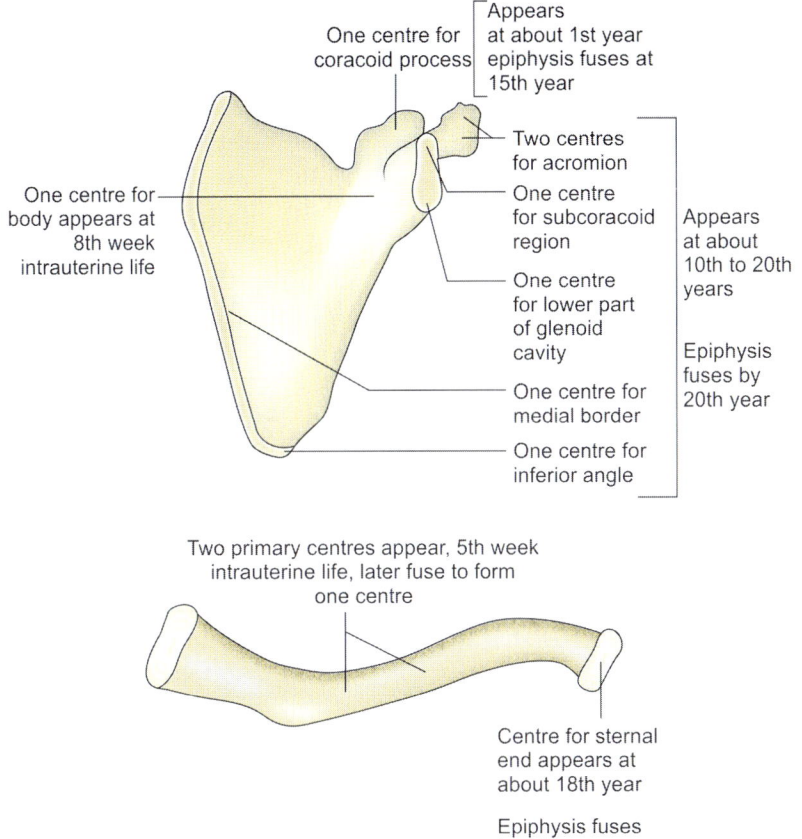

One centre for coracoid process | Appears at about 1st year epiphysis fuses at 15th year

Two centres for acromion

One centre for body appears at 8th week intrauterine life

One centre for subcoracoid region

One centre for lower part of glenoid cavity

One centre for medial border

One centre for inferior angle

Appears at about 10th to 20th years

Epiphysis fuses by 20th year

Two primary centres appear, 5th week intrauterine life, later fuse to form one centre

Centre for sternal end appears at about 18th year

Epiphysis fuses by 25th year

Fig. 3.15: Ossification of scapula and clavicle

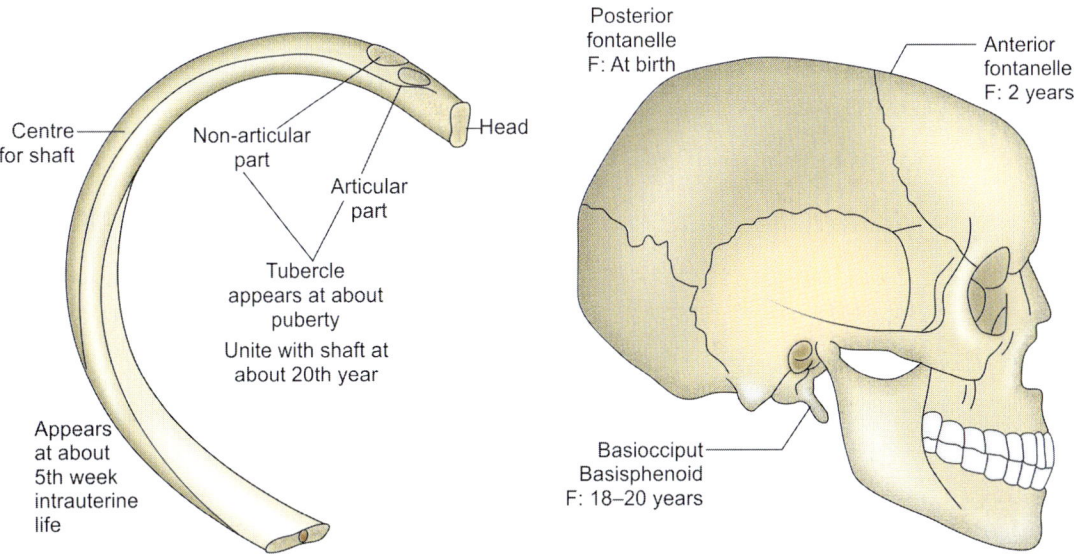

Centre for shaft

Non-articular part

Head

Articular part

Tubercle appears at about puberty

Unite with shaft at about 20th year

Appears at about 5th week intrauterine life

Posterior fontanelle F: At birth

Anterior fontanelle F: 2 years

Basiocciput
Basisphenoid
F: 18–20 years

Fig. 3.16: Ossification of ribs (typical)   Fig. 3.17: Ossification of skull by sutural closure

attaining the maximum height. The height of a person is more after relaxation in early morning and by late evening, it becomes less. The variation can be up to 1.5–2 cm. Teeth are very important tools in the assessment of age, during childhood, adolescents and even during old age.

Race

Due to the frequent shifting and inter-mingling of people around world for various needs such as migration after marriage or good job, official transfer, etc.; people of different races are likely to be present in any part of the world.

Caucasians, Mongols and Negroes are three main ethnic groups in the world. Mongoloid hair is almost circular in cross section. Most of the Indians show Caucasoid features. Nowadays, Indians are called coloured people.

Mongoloid features are more common in north east. Negroid features are more common towards deep south.

The skull is the most useful part of the body for race determination. Caucasians show long and narrow nasal aperture. Negroes show broad nasal aperture at the lower part.

The lower nasal borders are sharply defined in Caucasians. In Negroes, the lower nasal borders are smooth and scooped out,

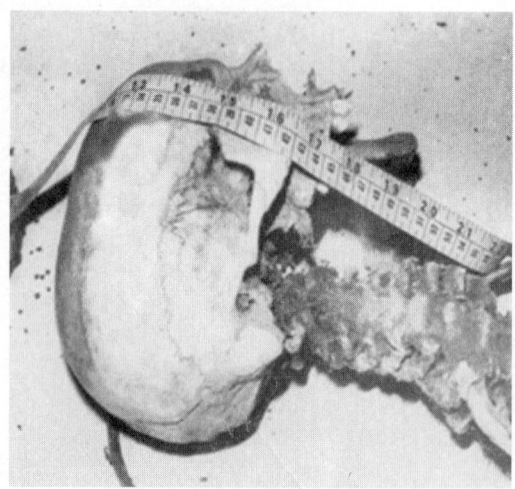

Fig. 3.19: Case of skeletal remains for examination

whereas the Mongols have features in between these two.

• The Mongoloids have prominent cheek bones. Negroes have rectangular orbits,

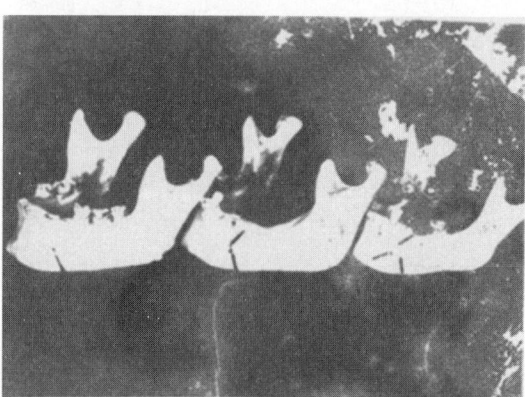

Fig. 3.20: Case of skeletal remains for examination

Mongols have round or oval orbits and Caucasians have triangular orbits. The lower jaw is more prominent in Negroes, the mid-facial skull is non-prominent in Mongols, Caucasians have prominent nose with vertical profile.

• The palate is wedge shaped in Caucasians, horseshoe shaped in Mongols, rectangular in Negroes.

Head hairs of the Caucasians are straight, of Negroes, tightly curled and oval or kidney shaped in cross section. Mongols show deeply pigmented, stout and coarse straight hair.

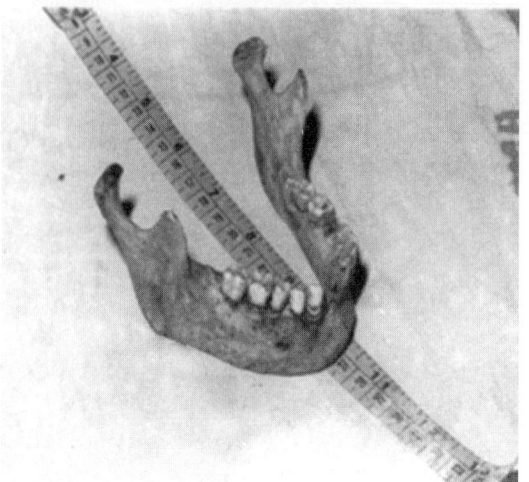

Fig. 3.18: Mandible with missing teeth

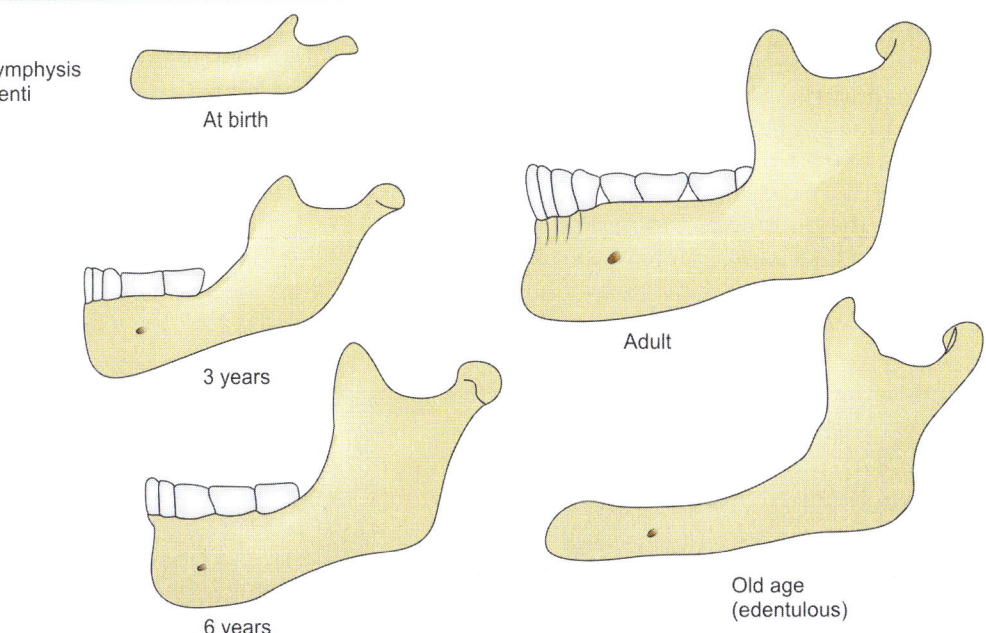

Symphysis menti

At birth

3 years

6 years

Adult

Old age (edentulous)

Fig. 3.21: Age changes in mandible

Temporary teeth are 20 in number and erupt between sixth months and 2 years. Permanent teeth are 32 in number and erupt between 6 years and 22 years. As the age advances due to wearing out, attrition, paradentosis, root transparency, secondary dentin formation, root resorption occur (Fig. 3.22).

Gosta Gustafson graded these characters from 0 to 4 for each and scoring of these data gives estimation of age from 30 years to old age. In late old age, the teeth fall off and gums recede. However, a third set of teeth may appear and remain beyond 100 years of survival.

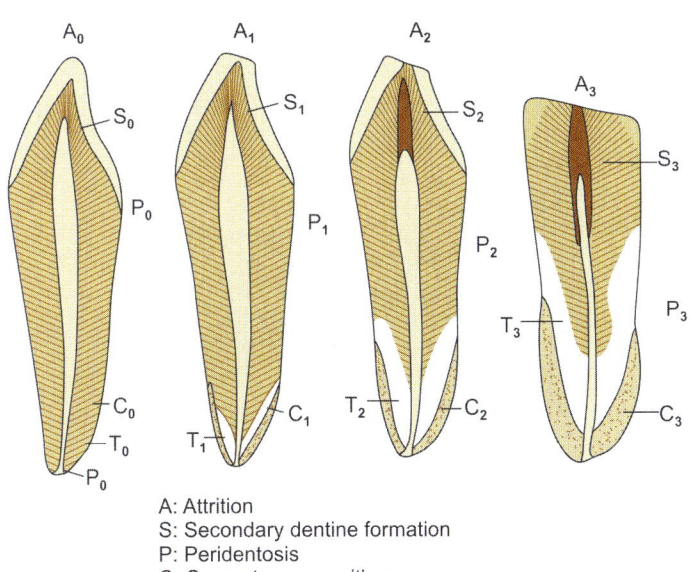

A: Attrition
S: Secondary dentine formation
P: Peridentosis
C: Cementum apposition
T: Transparency of root
R: Root resorption

Fig. 3.22: Gustafson's method

Superimposition

Superimposition photography is useful as tool of identification in cases where a close up front profile photograph of the person in question is available for comparison purpose (Figs 3.23 and 3.24). The principle involved here is to enlarge the photograph to natural size of the skull, to take X-ray photo of the skull and enlarged photograph of the skull of same size, taking a superimposed photograph of both of them and studying the matching of fixed and comparable data like superciliary arches, orbital margins, zygomatic prominences, tip of the chin, interpupillary distance, etc. If these comparable points are found matched, the presumption is in favour of accepting the skull in question to be the same of photograph provided.

If these data are not matching, then it can positively said that the skull (Fig. 3.25)

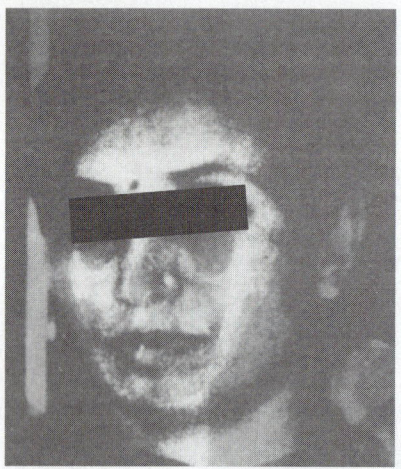

Fig. 3.23: Identification by superimposition technique

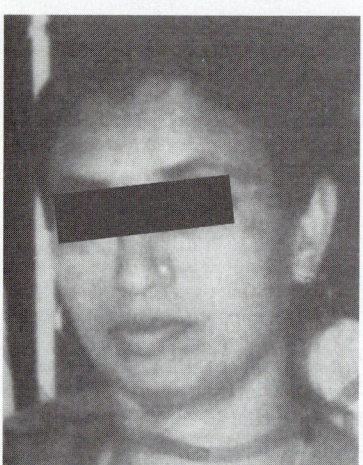

Fig. 3.24: Suspected victim

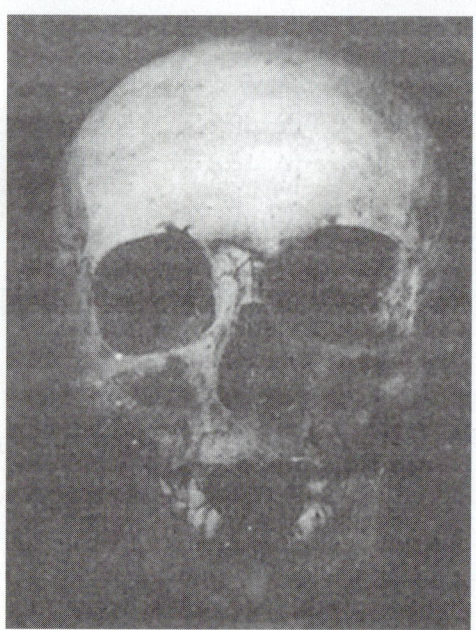

Fig. 3.25: Recovered skull—superimposition for identification

in question does not belong to the person in photograph (to obtain the natural photograph in original size. In the photograph, there may be possibility of having some material which can be obtained and cross checked with, like design of saree, shirt or button, etc.). As an advancement in this step, superimposed video photography and the superimposition on computer are being recommended nowadays as these procedures are technically more advanced.

Teeth

Teeth have a very important place in investigation of crime because they resist heat, they are not disturbed by decomposition, they present peculiarities and characters, that make them useful in pinpointing the identity many times (Fig. 3.26).

Types of Dentition

Temporary or deciduous containing 20 teeth with 5 in each quadrant of mouth comprising of 2 incisors, one canine and two molars. Incisors are cutting teeth, canines are tearing teeth and molars are grinding teeth (Fig. 3.27).

In the permanent set there are two incisors, one canine, two premolars and three molars in each quadrant.

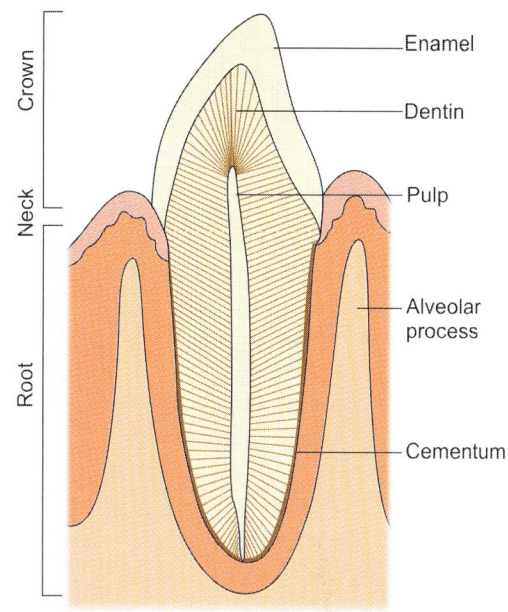

Fig. 3.26: Cross-section of tooth

There are no premolars in the temporary set but only two molars in the temporary set. The first permanent molar comes behind the second temporary molar and it is the first permanent tooth to erupt at around 6 years of age. The third molar is the last tooth to come, it erupts between 17 and 21 years. It is widely, popularly and wrongly refered to as wisdom tooth.

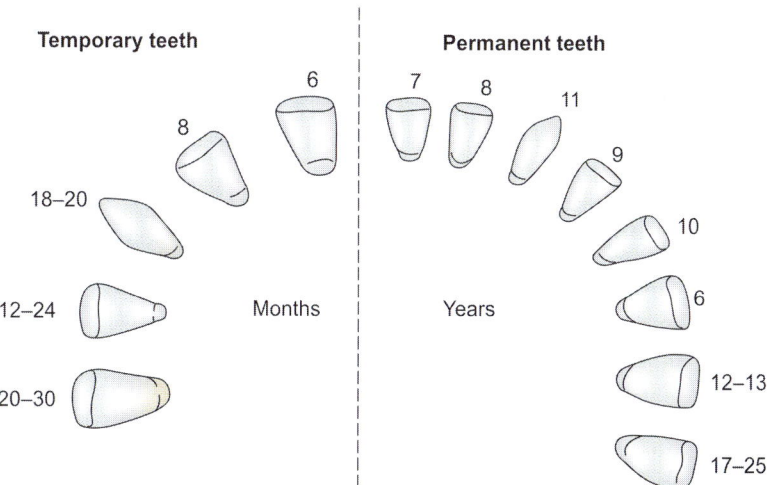

Fig. 3.27: Ages of eruption of teeth

The temporary set starts around six months and complete eruption comes by 24 months to 2 years. There is a mixed dentition figure showing both temporary and permanent teeth between 6 and 14 years (Fig. 3.27). During this period when a doctor is examining the teeth he should know whether the teeth are temporary or permanent. Temporary teeth are small, vertically placed, shiny white and show a notch between the junction of crown and neck.

Premolars have two cusps, molars have more than two cusps. Canine roots are longer than the incisor teeth. Temporary incisors show notches on the top of crown.

Peculiarities of teeth-like: Supernumerary teeth, broken, overlapping, malrotated, peg or shovel shaped teeth.

Gum abnormalities: Gingival hyperplasia.

Repaired and replaced teeth, root canal therapy, wiring dentures, etc.

• All required to be carefully noted while investigating a case.
• Up to 6% of the cases there may be congenital agenesis of one or more teeth without leaving any gap in between, so there is need for careful counting of the teeth.

Acquired absence of teeth is also seen when teeth are extracted or naturally fall off.

After all the teeth have erupted and root calcification completed, due to the daily use and misuse of teeth, there is a lot of wear and tear leading to progressive changes likely attraction, paradentosis, secondary dentin formation, root resorption, transparency of root and cementum apposition.

Attrition starts around 28 years of age and the various parameters are graded from 0 to 5 stages and a combination of the score helps in the determination of age from 28 years onwards. The error limit increases beyond 50 years of age. Transparency of the root does not occur before 30 years of age.

The resorption of root starts after 50 years. A normal healthy tooth shows a shining enamel, dentin and pulp cavity. Tooth has crown, neck and root. The determination of age after the secondary changes in the teeth goes by the name of Gosta Gustafson who streamlined and gave a scoring formula.

GUSTAFSON'S METHOD OF AGE ESTIMATION FROM TEETH: SIX CRITERIA

1. *Attrition*: Due to wear and tear from mastication, occlusal (upper surface of the teeth is destroyed gradually, first involving the enamel, then dentin and at last pulp is exposed in old age. It depends on the functional use of teeth and also upon the hardness of the enamel.

2. *Paradentosis*: Regression of the fumes and periodontal tissues surrounding the teeth taken place in advancing age, gradually exposing the necks and the adjacent part of roots, due to which the teeth become loose and fall of. Poor oral hygiene increases paradentosis.

3. *Secondary dentin*: It may develop from the walls within the pulp cavity, and decrease the size of the cavity. First it is deposited at the pulp chamber and gradually extends downwands to the apex, and may completely fill the pulp cavity. This is partly due to ageing and partly due to pathological conditions like caries, and paradentosis.

4. *Cementum apposition*: The cementum increases in thickness particularly due to changes in the tooth position, especially near the end of the root. Secondary cementum is slowly and continuously deposited throughout life, and forms incremental lines. Incremental lines (devised by Boyde) appear as cross-striations on the enamel of teeth due to cementum apposition, and are thought to represent daily increments of growth. The age can be calculated by counting the number of lines from the neonatal line onwards. This is mainly applicable to infants.

5. *Root resorption*: It involves both cementum and dentin which show characteristically sharp grooves. Absorption of the root starts first at the apex and extends upwards. It usually occurs in late age. It may be due to pathological process.

6. *Transparency of the root*: It is not seen until about 30 years of age. The canals in the dentin are at first wide. With age they are filled by mineral, so that they become invisible and the dentin becomes transparent. It is the most reliable of all criteria.

Medicolegal importance

- From the tooth one can access the age of a person.
- Sex from cells of pulp cavity.
- Identity from peculiarities and dental alterations.
- Diseases like fluorosis, caries, syphilis (Hutchinson's teeth), acid poisoning cases of H_2SO_4 and HNO_3.
- Drug use—brown in tetracyclines, yellowish due to excessive use of mouthwash.
- Depositions of poison like arsenic and mercury.
- Chromosomal studies and DNA analysis can be carried out from the teeth even after incineration, conflagration and decomposition.

Lip Prints (Cheiloscopy)

In view of the multi-coloured lipsticks being used, the chances of identifying the individual from the lipstick colour, the shape and the lines on the lips, are considered as important identification features. Chance lip prints may be found on the clothes, on the bodies, on left out fruits, glasses, cups, saucers, etc.

Ear Prints

The shapes of ear lobes and the tips of ears are of various types, some people have broad wing like upper lobe, some people have wide, loose hanging lower lobes, some people have whole ear tending to come forward, some people have ear nearer to occipital region, the lower lobe may be fixed to the face.

The helix is hard in some people and soft in some people. Similarly, the lobule is soft in majority of people but may be hard in some people. Overall, some ears are hard and some ears are soft. Hair on the ears, on the helix and tragus are seen in males (linked to Y chromosome).

Nose Prints

Nose prints are chance impression which may be found at the scene of offence or on the body of victim or accused on the mirrors, corners of walls, doors and so on. The lines on the nose and the shape of the tip are helpful in identification.

Palate Prints

Dental prosthesis of palates as made by dentists is made and when originally available, the moulds can be of help in identifying the persons from palate and palate prints. Palate can be high or low, broad and narrow with bony ridges and prominences and rugosity of the palate.

Dr. Sreenivas Method

The ECG pattern of individual vary from person to person. Dr. Sreenivas from Patna developed EVG method of identification from ECG and vector cardiogram.

Dr. Subrahmanyam from Surat has Described Namastae Technique for Identification (the Author)

When two hands are brought together like in 'Namastae' the digits and palm apposed to each other match well in a given person and do not match with any other person.

A decomposed hand up to wrist was brought for examination and identification. During the same period, there was a patient admitted in orthopaedic department of New Civil Hospital (NCH), Surat, with his (left) upper limb amputed up to level of middle of arm. The question arose as to whether this decomposed hand could belong to that person. Since the decomposed hand belonged to the same side of the amputed limb, the above principle was applied in this case by putting the decomposed hand in available normal hand of the patient and taking both the hands together and X-ray taken. The decomposed hand was put similarly over hands of Dr. Subrahmanyam, Dr. Sheikh and Dr. Tiwari and similar X-rays were taken.

The control and suspected material were examined in X-ray view box. The suspects hand matched well while the other hands did not. Thus, identity of the decomposed hand was established with that of the patient in orthopaedic ward who was deaf and dumb, somebody had cut his hand and threw near railway track.

Miscellaneous

Gait; mannerisms like trics, voice and occupational marks are also of help in the identification.

BONE DENSITY: USES

Dual X-ray absorptiometry (DEXA) quantifies bone mineral density (BMD) and bone

mineral content (BMC). This technique has rarely been used in Forensic Anthropology,

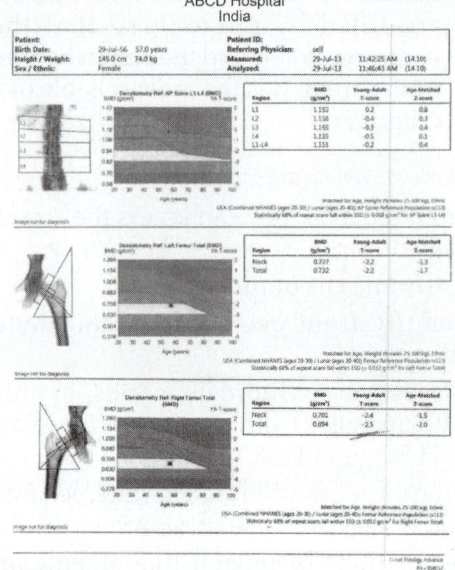

ABCD Hospital
India
DXA Bone Densitometry Report

Patient Rajeswari K completed a BMD test on 29-Jul-13 using the Lunar Prodigy Advance DXA system (analysis Version: 14.10) manufactured by GE Healthcare. The following summarizes the results of our evaluation.

Name:						
Patient ID:		Referring Physician:	Self		Height:	145.0 cm
Gender:	Female	Birth Date:	29-Jul-56, 57.0 years		Weight:	74.0 kg

RESULT

Site	Region	BMD	T-score	Z-score
AP spine	L1–L4	1.151 g/cm²	−0.2	0.4
Dual femur	Neck left	0.724 g/cm²	−2.2	−1.3
Dual femur	Neck right	0.701 g/cm²	−2.4	−1.5
Dual femur	Total left	0.732 g/cm²	−2.2	−1.7
Dual femur	Total right	0.694 g/cm²	−2.5	−2.0

ASSESSMENT:

The BMD measured at AP spine L1–L4 is 1.151 g/cm² with a T-score of −0.2 is normal, fractrue risk is low.
The BMD measured at femur neck left is 0.727 g/cm² with a T-score of −2.2 is low, fracture risk is high.
The BMD measured at femur neck right is 0.701 g/cm² with a T-score of −2.2 is low, fracture risk is high.
The BMD measured at femur total left is 0.732 g/cm² with a T-score of −2.2 is low, fracture risk is high.
The BMD measured at total right is 0.694 g/cm² with a T-score of −2.5 is low, fracture risk is high.

World Health Organization (WHO) criteria:
Normal: T-score at or above −1 SD
Osteopenia: T-score between −1 and −2.5 SD
Osteoporosis: T-score at or below −2.5 SD

FOLLOW-UP
Bsed on these results, a follow-up exam is recommended in July 2014
Exame Date: 29-Jul-13   Page 1 of 1   Patient: K. RAJESWARI

although its practical application has been demonstrated by various authors. Bone mineral density in the femoral neck, the trochanter, the intertrochanter, the proximal femur and Ward's triangle, in relation to anthropometric age and sex parameters. Bone mineral density is a useful technique for sex and age data in forensic anthropology, particularly in the measurements observed in the Ward's triangle area.

Bone mineral density is useful

- To determine the age of the individual
- To determine the sex of the individual
- To diagnose osteoporosis and risk of fracture.

A report of bone density MRI is shown as an example in pages 29–30.

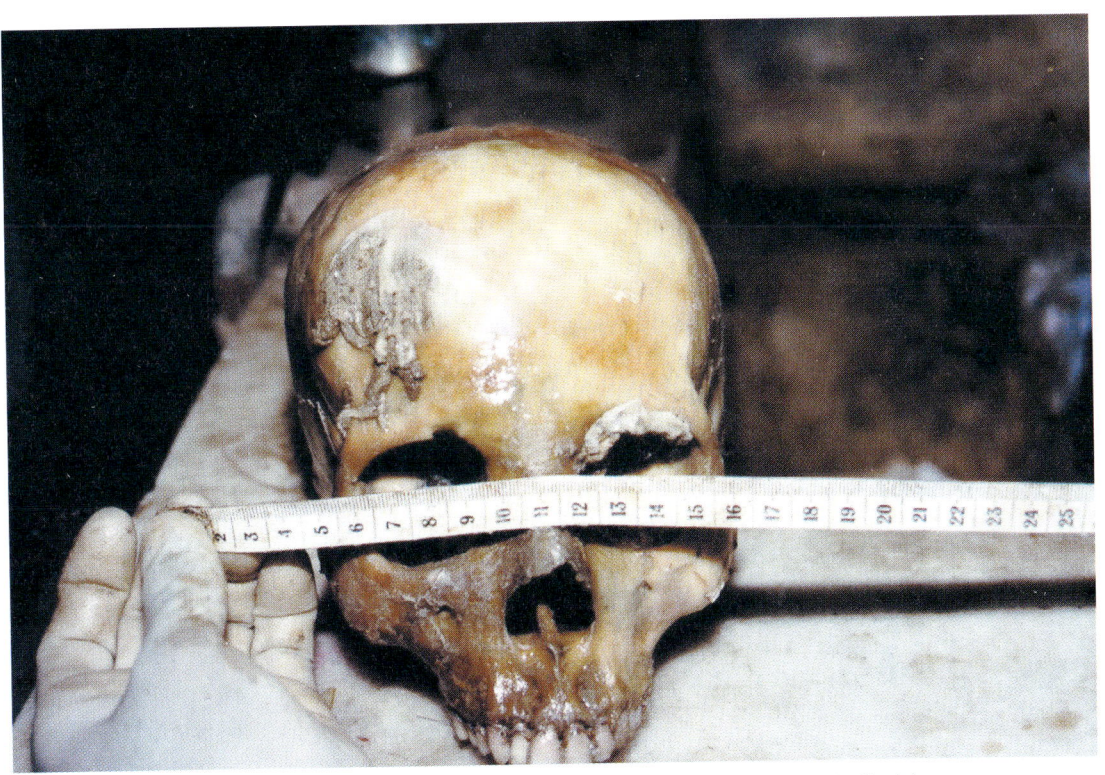

Skull for skeletal remain exam look at the orbital upper part on both sides

CHAPTER 4

Death and its Medicolegal Aspects

THANATOLOGY

It is the study of death in all its aspects (thanatos—death; logos—discourse).

Forensic thanatology is the subject dealing with medicolegal study of death, the chemistry of death, the conditions affecting the dead bodies and other facts about death that are applied in a Court of Law.

After the organ transplantation also the time cause of death, declaration of death, certification of death have assumed legal and clinical significance.

Traditionally, death has been defined as an irreversible cessation of functions of circulation, respiration and central nervous system. However, even with respiratory and circulatory failure, life activity may go on at the brain level. So, scientifically speaking the **brain stem death** is the death for all practical purposes and is diagnosed with the following conditions:

- The patient is in coma for at least 6 hours.
- All brain stem reflexes are absent.
  - The pupils are fixed in diameter.
  - No response to bright light.
  - Corneal reflex is absent.
  - Doll's head–eye movements (oculocephalic reflex absent).
  - Response to heat and cold (hot water and cold water) absent.
  - Vestibulo-ocular reflex absent.
- No motor response of any part of the body even after pinching.
- The gag reflex is absent.

- Respiratory movements are absent on withdrawal of mechanical respirator.

The moment of death is determined by the clinician by employing the stethoscope for at least 5 minutes in a noise-free environment and noting the absence of heartbeat.

For the purpose of transplantation surgery, the removal of the organs should be done within:

15 minutes	Liver
15–30 minutes	Lungs
Within 45 minutes	Kidneys
Within 1 hour	Heart
Within 2 hours	Cornea
Within 2–4 hours	Blood vessels
Within 6 hours	Bone

The death certifying team should be different from the organs removing team. The organ transplanting team should be different from organ removing team. Apparent death or suspended animations is the differential diagnosis of real death.

The causes of suspended animation are

- Electric shock
- Cataleptic/hypnotic trance
- Drowning
- Anaesthesia
- Cerebral contusion
- Newborn infant
- Vasovagal shock
- Sun stroke
- Typhoid
- Cholera
- Overdose of sedatives and hypnotics

Medicolegal Importance of Death (Fig. 4.1)

Declaration of death: If death is wrongly declared and body is transferred to mortuary, it can create a big problem.

Certification of death: A death certificate cannot be issued by a doctor unless death of the person is confirmed.

Disposal of the body: Mistakes in diagnosis of death cause a problem in the disposal.

Organ transplantation: Tissues for transplantation cannot be removed unless death is certified.

Presumption of death: If a person who lived for 30 years and now is not seen alive by nears and dears for a period of 7 years, a legal presumption of death and certification from Court of Law can be obtained by certification from nearest relatives.

MODES OF DEATH

The tripod life is said do consist of the activity of respiratory system, circulatory system and central nervous system. There are three modes of death. Traditionally called **Bichot's classification of death.**

Syncope
Asphyxia   Differences are given
Coma   in Table 4.1

Syncope

It is a mode of death brought about by the failure of action of heart.

It causes death due to cessation of heart actions.

- Sudden and excessive haemorrhage or bleeding as a result of injury to large blood vessels, injury to organs like lungs, spleen, liver, heart and rupture of aneurysms.
- Loss of large quantities of fluid component of blood as in cases of black water fever, cholera, burns, etc.
- Shock due to reflex inhibition of heart out of fear, blows on head, pit of stomach, spinal injuries, fluid or air embolism from uterus.
- Injury to carotid area of a the neck, cervix uteri, urethra, precordium, etc.

Clinical Features (Symptoms and Signs)

Pallor of lips, face, cold clammy skin, sweat, dilated pupils, restlessness, air hunger, low and sudden fall of blood pressure, weak or rapid pulse, delirium, convulsions and death.

Postmortem appearances: Heart chambers empty if it stops in systole. Chambers dilated and full if heart stops in diastole. Pallor of organs, lungs, brain, liver, spleen, etc., capillary congestion.

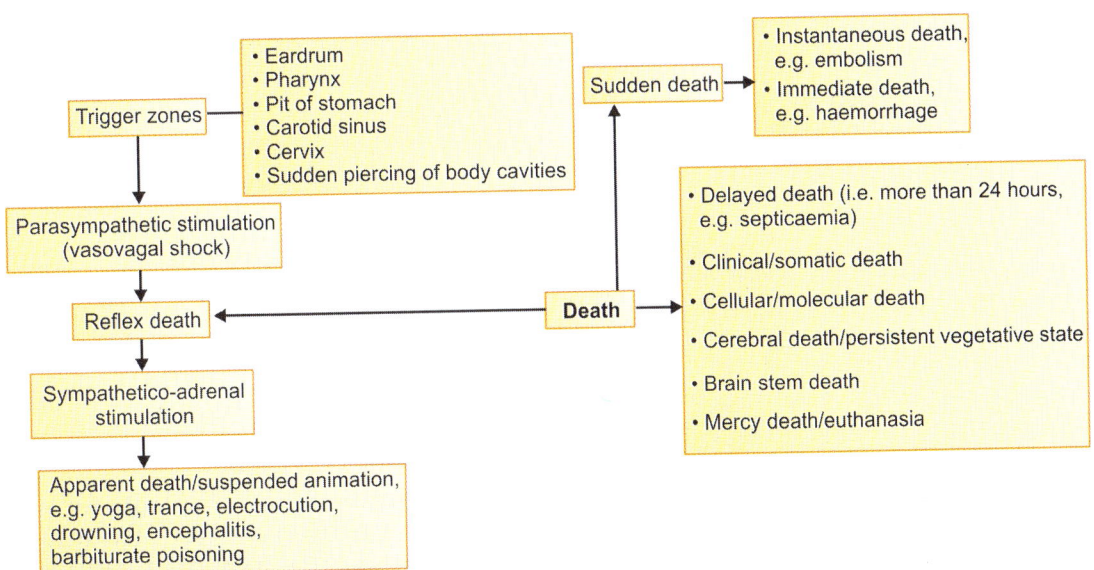

Fig. 4.1: Terminology related to death

Asphyxia

It is brought by the failure of respiration leading to death.

The word asphyxia (Greek word *a*—privation; *sphyzo*—to throb), which suggests absence of the throbbing or pulse. The term asphyxia however has been used widely for increased CO_2 and reduced oxygen followed by hypoxia or anoxia. Asphyxia is defined as mode of death due to deprivation of oxygen, leading to failure of respiratory function.

Causes

- Mechanical obstruction of respiratory passages from both within and without, e.g. closure of mouth and nostrils.
- Absence/lack of sufficient oxygen, e.g. high altitudes, CO, CO_2, HCN poisoning.
- Stoppage of chest movements due to pressure on the chest, paralysis of respiratory muscles (tetanus, strychnine poisoning).
- Collapse of lungs due to penetrating wounds of chest—lungs and pleura.

Symptoms and Signs

The stage of inspiratory dyspnea, the stage of expiratory dyspnea and convulsions, the stage of exhaustion and respiratory failure.

Postmortem Appearances

- Livid lips and nails.
- Congestion of viscera.
- Petechial haemorrhages.
- Deep postmortem staining.

Coma

It causes death by loss of consciousness and failure of the activities of central nervous system. The term coma is derived from Greek word *koma*—which means deep sleep. Coma means insensibility resulting in death. It involves the vital centres in brain stem so in the case of death from coma, all functions of brain stem cease permanently and irreversibly. Sometimes a person in coma goes into **persistent vegetative state (PVS)**. In PVS, the respiration is continued, there is a total loss of perception by senses, the person is in a stage of cerebral death, but not in a stage of brain stem death.

Causes of Coma

Head injuries : Subarachnoid haemorrhage, brain abscess, meningitis or encephalitis, space occupying lesions, embolism or thrombosis.

Poisons: Barbiturates, alcohol, opium and its derivatives.

Clinical states like: Uraemia, ketosis, diabetic coma, hepatocellular failure and coma.

Postmortem examination: The brain and membranes are congested. The injuries and haemorrhage are depending upon the cause are seen. Lungs are congested. Pooling of blood presents in venous system.

There is some overlapping of the modes of death sometimes. However, in majority of cases, there will not be any difficulty in ascertaining the mode of death.

In syncope, the cause of death is generally due to shock as a result of blood or fluid loss or vagal (inhibition) where there is a cardiac inhibition due to stimulation of vagus nerve because of triggering the vagal sensitive areas like tympanic membrane, carotid sinus, carotid body, solar plexus in the pit of the stomach, urethra, testes and cervix (Table 4.1).

Gordon's Classification of Mode of Death

Gordon felt that in all forms of death, the fundamental pathological changes are uniform in nature, and that is due to absence of oxygen supply to the tissues in whichever way it occurs.

Four types of anoxia have been recognized, they are

1. Anoxic anoxia.
2. Stagnant anoxia.
3. Anaemic anoxia.
4. Histotoxic/cellular anoxia.

Anoxic Anoxia

The amount of oxygen available for the purpose of respiration is reduced like in high altitudes or inspiration of inert gases like methane, H_2S or low oxygen content during

Table 4.1: Differences among syncope, asphyxia and coma

Syncope	Asphyxia	Coma
Circulatory distress and failure	Respiratory distress and failure	Central nervous system distress and failure
Conditions related to heart, blood vessels or blood present	Conditions related to larynx, trachea, bronchi and lungs present	Conditions related to meningitis, intracranial haemorrhages, infection of brain or space occupying lesion of brain present
Pallor of the organs generally seen Lesions related to cause	Congestion of the organs, petechial haemorrhages, cyanosis. Lesions related to cause	Visceral congestion, splanchnic pooling of blood. Lesions related to cause

anaesthesia or interference with respiratory function due to pressure over chest, paralysis of chest muscles due to failure of respiratory centre, due to interference in respiration by any mechanical obstruction like choking, gagging, drowning, throttling, hanging, strangulation, etc.

Stagnant anoxia: Occurs due to inefficient circulation of blood in tissues like heat stroke, shock, congestive cardiac failure.

Anaemic anoxia: Occurs due to reduction in oxygen carrying capacity of blood, e.g. anaemia due to any cause (haemorrhage), co-poisoning.

Histotoxic Anoxia

It is due to lack of tissue oxygenation and oxidation. It can be extracellular, cellular, intracellular, metabolic and substrate type:

Extracellular	Chloroform, ether
Cellular	Barbiturate
Intracellular	H_2S
Metabolic	Uraemia
Substrate	Hypoglycaemia

CLINICAL DEATH AND SEQUELAE OF DEATH

Every clinician has to certify death during his practice, though no one likes his patient to die. During the last moments of the life of the patient, the clinician cannot avoid the presence of anxious relatives. However, he should ensure that there is no noise in the vicinity of the patient. Most of the times just before a patient passes off, death rattle is observed. As the respiration becomes sluggish, accumulation of fluids in respiratory passages produces grunting noise which suddenly stops when the person takes his last breath.

The body tends to become cool, the sensations are lost, pupils become dilated and fixed, the pulse and heart clinical death. When the patient is declared dead, it is the duty of doctor attending at the time of death to issue the death certificate. The medical certificate of cause of death, should show the disease or condition directly leading to death. It should also show other significant conditions contributing to death though not related to the disease or condition causing death.

In clinical death, the body loses its life so it is called somatic death. In somatic death the signs are **stoppage of activity of the brain** which can be detected by flat ECG, if there is no electrical activity for 10 minutes in electroencephalogram we can presume death. **In stoppage of respiration,** as seen by the absence of respiratory movements, the surface of mirror held in front of mouth and nose is covered with moisture from a breathing person and not from a dead person. The **stoppage of circulation** as can be seen by absence of radial pulse, absence of heart-beats and absence of transillumination of vessels seen through the skin along the webs of the digits.

There is no sensation and there are no movements of the limbs. During this period, the person ceases to exist as a functional whole. On application of galvanic electric current, the muscles show contraction. On instilling atropine in eyes, pupils show dilation and on installation of physostigmine, the pupils show constriction.

During this stage of somatic death or clinical death, various tissues for the purpose of transplantation can be carried out under rules and regulations of **Organ Transplant Act.**

Cellular death follows somatic death. During this stage, the individual tissues and cells die, so it is also called molecular or cytological or cellular death. Cellular death occurs in nervous tissue rapidly and it is delayed in the muscles.

It is completed within about three hours after the clinical death. Following changes are seen on the body:

- Cadaveric spasm
- Heat loss in the body
- Changes in eye
- Changes in skin
- Changes in staining
- Postmortem staining
- Rigor mortis
- Putrefaction
- Mummification
- Adipocere formation.

Cadaveric Spasm

When a group of muscles are active at the time of death like trying to each weeds during drowning or holding a pistol or revolver in hand, these muscles continue to remain stiff as death overtakes the person. This stiffening of a small group of muscles, instantaneously, upon death is called **instantaneous rigor or cadaveric spasm.**

Cadavaric spasm continues through the stage of rigor mortis of the body and disappears only after the onset of secondary relaxation, e.g. a five rupee note was found clenched in outstretched hand of Deendayal Upadhyay, President of Jansangh, whose body was found near railway tracks of Mughul Sarai railway station. Professor I. Bhooshan Rao opined that it was in cadaveric spasm and that his death could have been due to accidental slipping from the train.

Medicolegal Importance of Cadaveric Spasm

- It indicates that the person was alive at the time of instantaneous rigor.

- The time of onset of instantaneous rigor suggests the moment of death or time of death.
- If some object belonging to assailant is found in victim's hand like hair, button, it suggests murder.
- If weeds are held in hand grasped in a drowned body, it suggests antemortem nature of the drowned body.
- If a knife is held in clasped hand of cut throat victim, suggests suicide.
- The exact mechanism of cadaveric spasm is not known.

Heat Loss in the Body

The normal body temperature at the time of death is more than that of the environment. The body temperature is maintained by thermoregulatory centre (TRC) of hypothalamus, which streamlines the variations. Once the person dies, the body starts losing heat until it reaches room temperature. The loss of heat occurs by conduction, convection and radiation. The average rate of temperature is 0.5–0.7°C/hour. However, it is governed by many factors like:

- Difference of body and environment temperature.
- Temperature of environment
- Clothing of a person
- Nutritional status
- Fat content
- Stature
- Age
- Sex
- Sickness at the time of death.

The greater the difference between the temperature of the body and surroundings, the faster is the rate of cooling. As the temperature starts approaching the temperature of atmosphere, the rate of cooling slows down. If the temperature of body is B and temperature of surrounding is S, the difference is S-B. In the first 2 hours, fall of temperature is S-B/2, in the next two hours, fall of temperature is S-B/4 and in the next two hours it is S-B/6. The body arrives at the surrounding temperature by 12–15 hours after death.

Postmortem caloricity (Post—after, mortem—death, caloricity—heat): Sometimes the body temperature instead of falling down, starts increasing. This increase in temperature after death of the body is called **postmortem caloricity.** It occurs in cases of *lobar pneumonia,* enteric fever, acute viral infections, sun stroke, brain stem haemorrhage.

Medicolegal importance of postmortem caloricity: Increase in temperature indicates infections are haemorrhage into the brain stem.

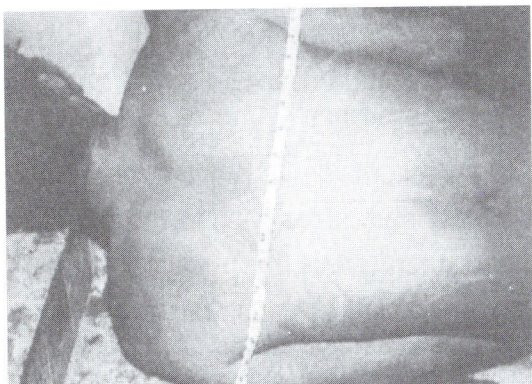

Fig. 4.2: Bluish coloured postmortem lividity on back. Note areas of contact flattening (pale areas)

Changes in Eye

After death, the corneal reflex is lost. The cornea becomes dry, cloudy and opaque. The intralocular tension falls. The eyeballs become flaccid. The eyeballs sink into the orbits. The optic disc becomes pale. Brownish area of discolouration appears on exposed parts of sclera when eyelids are open.

These are known as **taches noire scleroticus.** It is formed due to cellular debris and dust setting down.

Kevorkian Sign

When we look at the fundus, during life, the retinal blood vessels look like continuous red wavy lines. As soon as the death occurs, circulation becomes sluggish, there is stagnation of retinal blood columns, when we look at the fundus, the retinal blood columns look interrupted. This is known as **positive kevorkian sign** occurring soon or as early as 10 seconds of clinical death.

Jouelin, in 1967, felt that segmentation of retinal blood columns with **rail roading** movement of red cells resembling the movement of goods train wagons is a sign of cerebral death.

Changes in Skin

Living skin shows luster, elasticity and transparency (translucency). After death, the skin loses its elasticity, and due to stoppage of peripheral circulation it becomes dull, waxy and opaque.

Postmortem Staining

When a person is living and moving the circulating blood, pro-gravity and anti-gravity prevent collection of blood in any part of the body. However, when a person is lying on a bed, for a considerable time before death, due to sickness, there is a gradual sluggishness of circulation in the dependent parts of the body, leading to some amount of stasis of blood. Patches of discolouration generally of reddish colour occur sometimes in such cases like cholera, typhus, tuberculosis, asphyxia, congestive cardiac failure, uraemia and morphine poisoning.

After death of a person, the blood circulation stops, blood vessels lose their tone, blood continues to be in liquid state for some time. During this time the blood in toneless capillaries and veins of the body due to gravitational force gather blood. Because of this stasis of blood, we can see the discolouration of skin and organs. The colour of the staining will be the same as that of colour of the blood.

Normally, the discolouration is reddish. But in cases of asphyxia, it is purple in colour, in CO poisoning it is cherry red in colour, in HCN poisoning it is bright red in colour and in sodium nitrate poisoning it is chocolate brown in colour, in H_2S poisoning, it is green in colour.

To start with, it occurs in patches. Then it becomes continuous. It is well marked in about 4–6 hours. However, on the bony areas of the body, which are in touch with the surface, on which the body is lying, due to the pressure in the capillaries, the stasis of blood does not occur. So, these areas do not show postmortem staining or hypostasis. These areas like occiput, shoulder blades, buttocks, calf area, etc. are known as areas of contact flattening. In the same way due to similar mechanism, along the area of collar, waist band or under the belt or along the thread of the skirt, the staining is not seen in the early stages of formation of postmortem staining, if the position of body is shifted, due to the change of parts which are dependent, the staining develops in the new dependent parts. So, there may be two different areas of staining, sometimes opposite to each other suggesting the shifting of body position after death.

Postmortem staining: Resembles bruise or contusion. It also resembles congestion. Whenever there is a doubt, make a cut in the area. Blood in interstitial spaces, or collection of blood due to trauma, if can be differentiated. In hypostasis, blood is confined to the blood vessels while in contusion, blood is outside the blood vessels. In congestion due to inflammation associated inflammatory response like oedema and exudation are seen (Table 4.2).

Table 4.2: Postmortem staining: Causes and colour

Poisoning as cause of death	Colour of lividity
	Bluish pink followed by bluish purple
Normal aniline, CO_2	Deep blue
Copper sulphate $(CuSO_4)$ H_2S	Bluish green
Asphyxial death	Purple
Opium	Black
Death from septic abortion caused by *Clostridium perfringens*	Grayish brown
Phosphorus	Dark brown
Chlorate	Chocolate brown
Nitrates, nitrites, $KHCO_3$ (potassium bicarbonate), aniline	Red brown
CO, burn, cold, HCN, cyanide (KCN, NaCN)	Bright—cherry red, pink, brown

Medicolegal Importance of Hypostasis of Livor Mortis or Suggillation

- Hypostasis helps in estimation of time since death.
- From the distribution of hypostasis one can say whether the body was disturbed or not.
- From the colour, we can suggest the cause of death.
- Postmortem staining in hands and feet suggests hanging position of the body after death.

Hypostasis disappears with the onset and advancement of decomposition. The colour of hypostasis also changes as the decomposition advances due to destruction of capillary endothelial outline and chemical changes in disintegrating haemoglobin.

Vibices (Fig. 4.3) are the pale strips or bands due to compression by tight clothings, collar bands, tight neck-tie, skin folds of neck, etc.

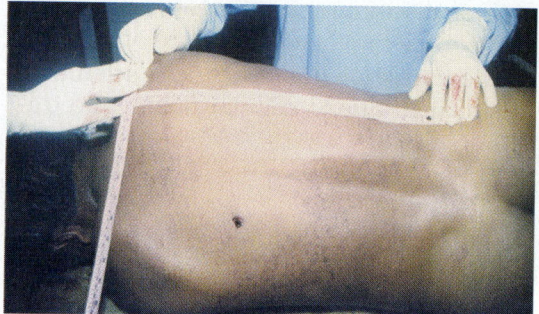

Fig. 4.3: Vibices

Patterned areas of pallor in between the areas of hypostasis are the vibices and they cause confusion, so one must be aware of vibices while noting the injuries on the dead body (Fig. 4.4).

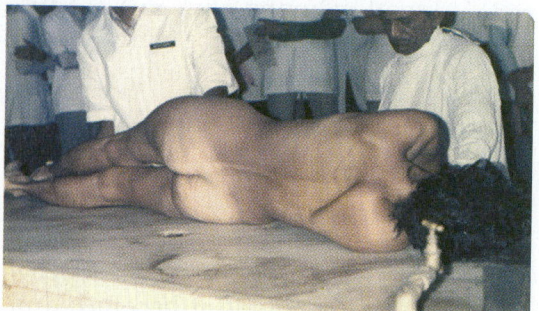

Fig. 4.4: Areas of contact flattening

Cause: Lividity Positions	
Cause	*Lividity positions*
Hanging	• Dependent lower limb • External genitalia • Lower part of forearm and hand
Drowning	• Head and uppermost part as body floats with face downwards • Does not develop in running water
Electrocution in water (bath tub)	• Lividity is sharply limited to horizontal line corresponding to the water level
Lying flat on back	• On back dependent portion of body • But it is not seen on back of shoulder blades, buttocks, and back of calves due to contact flattening (i.e. toneless capillaries are compressed and occluded by weight and pressure of body)

Primary flaccidity: After death soon the whole body becomes limp. When we touch the lower jaw, it falls and does not take back its place. When we lift the hand it falls flat and flab. Eyelids loose their tension, joints become easily flexible. This flaccid stage of the body lasts for about 2 hours. During this

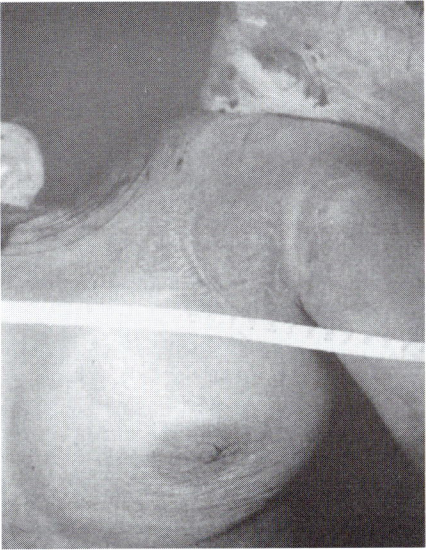

Fig. 4.5: Vibices due to pressure of bra

stage the sphincters relax and can cause urination and defecation, seminal emission and so on. Because of loss of muscle tone, the parts of the body subjected to pressure become flat like buttock, calf muscles, causing areas of contact flattening.

Rigor Mortis (Rigor—Rigidity; Mortis—of Death)

Rigor mortis is the rigidity of the body occurring after death. This occurs after the stage of primary flaccidity. It involves both voluntary and involuntary muscles of the body. When it is fully developed in skeletal muscles of the body, whole body becomes a log of wood and assumes board like rigidity.

Mechanism of Rigor Mortis

The human muscle consists of contractile myofibrils through the length of muscle fibre. The myofibrils consist of act in and myosin which are the muscle proteins. When a nerve impulse brings about muscle contraction, the actin–myosin filaments interdigitate like pistons into cylinders. During the stage of muscular relaxation, the interdigitating filaments move apart. Individually actin and myosin do not have power of contraction and relaxation. The combined form of actin and myosin is capable of contracting and relaxing in presence of an adequate quantity of adenosine triphosphate (ATP). During the resting stage of muscle, actomyosin is inactive and a high concentration of ATP is absorbed to it. When the muscle is stimulated the ATP is activated and muscle contracts. After death, there is fall of ATP and ATP finally disappears. Glycogen also disappears. There is an increase of inosine phosphate and accumlation of acid metabolites like carbon dioxide, lactic acid and phosphoric acid. With the result that actomyosin is converted into a stiff dehydrated gel. The muscles become rigid. Thus, rigor mortis occurs. As a part of the process of putrefaction, the acidity of the muscles increases and the myosin is dissolved leading to gradual disappearance of rigor mortis.

Secondary flaccidity: It occurs after the passage of rigor mortis. During this stage, there is no muscular response to electrical stimulation. Secondary flaccidity occurs in the same sequence like the appearance of rigor mortis. It takes about 12 hours for the complete setting of secondary flaccidity.

Breaking of Rigor

Due to handling of the dead body using force, the stiff joints become loosened and then the limb becomes flaccid. When breaking of the rigor occurs in this way, the muscles do not resume rigor again. The first voluntary muscle to develop rigor mortis is muscles of eyelids. Then it spreads to face, neck, trunk, upper extremities, lower extremities. Feet develop rigor in the end. Rigor mortis follows a proximodistal progression. Rigor mortis passes off first in the face and last in the feet. This progression of rigor mortis is said to be apparent and not real because rigor mortis occurs in all the muscle simultaneously.

Primary flaccidity	3–6 hours
Spread of rigor mortis	6–12 hours
State of rigor mortis	12–24 hours
Disappearance of rigor mortis	24–36 hours
Secondary flaccidity	12 hours after it starts to develop full relaxation

The rigor mortis is also seen in involuntary muscles of heart, occurs in 1 hour of death, left side is involved more than right side.

Factors Affecting the Rigor Mortis

Age
- In children and old people, rigor onset is quicker.
- In adults, the onset is slow.

Sex

In muscular males, rigor starts slowly and stays longer.

Temperature of environment
- In the winter, there is delay in onset.
- In the summer, it occurs fast and disappears fast.

Condition of body

If the person is emaciated, it will appear early and pass off early.

Condition of muscles before death
- If the muscles are relaxed, rigor sets late.
- If the muscles are exhausted, the rigor sets and passes off early.
- If muscles are in convulsion before death, onset is early but duration is longer.

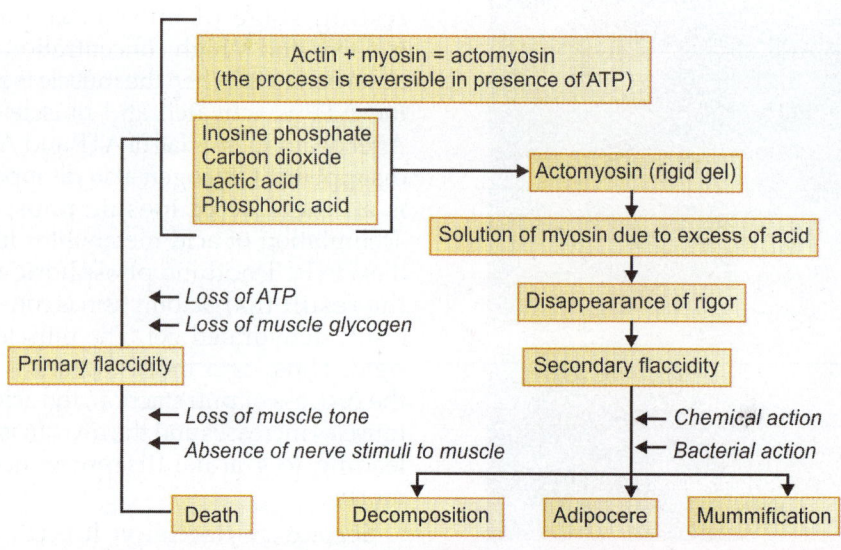

Fig. 4.6: Death and changes after death

Mode of death

In cases of tetanus, epilepsy, etc. onset is early and lasts short.

Causes of death

- Early onset is seen in typhoid, tuberculosis plague, cholera.
- Delayed onset occurs in cases of asphyxia, pneumonia, apoplexy, poisoning by arsenic and mercury, etc.

Differential Diagnosis

Cadaveric spasm: Seen in groups of muscles and not in whole body.

Cold stiffening: When the body is exposed to freez temperature below 3.5°C, due to solidification of muscle fat and body fluids, stiffening of the body occurs. Here the body is cold, crepitus (crackling noise) is felt in the joints due to breaking of frozen fluid of joints. When the body temperature is brought to environment temperature rigor mortis develops in these cases.

Heat stiffening: When the body is exposed to temperature above 70°C, heat stiffening occurs due to coagulation of muscle proteins. The muscles exposed to heat stiffening does not develop rigor mortis. They directly enter into decomposition stage.

Gas stiffening: It is due to gases of decomposition, making the joints stiff and swollen. The body is foul smelling with other decompositional changes.

Medicolegal Importance of Rigor Mortis

Helps in determination of time since death. The development of rigor mortis and its disappearance takes time in multiple divisions of 12 and so a rough guide of rule of dozen is used as postmortem clock timing using rigor mortis.

Posture of the body after death: The rigor mortis develops in undisturbed body after death in the same posture in which it is lying; so therefore, from the position of the body in the fully developed state of rigor mortis, it is possible to tell the position of the body after death.

Onset of rigor mortis removes any confusion about the diagnosis of death.

Putrefaction

Putrefaction/decomposition is a postmortem process of breaking down of tissue from complex organic state to simple inorganic ones. It is considered to be surest sign of death. Though, nobody waits for this to occur, to declare death.

Mechanism

Putrefaction is brought about by two processes:

1. **Autolysis:** During the process of autolysis, the body tissues undergo softening and liquefaction due to release of enzymes from cells after death. Autolysis starts from 3–4 hours after death and continues up to 2–3 days.
2. **Bacterial action:** As a result of bacterial action by both aerobic and anaerobic organisms like staphylococci, *Streptococcus viridans*, non-haemolytic streptococci.

Diphtheroids, *B. proteus, Clostridium welchii*, etc. (organisms of putrefaction) produce proteolytic and other enzymes break down proteins and carbohydrates of the intestine of the body itself. In the presence of warmth, moisture and air, decomposition is initiated by *Clostridium welchii*.

The Products of Putrefaction and Chemical Substances

Acids: Acetic, palmitic, oxalic, succinic, lactic acid, etc.

Amines and amino acids: Leucine, tyrosine, putrisine, cadaverine.

Aromatic and amino acids: Indol, skatol.

Mercaptans

Gases of decomposition: Hydrogen sulphide (H_2S), sulpur dioxide (SO_2), carbon monoxide (CO), carbon dioxide (CO_2), ammonia (NH_3), phosphine (PH_3) and methane (CH_4).

Enzyme levels: A steady increase in the levels of serum glutamic-oxaloacetic transaminase (SGOT), lactic dehydrogenase (LDH).

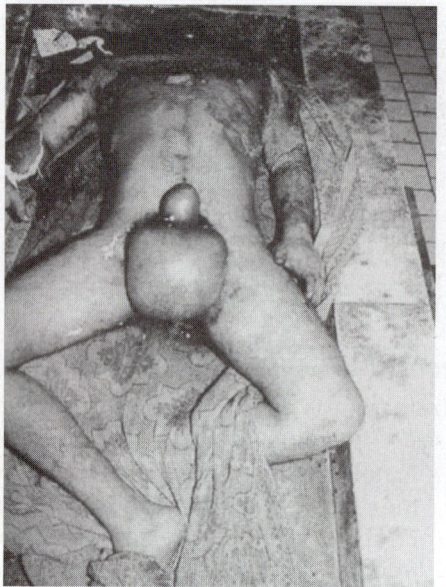

Fig. 4.7: Scrotal swelling due to gases of decomposition

Colour Changes

The earliest colour change to occur is over the right iliac region. The postmortem discolouration varies in colour from green to black. Haemoglobin changes to sulphmethaemoglobin in the presence of hydrogen sulphide (H_2S). This sulphmethaemoglobin gives rise to the colour changes of putrefaction. Flanks of abdomen show discolouration in about 24 hours. In beginning, it occurs in patches, which later unite, till the whole body discolours in around 2 days time.

Marbling: It is the mosaic pattern of the veins seen on the skin after death in the beginning stages of decomposition due to decomposition of blood inside. It occurs in 1–2 days. Earlier in summer, later in winter.

Blisters/blebs/bullae: The postmortem blisters are due to accumulation of gases in patches under the skin. They start as small blebs and enlarge by merger into bigger sizes. These blisters contain the gases and serosanguineous material of decomposition. They do not contain albumen or chloride-rich fluid and do not show a rim of inflammation. Thus, they can be differentiated from blisters of antemortem burns. They take about 36 hours to develop after death.

Peeling of the skin: It occurs in putrefaction. Sometimes the skin of the hands and feet may come out like gloves and stockings. This is seen in about 48–72 hours after death.

General Features

General features are bloated due to filling up of gases. Then the identification becomes difficult, if not impossible. The eyeballs and tongue protrude. There is bloating of penis, breasts and abdomen. Gases occupy inside and develop lot of pressure. So, when we make a cut on abdomen, gases come out with big noise and spread foul smell around. Through mouth and nostrils, froth and regurgitated stomach contents come out. The heart is emptied. There may be delivery of a foetus from pregnant uterus. Gas occupying liver makes it spongy or foamy; called as foamy or spongy liver. On cut section, the gases escape and the remaining architecture presents honeycomb appearance.

The decomposed body floats in water because of the accumulation of large gases of decomposition which make the body lighter.

Table 4.3: Order of putrefaction

1. Larynx and trachea
2. Infant brain
3. Stomach, intestine, spleen
4. Liver, lung
5. Brain
6. Heart
7. Kidney, bladder
8. Prostate, virgin uterus
9. Skin, muscle, tendon
10. Bone (last)

Entomology of the Dead

Common files are attracted to the body after death. They lay eggs in the moist places and orifices like mouth, nose, axilla, groin. These ova/eggs are seen in 18–36 hours. The eggs hatch into maggots in another 24 hours. Maggots become pupae in 4–5 days. Pupae become adults in another 4–5 days.

Hair become loose and can be easily pulled out. The nails become loose and easily fall down. This occurs in 48–72 hours. At the same time, uterus and rectum prolapse from the body.

Colliquative putrefaction commences by 5 days and gets completed by 10 days. This includes liquefaction of tissues, abdominal wall bursts with protrusion of stomach and intestines. The tissues become soft, loose and become like a gruel. The bones are separated from soft tissues and get exposed. Internally also the organs show decomposition changes. Organs which decompose fast are baby brain, adult brain, liver, spleen, stomach, intestines, mentum, mesentery. Slowly decomposing organs are heart, lungs, kidney, bladder, oesophagus, blood vessels, pancreas, etc.

Organs which resist decomposition for long time are virgin uterus and prostate, even when the rest of the body is highly putrefied.

Factors Affecting Decomposition

Stature of the body: Bodies of infants show delayed onset of decomposition. In a healthy muscular adult, when death is not due to disease, there is delay in decomposition. Fatty bodies are insulated from the environment; so the environmental effect decomposition is delayed in such cases.

Mode of death: In cases of death from bacteraemia/septicaemia decomposition is rapid. In deaths like arsenic poisoning, decomposition is delayed and retarded.

Environmental temperature: Around room temperature, decomposition is faster. When the temperature is more than 50°C, bacterial growth stops and putrefaction is arrested. When the temperature goes down to freezing points, putrefaction is arrested.

Humidity: When moisture is more in atmosphere, decomposition is faster than when the organs are dry. Moisture content of brain is high, so it liquefies fast. Teeth, bones, nails are dry structures and decomposition. Muscular organs also resist decomposition, e.g. heart.

Clothing (nature and number): Clothing hastens putrefaction because in tries to retain the temperature and facilitates bacterial action.

Location of the body: When body is present in moist and marshy places, the decomposition is delayed and may be modified into adipocere formation. When the atmosphere is dry and associated with blowing winds, decomposition is delayed and even modified to mummification.

Mummification

It is process of postmortem dehydration and desiccation of the body due to exposure to relatively high atmospheric temperature, dry air and blowing winds. The body dries up losing its moisture. First the exposed parts of the body, lips, fingers, toes become stiff, shriveled, dry leathery and then the process involves the remaining body also.

A mummified body is dry, leathery, shrunken with skin (gangrene to the skeleton. It is brownish black in colour. The features are preserved. Wounds are recognizable. Internal organs are also hard, shrunken but well preserved. It may take up to one year for mummification to be total.

Medicolegal Importance

- Identity is possible due to preserved features.
- Wounds can be appreciated, so nature of injuries can be assessed.
- Since internal tissues can also be rehydrated, histopathology can detect tissue pathology.
- Time of death can be estimated.
- The location of the body can be explained.

Adipocere Formation

Adipocere is a postmortem phenomenon of saponification of body fats or postmortem hydrogenation of body fats and hydrolysis into fatty acids aided by fat splitting enzyme lecithinase of *Clostridium welchii* in a marshy area. It occurs in moist, humid environment, when a limb is inside water with rest of the body out, local adipocere formation occurs so also if buttocks are touching water and rest of the body is dry, adipocere is seen in buttocks. It is more common in fatty people and women especially over breast, buttock and abdomen. The name adipocere is derived from French (*adipes*—fat; *cera*—wax), i.e. fat is converted into wax like substance. This term was given by a French man in 1879, AF Fourcroy.

Adipocere is a white or yellowish white waxy material with disagreeable rancid odour. It cuts easily, floats in water and melts easily on heating. When it burns, it emanates cheesy odour. It gives off ammonia and sulphur compounds. In adipocere unsaturated fatty acids like oleic acid are converted into saturated fatty acids like stearic, palmitic acid by hydrogenation.

Adipocere consists of calcium soap, proteins, glycerine, saturated fatty acids like palmitic acid, stearic acid, hydrostearic acid. In an adipocere area of the body, features are preserved and retained. Wounds are recognizable. The internal organs are also well preserved. Adipocere can occur from 3 days to 30 days time.

Medicolegal Importance

- Identity is possible.
- Wounds are preserved and how they are caused can be found out.
- Cause of death can be determined.
- Time since death can be ascertained.
- Location of body after death cab be explained.

TIME SINCE DEATH/TIME ELAPSED AFTER DEATH

One of the main jobs of the doctor is to give opinion about time since death in cases brought for postmortem examination. In hot climates, the criteria for time assessment starts appearing faster, than in colder climates.

Intemperate climates, the duration taken is almost the middle of extremes of cold and heat. The postmortem interval is the interval from the time of death till examination of the body by the doctor doing postmortem examination.

So, the doctor doing autopsy has to take note of various external factors helpful in assessment of time since death. If the body is kept in cold storage room, the features which exist before keeping it in the cold room continue to be present same as it is. When no eyewitnesses are available for the incident and the death has occurred unnoticed, the medical assessment assumes a lot of importance in investigation of the offence. It helps in eliminating the innocent persons from suspects list. The opinion about time since death is based on the following data:

- Postmortem cooling
- Rigor mortis
- Postmortem staining
- Putrefactive changes
- Adipocere
- Mummification
- Entomology on the body
- Hair growth over face
- Condition of plants beneath the body.
- Status of stomach contents.
- Contents of large intestine and bladder.
- Biochemical examination of blood, CSF, vitreous humour.

Postmortem cooling: It takes place at the rate of 1°C/hour on land and 1.5°C/hour in water. In cold months the process is

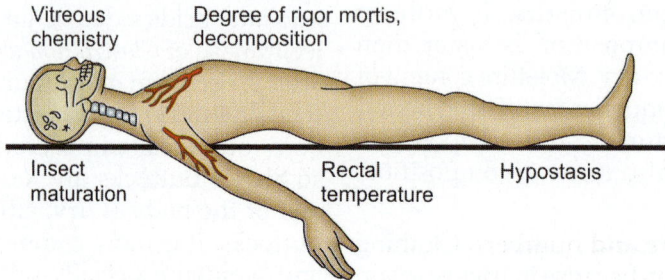

Fig. 4.8: Factors useful in assessment of time since death

delayed and in hot months the process is hastened.

Rigor mortis: The state of primary flaccidity lasts between 1 and 3 hours. Rigor mortis starts in 3–6 hours, develops in 6–12 hours, remains for 12–18 hours and passes off in 18–36 hours. Appearance of rigor starts from face, spreads to arms and trunks reaching to legs with disappearance occurring in same fashion.

Postmortem staining: It is seen in 4–6 hours after death. It continues to remain till decomposition is superadded and the lividity is masked.

Putrefactive changes: Greenish discolouration over right iliac region is seen in 18–24 hours. The flanks become discoloured or become green in about 36 hours. Marbling of the skin is seen by 36 hours and is completed by 2 days (48 hours). The body may be bloated and swollen with gases and the skin presents postmortem blisters or blebs within 36–48 hours. Distension of the abdomen with marked body swelling, all organs disrupted by gas, blisters filled with putrefactive gases occur in 2–4 days.

Bulging eyeballs, bursting organs and cavities, protrusion of tongue, extreme disfiguration occur in 3–5 days.

Colliquative necrosis, general liquefaction and soft tissue separation occur in 5–7 days.

Organs become crepitant, hair easily wiped away, nails easily pulled away, glove and stocking separation of hand and feet occur in 5–7 days.

Loosening of ligaments, exposure and separation of bones is sen in 1–2 weeks.

Adipocere formation: Adipocere formation can occur between 3 days to 3 months.

Mummification: It occurs between 3 months to 1 year.

Entomology of the dead: Maggots are seen over the body within 24–36 hours of death. These maggots get converted to pupae in 4–5 days and then into adult flies in next 3–4 days.

Hair growth over face: Hair does not grow after death. During life it grows at the rate of 0.4 mm/day. So, from the length of hair of the beard, the timing of last shave can be assessed.

Condition of plants beneath the body: The place where the body is lying may show plant materials like grass, flowers, etc. The flora surrounding the body continue to be fresh but those under the body show dryness, withering, etc. This also gives a rough guess about duration of the body lying at that place.

Status of stomach contents: Digestion of food stops after death of the person. However, autolytic changes acting on the stomach mucous membrane can bring some alteration in the contents of the stomach. If fresh pieces of bread are seen in the stomach, probably the patient died after breakfast. If dal, rice, sabji is seen, he might have died after a meal. Undigested food particles can be seen up to two hours after food intake. After two hours, the digested food and partly digested food are seen. Stomach digestion causing soft pulpy food can occur in 3–4 hours. Stomach emptying occurs in 5 hours. If someone ate 500 gm of food, after 30 minutes it becomes 250 gm. Every 30 minutes this is halved. However, the stomach emptying depends on whether it contains fat/carbohydrates, general health of the person and the digestive system.

Contents of large intestine and bladder: Before defaecation, large intestine may show formed faecal matter. So, if the person is dead before he wakes up presence of faecal matter helps in assessment of time.

If the urinary bladder is full, then again the person might have died before he woke up in the morning.

Biochemical examination of blood, cerebrospinal fluid and vitreous: Postmortem increase of levels of lactic acid, amino acids and nonprotein nitrogen substances is known. Up to 15 hours after death, these values are helpful for blood and CSF examination.

The K^+ level steadily increases between 12 and 72 hours (= 0.152 mEq/c/hr).

Thus, by listing all the points and knowing their status, we can arrive at time since death. The decomposition changes occur in the ratio of 1:2:8 in relation to air, water and soil as per the **Casper's dictum.** So, the variation factors must be kept in mind before giving time since death.

Complete skeletonisation of the body without any external interference occurs in about a years time in a deep grave and on exposure to atmosphere in about a month.

SUDDEN DEATH

It is defined as a death occurring suddenly and unexpectedly and not due to apparent trauma or intoxication or poisoning.

When an apparently healthy person dies under circumstances, when his death is not expected and dies suddenly, it is called **sudden death.** Ordinarily the terminal event is <24 hours before death or the person is not seriously ill during the 24 hours before death. Because the death occurs all of a sudden, there is a possibility of suspicion of foul play. If the last attending physician is satisfied with the terminal event he may issue the death certificate. If he has any doubt or suspicion, then it becomes necessary for him to get an inquest made and proceed in the direction of performing an autopsy.

The important causes of sudden death are

- Cardiac causes.
- Respiratory causes.
- Neural causes.
- Alimentary causes.
- Miscellaneous.

Cardiac Causes

Sudden cardiac death (SCD) is defined by Mayer and Castellani as a natural death due to cardiac causes by abrupt loss of consciousness within one hour of onset of acute symptoms with or without known existing heart disease, in an unexpected mode and at an unexpected time.

In about 80% of cases, examination of the heart at autopsies shows significant coronary artery disease. The remaining cases show structural heart diseases like hypertrophic cardiomyopathy, aortic stenosis, pulmonary hypertension, etc. sometimes an apparently normal heart is seen. More than 75% of sudden involving two or more vessels. In some cases, old scars of earlier infarction are seen.

Acute lesions in the coronary arteries are plaque, fissures, platelet clumps, organizing thrombus (coronary artery spasm), left ventricular hypertrophy, acute infarct, healing infarct, healed infarct, ventricular dilation, infectious myocarditis (viral).

Respiratory Causes

Pulmonary embolism, acute oedema of glottis, bronchial asthma, pneumonia, massive haemoptysis, spontaneous pneumothorax.

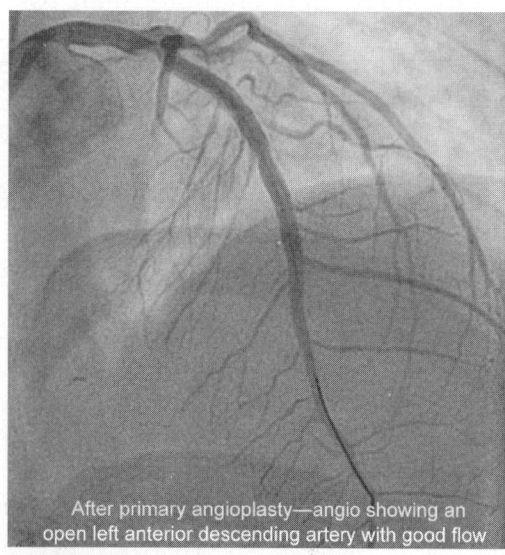

Before primary angioplasty—angio showing an occluded left anterior descending artery

After primary angioplasty—angio showing an open left anterior descending artery with good flow

Fig. 4.9: Anterior descending artery before and after primary angioplasty

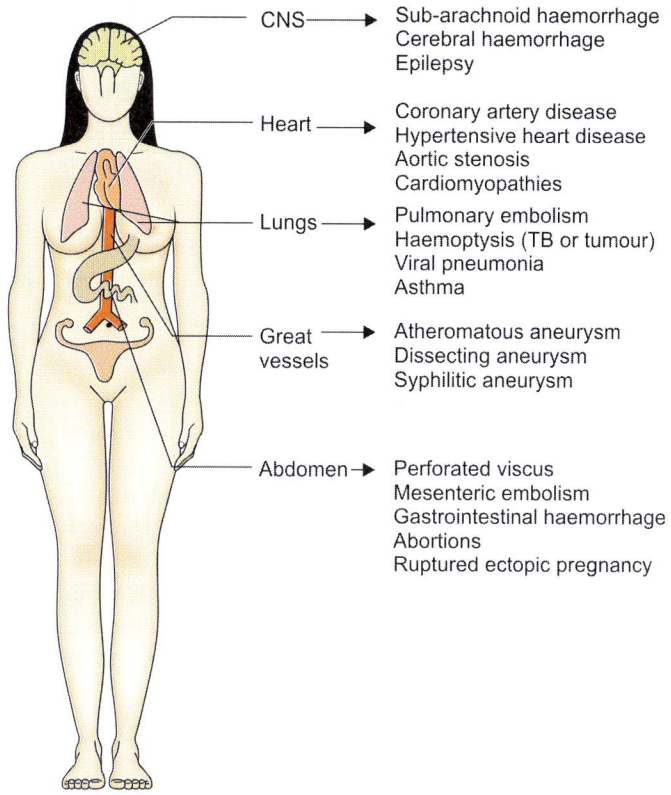

CNS → Sub-arachnoid haemorrhage
Cerebral haemorrhage
Epilepsy

Heart → Coronary artery disease
Hypertensive heart disease
Aortic stenosis
Cardiomyopathies

Lungs → Pulmonary embolism
Haemoptysis (TB or tumour)
Viral pneumonia
Asthma

Great vessels → Atheromatous aneurysm
Dissecting aneurysm
Syphilitic aneurysm

Abdomen → Perforated viscus
Mesenteric embolism
Gastrointestinal haemorrhage
Abortions
Ruptured ectopic pregnancy

Fig. 4.10: Sudden death—common causes

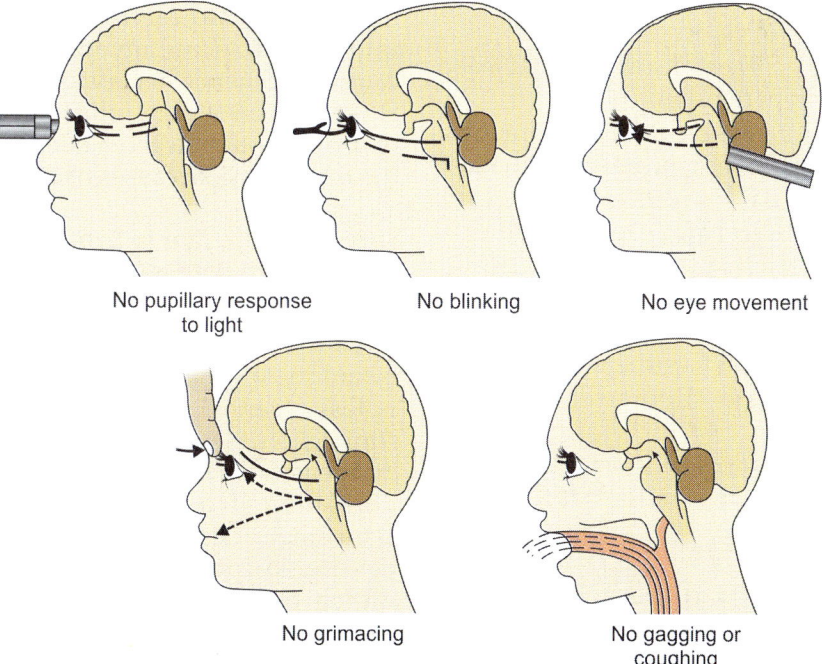

No pupillary response to light   No blinking   No eye movement

No grimacing   No gagging or coughing

Fig. 4.11: Sudden natural death: Signs of brain stem death

Neural Causes

Vagal inhibition, epilepsy (idiopathic or post-traumatic), nontraumatic subarachnoid haemorrhage (Berry aneurysm rupture), intracerebral (hypertension), cerebral infarction (ischaemic stroke), primary undiagonosed brain tumour, meningitis, meningococcaemia (rapid **fulminant** death within 12 hours of onset of symptoms), hydrocephalus.

Alimentary Causes

Massive haematemesis (oesophageal varices), gastrointestinal haemorrhage (gastric/duodenal ulcer, erosion in artery), strangulated hernia, perforation of gastric/duodenal ulcer, fulminant haemorrhagic pancreatitis, diabetic coma.

Hepatocellular failure and hepatic coma, adrenal crisis (phaeochromocytoma), rupture of spleen (malaria).

Miscellaneous

- Sickle cell disease (haemoglobinopathy).
- Ruptured tubal pregnancy.

Sudden Deaths in Infants and Paediatric Age Group

Cardiac causes: Pericarditis due to rheumatic fever or bacterial cause.

Vascular causes: Kawasaki disease, pulmonary hypertension.

Respiratory causes: Status asthmaticus bronchitis, acute bronchopneumonia, pneumothorax.

Neural cause: Meningoencephalitis (Japanese).

Haematological: Acute leukaemia, bleeding diathesis, sickle cell haemoglobinopathy.

Gastrointestinal: Gastroenteritis.

Genitourinary: Glomerulonephritis, pyelonephritis.

Metabolic disorders: Reye's syndrome, sudden infant death syndrome (SIDS).

Vagal Inhibition

It is also called reflex death. In vagal inhibition, death occurs all of a sudden as a result of reflex vagal stimulation leading to cardiac inhibition.

Causes of vagal inhibition are

- Sudden fear/emotion
- Injury to trigger areas
- Carotid body and carotid sinus in the neck
- Solar plexus (pit of the stomach)
- Precardium
- Tympanic membrane
- Other serous membranes
- Cervix uteri
- Testes
- Urethra

Stimulation of the trigger area brings about cardiac inhibition. Even a trifle injury or **microtrauma** to the receptor nerve endings in these trigger areas leads to death. The vasovagal reflex is may be some pallor and death due to sudden cardiac asystole. At autopsy, no organic disease is discovered. The autopsy findings are negative. Vagal inhibition is an example of functional death. The circumstances of death can be application of pressure on the neck, foreign bodies in the air passages (e.g. sudden impaction of food in the glottis), puncture of pleural cavity, passing urethral sound, distension of hollow organs (e.g. attempt at criminal abortion through passing instruments into cervix, fluids introduced into uterus), acute myocardial infarction causing ischaemic denervation of SA node.

An opinion of vagal inhibition as the cause of death should be given after excluding all the other possible causes of death.

Sudden Death due to Sympathetico-adrenal Stimulation (SASA)

Reflex death due to vagal inhibition is well known. However, sudden fatal circulatory failure due to sympathetico-adrenal stimulation is less stressed. In sympathetic adrenal stimulation, there is an increased myocardial and ventricular fibrillation. Acute ventricular fibrillation gives rise to rapid death. This sympathetic death takes several minutes to develop in comparison to vagal inhibition which occurs instantaneously. Before death patient shows features of hyperacute cardiovascular failure, e.g. dyspnea, pulmonary oedema, etc. are seen.

At autopsy, coronary artery sclerosis, fatty changes in myocardium, chronic valvular disease may be seen, marked pulmonary oedema is seen. Pleural petechial haemorrhages are seen. Difference between SDSA and vagal inhibition is given in Table 4.4.

MEDICOLEGAL POSTMORTEM EXAMINATION

The word autopsy is derived form Greek word *Autopsia* meaning "seeing with one's own eyes".

Every doctor doing the postmortem examination must see the whole case with his own eyes, make his own observations and record them as the autopsy report.

Postmortem examination consists of external and internal examinations.

Postmortem examinations are carried out at the request of treating doctors who are unable to arrive at a clinical diagnosis before death with a view to know final diagnosis and alternative cause of death. This autopsy examination is called **clinical autopsy.** For conducting clinical autopsy, consent must be taken from the patient at the time of admission into the hospital or from the relatives after the death of the patient.

Postmortem examination is also carried out on a written request from a police officer or a magistrate after the completion of a police or magistrate inquest.

The aims of a medicolegal autopsy and its objectives are:

- To know the causes of death.
- To know the time since death.
- To know the manner of death.
- To establish the identity of the person.
- Incases of infanticide, to know whether the baby was live born or dead born; to know whether the baby had achieved the viability or not.

A medicolegal autopsy is, in other words, a clinical autopsy plus legal issues connected with death.

Postmortem examinations should not be carried out without proper requisition. The cases coming away from the jurisdiction should not be conducted unless the concerned area superintendent of police and district magistrate ask for the same in writing with necessary justification. After valid papers are received, the doctor should make a careful general examination of the body from top of head to bottom of the toe on front, back and sides of the body.

Every medicolegal autopsy requires same amount of attention. No case is less or more important than other case.

The doctor should examine the right body and not the wrong body. This should be done by and by asking the police constable incharge of the body and by asking him to sign on the postmortem report identifying the body brought by him. Once the accompanying police identifies the body, the doctor can proceed further.

External Examination

In the external examination, note should be made of temperature, postmortem staining,

Table 4.4: Difference between sympathetico-adrenal stimulation and vagal inhibition

Sympathetico-adrenal stimulation	*Vagal inhibition*
• Cardiac disease may be present	• Apparently healthy
• Myocardial irritability occurs (ventricular fibrillation)	• Reflex death
• Pulmonary oedema	• Instantaneous
• Pulmonary congestion	• Negative autopsy
• Evidence of hyperacute congestive cardiac failure	• Functional death
• Cyanosis	• Microtrauma or no evidence of trauma
• Intravenous injection of adrenaline	• Pallor
	• Stimulation of urethra, cervix, precordium, other synovial membrane, testes, etc.

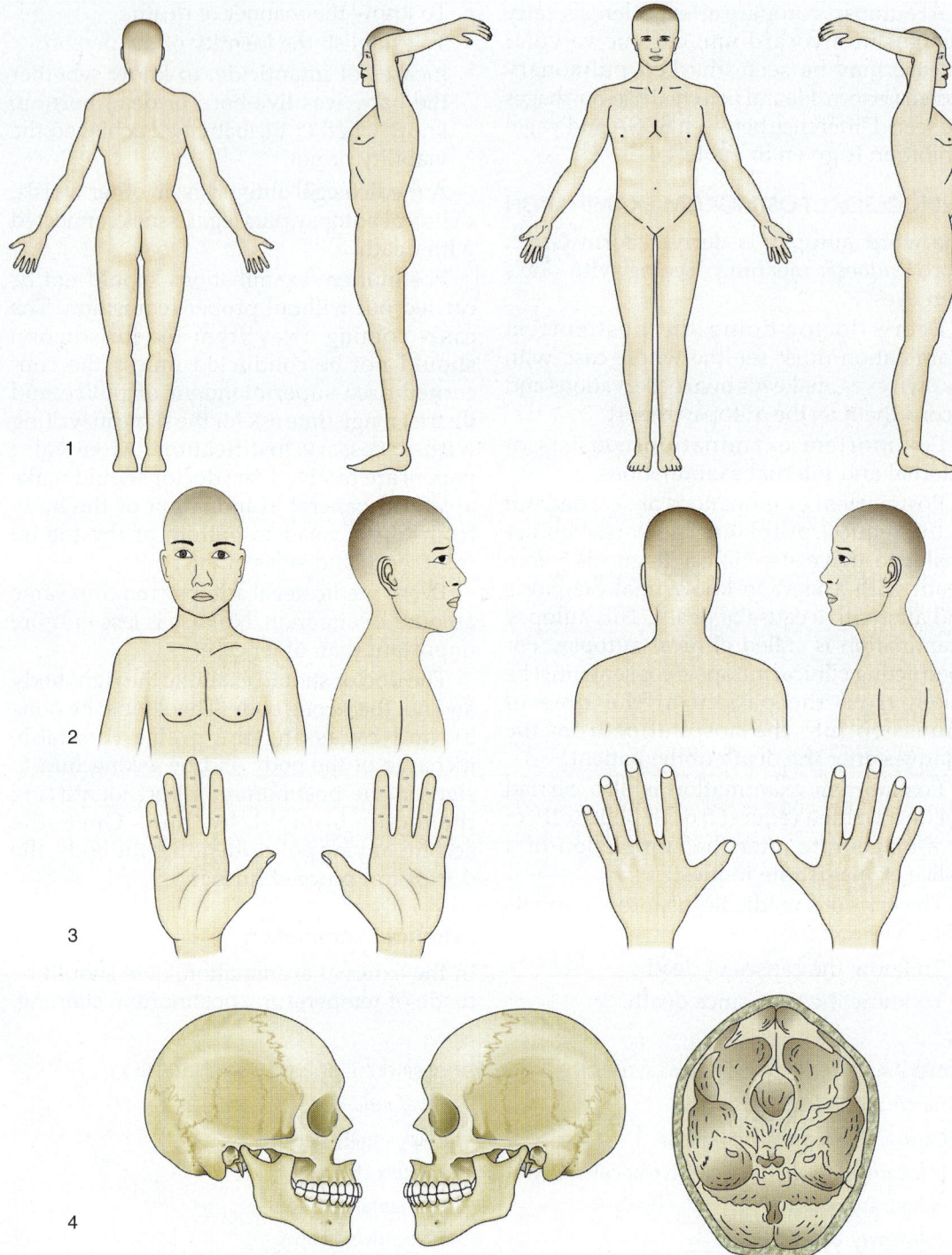

Fig. 4.12: Medicolegal autopsy (1, 2, 3, 4—examination features at autopsy)

rigor mortis, features of decomposition, external appearance of the body, the position of the body. The orifices, eyes, ears, nostril, urethra, vagina and anus should be examined for presence of signs of any intervention, infection, trauma, etc.

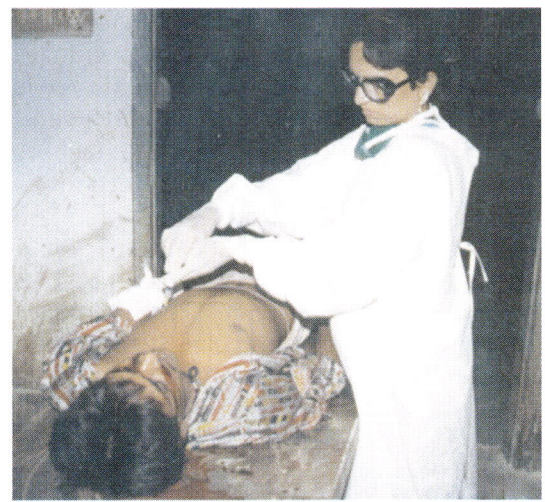

Fig. 4.13: Mortician dissecting the body

The clothes on the body of the person, their type, nature, normal or showing struggle like tears, button loss, etc.; stains like blood, faecal, seminal, etc.; injuries on the clothes, burning, soot deposition, blackening, grease marks, mud/faecal matter, etc. should be looked for and noted.

Dental formula should be noted. When there are tears or holes or cuts or slashes on the clothes, whether corresponding injuries are present or not on the body, should be noted.

Photography of the body and clothes is carried out to preserve the evidential value of the injuries noted. X-ray examination of the neck structures, head and neck, all areas of suspected trauma are carried out. Description of the injuries on the clothes should be recorded. All findings mentioned in the inquest report should be carefully reviewed and if there are contradictions, it should be shown to the police officer or the magistrate and their signature obtained on the postmortem report.

Ordinarily postmortem examinations are carried out during daylight because a postmortem examination is not a medical or surgical emergency and during prescribed hours. However, in case of deaths due to police firing in curfew imposed cities, autopsy examination can be carried out at odd hours on request of a District Magistrate, only to maintain public tranquility. The clothes should be removed by cutting them with scissors and retaining the shape of the clothes and evidence on the clothes. The clothes should be packed, sealed, signed and handed over to the police.

The body should be washed under running water before the autopsy examination is started. The doctor should look for whether the body is hot or cold, whether rigor mortis has set in, its status, presence, colour and distribution of postmortem lividity, eyeballs closed or open, pupils dilated or contracted, sclera, conjunctiva and lens; presence of discharge from nose, serodischarge in decomposition, lathery froth in drowning, colourless saliva trickling in antemortem hanging, congested face in cases of pressure on the neck, pallor in cases of exsanguinations (blood loss), yellowish discolouration of jaundice, tongue protrusion, caught between

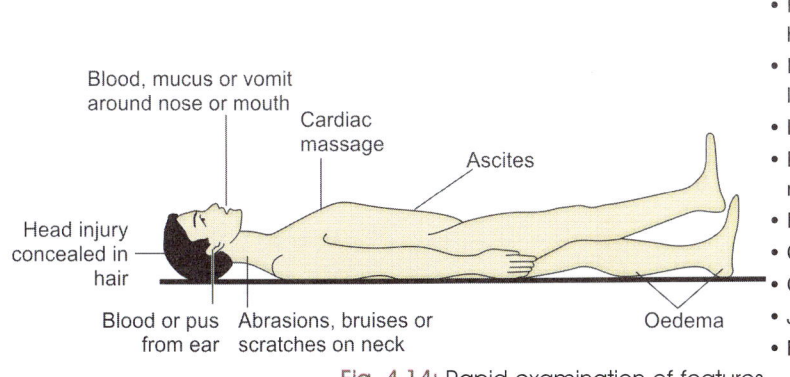

Blood, mucus or vomit around nose or mouth

Cardiac massage

Ascites

Head injury concealed in hair

Blood or pus from ear

Abrasions, bruises or scratches on neck

Oedema

Other Features
• Presence, position and colour of hypostasis, cyanosis
• Injuries, fracture or deformities of limbs or trunk
• Lip, skin or conjunctival petechiae
• Distribution and degree of rigor mortis
• Pinkness due to carbon monoxide
• Congestion on the face
• Gangrene
• Jaundice
• Bruising

Fig. 4.14: Rapid examination of features

teeth or not, cyanosis of ear lobes, lips, tip of nose, etc. Rigor mortis should be examined by bending at the joints; postmortem lividity should be tested by pressure of thumb to know whether blanching occurs or not, pallor of areas of contact flattening, congenital abnormalities like extra fingers or toes, deformed hands, feet, etc.

Internal Examination

It is a good practice to begin autopsy with the exposure and removal of brain. All organs should be weighed before they are dissected. The scalp should be dissected up to the eyebrows on the front and below the mastoids on the back. The anterior and posterior flaps should then be examined carefully. The vault of skull should then be removed and examined by stretching it in both sagittal and coronal planes. This exposes any fracture, if present. The extradural space should then be examined followed by subdural space. If there is subdural haemorrhage, it should be removed and looked for presence of subarachnoid haemorrhage. Brain is then removed and then placed on its vault to expose the basal surfaces. This exposed surface is then examined. The circle of Willis is dissected out and examined *in situ*. Then it is turned to rest on its base. Each stage of brain is dissected. The base of skull along with the meninges should be examined before and after wiping its surface. The basal meninges should be stripped off. The stretch force is applied to base of skull in its sagittal and coronal planes to expose any type of fracture.

Next, to open the body, from chin to symphysis pubis dissection is made to expose the abdominal cavity. The neck and chest wall are dissected to their extreme sides to expose the front as wide as possible. This widely exposed neck and chest wall should be examined. The cupped palm should be gently dipped into the pelvic cavity and raised. If there is blood, it will be seen in the palm. If palm is empty, then there is no blood in the pelvic cavity which excludes bleeding from injury to the visceral organs of the abdomen. The sternum is cut at costal cartilages. The removed sternum should then be bent in both the planes to expose any fracture. The hand is checked for pleural cavity to rule out any bleeding injury. The pericardium with heart *in situ* should be examined. The heart is exposed *in situ* after wiping the pericardial sac.

Brain

The surface of brain—cerebrum, cerebellum, pons, medulla examined for presence of:
• Widening of gyri and flattening of sulci characteristic of cerebral oedema.
• Petechial haemorrhages should be noted.

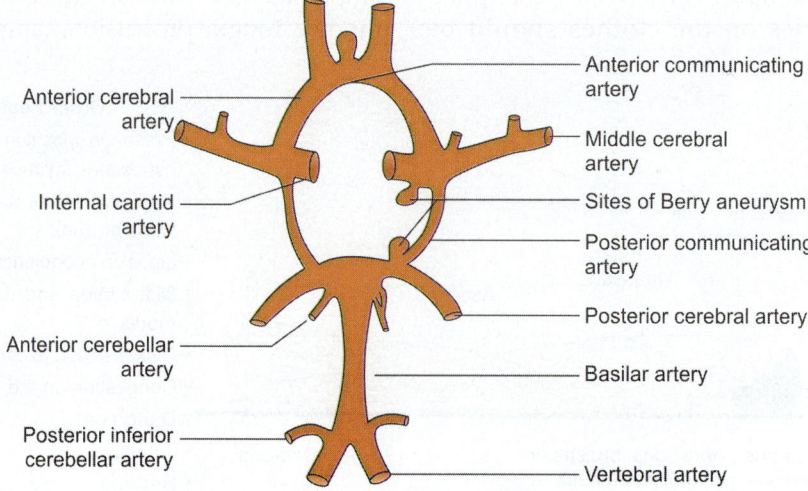

Fig. 4.15: Berry aneurysm—circle of Willis

Subdural and subarachnoid haemorrhages can be differentiated by directing a thin stream of water on the haemorrhage. Subdural haemorrhage can be washed, whereas subarachnoid haemorrhage cannot be washed. Subdural haemorrhage involves one or both of the cerebral hemispheres. Subarachnoid haemorrhage is diffuse in distribution. Extradural haemorrhage is well defined and can be scraped even by hands, intraventricular haemorrhage gives blood stain to the cerebrospinal fluid. The brain is kept with the bottom up, holding the medulla oblongata and pons along with cerebellum. A transverse cut is made as high up as possible in midbrain. The separated cerebrum is put on the dissection table. Coronal sections are made on one side, sagittal sections are made on other side cutting from above downwards about 0.5 cm thick slices. The cut surfaces are consequentially examined for presence of softening, cystic degeneration, petechial haemorrhages, space occupying lesions, etc.

The cerebellum is held in one hand and separated from the midbrain, pons and medulla and spinal cord. The cerebellum again is kept on the dissection board. The slices are made perpendicular to the cerebellar grooves. The cut sections are again

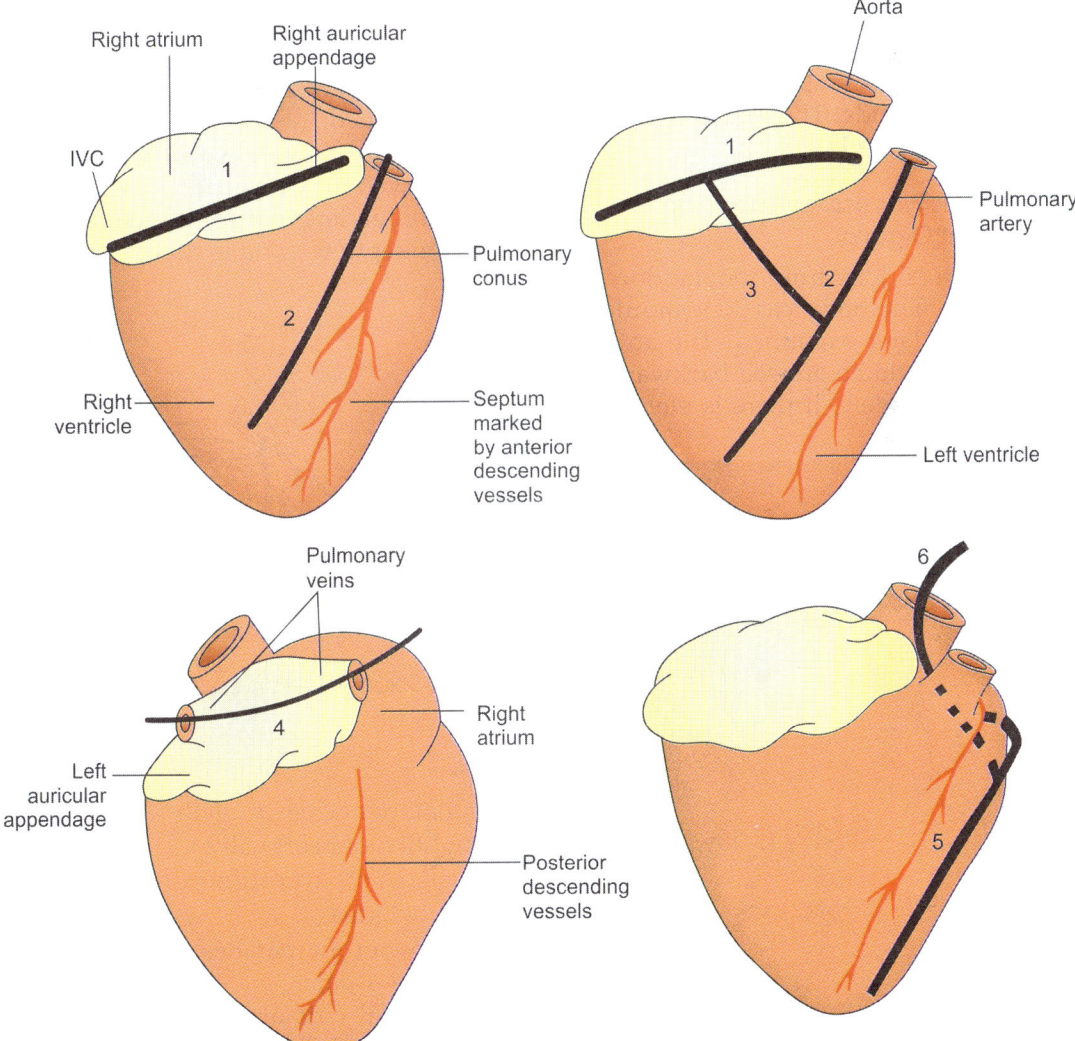

Fig. 4.16: 1, 2, 3, 4, 5, 6 Order of disection of heart

examined consequentially for softening, cystic degeneration, petechial haemorrhage, etc. The medulla and pons are kept on slicing board. Transverse cuts are made and sections examined for haemorrhages, etc.

Neck

The superficial muscles of neck should be exposed and examined. Then the superficial muscles of neck are removed with a little dissection of deep muscles. This will partly expose the hyoid bone.

The hyoid bone is examined *in situ* by slight adduction and abduction of greater cornua of hyoid bone. This manoeuvre shows inward and outward compression fractures, if present.

The deep muscles of neck are removed to expose the larynx, submandibular glands and thyroid glands. The exposed surfaces should be examined.

Evisceration Process (Evisceration Means Removal of Organs)

Evisceration is done from tongue down to the rectum. The body cavities should be cleaned and later examined. The anterior chest wall should be pressed backwards on each side separately. If there is yielding, it indicates fracture of ribs and that area should be examined. The aorta should be examined before the visceral organs are separated. The intima of aorta should be examined. The posterior surface of pharynx and the oesophagus should be looked for presence of blood.

The oesophagus is opened up to its cardiac end and examined.

The larynx and trachea should be opened and examined.

Heart

The heart should be weighed before and after dissection, after removing the clots.

The opening of heart is done following the direction of blood flow. First the right atrium and right ventricle along lateral border; then along the interventricular septum, pulmonary artery is opened.

Next pulmonary veins are opened and then followed into left atrium along the left lateral border, left ventricle is opened. Next along the septum, aorta is cut open.

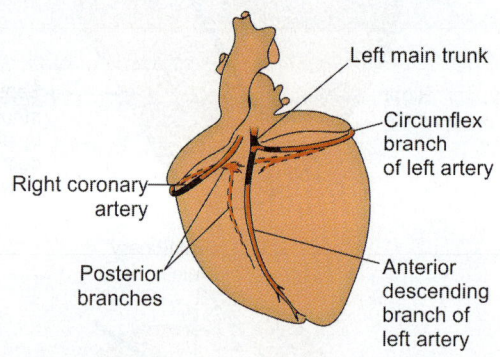

Fig. 4.18: Coronary artery branches: Common sites of thrombosis

Look for

- Antemortem clots in cavity
- Condition of heart valves
- Thickness of myocardium
- Infarcted area
- Atherosclerotic patches over aorta and coronary ostia.

Next serial cuts are made over all the three vessels at a distance of 3–5 mm to look for block.

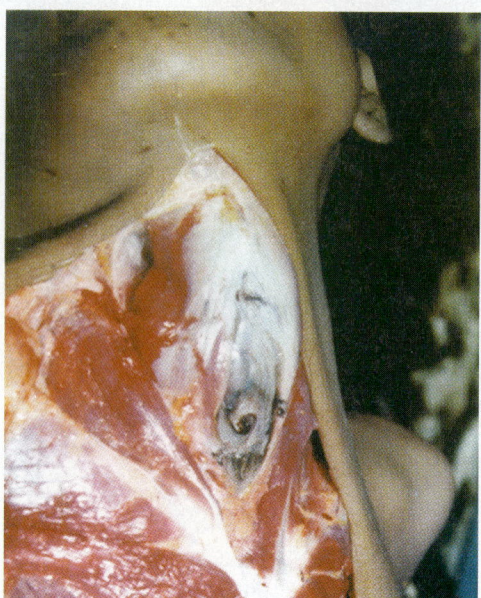

Fig. 4.17: Dissection of neck

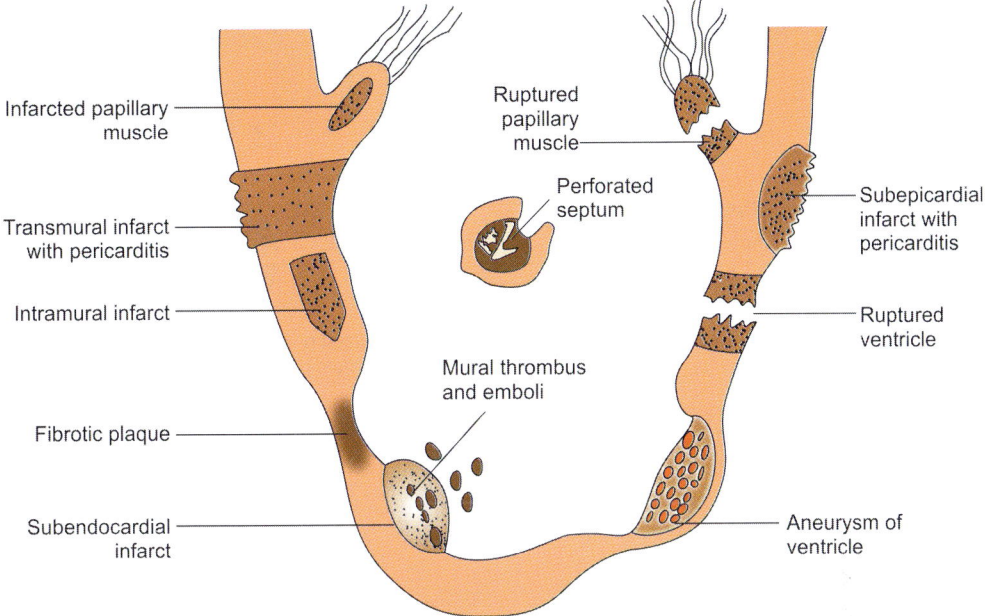

Fig. 4.19: Complications of myocardial infarct

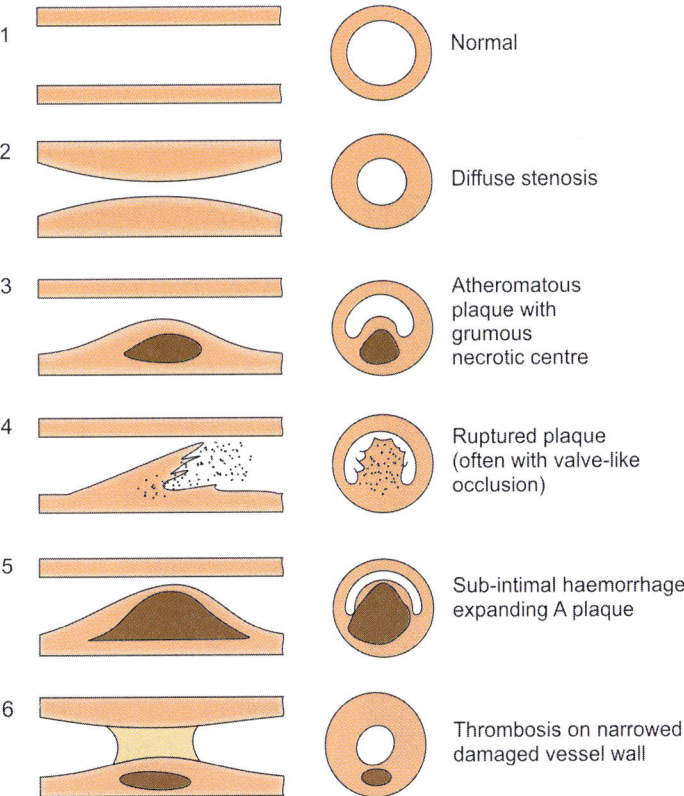

Fig. 4.20: Cross-section of normal (1); Diffuse stenosis (2); Atherosclerosis and its fate (3, 4, 5, 6)

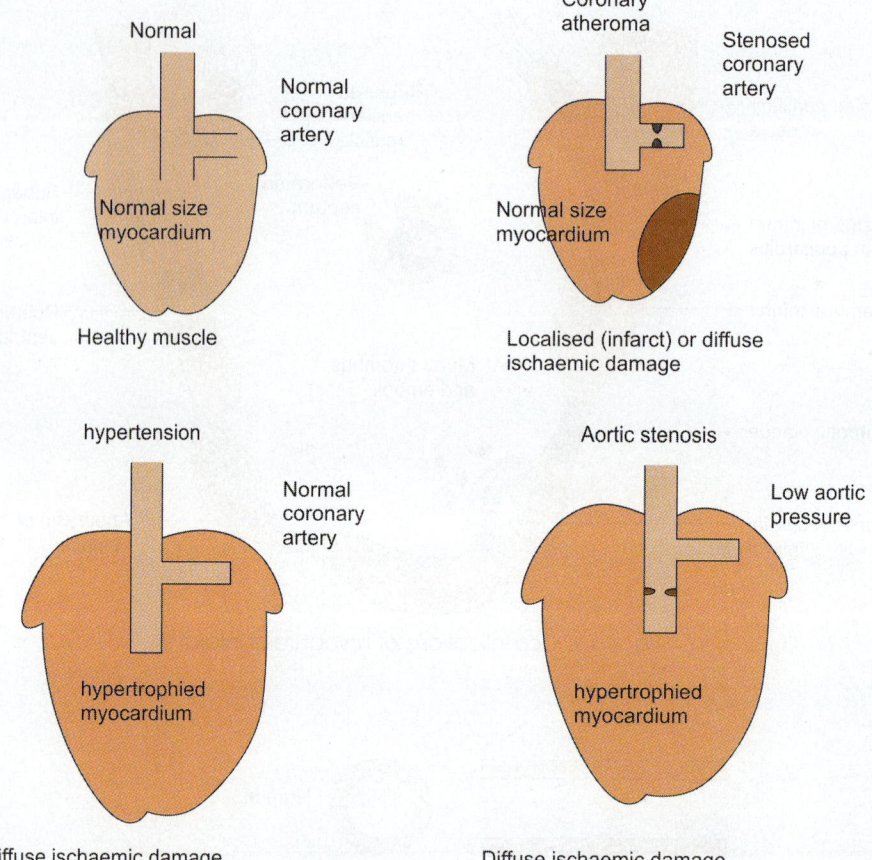

Fig. 4.21: Schematic representation of heart muscle changes

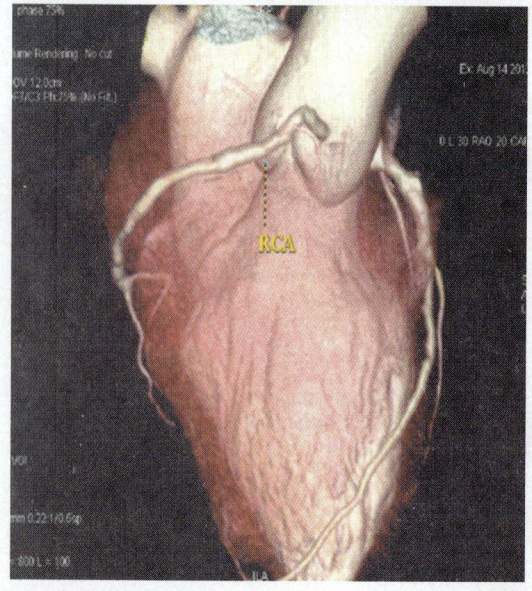

Fig. 4.22: Displaying position of right coronary arteries origin

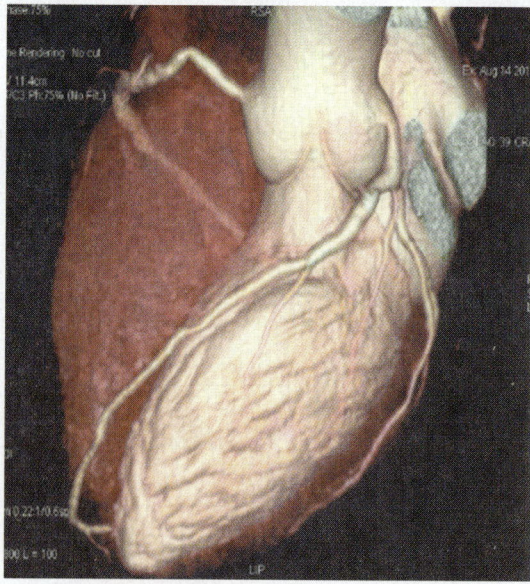

Fig. 4.23: Displaying coronary arteries

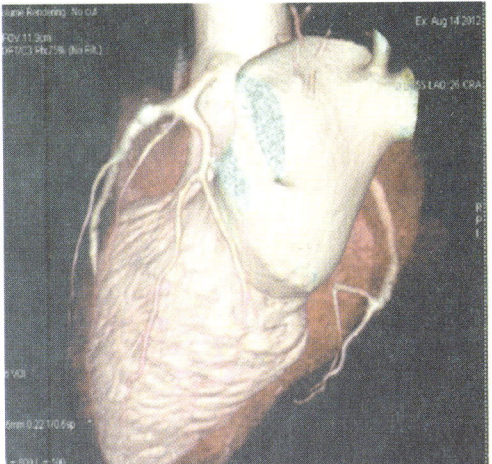

Fig. 4.24: Coronary at the margins

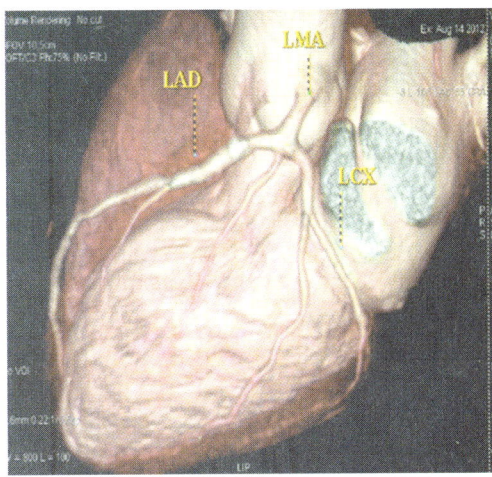

Fig. 4.25: Left anterior descending and left main artery

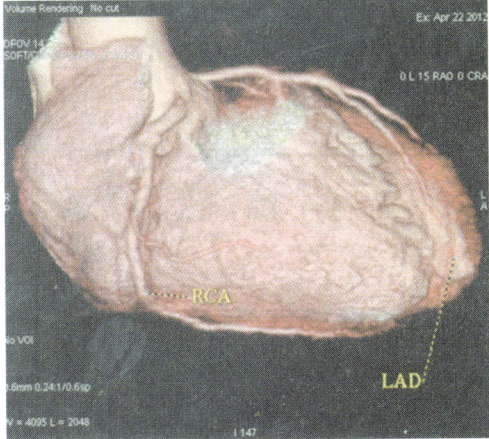

Fig. 4.26: Right coronary artery and left anterior descending artery

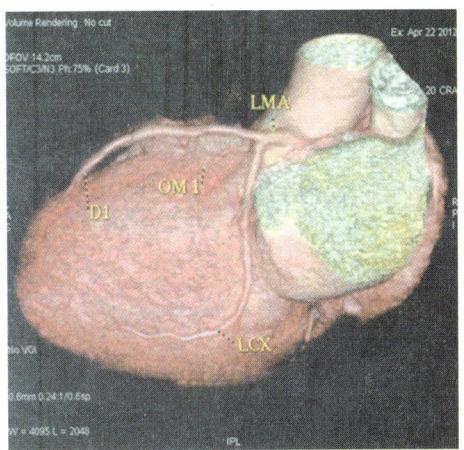

Fig. 4.27: Left main artery and left circumflex artery

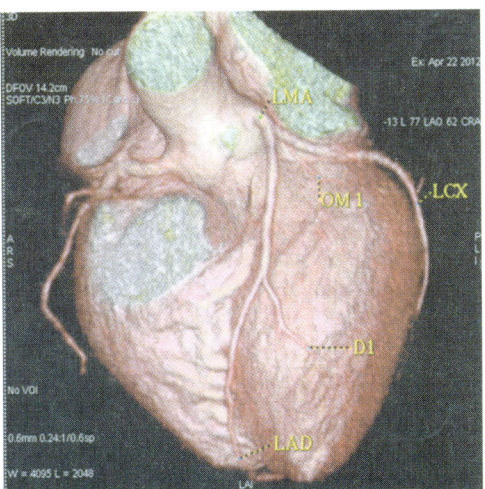

Fig. 4.28: Left main artery, left circumflex artery and left anterior descending artery

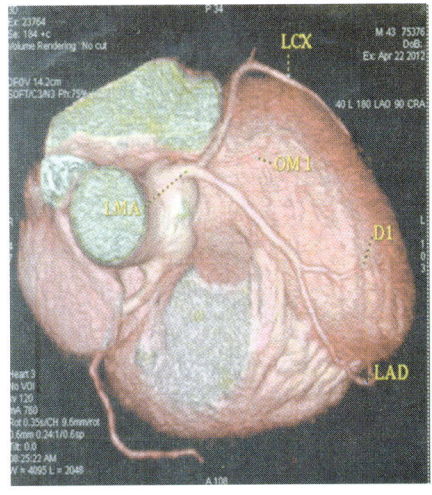

Fig. 4.29: Left main artery, left circumflex artery and left anterior descending artery

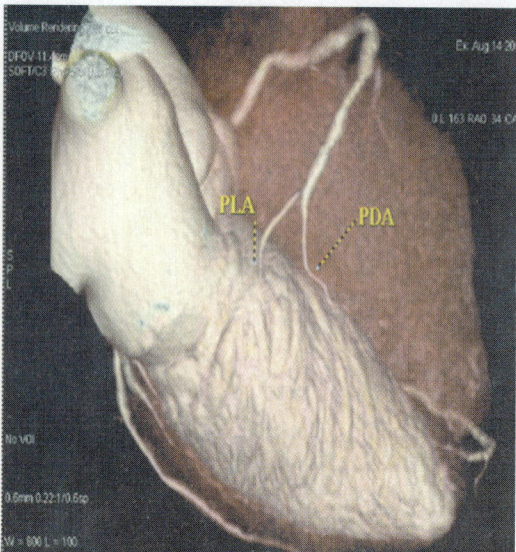

Fig. 4.30: Posterior left artery and posterior descending artery

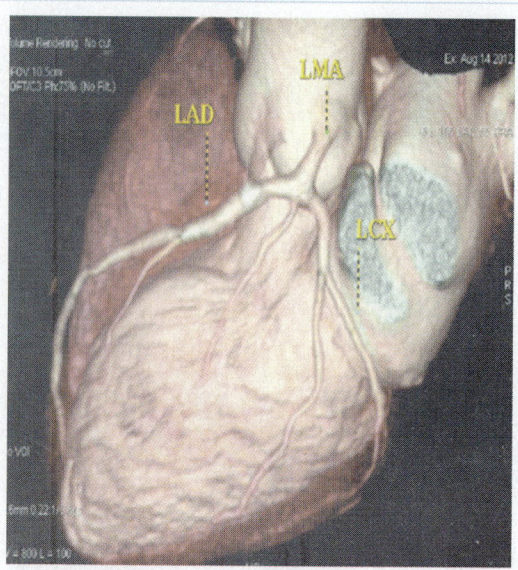

Fig. 4.31: Left anterior descending artery, left main artery and left circumflex artery

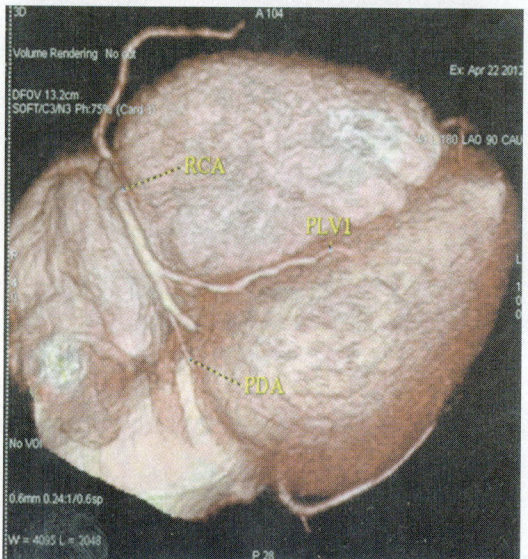

Fig. 4.32: Right coronary artery, posterior left ventricular artery and posterior descending artery

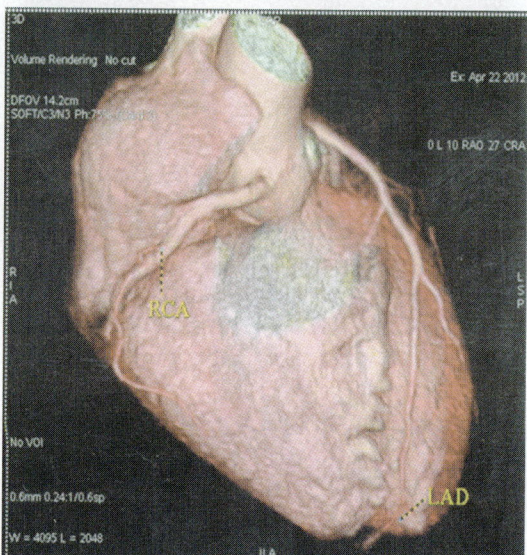

Fig. 4.33: Right coronary artery and left anterior descending artery

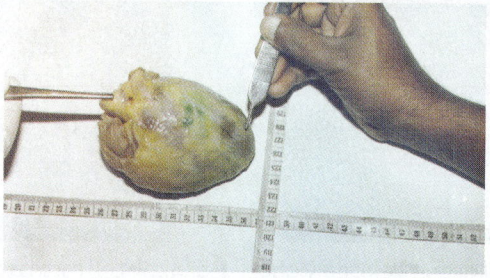

Fig. 4.34: Cardiac contusion

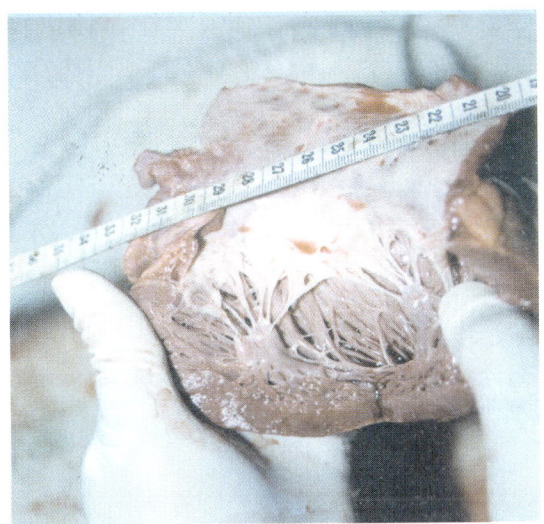

Fig. 4.35: Subendocardial haemorrhages

Stomach

It should be opened between ligature on the front, midway between the greater and lesser curvatures. Both sphincters should be examined. The mucous membrane is examined for the rugae congestion, pallor, ulceration, thinning out due to autolysis, characteristic odours, nature and quantity of stomach contents, should be examined. Look whether the food is undigested, partly digested or chyme.

Liver

The liver is dissected like the loaves of bread at half centimeter intervals along the axis from outside to inside. The gall bladder is slit open along the duct to the body and

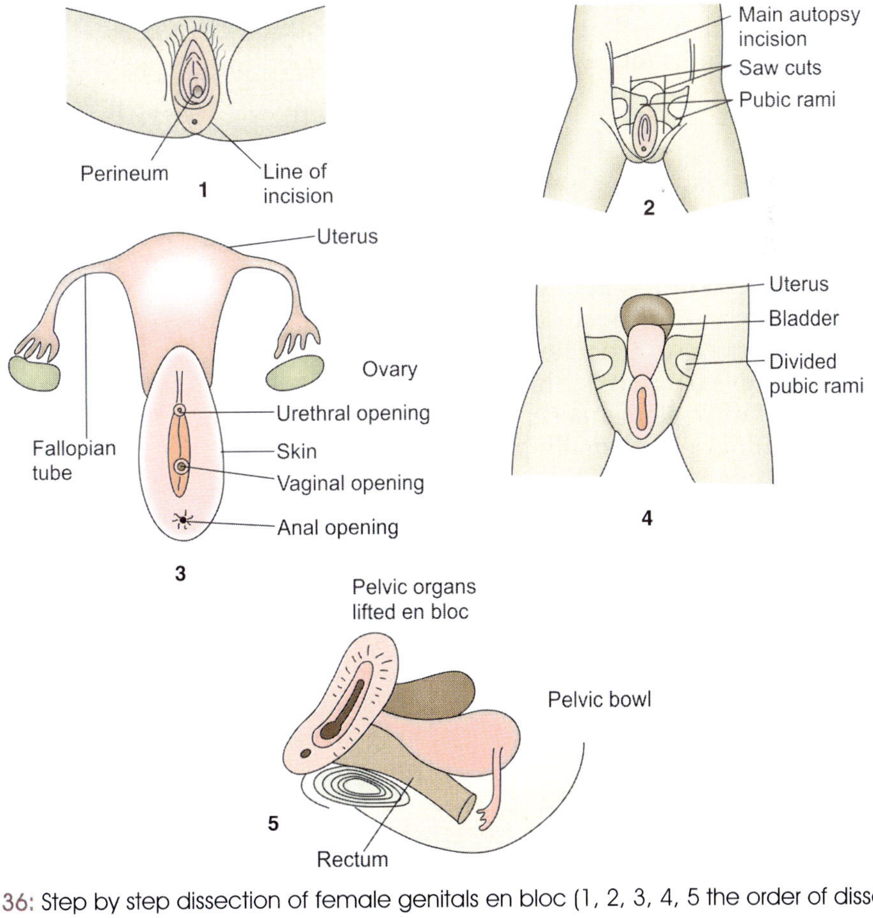

Perineum   Line of
          1   incision

Main autopsy incision
Saw cuts
Pubic rami

2

Uterus
Ovary
Urethral opening
Fallopian tube   Skin
Vaginal opening
Anal opening

3

Uterus
Bladder
Divided pubic rami

4

Pelvic organs lifted en bloc

Pelvic bowl

5

Rectum

Fig. 4.36: Step by step dissection of female genitals en bloc (1, 2, 3, 4, 5 the order of dissection)

examined for the quantity and quality of bile, presence or absence of gall stones. The surface of the liver should be examined for nutmeg appearance, congestion and pallor suggestive of chronic venous congestion. Fatty changes of the liver can be noted by the colour of the liver. Honeycombing of the liver should be noted when present. Shrunk and difficult to cut liver suggests cirrhosis of posthepatic type.

Big liver with soapy feeling while cutting suggests chronic alcoholic cirrhosis. Primary hepatoma of liver presents great difficulty in cutting. Surface of liver presents small nodules, big nodules, umbilicated nodules. Necrosed liver is soft and tends to cut easily. Liver may be studded with multiple hard nodules in secondaries.

Spleen

Spleen is cut along the long axis from hilum outwards. Huge spleens show areas of infarction. Chronic malaria is the commonest cause of big spleen in India followed by kala-azar in West Bengal.

Kidneys

They are held in palm of left hand, hilum facing the palm. Then into two equal halves up to hilum to expose the pelvis. The outer capsule is stripped with the help of right index and thumb noting decortication while stripping. Surface scars on the kidney are seen in chronic pyelonephritis. Shrunken kidneys suggest chronic glomerulonephritis. Pyelonephritic kidneys are usually bigger with hydronephrotic changes. The cortex and medulla of the kidney should be looked carefully with the help of a hand lens.

Pancreas

Dissected along the long axis from tail to head and looked for presence of cysts, calculi, necrotic areas and tumour near the head.

Testes

Also can be examined without making any cut on the scrotum by pulling them from inguinal canal and examined by making a cut section along long axis of each.

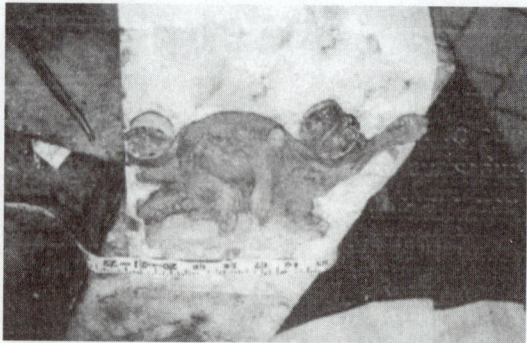

Fig. 4.37: Demonstrating cut open section of female genitalia at autopsy

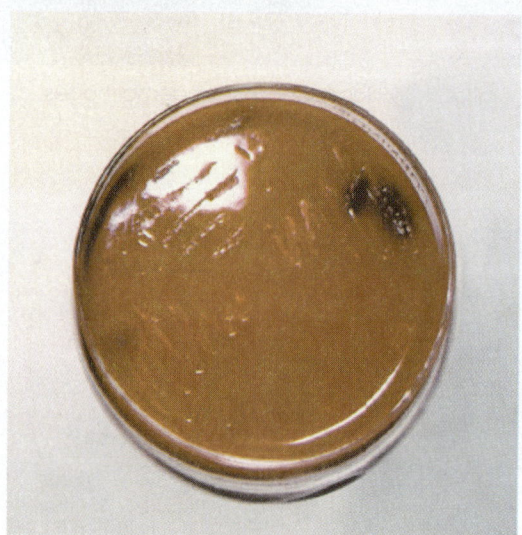

Fig. 4.38: Blood culture for plague organism

Healthy seminal tubules can be lifted by toothless pointed forceps like thin long filaments.

Lungs

They are dissected from hilum outwards along the bronchial tree. Pressed from periphery inwards and looked for presence of froth and its colour. Lungs are generally found congested at autopsy except in cases of exsanguinations. Consolidated zones of lungs feel like liver and break on thumb pressure (Fig. 4.39).

Tissues for histopathology examination should be sent in 10% formalin from the suspected zones of pathology. Viscera for chemical analysis in cases of poisoning are

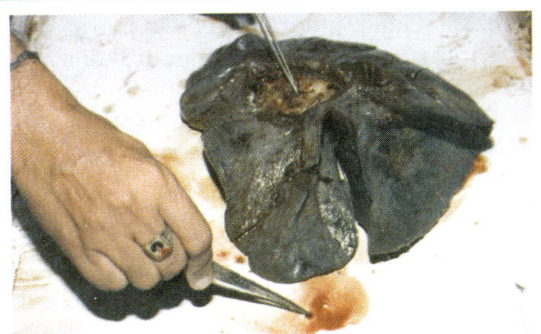

Fig. 4.39: Lung consolidation

collected, preserved and transmitted as described in appendix. Subcortical steaky haemorrhages are seen in acute renal shutdown.

Suprarenals

The suprarenals are dissected along the long axis like pages of a book. The suprarenal haemorrhages should be looked for.

Urinary Bladder

It is opened from the pelvic surface to visualize the trigone *in situ*.

Uterus with Adnexae in Women

This is dissected by lifting them carefully downwards towards cervix and as low down as possible and a circular nick is made to bring out the vagina along with the cervix. The whole reproductive system is then opened up to long axis and from the body towards the fallopian tubes and ovary. The ovaries are sectioned along their long axis and looked for the presence of corpus luteum, haemorrhages, tumours etc.

Precautions during Autopsy

Precautions must be taken whenever autopsies are done to see that the doctor and paramedical staff do not get infected from autopsies with:
- HBsAg (hepatitis)
- HIV (AIDS)
- Tuberculosis
- Plague
- Anthrax, etc.

In these cases, before and after autopsy, instruments should be washed in 10% sodium hypochloride solution and/or 6% carbolic acid solution.

Gloves should be worn up to the elbow level. Eye should be protected by plain goggles fully covering the orbits. Gum boots should be worn. Mask also should be kept and the apron-like in operation theatre should be worn.

Postmortem operation theatres should be maintained disinfected by 10% bleaching powder sprayed up to 6 feet on walls and floors.

All postmortem team members should get immunized against tetanus, hepatitis B, tuberculosis depending upon the needs of work.

Photography, radiography and videography have to be meticulously carried out to keep the data preserved.

During videography doctor's photo- and videography is not advised.

Preservations of Viscera After Autopsy

- Tissues are preserved for histopathology examination in blocks of 1 cm thickness and 2 cm length and width. Preserved in 10% formalin are sent for histopatholgy examination. Whenever required control tissue samples also can be sent.
- For microbiological examinations, the materials are transmitted in sterile tubes and swab obtained from the microbiology departments.
- Tissues for DNA examination like hair, bone and bloodstained clothes can be transmitted as they are. In the remaining cases, the material should be transmitted in frozen state (–20°C).
- For forensic science laboratory chemical analysis.
    - Stomach and its contents in one bottle (wide mouthed-glass capped): Liver (500 gm) and kidney (one or half of each) in one bottle.
    - Bloodstained gauzepiece.
- Urine (100 ml) or whatever the quantity if below 100 ml.

- Sample packet of common salt used. The bottles are to be labeled and sealed and handed over to the police as soon as the autopsy is over.

Saturated solution of sodium chloride is made by keeping on pouring the salt into water and stirring vigorously till some quantity remains at the bottom. The tissues are put in the bottle and the preservative is poured up to 2/3rds of the level leaving 1/3rd empty so that if gas formation occurs, the stopper is not disturbed due to inbuilt pressure.

Common salt should not be used in following cases

- Acid poisoning except carbolic acid
- Aconite
- Vegetable poisons

In these cases, rectified spirit should be used.

Alcohol should not be used in

- Alcohol poisoning
- Phosphorus poisoning
- Paraldehyde poisoning
- Kerosene poisoning
- Carbolic acid poisoning
- Acetic acid poisoning

Viscera transmission

Viscera boxes specially made are used for the transmission of viscera. The key of viscera box should be sealed and given to the police officer. The chemical analyzer will check the seal and open the viscera box.

The completed postmortem reports should by handed over to the police as soon as the autopsy is over.

To prevent doing autopsies on wrong bodies, doctor should always get the body identified by relatives and the police before the start of autopsy. The dead body is always under the custody of police and the constable accompanying the body should be present at the time of autopsy, outside.

When death is suspected to be due to poisoning, the medical officer should reserve his opinion, till he receives and pursues the chemical analysis report from forensic science laboratory. Even in a case of poisoning sometimes, the chemical analysis may turn out to be negative due to:

- The poison is in such insignificant quantity that analysis is unable to detect.
- The poison is so obscure that its presence is not detected.
- The poison is vomited or excreted.
- The poison is neutralized or metabolized or rendered innocuous.

EMBALMING

- Embalming is done in a dead body with antiseptics and preservatives to prevent putrefaction and facilitate preservation. Embalming of chemical stiffening similar to rigor mortis but normal rigor does not develop. Embalming rigidity is permanent.
- It coagulates protein, fixes tissues, bleaches and hardens organs and converts blood in brownish mass. Decomposition is inhibited for many months if injection is made shortly after death (<6 hours) and if done several hours after death body will show mixture of bacterial decomposition and mummification and will disintegrate in a few months.
- 70 bodies require 10 litres fluid. About 10% of it will be lost through venous drainage, purging, etc.
- Arterial embalming is forcing of fluid in an artery to reach the tissues through arterioles and capillaries. The nearer the vessel to heart, the better the result. However, multiple site '6 point' injection involves right and left common carotid arteries (for head and neck), both left axillary arteries (for upper limbs) and both left femoral arteries (for lower limbs).
- Cavity embalming is recommended after ½–1 hour which will allow for hardening of viscera.

Disadvantages of Embalming

- Alters appearance of body, tissue and organs, making it difficult to interpret any injury or disease.
- Completely destroys cyanide and alcohol. As most embalming fluids contain methyl

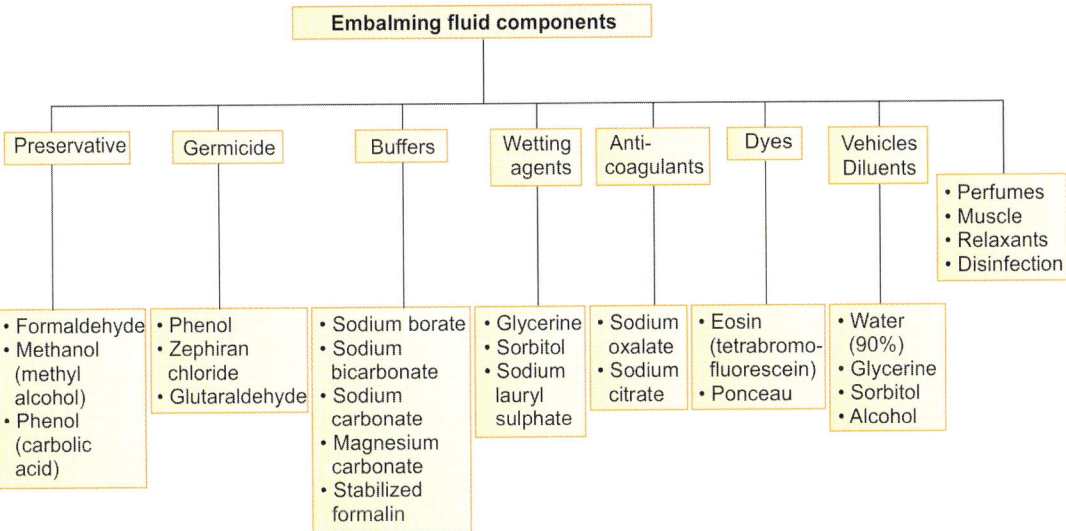

Fig. 4.40: Embalming fluid components

or ethyl alcohol or both so that analysis for these substances is rendered meaningless, and cyanide reacts chemically with formalin.

- Determination of presence of many alkaloids, organic poisons and volatile poisons becomes very difficult.
- The fixation process makes it difficult to extract drugs.
- Blood grouping cannot be made out.
- Thrombi and emboli are dislocated and washed away.
- In already embalmed bodies it is desirable to take a sample of embalming fluid, used as control. Tissues from buttock muscle, centre of liver, vitreous fluid should be retained for analysis as they are least affected.

PRACTICAL PERSPECTIVES OF MEDICOLEGAL AUTOPSY

There are many differences between medico-legal autopsies and hospital autopsies done strictly for clinical scientific purposes. Some practical observations on medicolegal decision-making, the preservation of evidence, and courtroom testimony by forensic pathologists concern the findings of a medicolegal autopsy. Determining the causes of death is not the end of medico-legal investigation. In fact, determining the cause of the death is many times simple and least controversial part of the investigation.

The two procedures are performed under different authorizations for different reasons. Some important medicolegal questions, such as identity of the decedent, time and place of death, and postinjury incapacitation and survical interval, never arise in hospital autopsies. Beyond these obvious differences, however, there is a conspicuous dissimilarity in the procedural and intellectual focus of the person performing the autopsy. In the typical hospital postmortem, external examination of the body is a perfunctory prelude to "getting on" with the primary business of determining the cause and mechanism of death and of evaluating medical, surgical, and radiological diagnosis and treatment.

It is just that in and of itself the medical evidence usually does not establish the guilt or innocence of the defendant, nor does it independently establish a drgree of fuilt. What it really is all about in a majority of instances is to provide expert opinions bases upon objective, indisputable facts that help to evaluate the reliability and credibility of the cadaver and the testimony of persons whose version of the fatal episode is a matter of deliberation in the Court of Law.

Table 4.5: Differences between hospital autopsy (HA) and medicolegal autopsy (MLA)

S. No.		HA (Synonym: Clinical autopsy)	MLA
1.	Demand	From doctors	From law enforcing agencies
2.	Consent of relatives	Required	Not required
3.	Authorization	–	From police/magistrate
4.	Aim	To know cause of death	To know cause of death and the circumstances connected cites death and manner of death live suicide/homicide/accident, etc.
5.	Implication	Diagnosis	Diagnosis and medicolegal
6.	Style of study	In depth organ study	Organs study to correlate circumstances of death
7.	Scene of (crime) death	–	Important for correlation with findings
8.	External examination	General	Particularly about death, postmortem changes, and evidence of trauma, poisoning, violence, etc.
9.	Examination of clothes	Not specific	Specific and useful in correlation of firearm, stab injuries
10.	Preservation of evidence	Not specific except needs of diagnosis	Specific and particular liver, blood, semen, hair, saliva, nails, etc.

Complete autopsies on victims of apparent violence, whose deaths were surrounded by seemingly suspicious circumstances, commonly disclose that the fatalities resulted from natural causes. In some of these instances, the police arrest suspects prior the autopsy on the basis of reasonable inferences drawn from their observations at the scene of death and from the external appearance of the deceased. "Medicolegal masquerades" of this nature often are characterized by the clumsiness, carelessness, fragility, and convoluted domestic relations of alcoholic persons. The classic example is that of a dead alcoholic woman with multiple bruises whose spouse admits that he occasionally "whacked her around". At the scene, the police find blood stains in several rooms. Presumption of homicide and their willingness to accept the husband-assailant's admission of responsibility for her injuries are perfectly understandable.

The usual autopsy findings in such instances consist of multiple bruises of multiple ages on the extremities and trunk with a distribution suggesting that they probable are caused by stumbling into objects or falling. Facial contusions, consistent with spouse-abuse, complete the mistaken external appearance of a homicidal assault. It is not possible to detect all aspects of such a death without a complete autopsy.

The medicolegal autopsy should include appropriate chemical studies and examinations of the brain and neck as well as the thoracic and abdominal viscera. In medicolegal circumstances, partial autopsies are undesirable and are mentioned here only for the purpose of condemnation; they leave reasonable questions unanswered and erect an unwarranted façade of scientific validity.

Pseudoviolent deaths demand the best of us; they test our independence and open-mindedness.

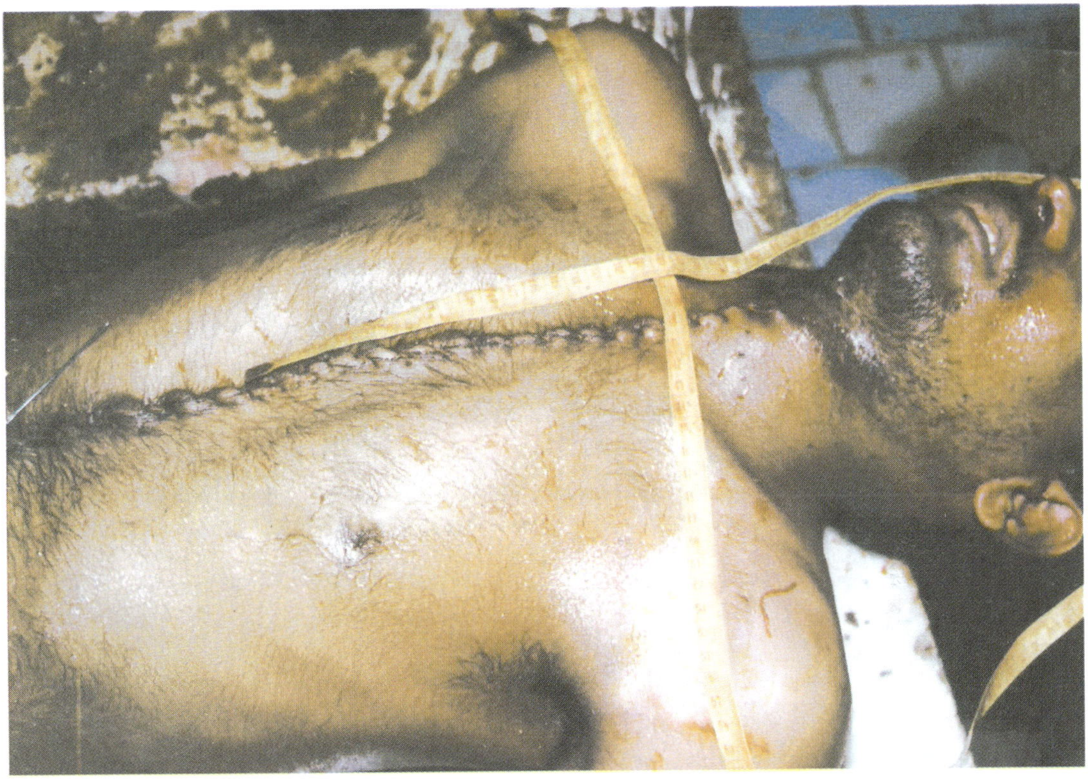

Body sutured after postmortem

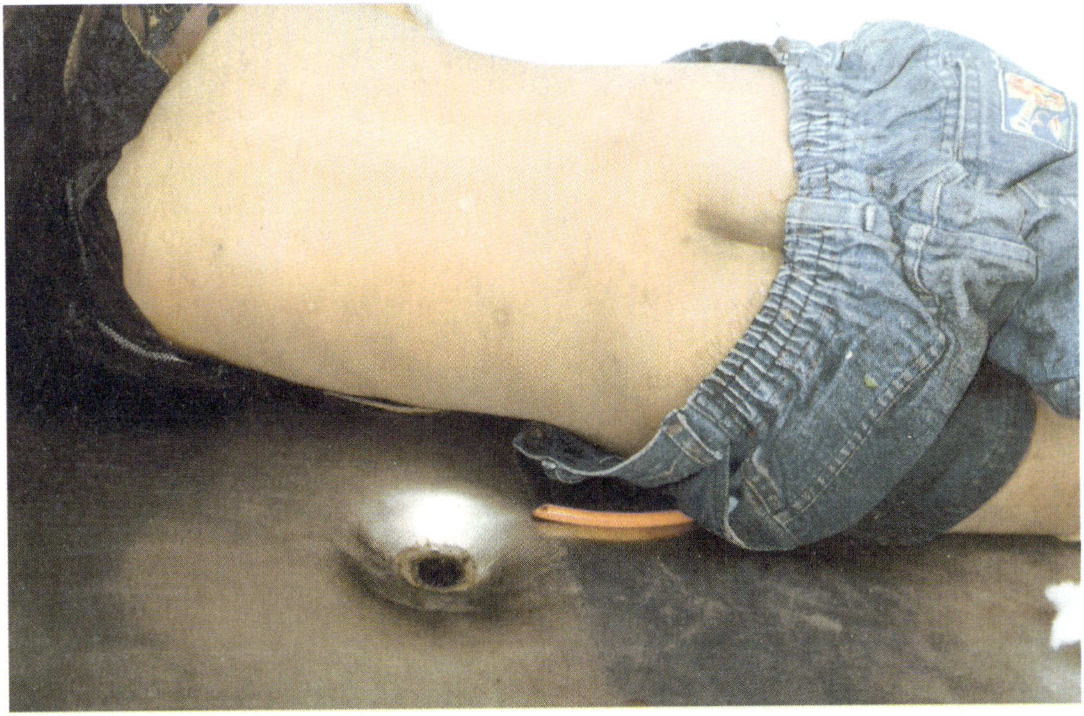

Elastic under wear *in situ*

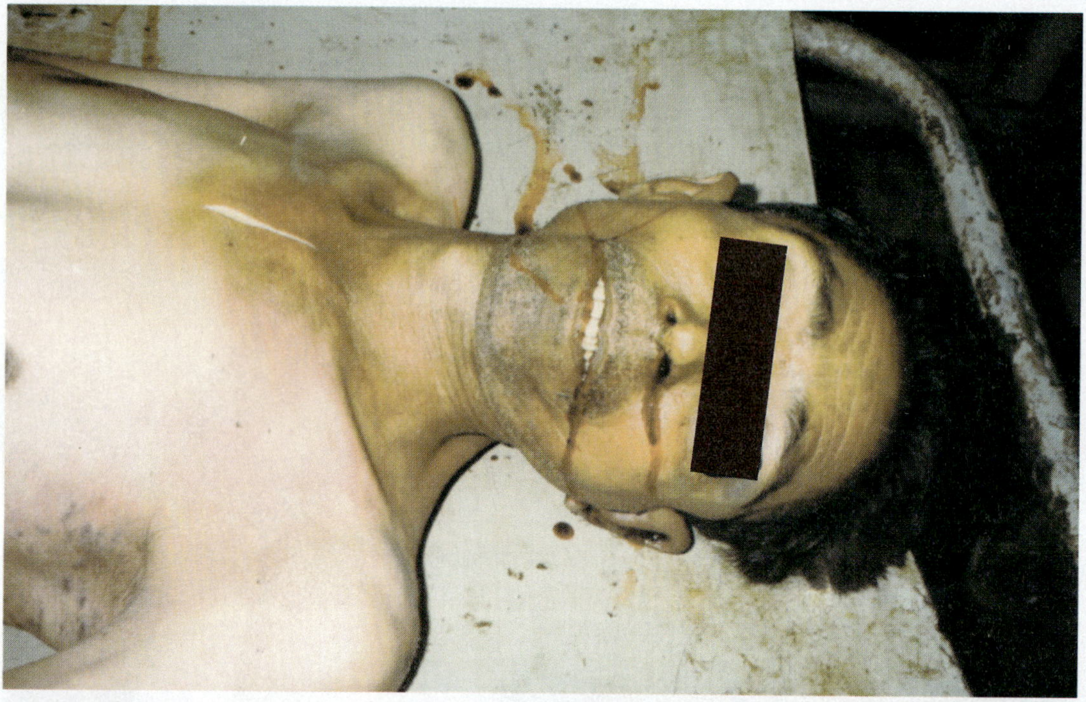

Serosanguineous discharge from mouth and nostrils, *note* PM cut to look for contusion

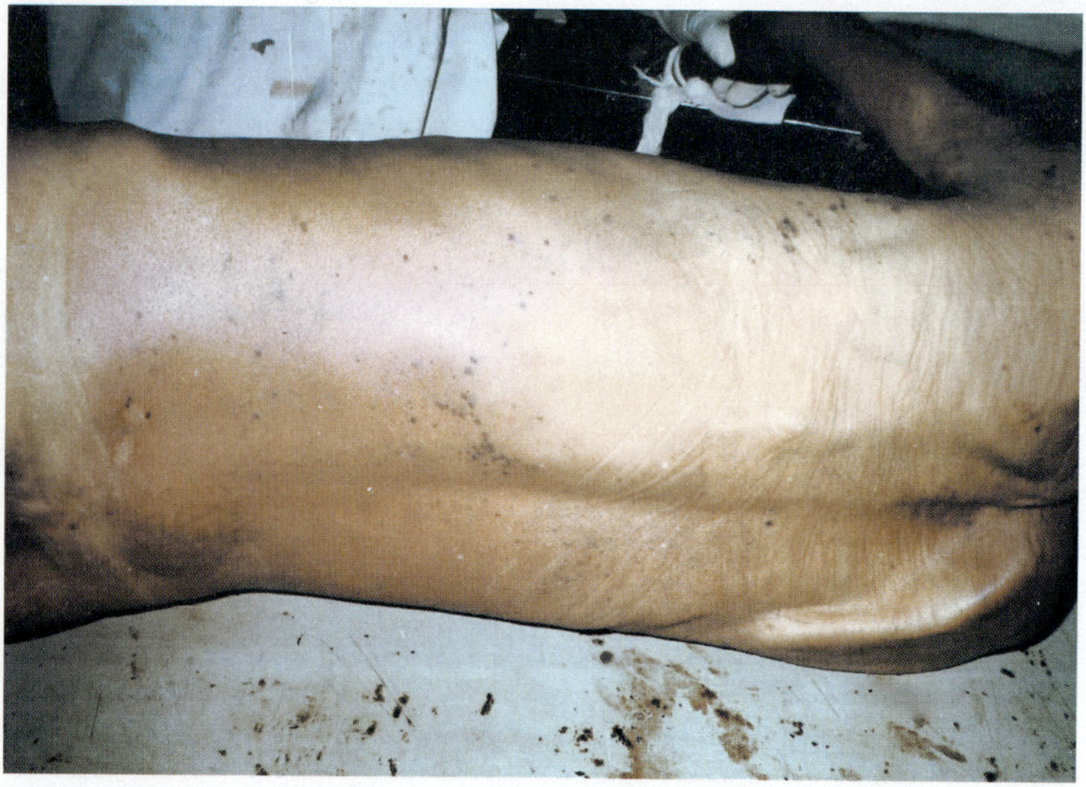

Demonstrating postmortem staining and antemortem small multiple contusions

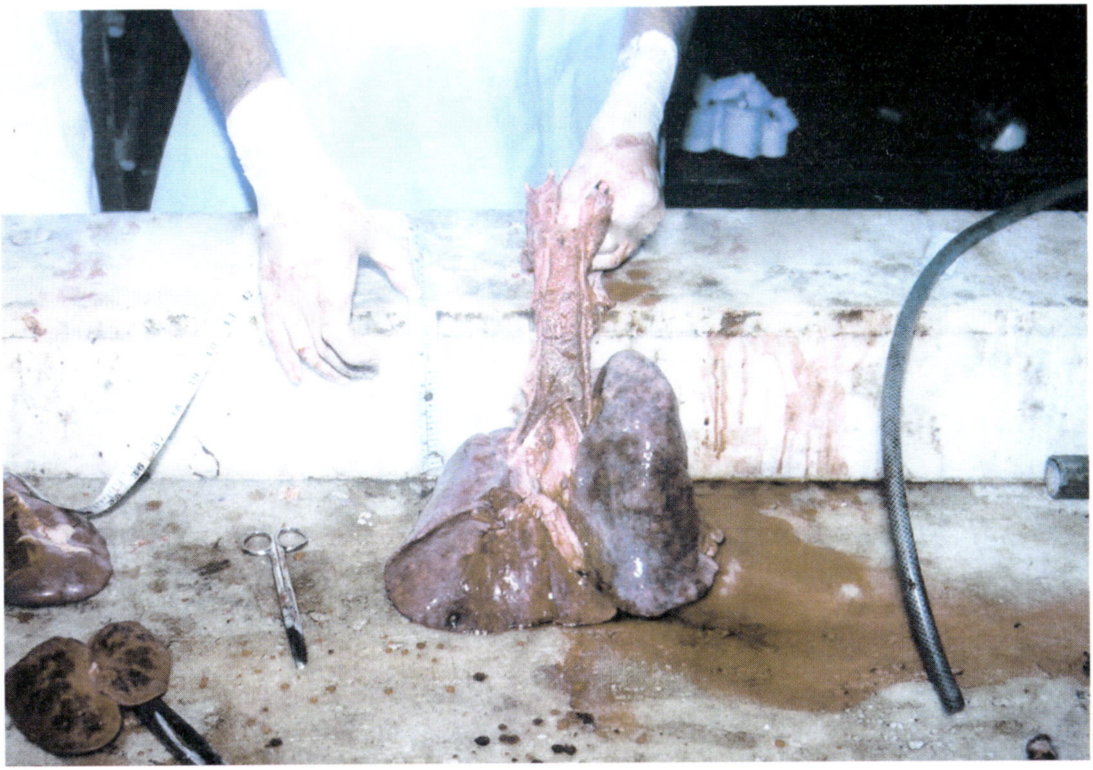

Demonstrating lungs and upper respiratory tract

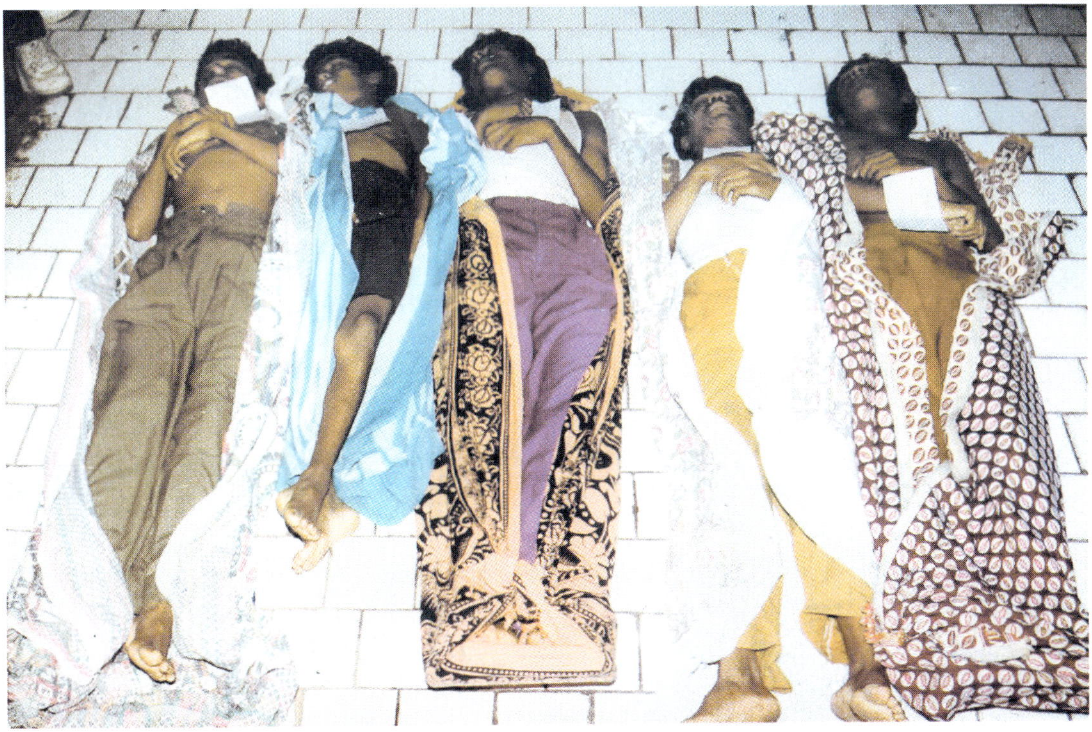

PACT suicide

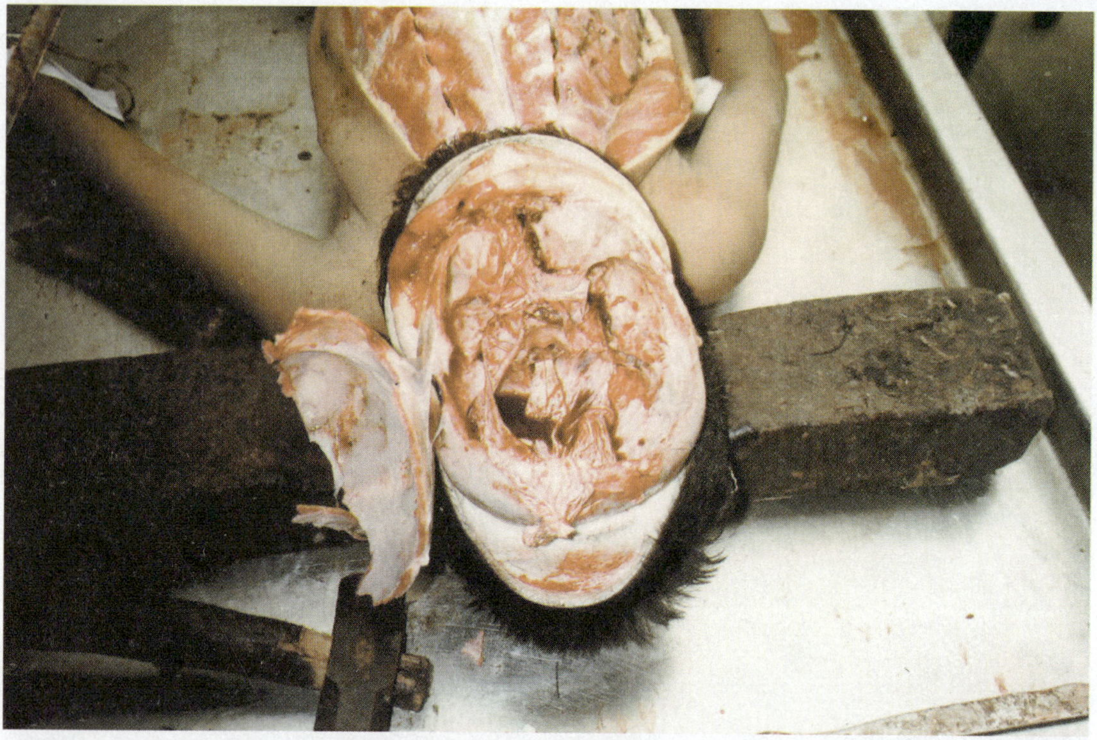

Demonstrating chest and head dissection

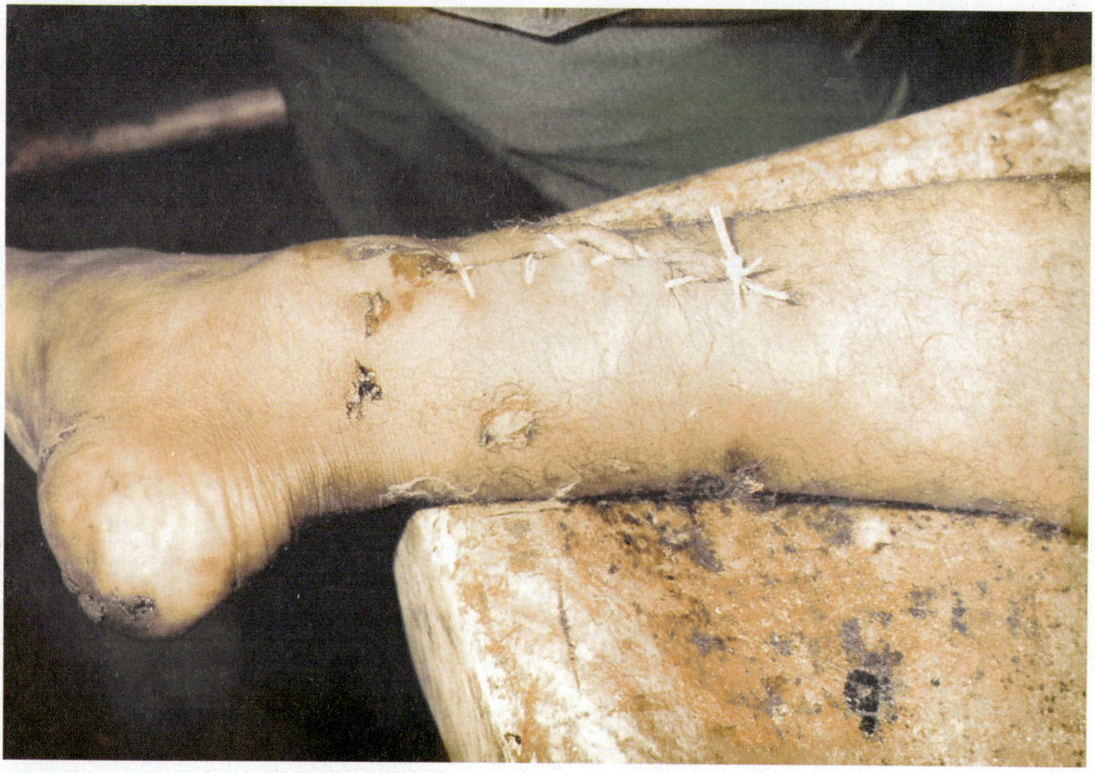

Firearm injury wound of entry (*Courtesy* by Dr PH Barai)

CHAPTER 5

Forensic Traumatology

WOUNDS

Wound is the interruption in continuity of any tissue of the body.

Causes of Wounds

Mechanical (e.g. contusion, abrasion, laceration, stab wounds, firearm wounds, incised wounds, fractures).

Physical (e.g. heat, cold, electricity, lightning).

Chemical (e.g. corrosive acids or alkalies, irritant juices) (Fig. 5.1).

Radiation (e.g. X-ray, ultraviolet, infrared, ionizing radiation).

MECHANICAL INJURIES

Mechanical trauma occurs due to a mechanical force acting on a person:

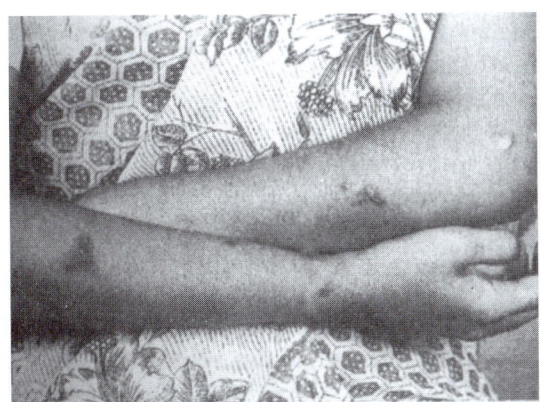

Fig. 5.1: Dermal bullae due to exposure to bromine gas

- The person may be stationary and the force is moving.
- The person is moving but force is stationary.
- The person and force, both are moving.

ABRASION

It is a mechanical injury involving the superficial layers of the epidermis. This is the simplest type of injury. There may be a little or no bleeding and it heals rapidly. When the healing has been completed, it does not leave any scar except the case where deeper layers of dermis are involved. Healing is completed in 5–7 days time.

Types of Abrasion

1. Graze abrasion.
2. Scratch abrasion.
3. Pressure abrasion.
4. Imprint abrasion.

Graze Abrasion

Graze is caused when a wide rough object slides or scraps or grinds through the surface of the skin. The beginning of the wound is clean; the end of the wound presents serrated border and heaping up of epithelium. When a man falls on the road or when a moving vehicle passes over a man, grazes are caused.

Scratch Abrasion

Scratch is a linear abrasion caused by a pin or a thorn or any other pointed moving object passing along the skin (Fig. 5.2).

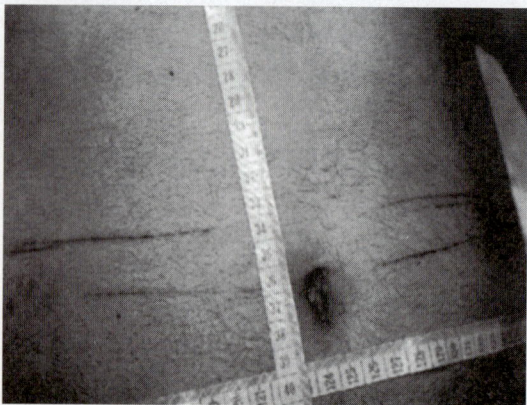

Fig. 5.2: Scratch abrasion (produced by tip of a pointed weapon)

It causes long epithelial tear. Nails also cause scratches.

Pressure Abrasions

They are caused by a continuous pressure exerted by the force leaving the impression of the object on the area pressed. Pressure abrasion can show the pattern (Fig. 5.4) of the pressing object on the pressed area. Ligature marks of hanging, strangulation, etc. are examples of pressure abrasion.

Impact Abrasion

When an object strikes or impacts with force suddenly on the body, it causes the replica

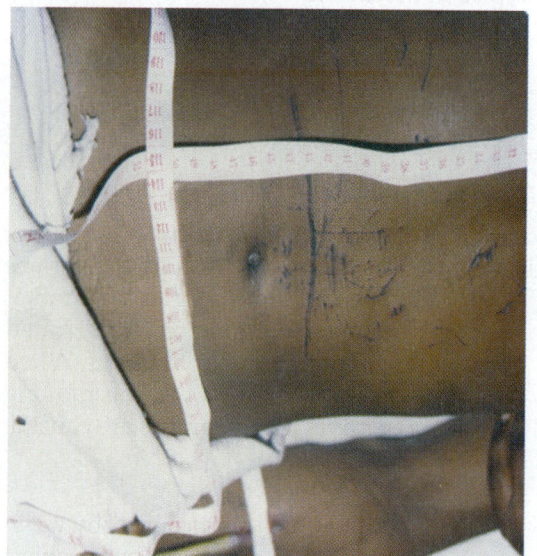

Fig. 5.3: Self-inflicted injuries

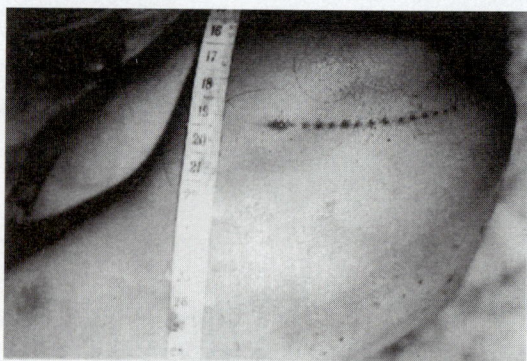

Fig. 5.4: Pattern of pressure abrasion due to beaded male

of the object on the body. This is due to sudden forceful impact, e.g. radiator of a car, headlight of a car.

Healing of Abrasion

- Fresh abrasion is red in colour.
- A crust is formed in about 12–18 hours consisting of lymph, epithelial and atmospheric debris.
- A scab is formed in 18–24 hours. Fresh scab is red in colour, it consists of dried blood, lymph and epithelial debris.
- Dry reddish brown scab is formed in 3 days.
- Abrasion heals from periphery towards centre in case of scab.
- The new epithelium is formed in about 5–7 days.
- Itching occurs between 5 and 7 days forcing the person to remove the scab. This exposes the new epithelium.

The new epithelium assumes the colour of skin in 7–14 days.

Microscopy	
Scab formation	12–18 hours
Epithelial regeneration	30–72 hours
Subepidermal granulation	5–8 days
Keratinization of new epithelia	9–12 days
Regression	After 12 days

Medicolegal Importance of Abrasion

Abrasion is the most superficial injury which heals without leaving any scar, but it is an important injury before it heals, for medicolegal purposes.

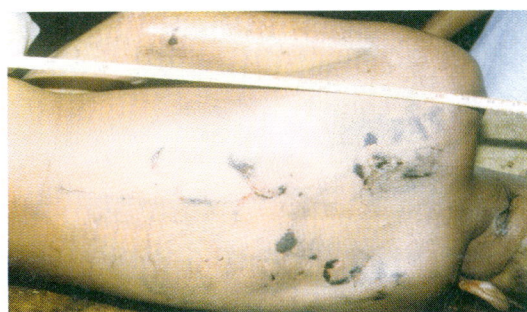

Fig. 5.5: Irregular healing abraded contusions

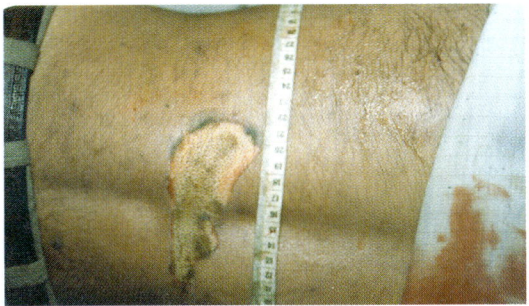

Fig. 5.6: Irregular scar fresh

- In case of hanging, pressure abrasion is seen on the neck with gap below the ear or on the nape of the neck, at the place of knot.
- In strangulation, pressure abrasion is seen all round the neck.
- In throttling, fingernail marks (scratches), (crescentric abrasions) are seen on either side of the neck, in the front or the back. From the position of thumb and nail marks; it can also be suggested that whether the person is throttled from front or back.
- In smothering cases, fingernail marks are seen around mouth and nostrils.
- Crescentric abrasions on the breast, inner aspects of the thighs suggest sexual violation.
- Nail marks around the arms and perianal region suggest anal violation.
- Heaped up epithelium indicates end of abrasion.
- Grazes are seen in traffic accidents.
- Teeth bite marks seen on the breasts and buttocks indicate sexual violation.
- Teeth bite marks on the hands of the accused may suggest resistance of an attack by the victim.

- Tyre thread marks suggest vehicular accident and the nature of the vehicle.
- Stage of healing of the abrasion suggests time since injury.
- Abrasion may indicate the possible location of deeper injuries.

Differential Diagnosis of Abrasion

Ant bite marks: Crowded, close, multiple ant bites in an area look like an abrasion. Close look with a hand lens clearly presents multiple meniscus sand like bite marks of ants. Each one is separated by normal skin.

Postmortem abrasion: The exposed parts of the body dragged after death scrap the superficial layers of skin showing lifeless pale abraded areas.

Postmortem peeling of the skin: Skin is peeled off at many places as a process of decomposition. The peeled areas are white, dry, devoid of any red margins.

CONTUSION

It is a wound caused by blunt force mechanical trauma causing disruption in the subcutaneous tissues keeping the skin intact. The subcutaneous vessels are ruptured causing escape of blood into the tissues. The skin above the contusion is generally raised due to the blood collection underneath. The blood disintegrates by haemolysis, it liberates haemoglobin, which is broken down into haemosiderin, haematoidin and bilirubin. This is caused by tissue histiocytes and tissue enzymes. These liberated pigments

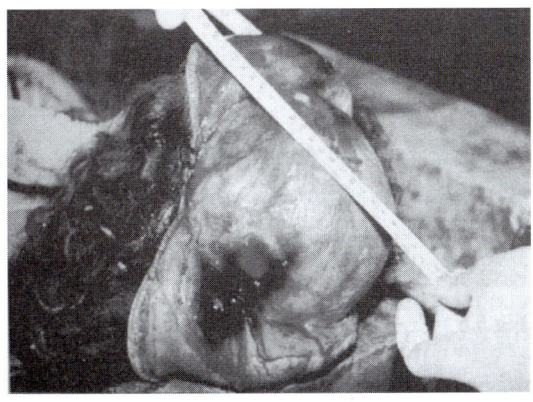

Fig. 5.7: Scalp lifted, haematoma exposed

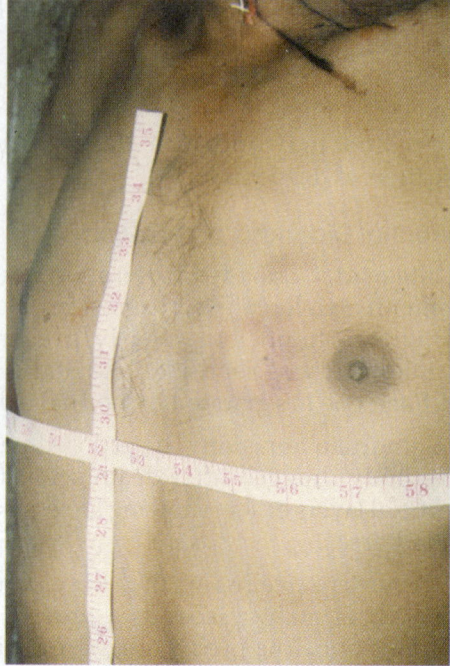

Fig. 5.8: Patterned abraded contusion

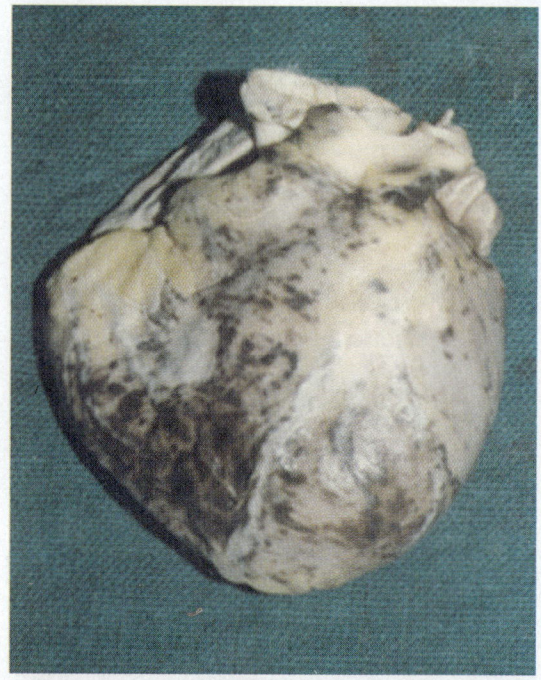

Fig. 5.9: Contusion of heart—blunt force pre-cardial trauma in a road accident

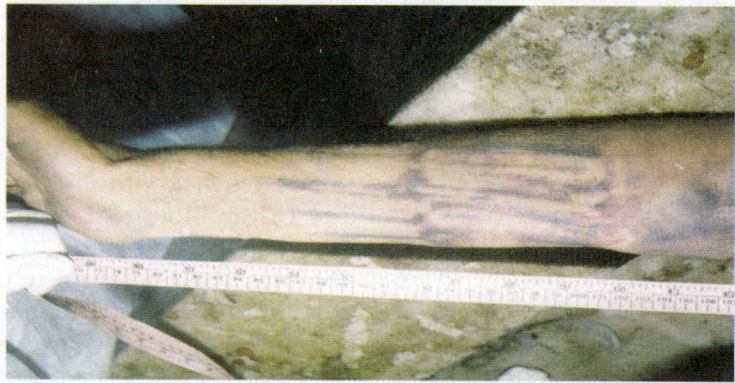

Fig. 5.10: Linear abraded contusions

impart colour to the bruise which can be seen intact on skin.

- Fresh contusion is red
- By 1st day, becomes blue
- By 3 days, becomes brown
- By 5 days, becomes green
- By 7 days, becomes yellow
- By two weeks, normal skin colour.

When the contusion is deep seated, colour changes may not be appreciated. The size and shape of the contusion roughly resemble

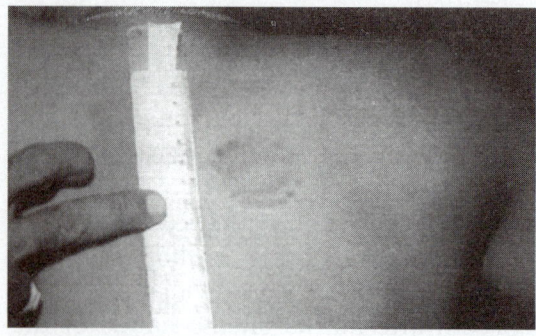

Fig. 5.11: Love-bite suction contusion with teeth bite marks

the causative agent with the lapse of time, the contusion becomes more diffused. The amount of blood collected in a contusion depends upon the:

- Site of impact
- Vascularity of the part
- Amount of force causing injury
- Age and sex of victim
- Bleeding disorders in the victim.

Eyelids and scrotum show more blood collection due to loose skin. Palms and soles show less blood collection. Same force causes more blood collection in women. Children and old people also show more blood collection. People with bleeding disorders like haemophilia, vitamin C deficiency, etc. bleed more with trivial trauma also.

Differential Diagnosis

- Contusion may be mistaken for congestion in cases of internal organs. Congestion is inside the organ, whereas contusion is in the interstitial spaces. Contusion shows breakdown of cells, whereas congestion shows inflammatory cells. Contusion is localized, whereas congestion is generalized.
- Contusion may also be mistaken for hypostasis. Hypostasis is seen in dependent parts.

Contusion is seen in injected area in any part. After making a dissection, traumatic collection of blood in contusion is seen. Postmortem staining is confined to the vessels.

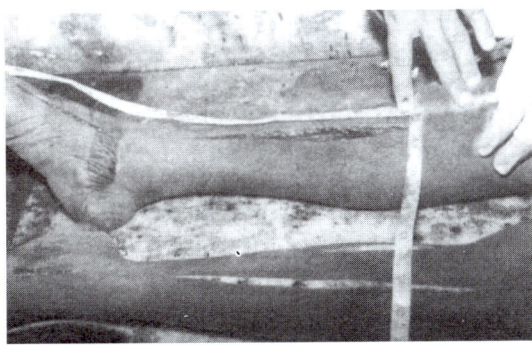

Fig. 5.12: Practical demonstration differentiating hypostasis and contusion

Pseudobruise

Pseudobruise or artificial bruise is caused by juice of marking nut. Here the skin is involved, surrounding area of discolouration show satellite pseudobruises. On scratching, tracking of pseudobruise (vesicles) occurs along the track.

Shifting of the Bruise/Ectopic Bruise

Example: *Black eye*—black eye may occur when there is injury inside the cranial cavity or scalp injury and the blood gets collected inside the orbit.

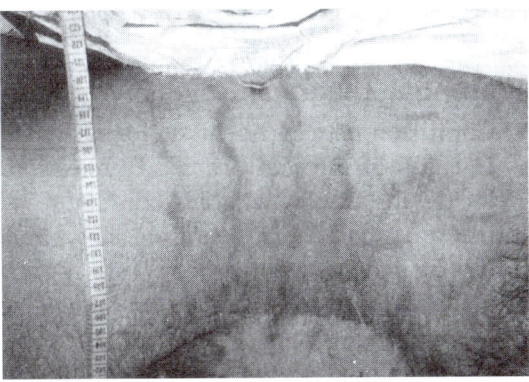

Fig. 5.13: Patterned contusion (tyre marks appearance in run over accident)

Patterned bruise: Contusions show the pattern of the object causing them facilitating the identification of causative agent, e.g. tyre marks.

Rail track bruise: Two linear parallel bruises adjacent to each other with normal skin in between looking like parallel rail lines is seen in cases of trauma caused by canes (flexible stem).

Medicolegal Importance

- From the size and shape of bruise causative agent can be presumed.
- From the colour changes, time since causation of bruise may be approximated.
- From the location of bruises, certain causes can be assessed like the following:
  - Bruises over nose and mouth—smothering.
  - Bruises on front of neck—throttling.

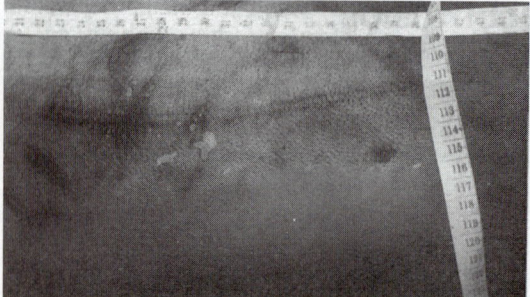

Fig. 5.14: Road or railway track contusion

- Bruises on inner aspects of thigh and genitalia—sexual violation.
- Bruises in anal region—anal violation.
- The amount of blood collected under the bruises when there are plenty of contusions involving upper limbs and lower limbs, back of the body, can be sufficient enough to cause of death in ordinary course of nature due to haemorrhagic shock.
- In the case of dark skinned people, many contusions are likely to be missed unless multiple incisions are made. Therefore, without hesitation multiple cuts should be made and looked for such contusion.

LACERATED WOUND

When a blunt force injuries the skin and deeper tissues, a lacerated wound results.

A lacerated wound is caused by blunt force trauma leading to rupture or tear of skin and underlying tissues. The length is more than the breadth, the edges are contused, irregular, tags of tissues sometimes hang along the edges. Unattended, infections are common. Hence, delayed repair by secondary union is more common. The blood vessels are crushed.

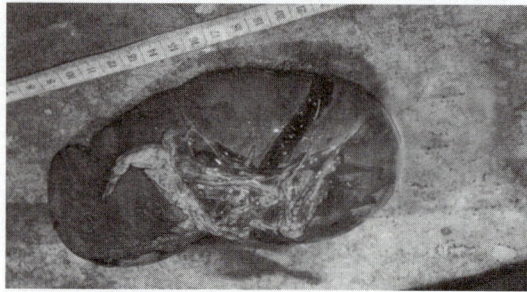

Fig. 5.15: Splenic tear/laceration produced by blunt trauma of abdomen

Types of Lacerated Wounds

- Stretch laceration
- Split laceration
- Avulsion
- Cut laceration

Stretch laceration: When the blunt force overstretches the skin to a breaking point to cause the laceration, stretch laceration occurs.

Split laceration: When the blunt force splits the skin, where there is bone underneath the skin, split laceration occurs. Cheek bones, lower jaw, scalp, chin are common sites.

Avulsion: It is lifting and pulling the skin due to grinding compression of a weight leading to tearing away of the skin causing avulsion, e.g. scrotal skin, when a tyre lifts it. Avulsion of scalp when the hair get caught in a moving belt of machinery.

Cut laceration: When a heavy cutting instrument causes the wound on the skull, the skin is cut but the edges are abraded and contused. This type of wound is called chop wound caused by weapons like axe.

AVULSION INJURY OF FACE (Fig. 5.16a to c)

- A 35-year-old female presents with accidental falling of metal sheet over face with facial trauma.
- Involving entire left hemi face with fracture of left maxilla, palate.

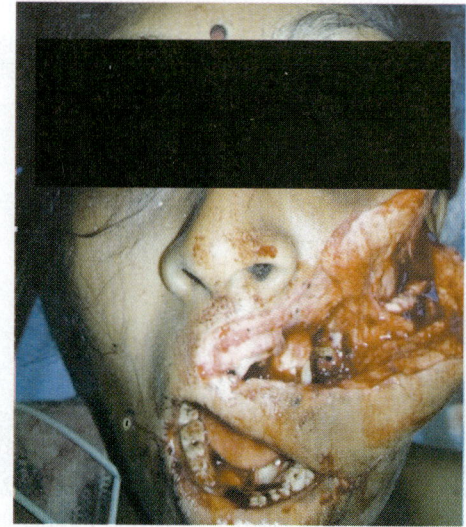

a

Fig. 5.16a: Preoperative

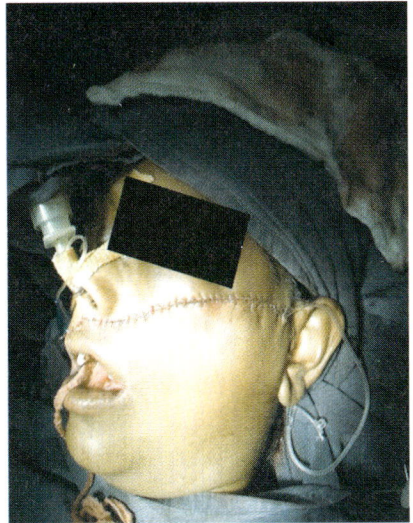

b

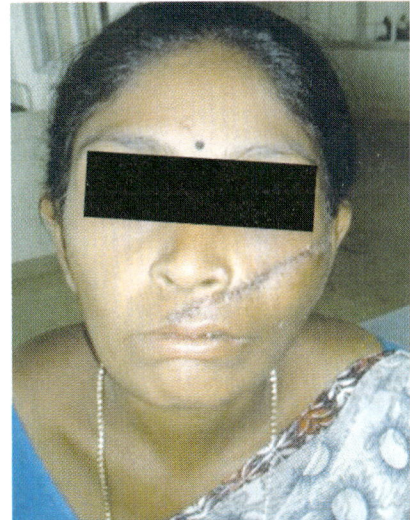

c

Fig. 5.16b and c: Postoperative and follow-up view

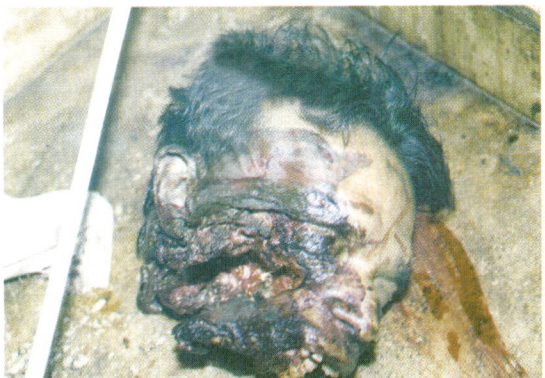

Fig. 5.17: Deep irregular slash

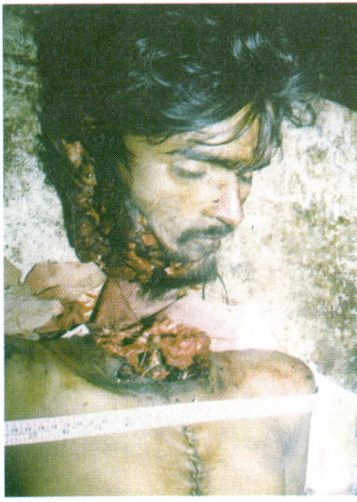

Fig. 5.18: Homicidal cut throat

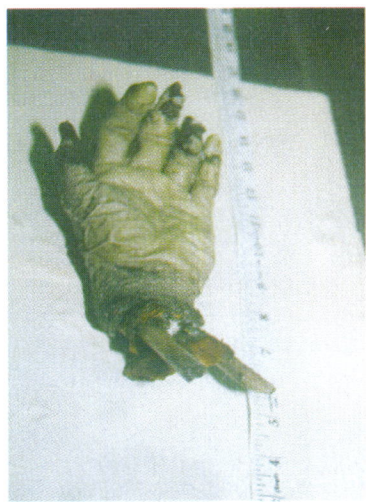

Fig. 5.19: An irregularly crushed decomposed left hand

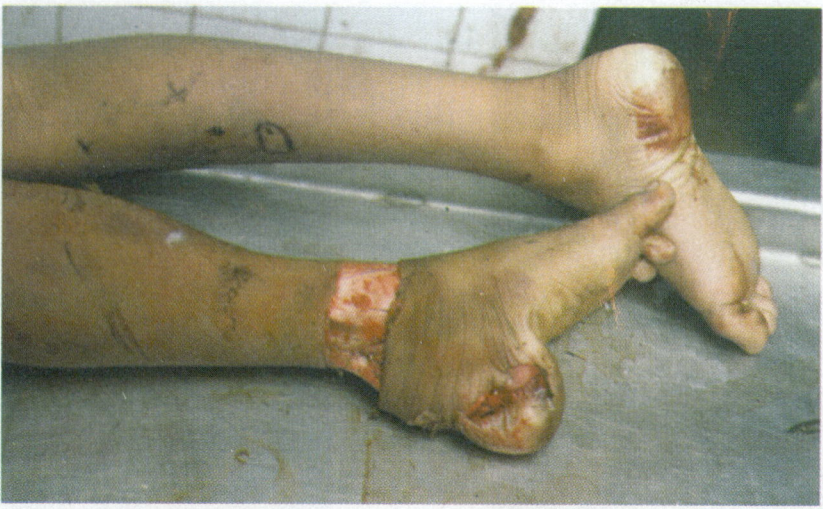

Fig. 5.20: Laceration in a traffic case

Incised-like Lacerated Wound

Incised-like wound looks like an incised wound or a cut. It is caused by a blunt force hitting on skull forehead, bony prominences, skin, etc. It is due to the split of the skin. At a cursory glance, the injury looks like incised wound but on closer look, absence of clear cut margins become obvious.

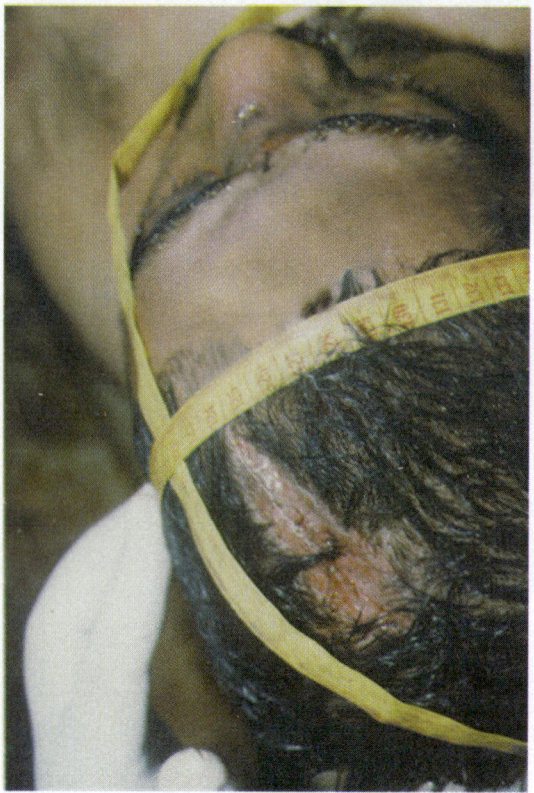

Fig. 5.21a: Laceration scalp

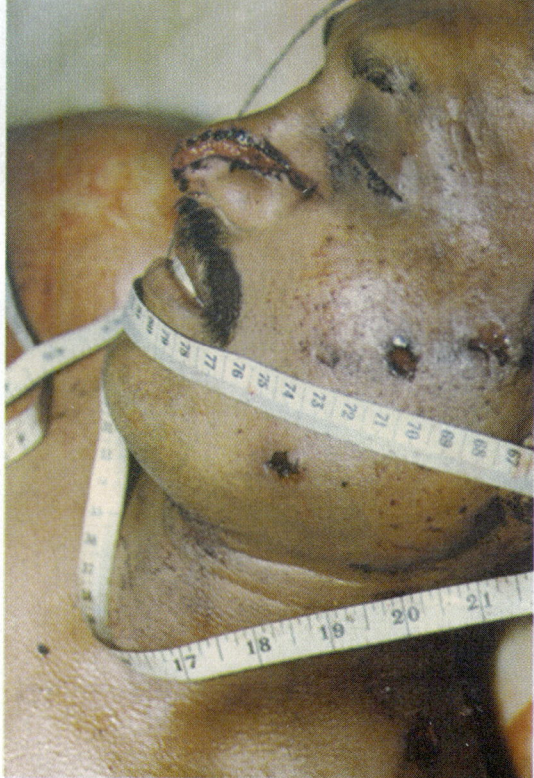

Fig. 5.21b: Three puncture marks. Nose lacerated

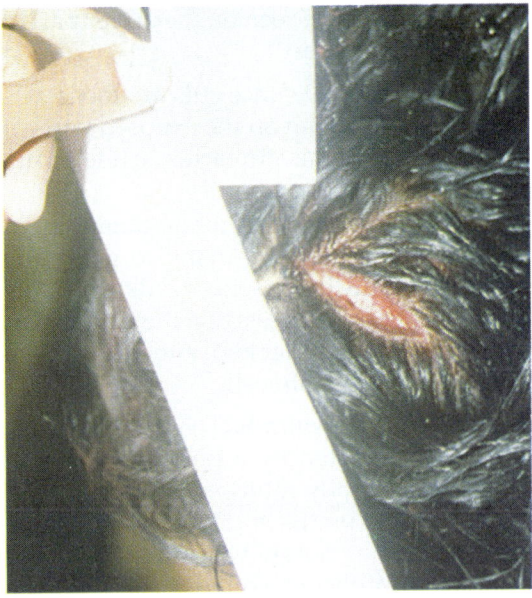

Fig. 5.22a: Sutured scalp wound

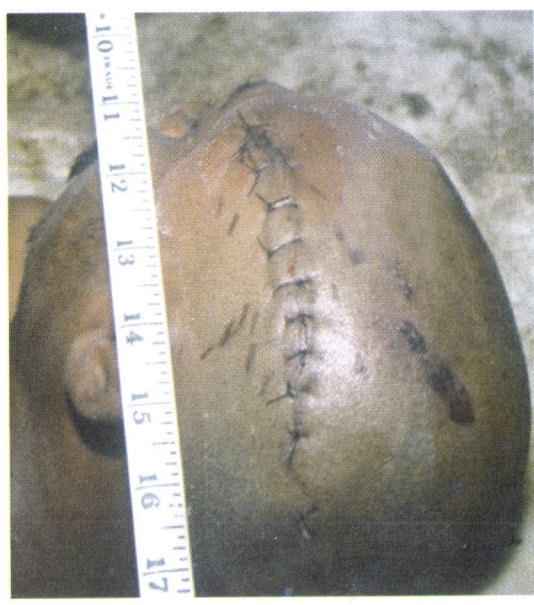

Fig. 5.22b: Postmortem laceration

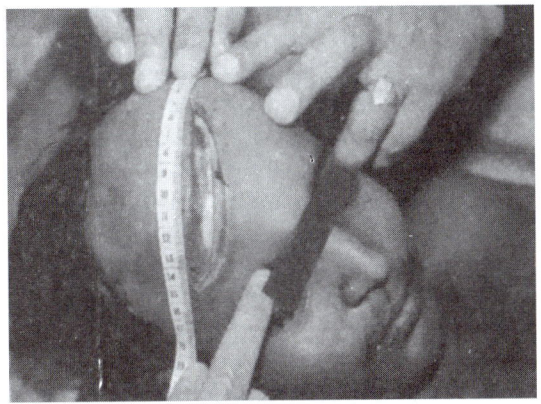

Fig. 5.23: Incised wound over forehead (*note* the clean cut margins and the cut over skull bone)

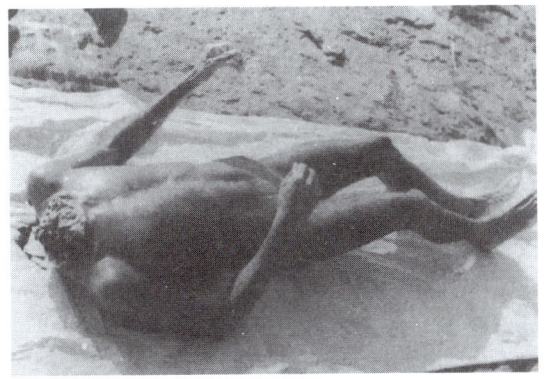

Fig. 5.24: Decapitation

Age of the laceration: Complete healing of the laceration with scar formation takes 1–2 weeks.

Medicolegal Importance

- Lacerated wounds are due to blunt force from the size and shape of the wound, nature of causative agent can be determined, e.g. axe.
- Avulsions of scrotum with associated tyre marks suggest road accidents.
- Chop wounds are caused by cutting implements with rough edges.

INCISED WOUND

An incised wound is caused by a sharp cutting weapon. It is deeper at the beginning and tapers at the end. The margins are clean cut. It bleeds freely and heels quickly. The repair is by primary union. It leaves a linear scar. There is gaping of the wound. Maximum retraction is seen at the middle of the wound. The edges are clean cut and regular. There is no contusion of the margins. Incised wounds are longer instead of wide and deep.

Medicolegal Importance

- Nature of the weapon—sharp cutting weapon.

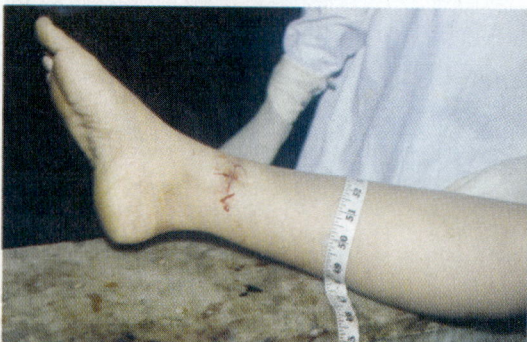

Fig. 5.25: Venesection-sutured wound

- Tapering and tailing of the wound—direction of the wound.
- Multiple incised wounds in inaccessible parts of the body—homicide.
- Incised wounds in reachable parts of the body with small cuts at the beginning of the wound—suicide.

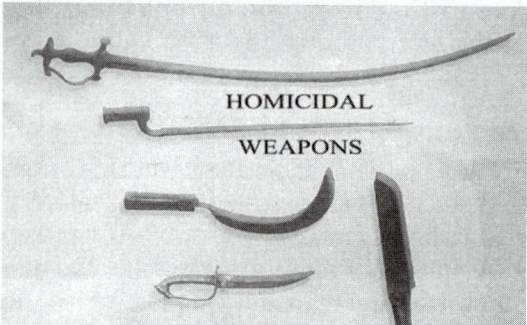

Fig. 5.26: Dangerous weapons: Instrument used for cutting, shooting or stabing (Section 325 of IPC)

Differential Diagnosis

Lacerated wound: Incised wound is easy to diagnose because of its clean cut margins. In case of doubt a magnifying glass should be used.

Hesitation cuts: Hesitation cuts are hesitation marks superficial, multiple, parallel or crisscross cuts or slashes or exploratory cuts made by a person committing suicide before he finally summons enough courage to deal a final fatal blow:

- These are commonly seen on the neck, at beginning of cut throat wounds.
- They can also be seen on the wrists.

- They can also be seen on the upper part of abdomen or chest.

Defence cuts: Defence cuts are those cuts caused on the victim on the exposed parts of the body like palms, forearms, while trying to ward off an attack.

They are also caused while defending a pouncing attacker and trying to grasp the weapon of attack. Presence of defence cuts on victims body suggests that the person was conscious when attacked and he tried to defend or protect himself.

Self-inflicted wounds: There are wounds, which are inflicted by a person upon self. They are generally multiple and superficial and are found on the chest or the abdomen. The clothes may not show any injury. People resort to self-inflicted wounds to derive some advantages like to make false allegations.

Fabricated wounds: These wounds are self-inflicted wounds, may be injuries or false injuries. Artificial bruise is an example of fabricated wound. Most of the time, they are false or fictitious wounds and may be caused by some other person on the body of victim with consent to derive mutual benefit.

An existing simple injury may be modified and fabricated. Similarly, a hymenal bruise or tear is fabricated by mother or father to bring a false charge or rape on child (artificial bruise, see under bruise).

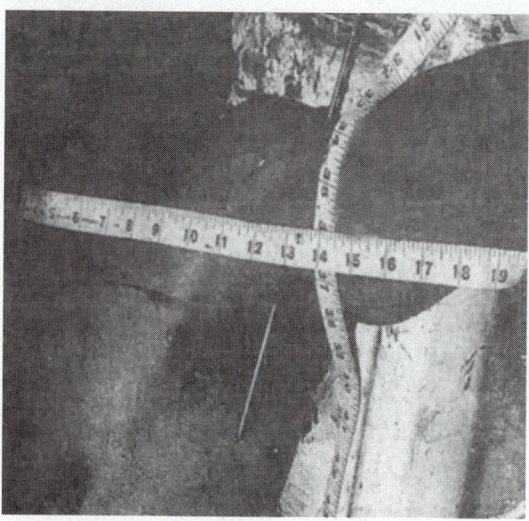

Fig. 5.27: Perforating injury through left axilla

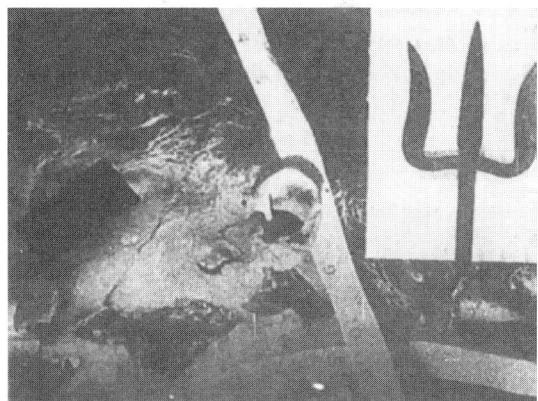

Fig. 5.28: Trident injury over face

STAB WOUND

Stab wounds are those wounds caused by cutting, stabbing or shooting implements producing deeper injuries.

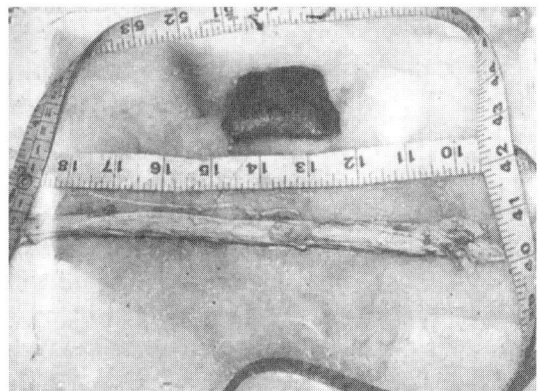

Fig. 5.29: Spinal cord injury (the skin piece above shows injury)

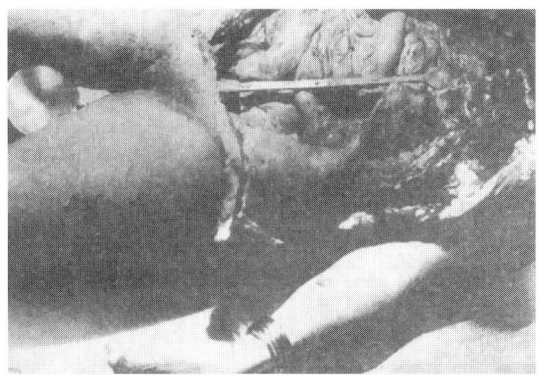

Fig. 5.30: *Kalchu* in the stomach passed through the vagina

Stab injury is penetrating and perforating injury when it enters and exits through a body cavity or hollow organ.

In other words, perforating wounds show entry and exit, while penetrating injury shows only entrance wound. *Stab injury is a convergent injury, whereas firearm injury is a divergent injury.*

The edges of wound of entrance in a perforated wound are inverted. The edges are everted in the case of the exit wound. Clothes or tissues are pushed in or stucked in entry wound. The clothes may or may not be involved in the exit. The tissues and the fabrics are pushed out of exit wound when involved.

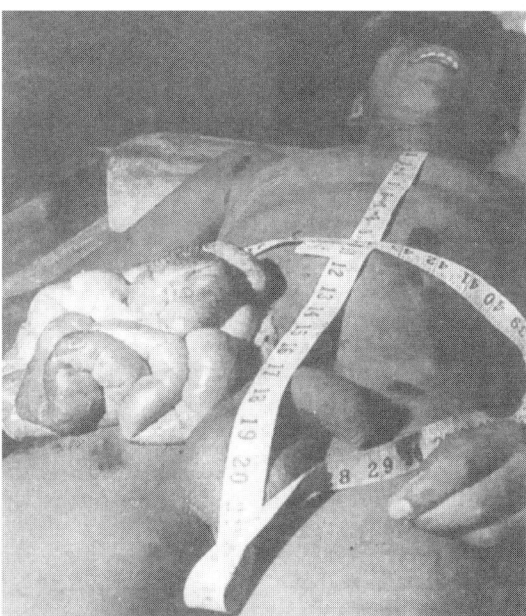

Fig. 5.31: Intestinal coils protruded through stab wound over front of abdomen

The shape of the entrance depends upon whether the weapon has both sides sharp edges or one blunt and one sharp edge. Double-edged weapon causes elliptical wound, single-edged weapon causes wedge-shaped wound. The blunt edge shows contused area. When the weapon enters at right angles, there is no beveling or overhanging. If there is an oblique entrance, the entering side edge is beveled and the opposing edge overhangs. The inside tissue shows pouting when the entry is straight.

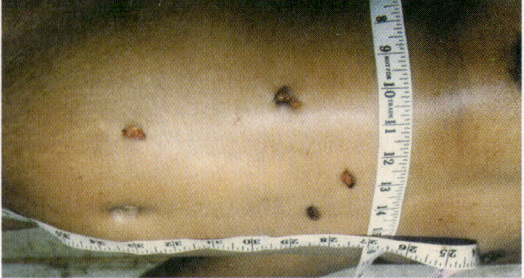

Fig. 5.32: punctured wounds

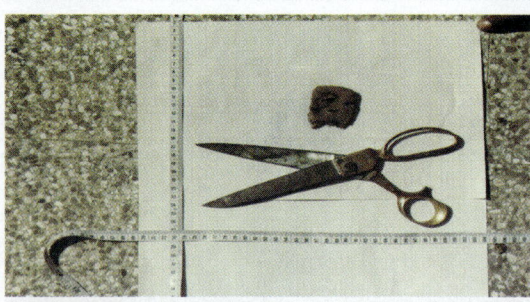

Fig. 5.33: Scissors—skin piece showing wound caused by scissors

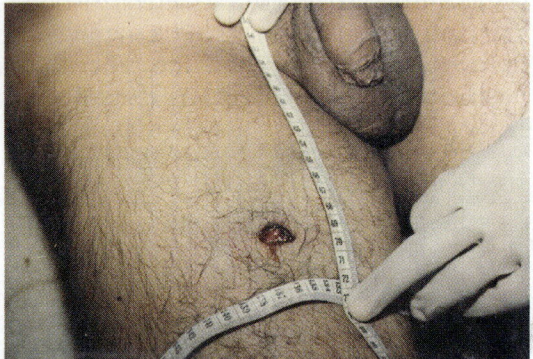

Fig. 5.34: Stab wound on thigh

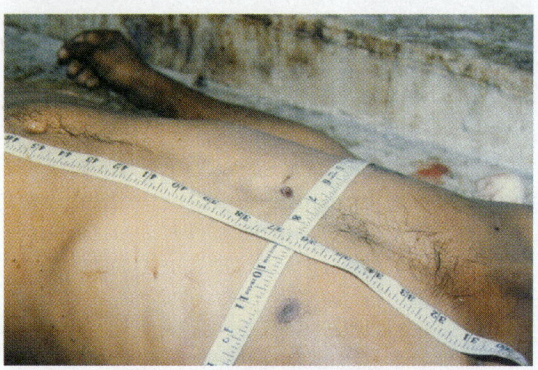

Fig. 5.35: Firearm wounds entry

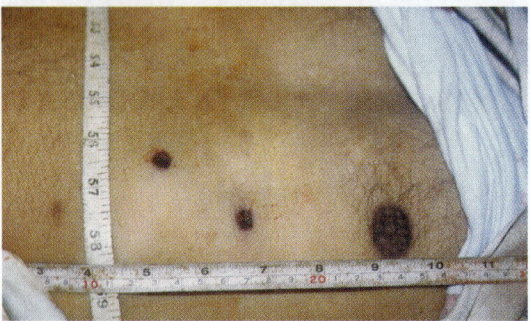

Fig. 5.36: Stab wounds—entry cuts

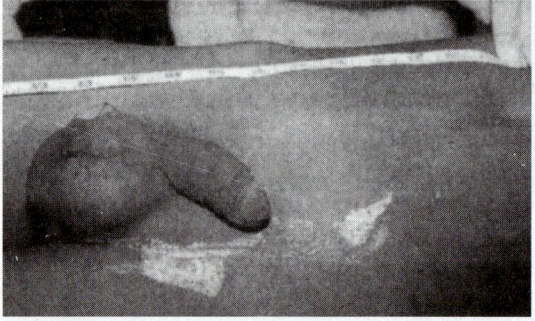

Fig. 5.37: Scrotal contusion with concealed puncture wound

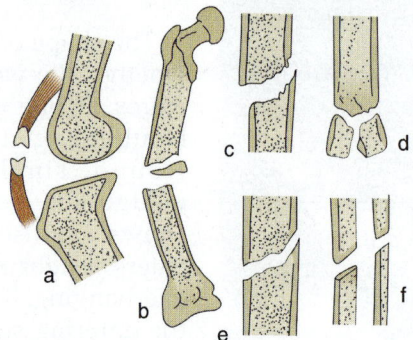

Fig. 5.38: Types of fractures: (a) Avulsion fracture; (b) Wedge fracture; (c) Oblique fracture; (d) Multiple fractures; (e) Oblique undisplaced fracture; (f) Double fracture

Medicolegal Importance of Stab Wounds

- Nature of the weapon:
  - Single edged or double edged.
  - Blunt or sharp edged can be known.
  - The direction of the wound can be known.
  - The depth can be known in cases where the hilt strikes and produces an imprint (abrasion or abraded contusion).
  - Trickling of blood at the entrance suggests the position of the victim. When the victim is standing, blood trickles towards the feet, when the victim is lying the blood trickles along the sides of the body.
  - In the case of postmortem stab injuries, the active bleeding in the form of spurting, and thick staining is absent. However, oozing may be seen.
  - Gaping is the characteristic feature of antemortem injury because of retraction occurring due to elasticity of skin.

FRACTURE OF BONE

Fracture is breaking or crack in the continuity of bone due to blunt force trauma. The various fractures are:

- Greenstick fracture
- Pond fracture
- Simple fracture

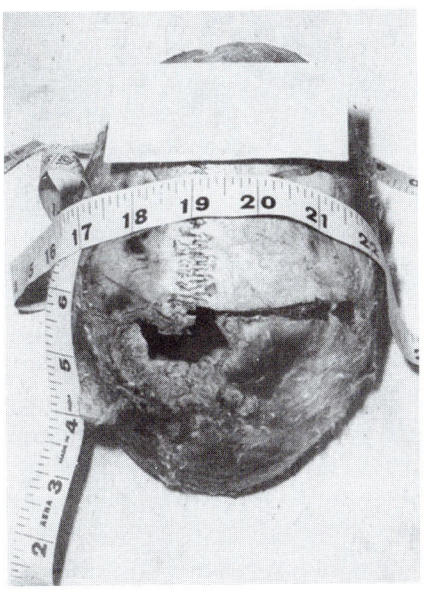

Fig. 5.39: Signature fracture of skull

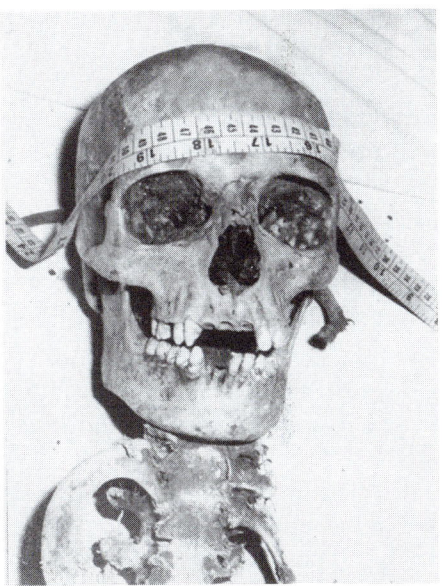

Fig. 5.40: Nose bridge fracture

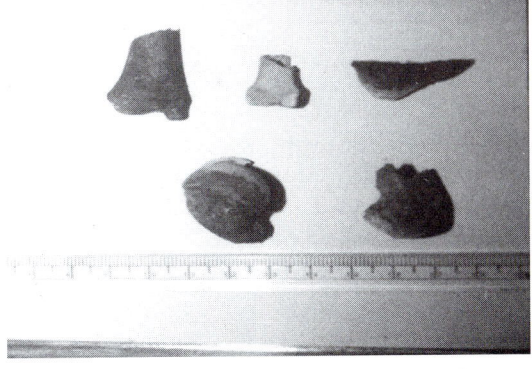

Fig. 5.41: Skeletal remains for examination

- Compound fracture
- Complicated or complex fracture
- Comminuted fracture
- Depressed fracture
- Diastatic fracture
- Gutter fracture
- Direct fracture
- Indirect fracture
- Transmitted fracture
- Transverse fracture
- Spiral fracture
- Oblique fracture
- Ring fracture
- Signature fracture
- Fissure fracture
- Displaced or dislocation fracture
- Fracture *in situ*
- Avulsion fracture
- Epiphyseal fracture
- Stress fracture or March fracture or fatigue fracture
- Pathological fracture
- Spontaneous fracture
- Dentate fracture
- Stellate fracture
- Wedge fracture

Greenstick fracture: When the bone bends but does not break, it is called greenstick fracture. It is more common among young children.

Pond fracture: It occurs due to a pressure on the skull bone of a foetus or an infant, when the pressure applied is similar to the pressure applied on a ping-pong ball.

Simple fracture: Simple fracture is a fracture where there is no displacement of the fractured ends, there is no involvement of any tissue in the fracture (e.g. vessel or nerve), there is no communication between fractured ends and outside.

Compound fracture (communicated fracture): When there is a communication between the fracture and outside body, through opening in the skin, it is called compound fracture.

Complicated fracture: It is a fracture where there is involvement of vessels or nerves within the fracture.

Comminuted fracture: When the bone breaks into more than two pieces, it is called comminuted fracture.

Depressed fracture: When the fracture site is depressed from rest of the surrounding area of bone as in case of skull, it is called depressed fracture.

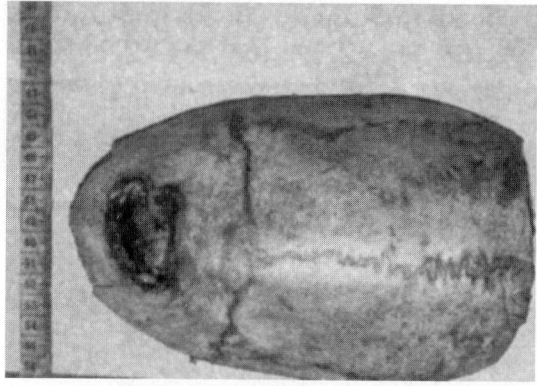
Fig. 5.42: Depressed fracture

Diastatic fracture: When the fracture causes separation of sutures, or when the fracture occurs due to separation of suture, diastatic fracture occurs. When there is pure sutural separation, it is pure diastatic fracture and when fracture ends in suture separation, it is **associated diastatic fracture.**

Gutter fracture: A glancing sword or a grazing bullet can cause grooving of the skull bone leading to a canal-shaped or gutter-shaped fracture.

Direct fracture: When the fracture site corresponds to the place of contact of force or weapon causing the fracture.

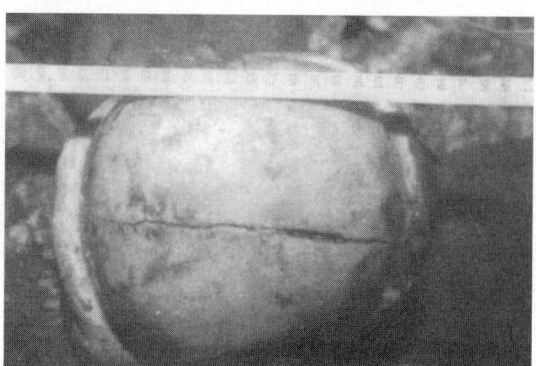
Fig. 5.43: Linear-cum-diastatic fracture

Indirect fracture: It is a fracture occurring away from the site of impact of the force or the weapon.

Transmitted fracture: A transmitted fracture differs from the indirect fracture in the sense that there is a transmission of the force causing fracture at the point of maximum transmitted force or at the weak point or process of transmission, e.g. breaking the base of skull while falling on the buttocks.

Transverse fracture: It is a fracture occurring along the axis perpendicular to the length of the bone. Generally it is due to a perpendicular striking force affecting a long bone.

Oblique fracture: When the bone is struck by a weapon at an angle, oblique fracture occurs.

Spiral fracture: It occurs due to twisting of bone along its own long axis, e.g. fracture of middle third shaft femur or humerus.

Ring fracture: Type of transmitted fracture affecting base of skull around foramen magnum, when the person falls on **vertex,** or both buttocks.

HINGE FRACTURES

Fractures which bisect the base of the skull and make a transverse hinge, are called hinge fractures. Hinge fractures are of three types. Type I run across the skull from one side of petrous part of temporal bone to the other side via sella turcica. Type II runs from front to the opposite back passing through sella turcica. Type III runs from side to side, but in front of sella turcica.

Signature fracture: When a fracture points out the nature of weapon or striking surface of the weapon, it is called signature fracture, e.g. hammer hit on the head showing disc-like shape.

Fissure fracture: When a linear force strikes on the head causing fissure of the skull, it produces fissure fracture. Beginning of the fracture is wider, whereas the terminal

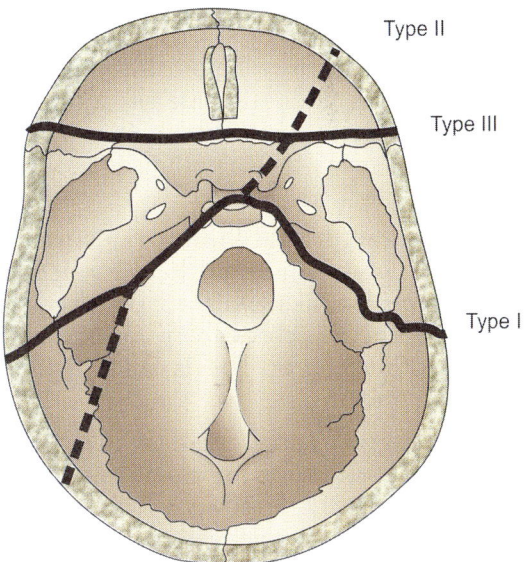

Fig. 5.45: Hinge fractures: Type I, II, and III

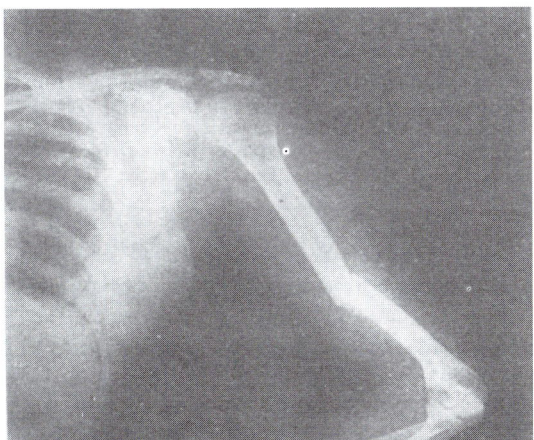

Fig. 5.44: Spiral fracture of middle third shaft humerus (grievous hurt, IPC, Section 320)

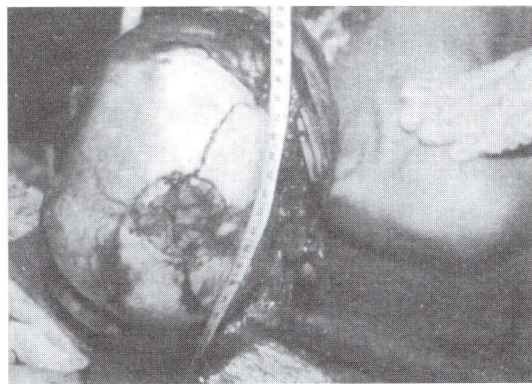

Fig. 5.46: Signature fracture—circular and depressed fracture of skull produced by hammer

part is narrower, so we get a clue for the direction of the injury.

Displaced fracture: When the fracture pieces are moved away from the place of the bone, one end protruding upon other causing projection or angulation, it is called displaced fracture.

Fracture *in situ*: The bone is broken but the pieces are not displaced or misplaced and remain where they are.

Avulsion fracture: Bones attached to muscles or tendon break due to a pull of the muscle leading to the broken piece being pulled along with the tendon or muscle along the direction of the pull, e.g. patella.

Epiphyseal fracture: Before the epiphyses and diaphyses unite they are separate, the epiphyses show tear or break in growing children. It is caused by a pulling or pushing force.

Stress fracture or March fracture or fatigue fracture: Normal healthy active vigorous persons like soldiers or police going along a route March develop fatigue and fracture of metatarsal. This is called fatigue or March fracture.

Pathological fracture: It occurs with minimum trauma due to pre-existing bone disease, e.g. osteoporosis, secondaries in body of vertebrae, osteomyelitis, osteomalacia.

Spontaneous fracture: When the bone breaks all of a sudden without obvious indication of trauma appearing as if it occurred on its own, it is called spontaneous fracture, e.g. osteoporosis.

Dentate fracture (bumper fracture): They occur due to trauma of variable force hitting the body.

Wedge fracture (bumper fracture): When bumper of vehicle strikes a pedestrian from front, the tibia suffers wedge fracture. A wedge of bone is separated from both ends.

All bumper fractures are not wedge fractures but all wedge fractures are bumper fractures.

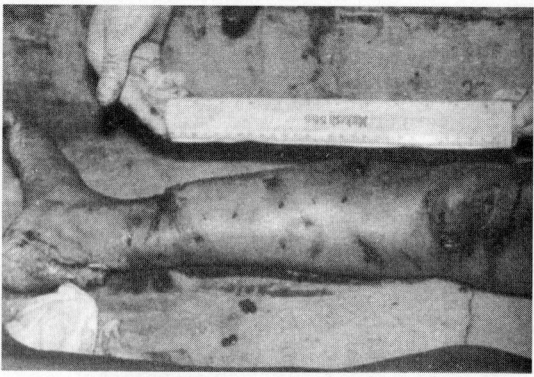

Fig. 5.47: Bumper fracture

Stellate fracture (spider fracture): Occurs due to disbursal of the force in all directions after impact as hit with a stone or pointed object occurs over skull. Also called spider fracture (Tables 5.1 and 5.2).

Medicolegal Importance of Fractures

- All fractures come under the category of grieveous hurt when caused by other persons.
- When a person is suffering from a disease and fracture occurs due to the pre-existing condition as a pathological fracture or due to an injury which would not have normally caused fracture in a normal bone, then in the absence of intention to cause a fracture, the resultant fracture does not come under the category of grieveous hurt.
- Fractures can cause loss of function and deformities. They may lead to permanent disability. Such patients may come for disability evaluation for compensation purposes.
- Fractures can cause death due to haemorrhage or fat embolism.
- From the stage of healing of the fracture, age of injury can be ascertained. As soon as the injury is caused there is haematoma associated with fracture. The patient suffers from pain, loss of movement, deformity, swelling, tenderness. Soft callus is formed in two weeks time. Callus gets completely ossified by 6–8 weeks and bone gets united by 8–10 weeks and excess bone resorption takes 2–3 years.

Table 5.1: Healing: Fracture of bone

Feature	Time
Haematoma formed around fracature is clotted	Within 12–24 hours
Clot organization, necrosis of bone ends and migration of polymorphs into necrotic tissue	Within 48 hours
Formation of osteoid matrix	– 3 days
Hyperemia and oedema	– 4 days
– New vessel formation and presence of numerous fibroblast	
– Osteoid matrix transforms into soft callus	
– Small areas of bone are laid down around blood vessels in irregular interwoven manner	7 days
Fibroblast lay down reticulin and then collagen which is well marked	By 10 days
Haematoma is absorbed	In 10–14 days
Callus formation is well advanced	10–12 days
Callus radiologically visible	3 weeks
Fracture (periosteal) gap is filled by callus	30 days
Callus is transformed into bone (hard callus): Bony union	6 weeks–2 months
Remodelling and reabsorption	6 months

Table 5.2: Healing of injury and loss of tooth

Bleeding stops and clot formed	12 days
Clot is obliterated by fibrous tissue	In about 14 days
Socket completely filled with new bone as seen on X-ray	1 year

FIREARM INJURIES: BALLISTICS

A firearm is a weapon consisting of a barrel through which the ammunition is fired at a target. It has a breech end towards the user, muzzle end towards the target, a cartridge consisting of the ammunition and the propellant of ammunition, i.e. gunpowder. The firing pin and ignites the propellant powder. The propellant powder produces gases under pressure due to heat generated and also flames and hot carbon particles. The common gases are oxides of nitrogen. The ignition mixture or detonator consists of mercury fulminate, lead azide, potassium chlorate, antimony sulphide. The propellant powder or gunpowder consists of nitrocellulose as smokeless powder and the black powder which produces lot of smoke consists of 15% charcoal, 75% potassium nitrate and 10% sulphur.

Black powder produces carbon dioxide, carbon monoxide, hydrogen sulphide, hydrogen and methane. It leaves a lot of residue consisting of ammonium carbonate, nitrates, sulphur, sulphides, sulphates, potassium carbonate, thiocyanate and thiosulphates.

The residue in smokeless powder is very little and consists of nitrates and nitrites. A mixture of 20% smokeless and 80% black powder is called semi-smokeless powder. The ammunition used is of two types:

1. Bullets
2. Pellets

Both are fitted to cartridges. The cartridges in smooth bore weapons consist of a metallic base, a plastic or a cardboard case. The ammunition is separated from the primer or igniting mixture and the projectile by wads. The wad which keeps the bullets in position is known as retaining wad, which is thinner than the main wad between the pellets and gunpowder. In the case of rifled firearms, cartridge, the base as well as the case are

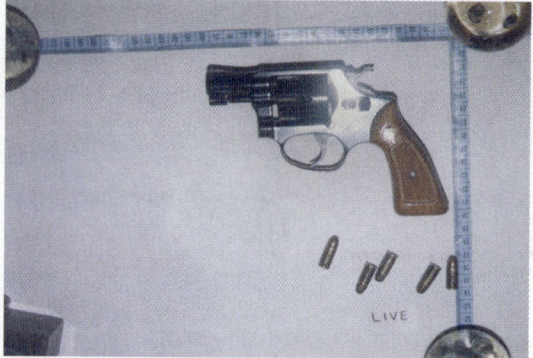

Fig. 5.48: Improvised (country made) revolver

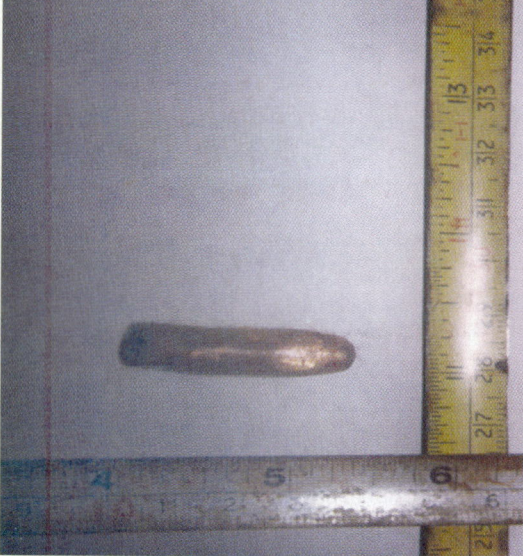

Fig. 5.49: Discoloured and distorted bullet

made up of metal. It is made of an alloy of copper and zinc. In the case of shotgun cartridge, the base is made of brass.

The bullet consists of a lead core with a coating alloy of copper and nickel. The bullet is conical in shape. The tip is called the nose.

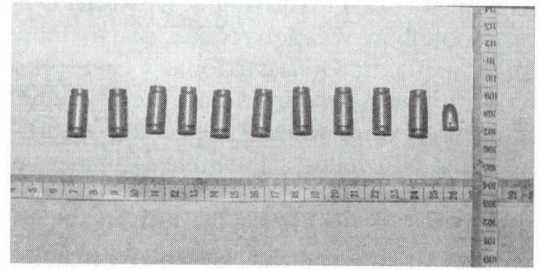

Fig. 5.50: Used bullet and bullet case

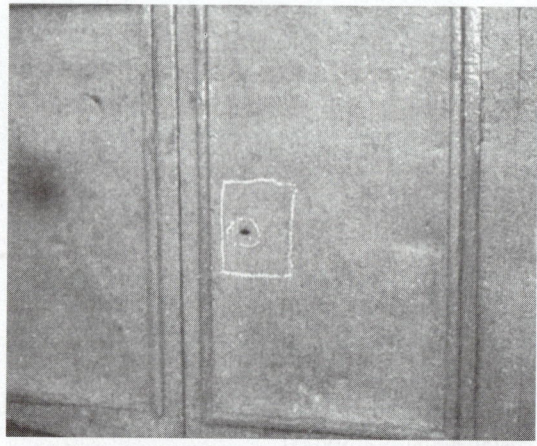

Fig. 5.51: Bullet hole at scene of offence

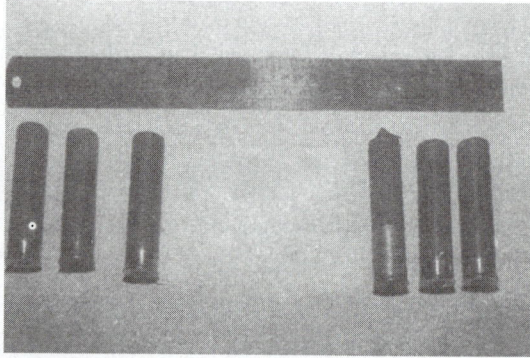

Fig. 5.52: Used and unused shotgun cartridges

The pellets in case of shotguns are made up of lead. The number of lead shots present inside the cartridge vary with the type of the

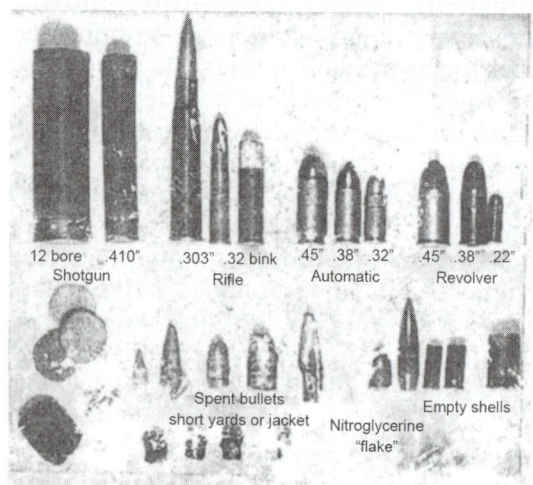

Fig. 5.53: Used and unused shotgun cartridges

shotgun. When a pound of lead is divided into 12 equal sizes of spherical lead balls and once such lead ball fits into the barrel of gun, the weapon is described as 12 boregun so the caliber of shotgun is described as 12 bore, 6 bore, etc. depending upon the number of lead balls made from one pound of lead and used in that particular type of weapon. The calibre of rifled firearm is equal to the distance between 2 lands inside the barrel of weapon. In the case of a rifled firearm the barrel is spirally etched like in a mechanical screw and the cross section of the barrel presents opposing elevated areas called lands and furrowed areas known as grooves.

The spiraling is either clockwise or anticlockwise. This process of spiraling is called rifling. Rifling gives spin to the bullet passing through the barrel of the gun with high pressured gases pushing the spinning bullet forward, as the bullet leaves the barrel of rifled firearm it achieves a gyroscopic trajectory, i.e. a steady movement along a line while spinning along its own axis. This gives greater penetrating power, higher velocity and a steadier trajectory for the bullet.

In the case of shotguns, the barrel of the gun is made narrower towards the distal end. When the pellets pass through the barrel pushed forward by the gases, it is pushed out with a greater force at the farther end as it is **chocked** by the narrowed farther end of the barrel. This process of narrowing the distal end of barrel is called **chocking.** It helps in increasing the velocity of the pellets coming out of the barrel of gun. In view of the choking, the pellets travel like a single mass resembling ball for some distance passing out of tunnel. This is called **balling of the shot.**

The study of projectiles and missiles and their transmission through firearms is called **ballistics.** The knowledge of ballistics required for purpose of administration of justice in a Court of Law is called **forensic ballistics.** The firearm, cartridge, ammunition and the study of the projectile and its travel up to the barrel of the gun is called **internal ballistics.**

The study of the projectile and its happenings after it leaves the barrel and before it strikes the target is called **external ballistics.**

The changes happening in the target, i.e. human body as far as we are concerned is called **terminal ballistics.**

The medical man is more interested in injuries and wounds. It is also called **wound ballistics.**

A typical shotgun cartridge consists of
• Metallic base with percussion cap
• Paper or plastic case

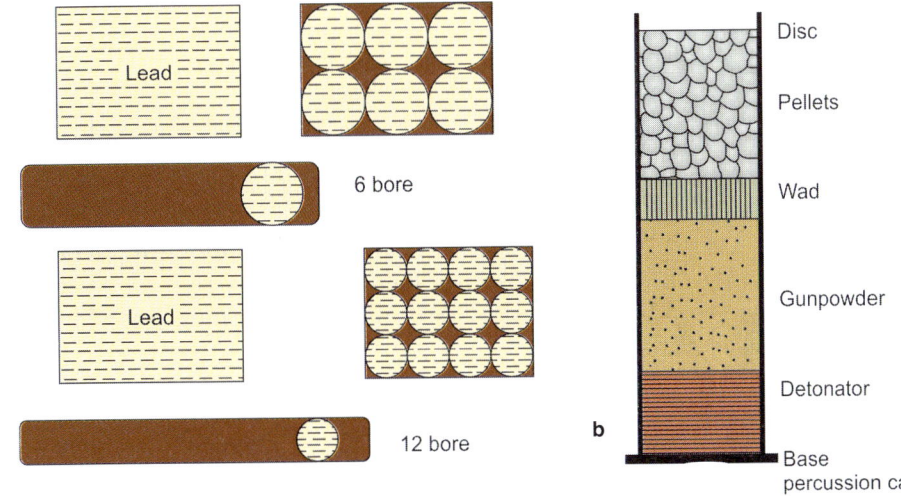

Fig. 5.54a and b: Calibre of shotgun indirect method; (b) Longitudinal section of shotgun cartridge with its structure

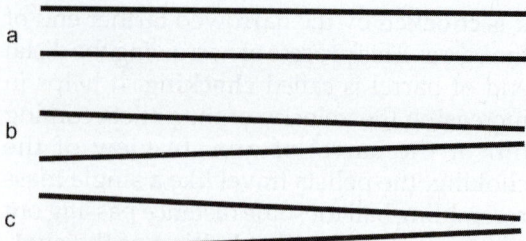

Fig. 5.55a to c: Choking of shotgun. (a) Non-choke; (b) Half choke; (c) Full choke

- Wad
- Retaining wad
- Primer or ignition mixture
- Gunpowder or propellant powder
- Pellets or lead shot.

A typical rifled firearm cartridge consists of

- Metallic base with percussion cap
- Metallic case (body)
- Gunpowder/propellant powder
- Primer/ignition mixture
- Cannelure
- Bullet

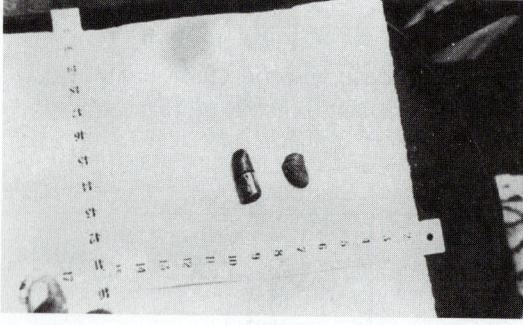

Fig. 5.56: Used bullet and fragment

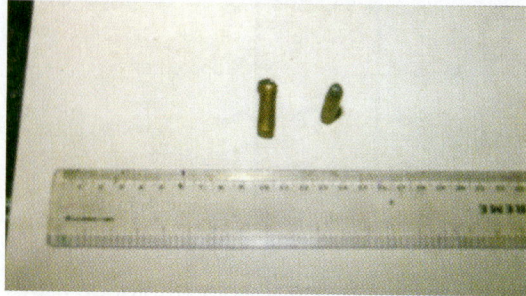

Fig. 5.57: Distorted bullet and fragment

Cannelure is the grooved surface of the body into which the bullet fits in the contents coming out of barrel of firearm:

- In shotgun:
  - Flame
  - Carbon particles
  - Gases (nitrogen, hydrogen, carbon dioxide, oxide of nitrogen, etc.)
  - Wad
  - Retaining head/disc
  - Pellets
  - Smoke
- In rifled firearm:
  - Flame
  - Smoke
  - Carbon particles
  - Gases
  - Bullet

Effect of the Contents on the Body

In case of rifled guns

- Smoke
  - Blackening of the skin (smudging)
- Flame
  - Singeing, burning (scorching)
- Carbon particles
  - Involuntary tattooing, peppering
- Grease
  - Grease collar
- Bullet
  - Abrasion collar
  - Contusion collar
  - Entry wound
  - Track
  - Exit wound

In case of shotguns

- Smoke
  - Blackening/smudging of skin
- Flame
  - Singeing, burning (scorching)
- Carbon particles
  - Involuntary tattooing, peppering
- Wad
  - Entry wound track
- Pellets
  - Single/multiple wounds track (single/multiple) exit, when present

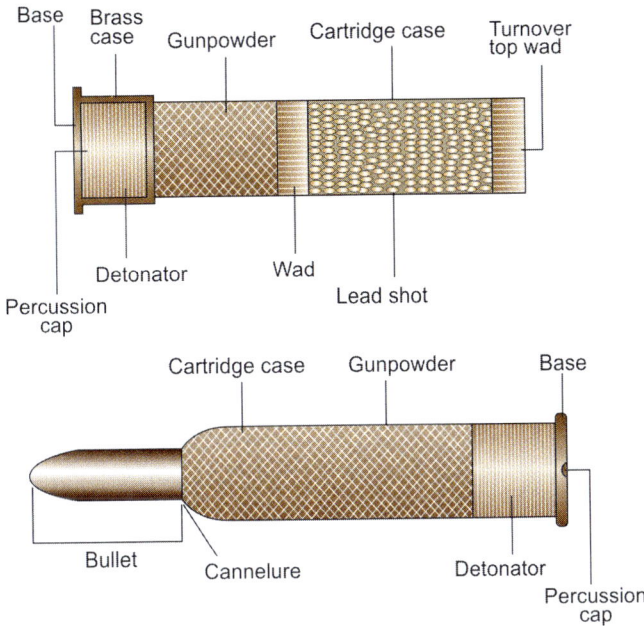

Fig. 5.58: Longitudinal section of shotgun cartridge and rifle firearm cartridge

In case of rifled guns, the effect is seen up to a distance of

- Flame effect/scorching burning: 15 cm
- Smoke effect/smudging: 30 cm
- Carbon particles/tattooing: 45–50 cm
- No smoke/tattooing: >50 cm

In case of shotgun injuries

- Flame effect/scorching: 45 cm
- Smoke/blackening: 30 cm
- Tattooing: 1 metre
- Single entrance wound: 1 metre

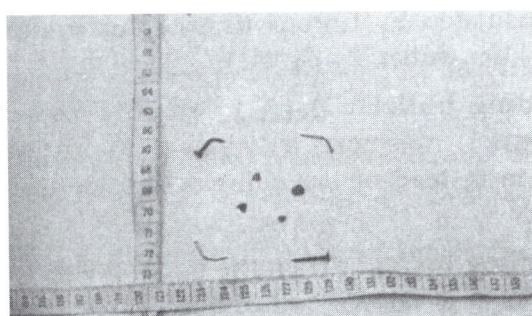

Fig. 5.60: Contents of a country made bomb

Typical wound of a firearm injury consists of

- The **entrance wound** surrounded by grease collar, tattooing/peppering, contusion and abrasion collar, smudging, scorching, singeing. The edges are pushed in, the border is clear cut or punched out.
- In an angular contact, abrasion collar is more at the first point of contact.
- The grease collar is due to the lubricant carried forward by the propelling bullet through the barrel. It is also called **dirt collar**.
- Deposition of smoke causes blackening or smudging. It can be wiped out with wet cotton swab.

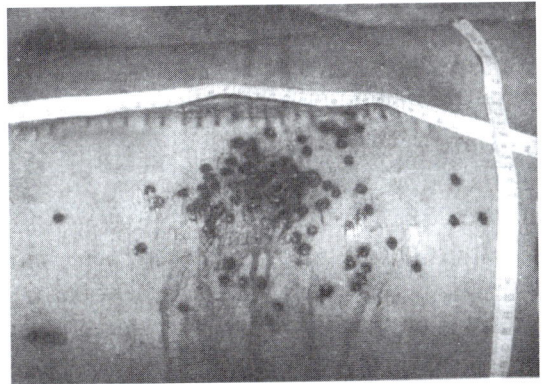

Fig. 5.59: Multiple pellets and wad entry wounds, wounds due to shotgun discharge

- Black powders cause more blackening. When clothes are present, blackening may occur on clothes and not on the wound.

When in doubt, the smoking can be seen through infrared or ultraviolet photography. Microscopic examination of the entrance wound, shows deposits of carbon, homogenization of dermal collagen and swelling.

A cherry red rim at the entrance wound due to carbon monoxide mixing with haemoglobin and producing carboxyhaemoglobin can be seen.

Due to intense heat, lead may be deposited at entrance wound. So with X-rays this radio-opaque material can be appreciated. Neutron activation analysis also helps in detecting the elements.

- **Exit wound** does not show grease collar, tattooing, blackening, burning, singeing, lead ring, cherry red ring due to carbon monoxide.
- The tissue of the exit wound protrudes outwards. The wound edges are also pushed out. Generally the exit wound is bigger than the entrance wound.
- Entrance wound is well defined; exit wound is irregular.
- Exit holes on the cloth may or may not be present. When present the fabric is pushed out.

In the case of shotgun entry wound within the range of shot, all these features including a single entrance hole is found. As the range increases beyond three feet, multiple holes appear due to dispersal of pellets. The farthest distance between two satellite wounds, measured in-between two satellite wounds, measured in inches give a rough range of firing in yards for, e.g. **8 inches to 8 yards.** By linking the exit wound towards the entrance wound, the direction of the travel of the missile can be traced. The track inside is variable due to expanding gases when the range is near. Also there is an expansion followed by a halo effect due to fast travel of missile inside the body.

In the case of contact firearm entrance wound, tattooing, burning, smoke, wad in case of shotgun all are found in the track inside the entrance wound. The wound is stellate.

In near contact wound, i.e. in point blank range, typical firearm entrance wound is found. When the firearm is fired so close to the target that there is no need for aiming the target, it is called **point blank range.**

In a distant range entrance wound, effects of smoking, scorching, tattooing are not seen. Size of the wound is larger than the size of bullet, margins are inverted.

A Typical Firearm Entrance Wound
They are caused by

- Bullets which are not of normal shape and size.
- When clothes interfere between the entering bullet and the body.
- When a bullet deviates from its path, gets distorted and deflected before entering the body, e.g. **ricochet phenomenon.**

Various Types of Bullets
Ricochet bullet: When a bullet alter sits path due to deflection before entering the target is called ricochet bullet. It can occur before entering the body also inside the body after entering, e.g. like in the skull where it may be changing its path many times while striking the hollow and protruding surfaces inside the skull (cranial cavity).

Tandem bullet: When one bullet behind the other enters the body through the same entrance wound, it is called tandem bullet. When a firearm is loaded and not used for a considerable time, on pressing the trigger the bullet may still stick to the barrel. When a second bullet is loaded and fired, the first and second bullets travel at tandem causing the tandem bullet phenomenon.

Dumdum bullet: When the nose of bullet is sawn off, it mushrooms out on striking the target producing an entrance wound larger than the size of bullet.

Frangible bullet: When the bullet breaks into multiple pieces before entering the target, it is called frangible bullet.

Rubber bullet: Solid, flexible, small, rubbermade, tapering, blunt shells used to control the rioting mob are called rubber bullets.

Souvenier bullet: When the bullet remains embedded in the body for a long time it is encapsulated by fibrous tissue. This is called souvenier bullet.

Yawning bullet: When the bullet loses its gyroscopic trajectory, it travels in an irregular fashion instead of traveling with nose to the front.

Tumbling bullet: When the bullet rotates end on end, it is known as tumbling bullet.

Karonlein shot: When a bullet passes through and through the skull and brain causing a bursting fracture of the skull, with external herination of brain matter, it is called **karonlein shot.**

LG cartridge: Consists of six lead shot inside the case of cartridge.

Buck shot: Six to nine large pellets in a twelve bore cartridge.

Dust shot: In this the twelve bore cartridge consists of nearly 600–1200 small lead balls.

AK 47-Kalashnikov rifle: It is an assault rifle which can fire nearly 600 rounds per minute.

Musket: It is smooth bore shoulder weapon used by military people.

Carbine: It is sawn off rifle.

Saloon pistol: They are short range toy pistols sufficient to kill people.

Air rifles: Lead shots are fired by using compressed air.

Stud gun: It is an industrial gun, used to fix metal studs on wood or metal.

Revolver: It is a hand weapon with a revolving circular magazine containing 5–6 cartridges.

Pistol: It is a hand weapon, with rifled bore.

To prove a firearm injury case, there is need for recovering bullets or pellets intact or broken. Wads, also help. All the materials connected with the firearm cartridge should be handled between thumb and fingers and not with any forceps. The recovered materials are dried before they are packed and sealed (Table 5.3).

1 yard = 90 cm.

Medicolegal Aspects

Firearm injuries can be suicidal, accidental or homicidal:

- A person committing suicide may fire random shots at the scene of incidence

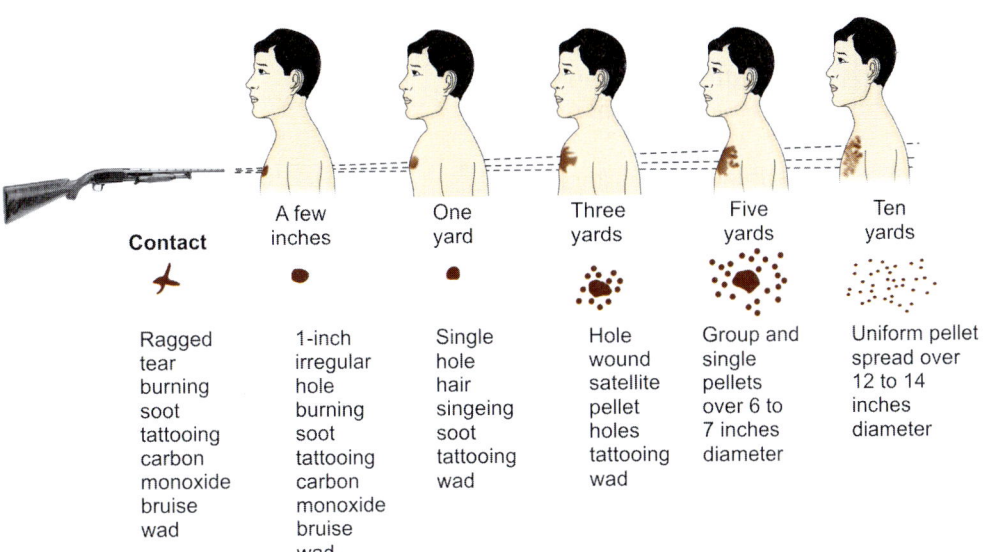

Fig. 5.61: Shotgun wounds: Range wise

Table 5.3: Firearms and ranges

Weapon	Effective range	Muzzle velocity
Shotgun	30–35 metres	240–00 m/s
Musket—shotgun (0.410)	90 metres	350–600 m/s
Revolver	100 metres	150–180 m/s
Automatic pistol	100 metres	300–360 m/s
Carbine (short barrel rifle)	300 metres	
Rifle (long barrel)	1000 metres	
Military rifle	3000 metres	800 m/s

before finding sufficient courage to fire at himself or herself. These are called hesitation shots.

- While looking for the firearm wounds, sometimes concealed firearm wounds may be seen. They are seen in mouth, nose, inner canthus of eye, occiput, armpits or groins, etc.
- When there are multiple injuries of entry and exit, if there are equal number of entry and exit wounds, the inference is that there are no bullets inside. If there are unequal entry and exit wounds, the chance of recovery of the bullet exists. This is called **odd and even rule** which works as thumb rule for autopsy surgeon.
- The person committing suicide leaves on his hand the gases leaking from the weapon.

Lunge's reagent gives blue colour to the washings of the hand. A paraffin cast of the hand helps in detecting nitrites in the dermal residues. This is called **dermal** nitrate test.

- Injuries over accessible parts of the body suggest suicide.
- Disorderly clothes show struggle.
- In suicide clothes may be spared of injuries.
- When the weapon is in (cadaveric spasm) hands of person, it suggests suicide.
- Multiple wounds suggest homicide.

Fallacies of Dermal Nitrate Test
- If a person wears gloves, the test is negative.
- If hand is contaminated with urine or cigarette smoke, there is a false positive test.

Classification of Firearms
a. Smooth Bore Weapons
Shotgun

Rifled weapons
- Rifle
- Pistol
- Revolver

b. Depending on Number of Barrels
- Single barrelled
- Double barrelled
- Triple barrelled
- Tetra barreled

Shotguns

c. Depending on Chocking
- Half choke
- One-fourth chocked
- Non-chocked (cylinder)

Shotguns

d. Depending on Mode of use
- Hand weapons
  - Revolver, pistol
- Shoulder weapons
  - Shotguns, rifles
- Mounted weapons
  - Bofor's gun (Howitzer)

e. Depending on Gunpowder used
- Smoke powder
- Semi-smokeless powder
- Smokeless powder

f. Depending on Velocity
- Low velocity—revolver, shotguns
- High velocity—pistol, rifle

g. Depending on Loading

- Muzzle loader (*Bharat Ka Bandook*)
- Breech loader (shotgun, rifle, etc.)

h. Depending on Operation

- Manual (rifle)
- Semi-automatic (pistol)
- Automatic [AK-47 Russian/AK-56 (Chinese version of Anitschkow)]

i. Depending on Length of Barrel

- Long barrelled.
- Short barrelled.

MEDICOLEGAL ASPECT OF WOUNDS

There have been instances of doctor's refusing to give the details of cases, i.e. their case record to the patients. As the patients feel the growing need for records of the doctors, the need for doctors to maintain proper records has assumed importance.

In the government setup, accident registers or medicolegal registers or EPR (emergency police report) are maintained in the casualty departments. The cases which need medicolegal action in terms of informing the police or magistrate or doubtful cases, regarding nature of trauma or disease, it becomes necessary to follow these records until discharge or death and postmortem examination, whatever happens. The medicolegal record keeping is better maintained by a medicolegal section of hospital under supervision of medicolegal officers or police surgeons or forensic medicine department personnel wherever possible. The register has details about the name, age, sex, address, history of the case, date, time and place of occurance of the incident, e.g. like accident. Consent for examination is taken. If the person is below 12 years then the consent of the accompanying person is taken. Examination of the person without consent should not be done except in cases when accused is brought under arrest. At least two identification marks are noted, as far as possible which are present on exposed parts of the body. Every injury is important from medicolegal point, from treatment angle

some injuries may not be that important. The site, size, shape, surrounding area and the dimensions of the wound in centimetres (metric system) should be noted.

Rough sketches can help in better description of injuries. Nontechnical and simple language is appreciated in the courts. When there are injuries on the clothes, they need to be labeled to know whether they correspond with body injuries or not. Stains on clothes and body require mention and identification, e.g. blood, mud, urine, saliva, hair, grease, semen, etc. The doctor examining the injuries is expected to give his opinion about nature of weapon, e.g. sharp cutting or firearm, etc. The nature of injuries whether simple or grievous needs to be mentioned. The injury certificate should be given to the police so that they can proceed further in the case. The injuries are simple or grievous.

Grievous Hurt is Detailed Under Section 320 of IPC

- **Emasculation:** It means that the masculine power of the male is deprived (cutting of the penis, injury or removal of testes, L_5S_1 spinal injury).
- Permanent privation of sight of either eye.
- Permanent privation of hearing of either ear.
- Permanent privation of function of any member or joint.
- Permanent disfiguration of face.
- Fracture or dislocation of bone or tooth.
- Any bodily injury which causes the person to be in severe bodily pain and unable to carryout his daily pursuits for at least 20 days.
- Permanent privation of any member or joint.

Explanation

- Here the loss of vision in one eye which is permanent is treated as grievous. A temporary loss is not grievous.
- In the same way, permanent loss of hearing even in one ear becomes grievous.

- When there is a destruction or loss of power of any part or organ or limb of the body, it becomes grievous in nature.
- When in injury causes disfiguration leading to the unpresentable features of head or face, then it becomes grievous.
- A visible scar on the face is an example of grievous hurt.
- When an injury causes breaking of bone or cartilage, it becomes grievous in nature.

When a bone or tooth is dislocated it is also considered as grievous hurt. Radiological examination in all suspected cases of fracture and dislocation is necessary. Injuries which cause danger for life or threat for life are treated as grievous in nature, e.g. injury to a major blood vessel.

- When a person suffers bodily pain which prevents him from carrying out his routine ordinary pursuits for a period of 20 days is considered as a grievous hurt. However, if a person is admitted under doctor's care for 20 days, it does not automatically become grievous hurt. Severe bodily pain or inability to carryout routine activities must be present before considering the grievous hurt.
- When there is a danger for life after the injury, such wound is a dangerous wound and is a grievous hurt. Many times the doctor is asked to give opinion about the weapon.

When the weapon is presented to him by the police officer, he should examine the weapon, its striking surface or area and whether the weapon produced by police officer can produce the injuries in question or not. The doctor can only certify that injuries on the body are possible by weapon produced by investigating officer. The weapon requires to be examined by forensic science laboratory and the doctor should accordingly instruct the *investigating officer.*

Any instrument which is used for shooting, stabbing or cutting or any instrument used as a weapon of offence and likely to cause death comes under the category of dangerous weapon.

Any injury seen on the body of the person after death requires to be designated. Whether it is caused before or after death, i.e. antemortem or postmortem in nature can be found out by the doctor by the presence of bleeding, clotting inflammatory response, colour changes on contusions, presence of infection and repair process. In cases of difficulty, microscopic examination may reveal extravasation of blood cells, leucocytic infiltration, oedema, fibrin formation, etc. If the person dies before visible changes take place, enzyme studies help. Study of enzymes like acid phosphatase, alkaline phosphatase, adenosine triphosphatase, aminopeptides help. Age of the injury requires to be assessed by the doctor.

Abrasions show scabs in about 12–24 hours. Redness, swelling occur in about 24–48 hours. Suppuration is seen after 48 hours. Healing by primary union is seen in 5–7 days. Granulation tissue is seen in about 1 week. Colour changes in contusion also help in dating injuries.

Fracture healing helps (look under fracture). Tooth injury bleeds into the socket. The bleeding stops in about 24 hours. The socket fills up in about a week. The gum heals completely in about 3 weeks after dislocation. X-ray examination can show socket filled up with new bone in a year's time. The adenosine triphosphatase activity helps in the first hour, aminopeptidase in two hours, acid phosphatase in 4 hours and alkaline phosphatase in about 8 hours.

There are many factors which modify healing process. Infection, low vitality, vitamin C and protein deficiency, calcium deficiency, etc. A wound which causes death is called fatal wound. Among the injuries, if there is a wound which appears to have been sufficient to cause death in ordinary course of nature, such an injury can be accepted as the fatal wound or injury. Doctor faces this question as to which of the injuries would have caused death. Injuries on vital organs like brain, heart, lungs, liver are likely to cause death. Sometimes vital organs may not be involved. The amount of bleeding that could have occurred from open or closed injuries and the rapidity with which it could have occurred can lead to death. *It is customarily said that at least one-third of the circulatory volume of the blood is required to the trapped in the wounded* areas or when lost from the body is sufficient **to cause death.** Small quantity of blood loss can cause death as in pontine haemorrhage, internal capsule haemorrhage or blood chocking the respiratory system (bleeding in respiration passage).

Period of survival: How long did a person survive after the injuries?

The person could have died instantaneously, immediately or after sometime. The survival time depends upon organ injury, involvement of the vital organ or vital centres on the brain.

Causes of the death from injuries

- Vagal inhibition, e.g. injury to trigger areas.
- Injury to vital organ → Primary neurogenic shock.
- Haemorrhage → External → Haemorrhagic shock.

   Internal → Asphyxia, e.g. cut-throat injury

Paralysis of vital centres, e.g. medullary haemorrhage	Cardiac tamponade, e.g. injury to heart	Cerebral compression, e.g. extradural haemorrhage

- Embolism → Fat embolism → Pulmonary
   ↓   ↓   fat embolism
   Air embolism Systemic fat
   ↓   embolism
   Pulmonary
   ↓
   Systemic

- Infection of the wound, e.g. septicaemia, tetanus.
- **Vagal inhibition** (already discussed in injury chapter).
- Injury to **vital organs** (discussed in injury to medicolegal aspects of injury).
- **Septic complications** (wound infections).
- When the wound is not clean, or the doctors attention was not available for considerable time, infections are likely

to be superadded. Common infections are tetanus and gas gangrene. Other infections like *E. coli,* Streptococci, Pseudomonas, also are common. The patient develops bacteremia followed by pyemia (septicaemia). In pyemia cases, abscesses may be present in liver, brain, kidney, etc. Toxaemia occurs in toxin producing organisms, e.g. *tetanus, gas gangrene, E. coli,* etc.

- Haemorrhage as cause of death is very common (discussed already).
- Embolism can be either air or fat embolism. Air embolism results when about 100 ml of air enters into circulation through arteries. Death can occur as qickly as 20–30 minutes. Pulmonary air embolism occurs:
  - During intravenous injection, air enters the veins (if not carefully observed through saline drip).
  - In cut-throat injuries, when jugular vein is cut, due to negative pressure created air is sucked into the veins.
  - When there is injury to superior sagittal sinus.
  - When air is injected under pressure into uterus for procuring criminal abortion, air finds way to the uterine, pelvic and paravertebral veins from where they are carried into the heart.
  - When fallopian tubes are filled up with air for the purpose of testing the patency of fallopian tubes.
  - When air enters into the lungs causing artificial pneumothorax.
  - While doing pneumoencephalography.
  - In cases of pulmonary embolism, death is due to the mechanical obstruction, because right ventricle is filled with foam of blood. It is also called **air locking embolism.**

During autopsy, when air embolism is suspected, the pericardium is filled up with water and then the heart is punctured. The right ventricle is distended and contains bright red froth.

Arterial air embolism can occur in coronary and cerebral arteries. Air bubbles are locked in the blood which can be seen through the arteries by gentle pressure with fingertips. When air enters pulmonary vein it is carried to the left side of heart and it can target different organs.

Fat embolism like air embolism is also of two types, pulmonary and systemic fat embolism.

Fat embolism occurs due to
- Fracture of long bones, e.g. femur, tibia.
- Crushing injuries involving fat, bone and muscle.
- Injury to adipose tissue
- Severe burns

Fat embolism occurs when fat is set-free from fat cells and enters the crushed veins. After entering the veins, the fat is carried through the veins. In the case of long bone fractures, marrow fat enters the haversian canal veins. Fat can also be introduced into the body by:
- Intravenous injection of fatty substances.
- Intrauterine injection of fatty substances.

Pulmonary Fat Embolism

In between the shoulder on the back of the body, petechial haeaemorrhages may be found. Petechial haemorrhages are seen on the surfaces of the lungs. Lungs are congested and oedematous. At autopsy, escaping fat droplets can be demonstrated by opening pulmonary artery underwater. Pulmonary capillaries are studded with fat droplets, which can be demonstrated by frozen sectioning and staining with osmium tetroxide, which imparts black colour to the embolus. Other fat stains are Sudan III, Sudan IV, Sherlock R, oil Red O, etc. In haematoxylene and eosin staining, fat is seen as empty area. Systemic fat embolism is seen in the target organs. Fat can be seen in suprarenals, spleen, kidney, pituitary, cerebral cortex and heart.

REGIONAL INJURIES
Head Injuries

The layers of scalp are:
- Skin
- Connective tissue
- Aponeurosis
- Loose areolar tissue
- Periosteum

The victims of attack very commonly suffer from head injuries. Blunt force attack with sticks, bamboos are very common.

Common Head Injuries
- Abrasions
- Contusions
- Laceration
- Fractures of the skull
- Extradural haemorrhage
- Subdural haemorrhage
- Intracerebral haemorrhage
- Cerebral contusions
- Subarachnoid haemorrhage
- Intraventricular haemorrhage
- Pontine haemorrhage
- Haemorrhage in internal capsule

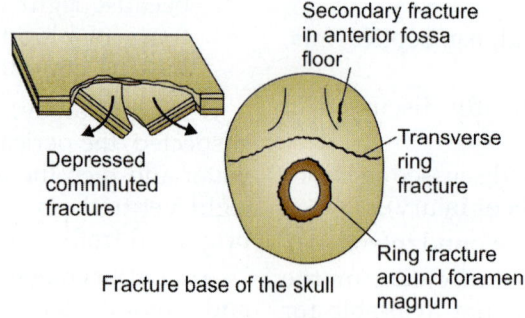

Fig. 5.62: Regional injuries

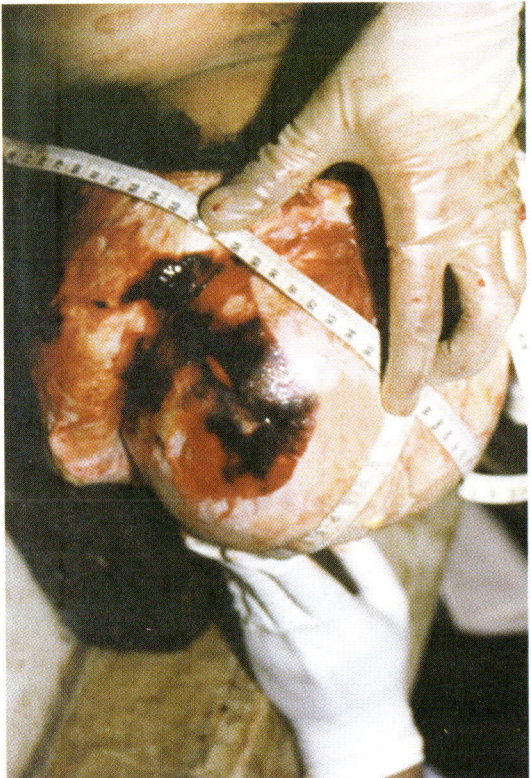

Fig. 5.63: Dissection showing contused laceration

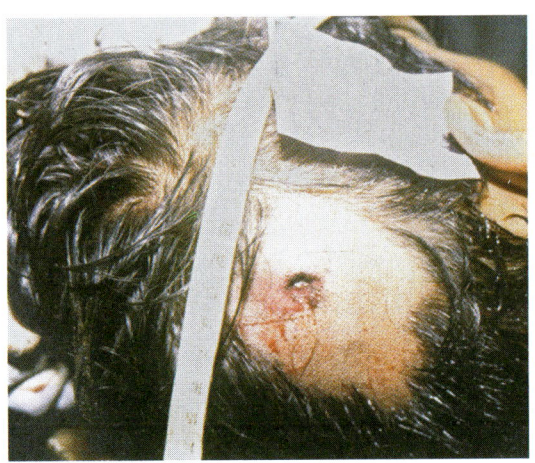 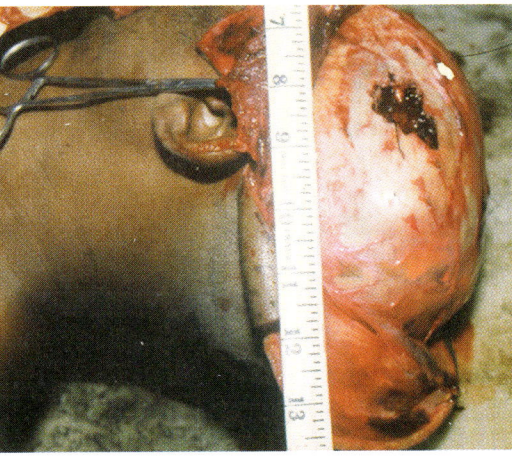

Figs 5.64 and 5.65: Scalp lifted showing depressed comminuted fracture (firearm injury)

The head injuries are direct head injuries or indirect head injuries. Direct head injuries occur under the impact. Indirect head injuries occur due to transmission of force to the head from another site of impact, feet, buttocks, etc.

Coup and Contrecoup Injuries

The contrecoup injuries occur away from the site of impact due to shearing and rotational strains. Avulsion of the scalp occurs when there is long hair trapped in a moving belt of a machine or when caught

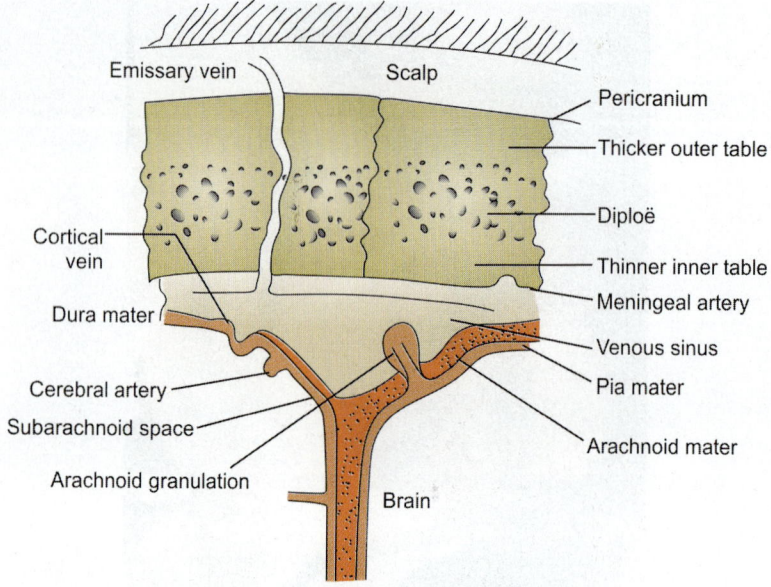

Fig. 5.66: Layers of skull: Scalp to brain

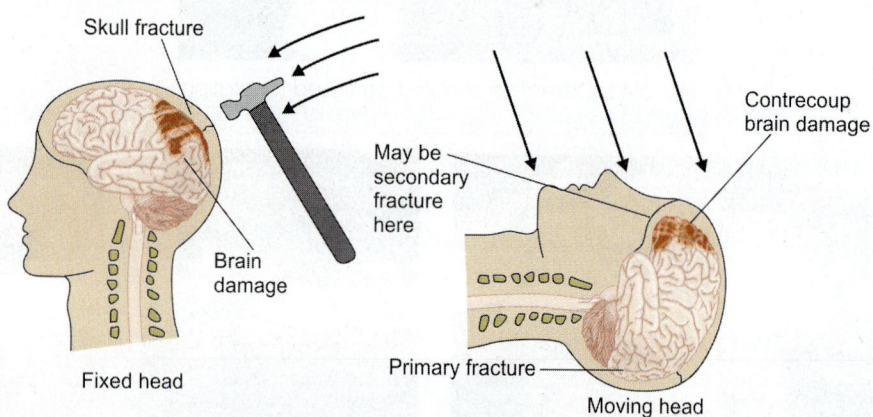

Fig. 5.67: Mechanism of coup and contrecoup injuries

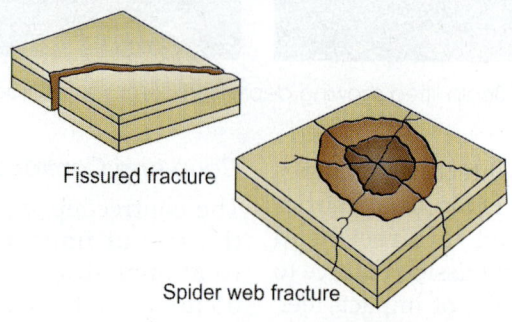

Fig. 5.68: Fractures of skull

under the wheels of a vehicle before coming to a halt.

CONTUSIONS OF BRAIN

There are six types of contusions of brain. They are coup contusions, contrecoup contusions, fracture contusions, intermediate contusions between the location of coup and contrecoup points in the deep structures of brain like brain stem, basal ganglia, corpus callosum, etc. along the line of impact, gliding contusions often associated with concussion/diffuse axonal injury, in frontal cortex and herniating contusion in temporal lobe or cerebellar tonsils getting herniated due to impact. A blow on head generally causes coup contusions. A fall on the head causes contrecoup contusions.

Fracture of Skull

The skull cap has two tables of bone separated by diploë. Some authors do not want to agree with diploë. The basic knowledge of anatomy of skull bones shows that there are diploic veins travelling between outer and inner table. Fractures may involve only outer table like the grazing fractures due to bullets or glancing swords. Tissue fractures also may involve outer table sometimes, especially the radiating portions form a stellate or cobweb fracture.

The fractures of vault are

- Fissure fracture
- Depressed fracture
- Depressed comminuted fracture
- Compound fracture
- Fracture a la signature (hammer head, axe).

Fractures of the base are

- Anterior cranial fossa fractures.
- Middle cranial fossa fractures.
- Posterior cranial fossa fractures.

Vault fractures are generally due to direct trauma. Base fractures can occur both due to direct and indirect trauma. Ring fracture of base of skull around foramen magnum is an **indirect transmitted fracture** due to fall of

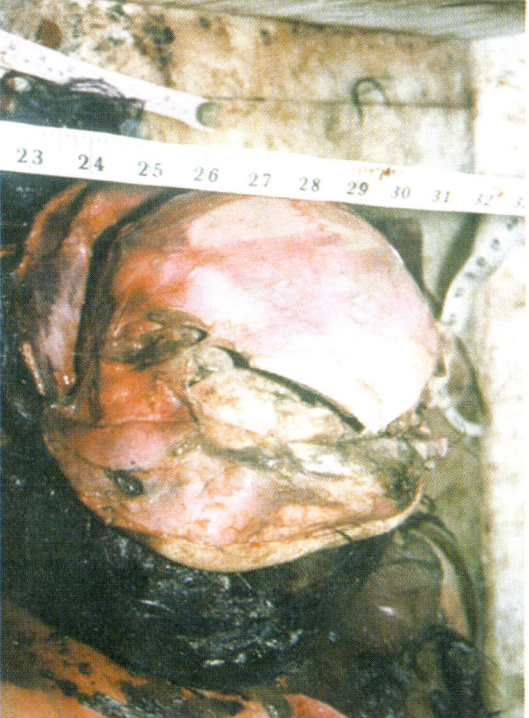

Fig. 5.69: Firearm entry with associated fracture

individual on buttocks. Contrecoup fractures occur due to shearing and rotational strains transmitted from the site of impact on the outside of the skull. For example, if the impact is on the frontal bone, it is transmitted inside and along the bone to the posterior part of the skull. The resultant trauma can be on the posterior part of the skull. Sometimes it is transmitted to the anterior part of the skull and the trauma may then be found on the anterior part of the skull.

Diastatic fractures are fractures separating the sutures. Sometimes, fractures pass through suture lines causing their separation.

Healing of Fracture of Skull

Healing of fracture of skull differs from other fractures. There is no visible callus formation. Because of injury to periosteal blood vessels, external callus development is delayed. Tissue fractures stick together in a week. The edges are slightly eroded. Undersurface of the skull shows pitting or deposition of lime salts in two weeks. Bands of bone tissue run across the fissure in 3–5 weeks. When there is a loss of bone, with a lot of gap, the gap is filled with fibrous tissue and may remain like that for a considerable time.

Intracranial haemorrhage

Intracranial haemorrhages can be:

- Extradural haemorrhage
- Subdural haemorrhage
- Subarachnoid haemorrhage
- Intracerebral haemorrhage
- Intraventricular haemorrhage
- Pontine haemorrhage
- Internal capsule haemorrhage.

By far the commonest haemorrhage due to trauma is the **extradural haemorrhage.** The dura mater is firmly attached to the skull. Emissary veins connect extracranial veins with the sinuses formed by the dura mater. When there is an impact of trauma, the dura mater is stripped from the bone. The vessels injured bleed and lead to the collection of blood between the dura and the cranium. Middle meningeal artery injury due to blow on the outer convexity of the head causes extradural haematoma. Extradural haematoma is seen more in adults than in children. The typical extradural haematoma as a result of trauma to the anterior branch of middle meningeal artery is a sharply defined clot, oval or circular, 10–20 cm in diameter, about 3 cm thick. It is adherent to the dura mater. It is seen in the temporoparietal area. It presses the motor cortex of cerebrum. Patients with extradural haematoma become unconscious as soon as the injury occurs. Later, the consciousness is regained before becoming unconscious again. The conscious state of lucid interval can be of a few hours to a few days duration depending on the pressure on the brain. Sometimes only the inner table of the skull may show fissure fracture causing difficulty in radiological diagnosis. **Extradural haematoma** is scrapped and weighed at autopsy.

Subdural Haemorrhage

Subdural haemorrhage occurs between dura mater and arachnoid mater. While the dura is thick, the arachnoid is a thin vascular meshwork. It is firmly in contact with inner surface of dura. The bridging cerebral veins cross the subdural space, to reach the sinuses. The dura and arachnoid are connected by venous sinuses and arachnoid granulations. *Subdural haemorrhage is more common in children and older people.* Subdural haemorrhages occur during quarrels, first fights or when somebody falls. It occurs when there is an impact on the head by a hard surface. Subdural haemorrhage occurs to rupture of:

- Bridging veins
- Dural venous sinuses
- Laceration of brain
- Laceration of dura and middle meningeal artery
- Rupture of inferior cerebral veins
- Injury to cortical veins.

There are three types of subdural haematoma

Acute: It is associated with laceration of the cerebrum. They are seen on the frontal and temporal poles. Bilateral subdural haemotoma is more common. The blood forms a thin layer of few millimetres to 2–3 cm.

Subacute: There may not be a brain damage in this type. The blood is thin.

Chronic: It is seen on parietal lobe in midline, bilateral or unilateral, occur as a widespread surface filling seen usually after 6 weeks of trauma.

Ageing subdural haematoma

- Fresh—fluid blood.
- Red cells seen—up to 48 hours.
- Brown blood—after 5 days.
- Fragile membrane—10–12 days; the membrane consists of fibroblasts and delicates membrane tissue. Encapsulated subdural haematoma is (cystic hygroma) converted into a cyst in a month or so.

Subarachnoid Haemorrhage

The pia mater is very thin; the subarachnoid space is between the arachnoid and pia mater. It follows the gyri and sulci. It is filled with cerebrospinal fluid. This is the

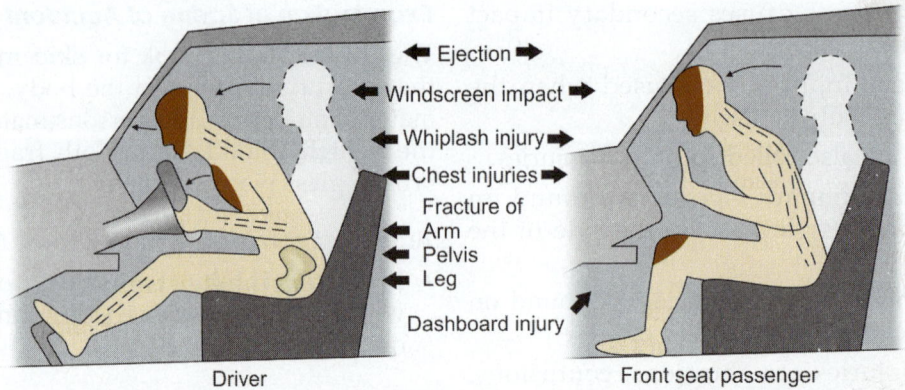

Fig. 5.73: Vehicular accident injuries to driver and side occupant

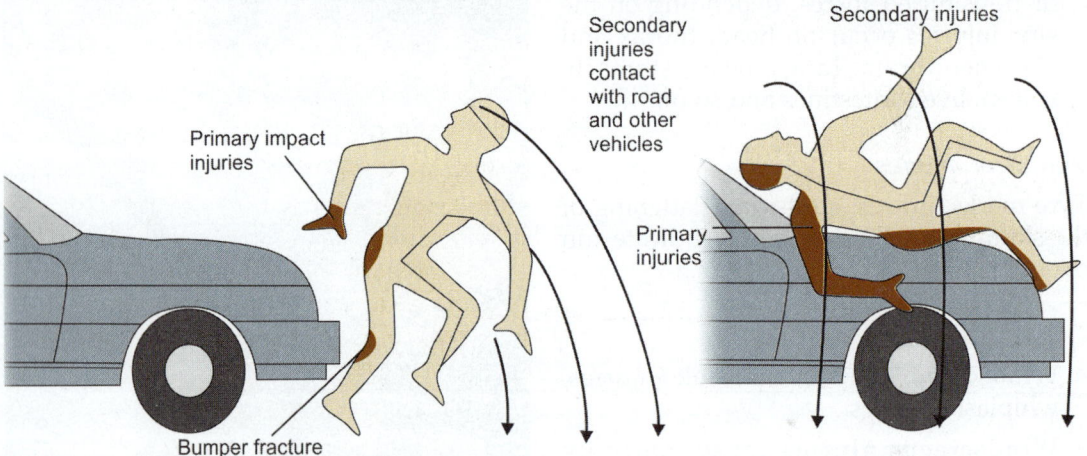

Fig. 5.74: Mechanism of occurrence of pedestrian injury

- The aircraft passengers sit with lap type safety belts. The injuries seen are:
  - **Hyperflexion injuries:** Facial injuries, fracture of thoracic spine, fracture of the base of skull, fracture of the lower legs, intrathoracic injuries, rupture or detachment of heart, rupture of liver, spleen, kidneys and abdominal aorta.
  - Generally death is due to burns or carbon monoxide poisoning.

Autopsy in air crash injuries

- Identification of bodies based on dental data, seat positions (e.g. when possible), tissue DNA typing, clothes and ID facilities like ID cards, passports, etc.
- Pre-travel biometric profiling is of immense help.

ROAD TRAFFIC ACCIDENTS

- Pedestrians
- Occupants
- Drivers

Pedestrian Injuries

- Primary impact
- Secondary impact
- Secondary injuries

Primary Impact Injuries

- They are the injuries found on the body part which receives the first blow.
- These depend upon whether the person is moving or stationary, hit from the front, sides or back.
- The person is hit on the presenting part.
- He then falls, moves or thrown away.

- This process causes secondary impact injuries.
- Tertiary injuries are caused when the victim finally lands.
- They are also called secondary injuries.
- Primary impact injuries are found on the knees or legs or on the side of the body.
- Secondary impact injuries are found on the head, shoulders, legs, etc.
- The injuries are abrasions, contusions, lacerations, fractures.
- Internal organs are injured due to impact or transmitted forces, depending on the site, injuries occur on head, thorax and abdomen, brain, lungs, heart, stomach, spleen, liver, intestines and so on.

Run Over Injuries

Tyre marks, grazes, avulsions, flattening of the skull, head, chest or pelvis indicate run over.

Occupant Injuries

- Windscreen injuries, seat belt injuries, whiplash injuries.
- **Windscreen injuries** cause injury by broken glass pieces. The front passengers may be thrown through the windscreen on the road.
- Whiplash injuries cause fracture dislocation of cervical spine, fracture dislocation of atlanto-occipital joint, V-shaped lacerations on head, multiple punctate lacerations on the face, basal fracture of petrous temporal bone and sella turcica.
- The driver sustains steering wheel impact.
- Transverse sternum fracture, heart rupture, aorta split, crush injury of liver, spleen or kidneys, lungs contused or lacerated, crushing of the throat. If right side impact is on the occupants injuries to right side are common, e.g. right arm and leg fractures, laceration of liver and right kidney. If impact is on left side, injuries are more on left side.

Examination of Scene of Accident

The doctor should look for skid marks of the tyres, tyre marks on the body, vehicle material on person and persons material on the vehicle, blood, hair, cloth fragments, broken glass pieces, paint, etc.

Autopsy Examination in Unknown Cases

- From the injury if possible to know whether the deceased is pedestrian, driver or occupant.

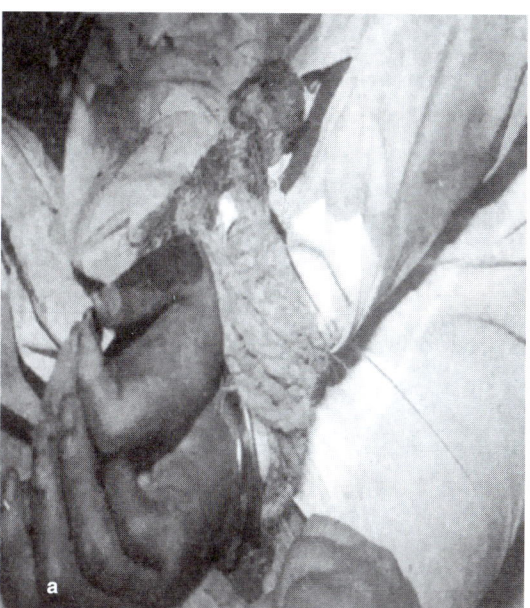

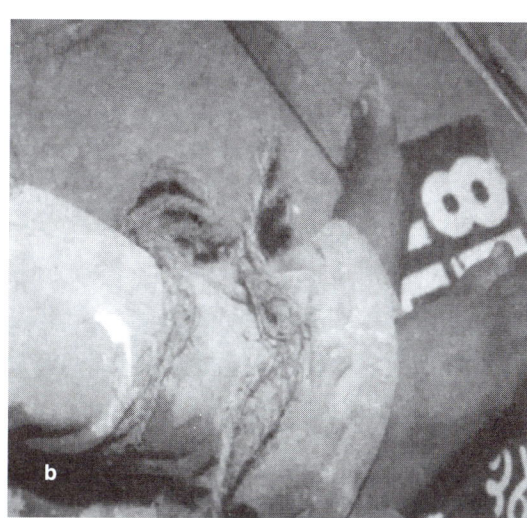

Fig. 5.75: Dead body found with tied hands (a) and tied feet (b) suggests homicide

- **To know nature of accident:** Hit and go, hit and run, etc.
- **Testing for alcohol and drugs** of the driver by subjecting blood samples for examination.
- **Postmortem run over:** The person might have been unconscious or dead and been run over by a vehicle.
- Postmortem nature of the injuries and postmortem burning marks suggest cause of death other than accident.

Homicide (Homo—Man: Cide—to Kill)

- Homicide: Killing of a human being by another human being.
- Infanticide: Means killing of an infant below one year.
- Patricide: Killing of father.
- Matricide: Killing of mother.
- Fratricide: Killing of brother/sister.

Homicide

Lawful   *Unlawful*

- Excusable   Culpable homicide   Culpable homicide
- Justifiable   Not amounting to murder   Amounting to murder

Excusable Homicide

It refers to death occurring due to an act done in good faith and for the good of the person by another person, without any intension to cause death, e.g. when a doctor performs an operation on a person in good faith for benefit of a person, the death occurring from operation is excusable homicide.

Justifiable Homicide

- It is the death happening in process of administration of justice, e.g. execution of death sentence passed by a judge, death occurring during judicial firing.
- Excusable and justifiable homicide are not punished in law.
- In culpable homicide not amounting to murder, the unlawful killing of a human being due to grave and sudden provocation.

- In this situation, there is no intention, deliberation, malice or a will to kill. There is no malice aforethought.

Murder

- It is homicide, willful, intentional, deliberate and accompanied by malice aforethought.
- Law does not differentiate between murder of an infant or child or adult.

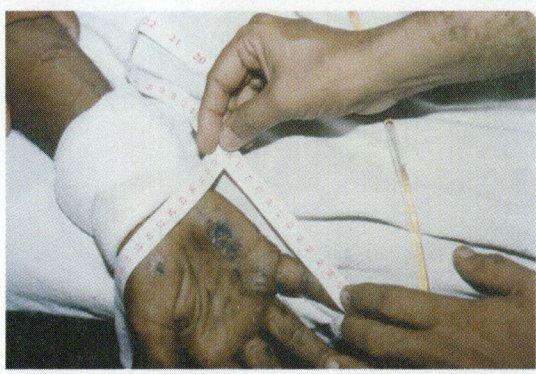

Fig. 5.76: Electrical entry wounds

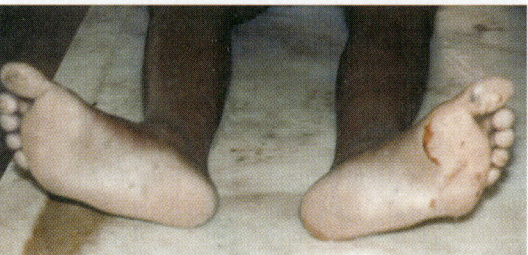

Fig. 5.77: Electrical injury sole

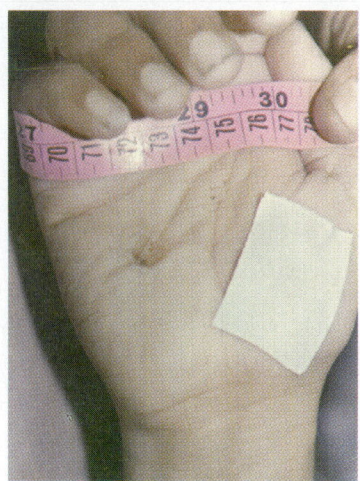

Fig. 5.78: Electrical entry wound

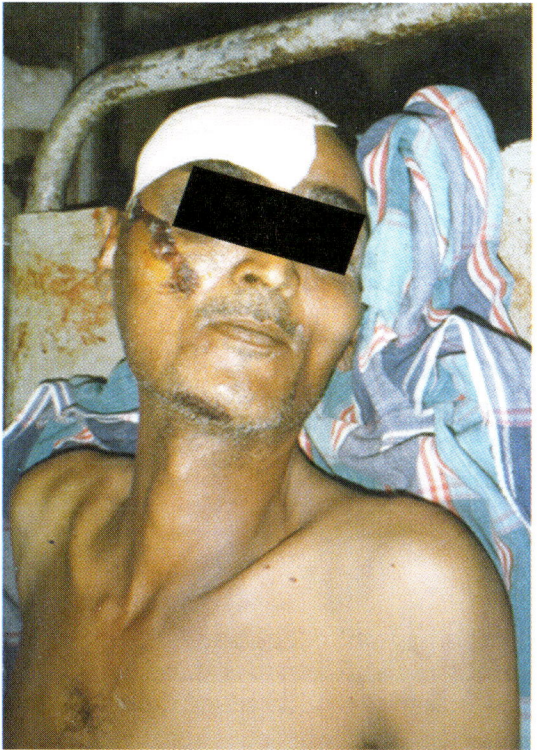

Fig. 5.79: Black eye and stitched wound—fall from electric pole

Suicide

- It is sometimes called **self homicide,** i.e. homicide of self upon self.
- An accidental death is one which occurs without intention and due to unforeseen reasons which are beyond the control of persons carrying out the Act.
- In accident there can be self death, death of other person or deaths of self and also other person.

Right of personal/self defense (RPD)

- When a girl is attacked by a man with the motive of sexual violence and when she understands that she is likely to be attacked, then in self defense if she attacks her attacker, to thwart sexual victimisation and associated injuries or even death, in this process if the attacker even dies it does not matter.
- It comes under the right of personal defence.
- In the same way, when any human being is attacked and he attacks the offender in self defence, the right of personal defence comes as a defence for him.

Section 299	Section 300
A person commits culpable homicide if the Act by which the death is caused is done:	Subject to certain exceptions culpable homicide is murder if the Act by which the death is caused is done:
INTENTION	
(a) With the intention of causing death; or	(1) With the intention of causing death; or
(b) With the intention of causing such bodily injury as is likely to cause death: or	(2) With the intention of causing such bodily injury as the offender knows to be likely to cause the death of the person to whom the harm is caused; or
	(3) With the intention of causing bodily injury to any person and the bodily injury intended to be inflicted is sufficient in the ordinary course of nature to cause death; or
KNOWLEDGE	
(c) With the knowledge that the Act is likely to cause death	(4) With the knowledge that the Act is so imminently dangerous that it must in all probability cause death or such bodily injury as is likely to cause death, and without any excuse for in curring the risk of causing death or such injury as is mentioned above

- The Indian Penal Code (Section 96) clearly stets that nothing is an offence which is done in the exercise of the right of private (personal) defence.

The other "CIDES" are

• Killing of insects	Insecticides
• Killing of adult insects	Adulticide, imagocide
• Killing of insect larvae	Larvicide
• Killing of insect eggs	Ovicide
• Killing of pests	Pesticide
• Killing of ants	Formicide, formicicide
• Killing of aphids	Aphidicide, aphicide
• Killing of bedbugs	Cimicide
• Killing of bees	Apicide
• Killing of fleas	Pulicide, pulicicide
• Killing of flies	Muscacide, muscicide
• Killing of gnats or mosquitoes	Culicicide
• Killing of lice	Lousicide, pediculicide
• Killing of mites	Acaricide, miticide
• Killing of mosquitoes	Mosquitocide
• Killing of spiders or scorpions	Arachnicide
• Killing of wasps	Vespacide

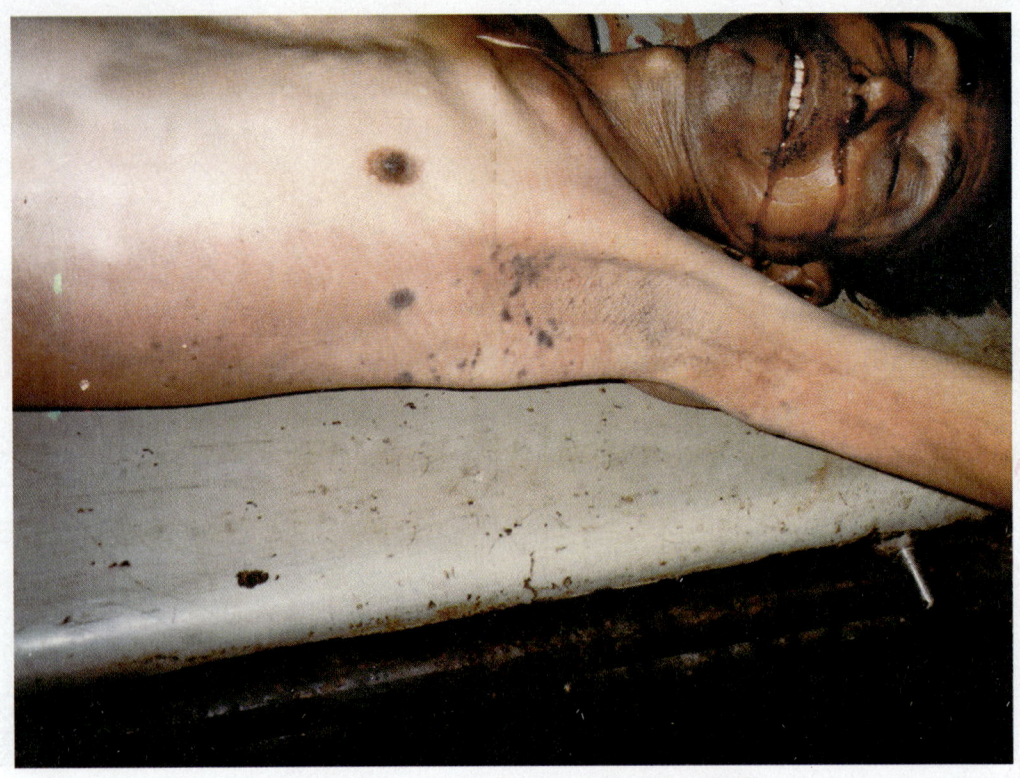

Obscure wound—multiple contusions in armpit

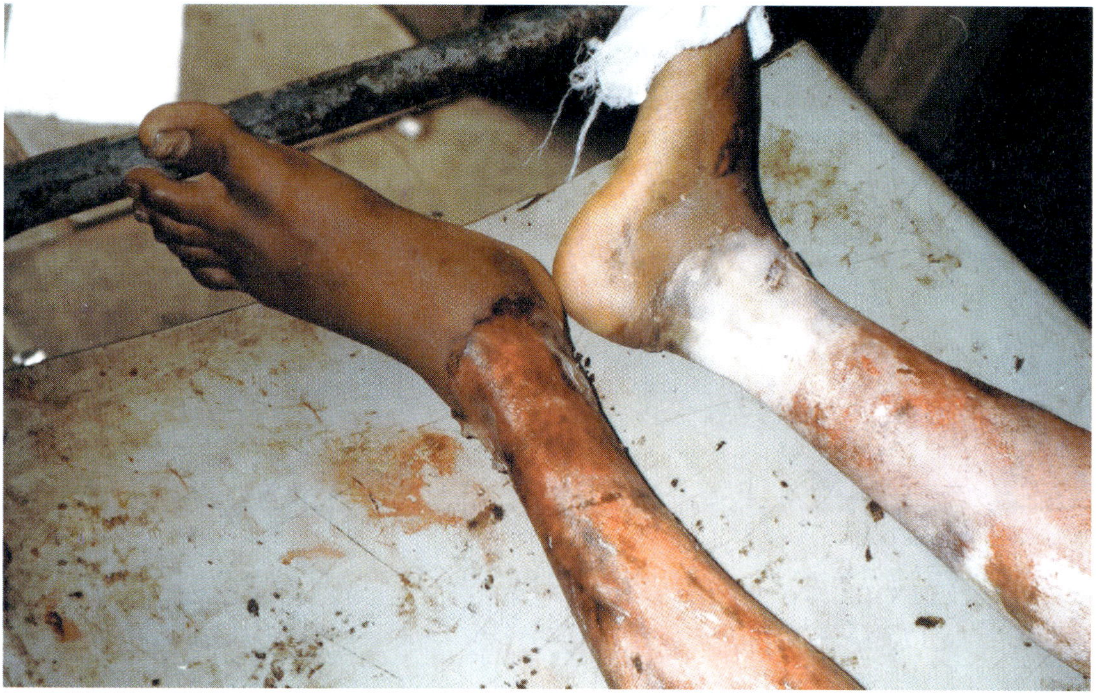

Lacerated wound with blunt force

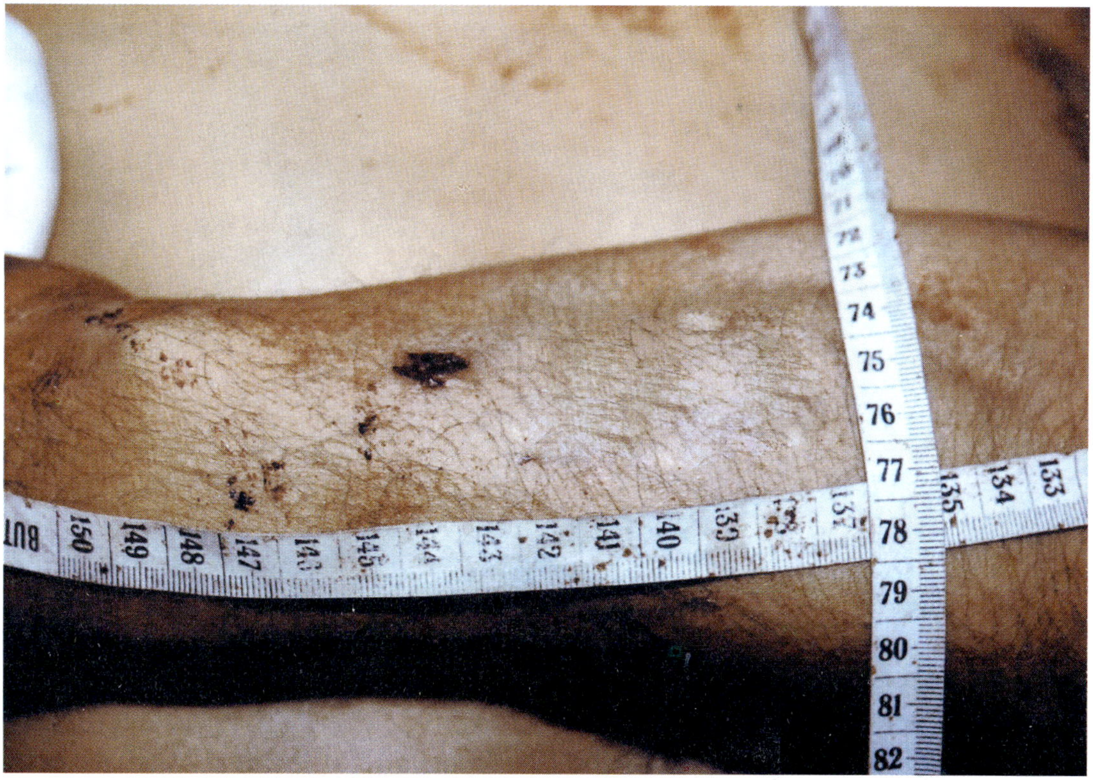

Abraded contused wound

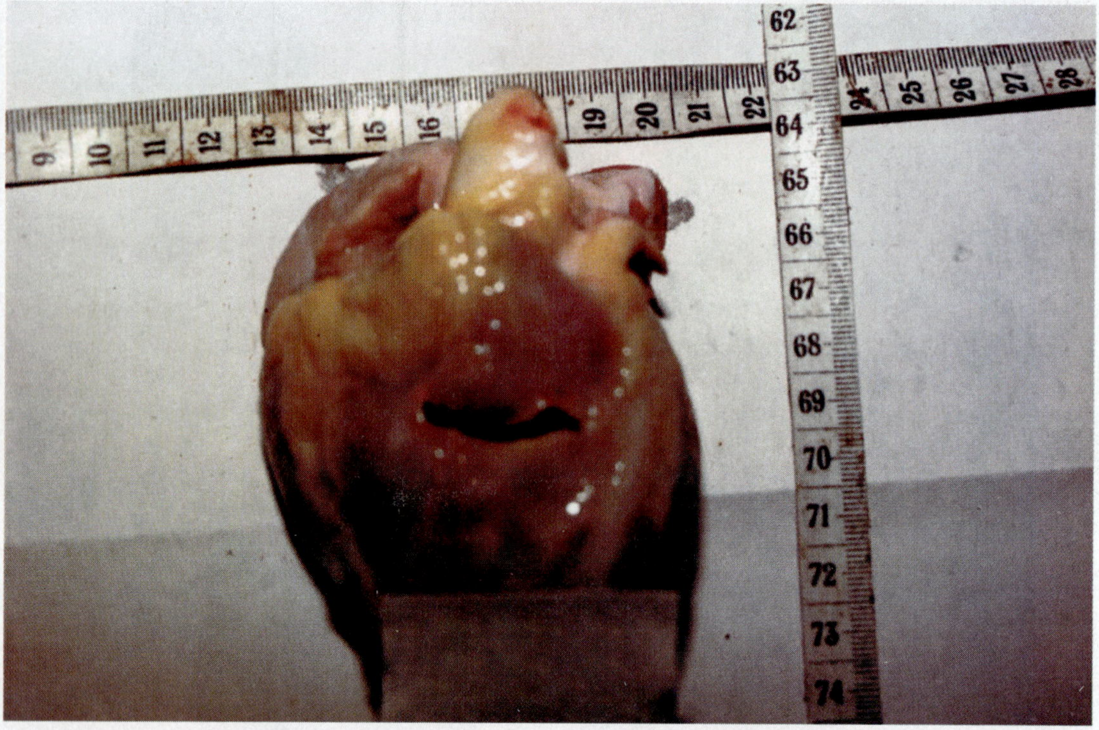

Stab injury heart with double-edged weapon

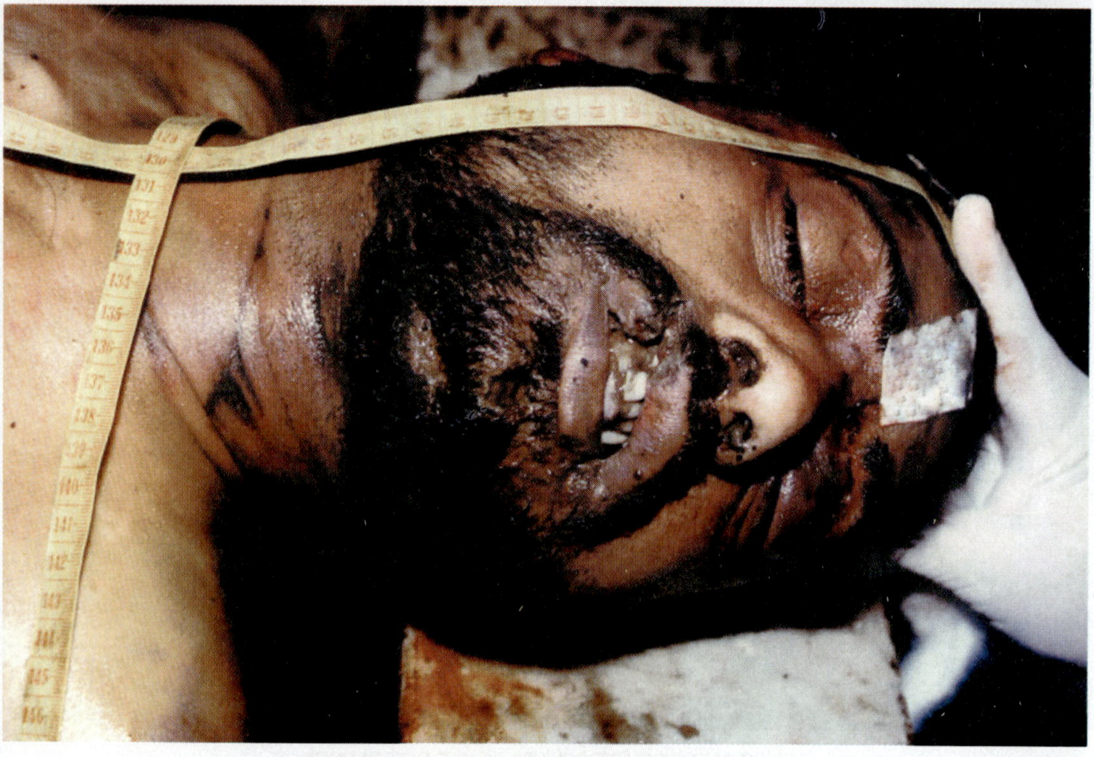

Note the injury to lips, eye and neck by blunt force

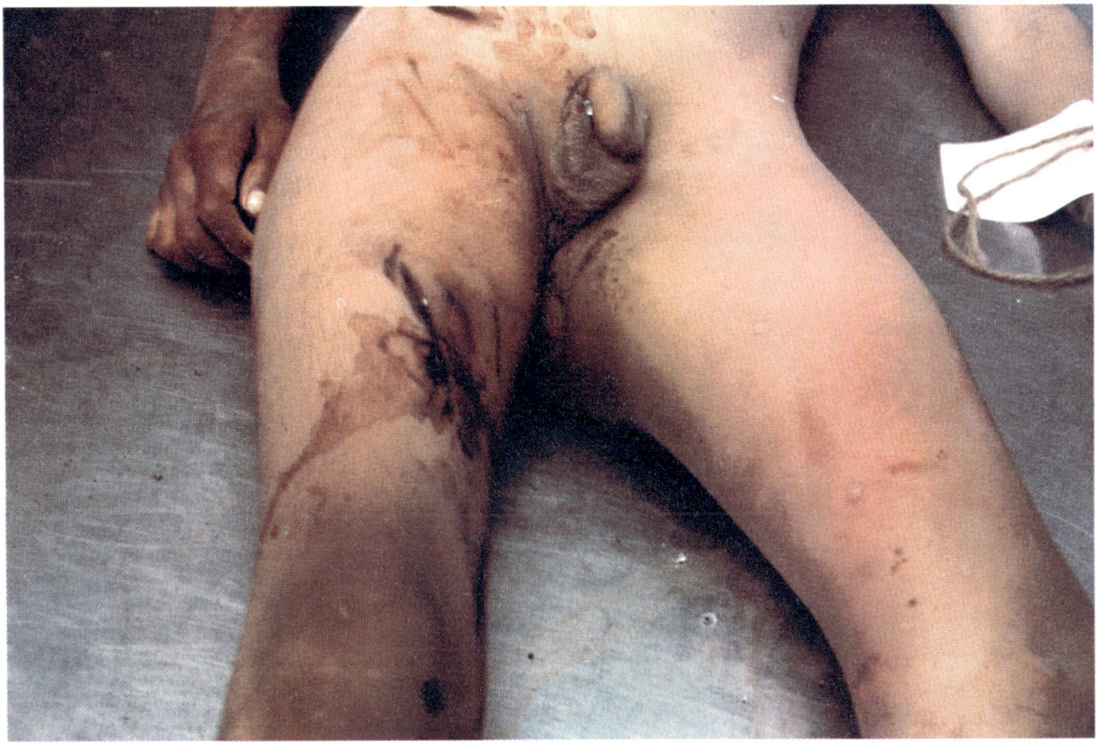

Scratch in road traffic accident

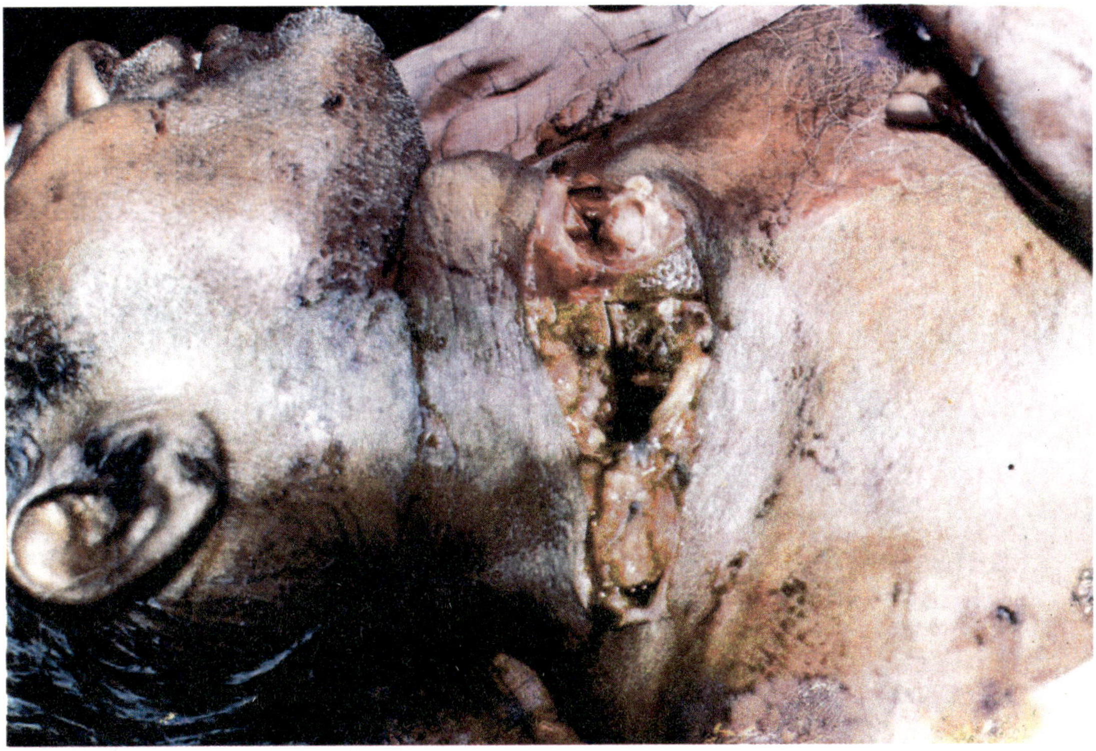

Heavy cutting force injury—lower part of neck

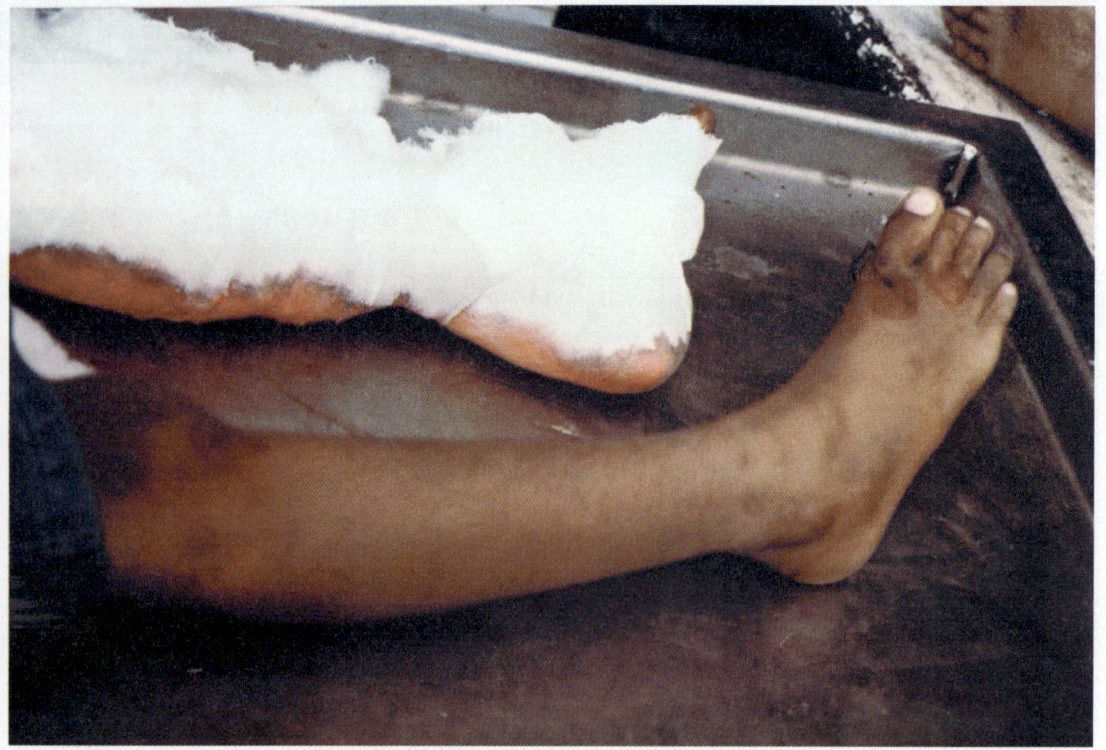

Superficial multiple suicidal cuts

Plastered fractured leg including foot

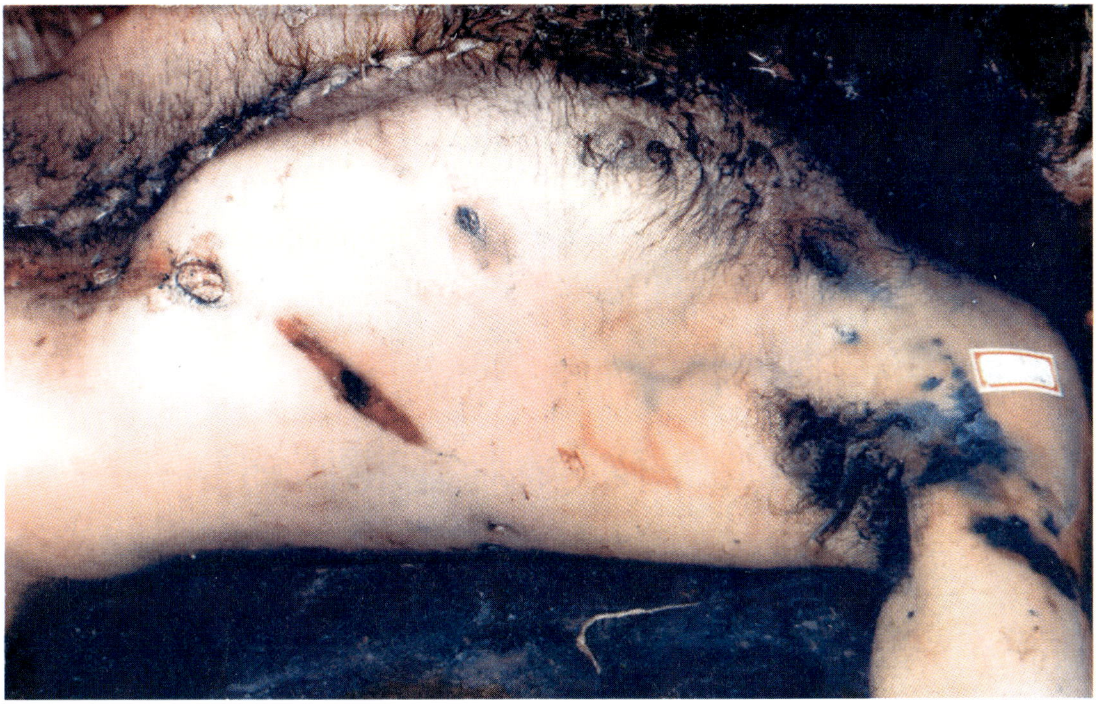

Firearm injury wound entry

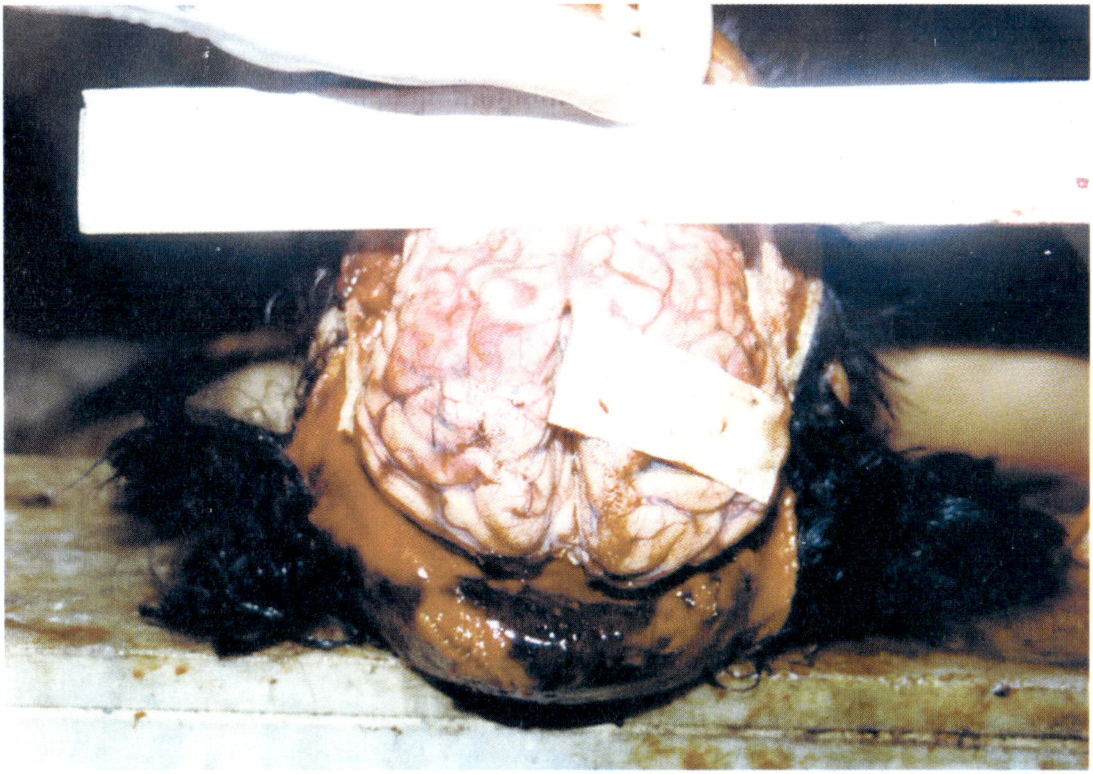

Cerebral oedema

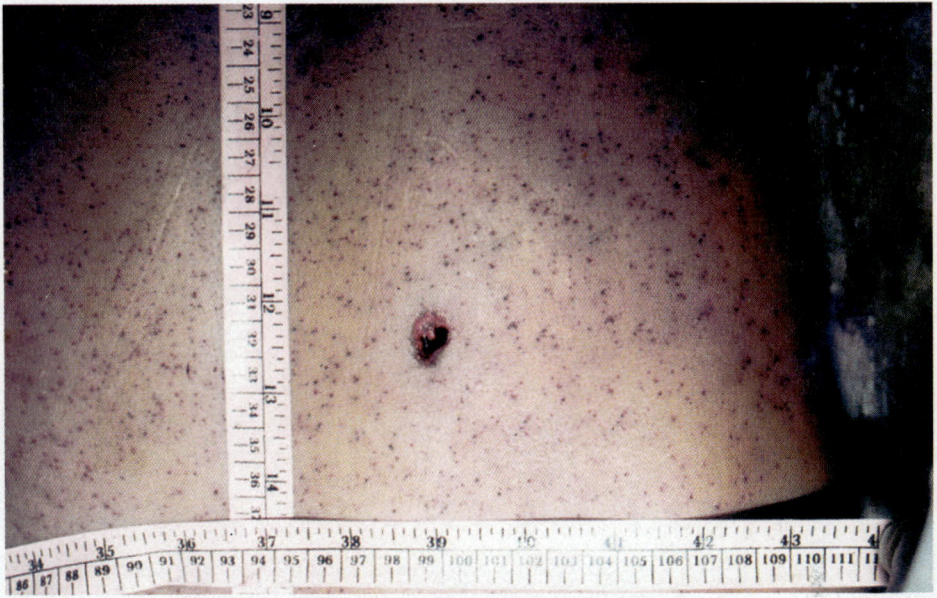

Firearm entry wound, *note* abraded contused collar

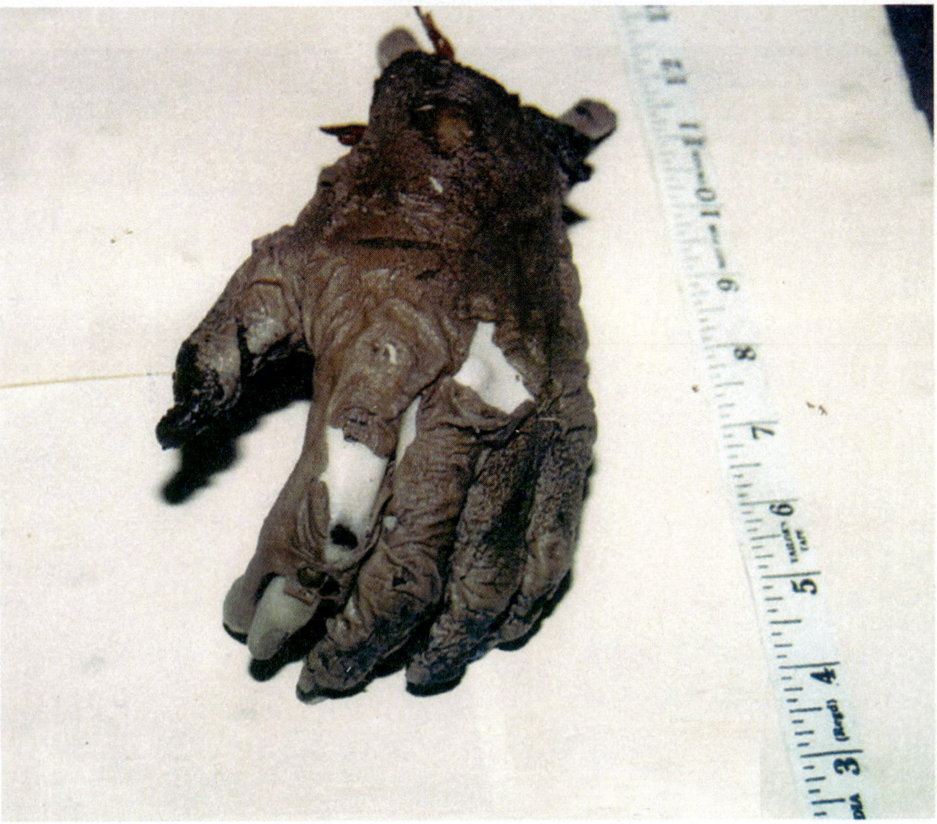

Irregular amputated decomposed hand

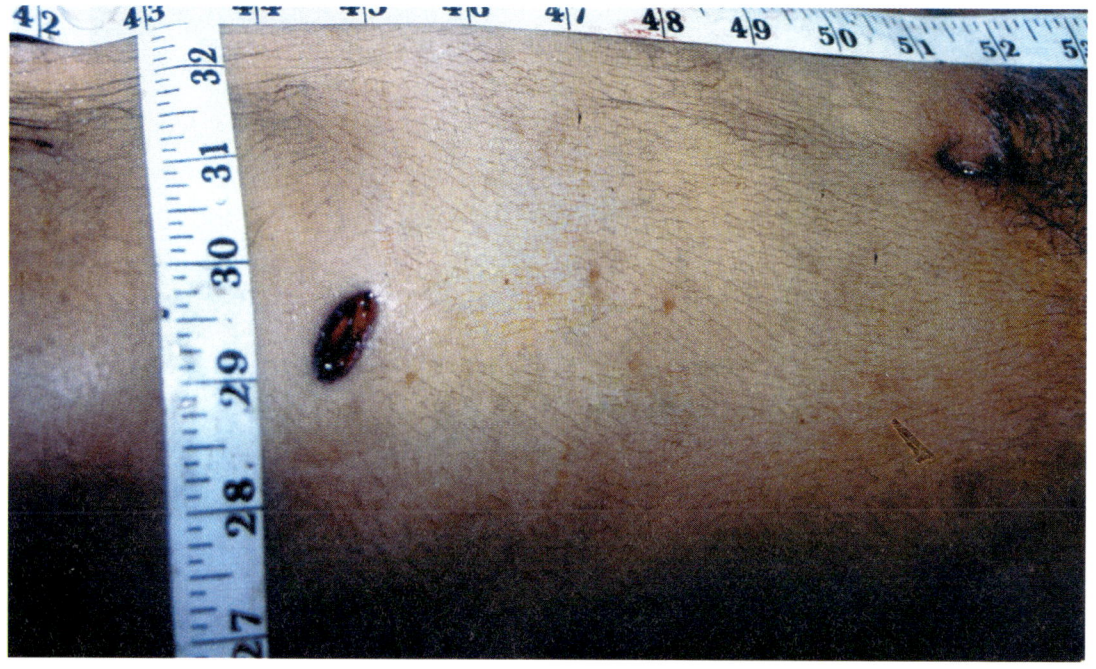

Stab injury with double-edged weapon, *note* hilt mark

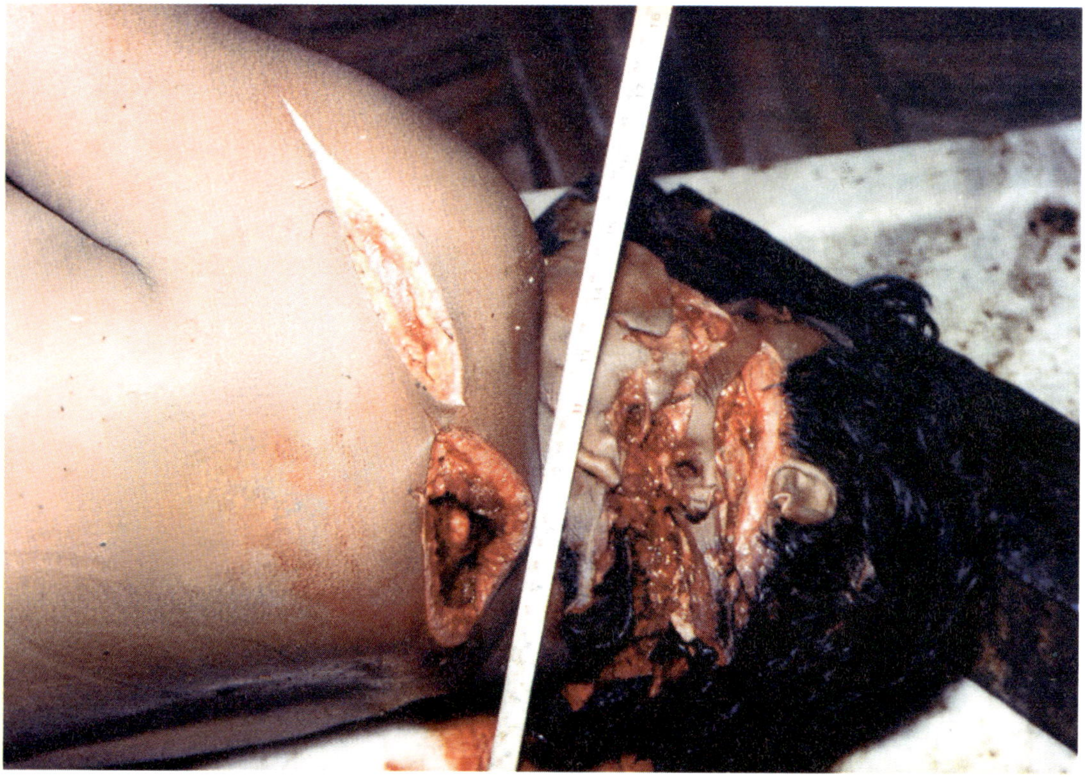

Postmortem incised wound stab injury

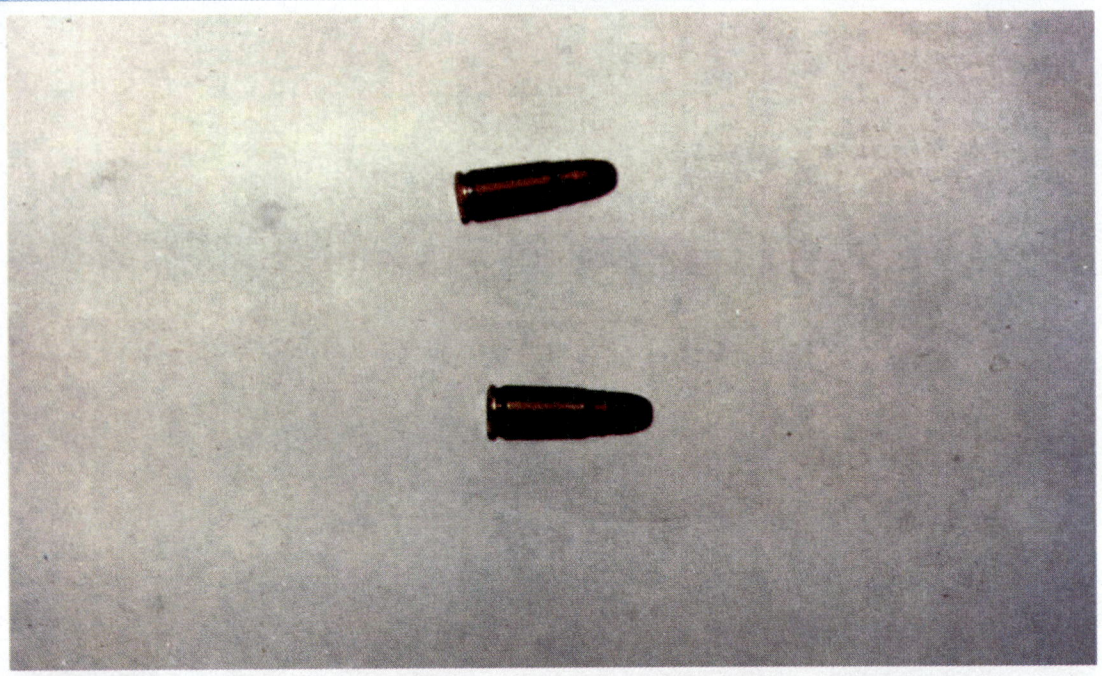

Two bullets recovered from scene of crime

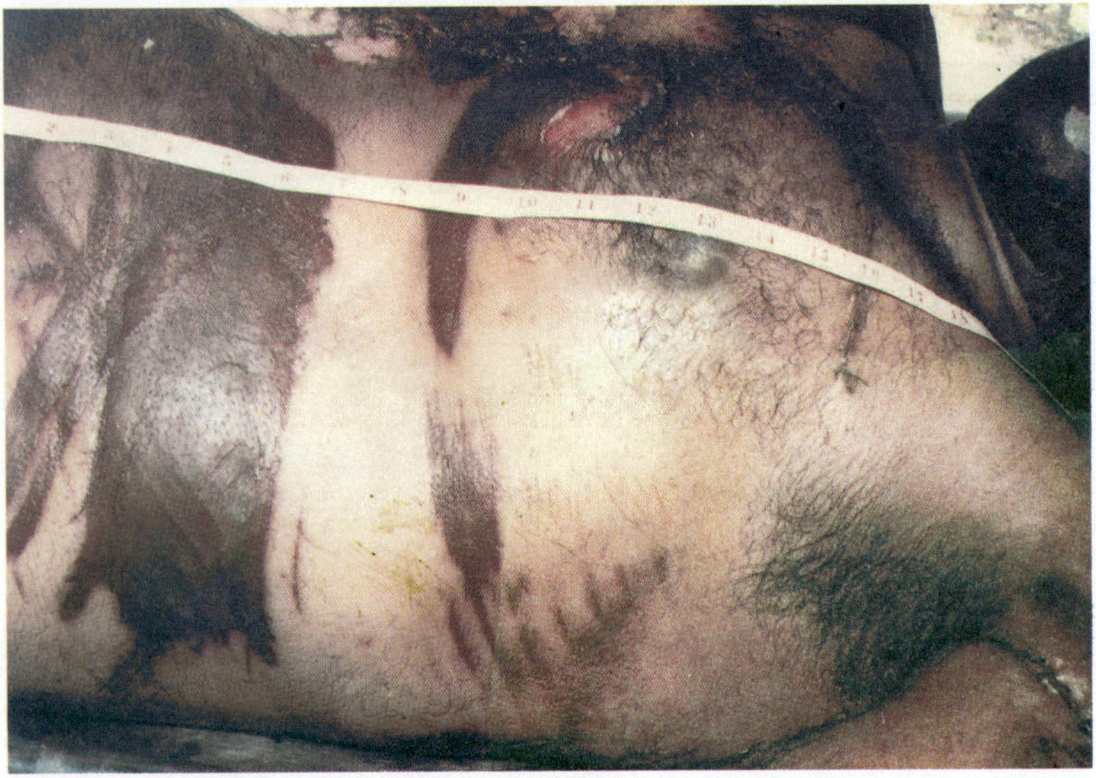

Tyre tread marks

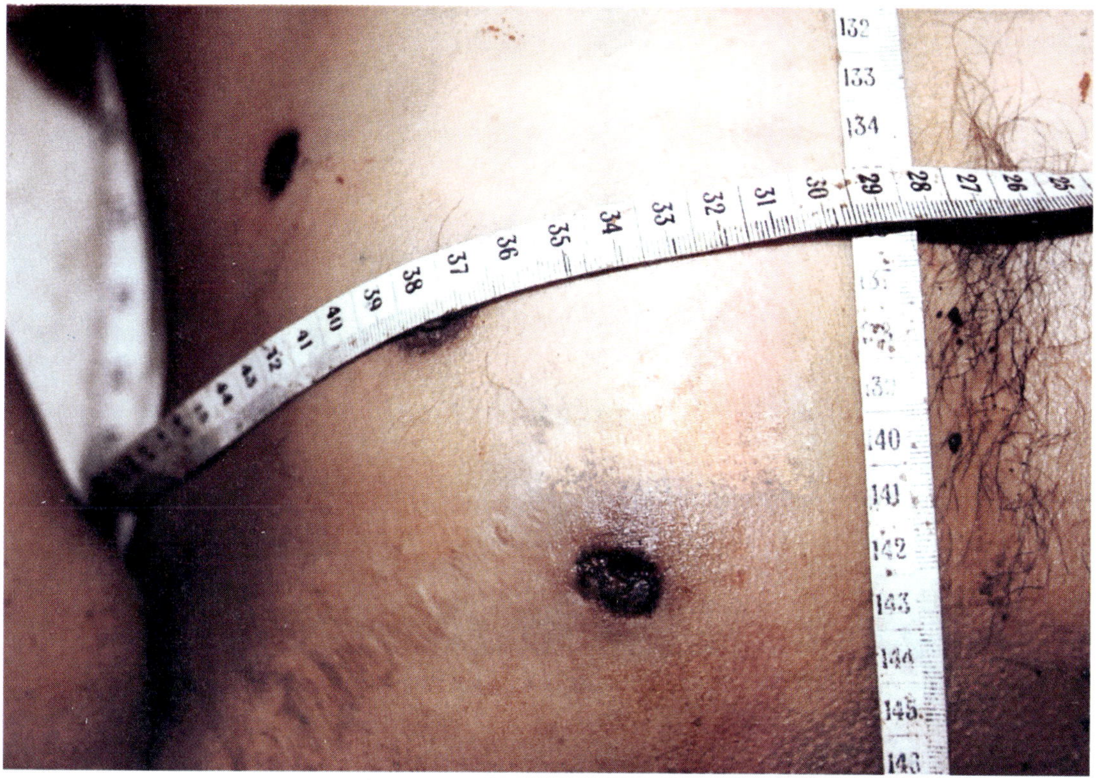

Firearm entry and exit wounds

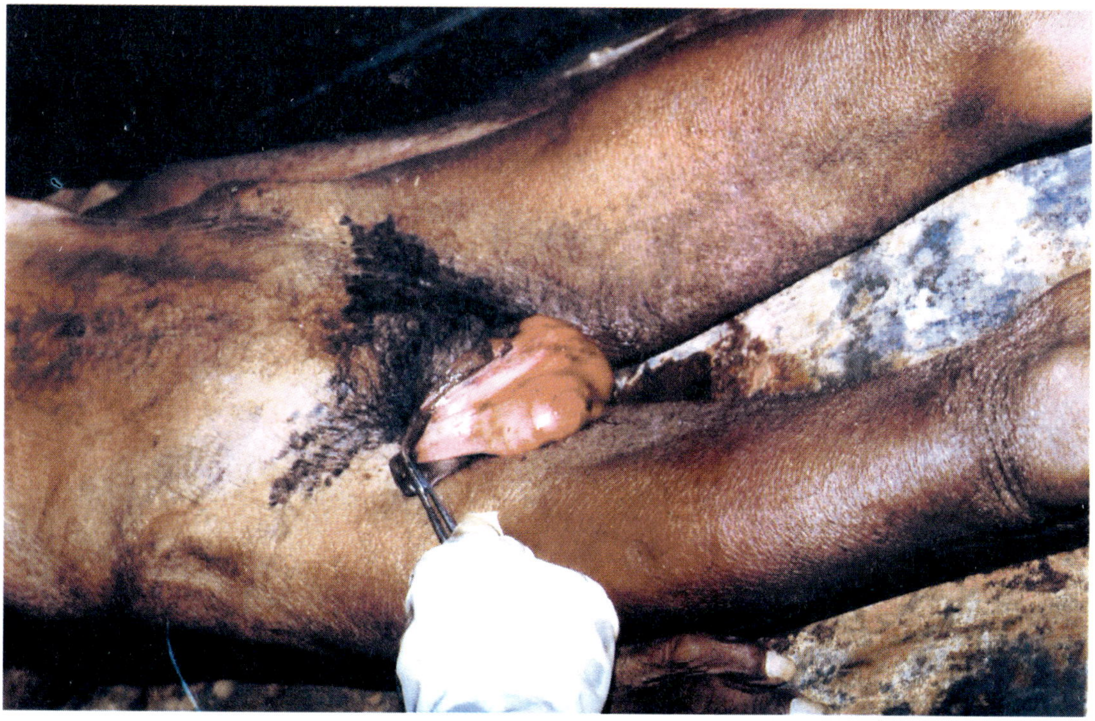

Avulsion of scrotum–testis exposed: Road accident

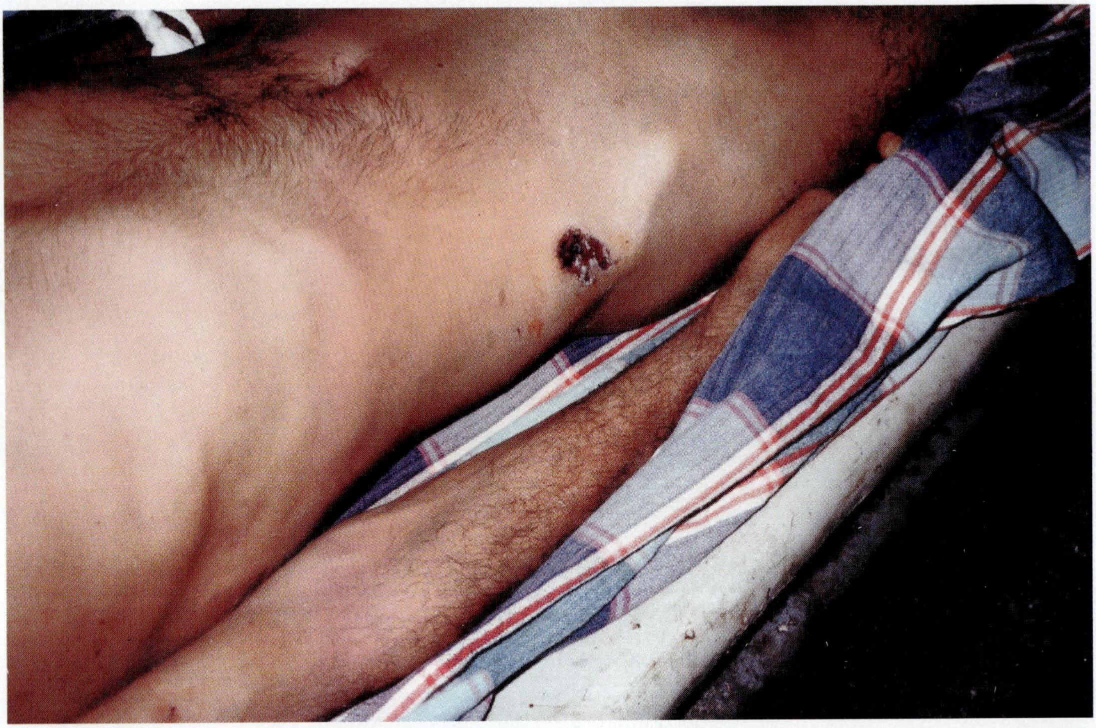

Firearm entry wound showing abrasion collar

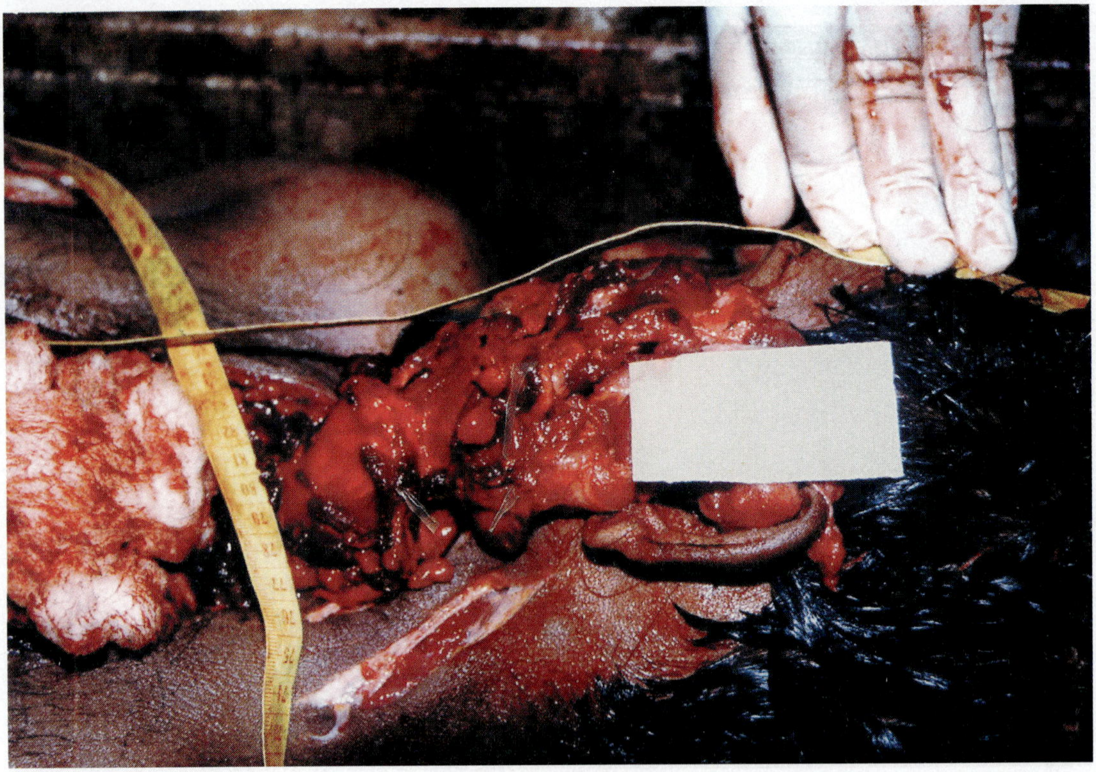

Multiple contusions

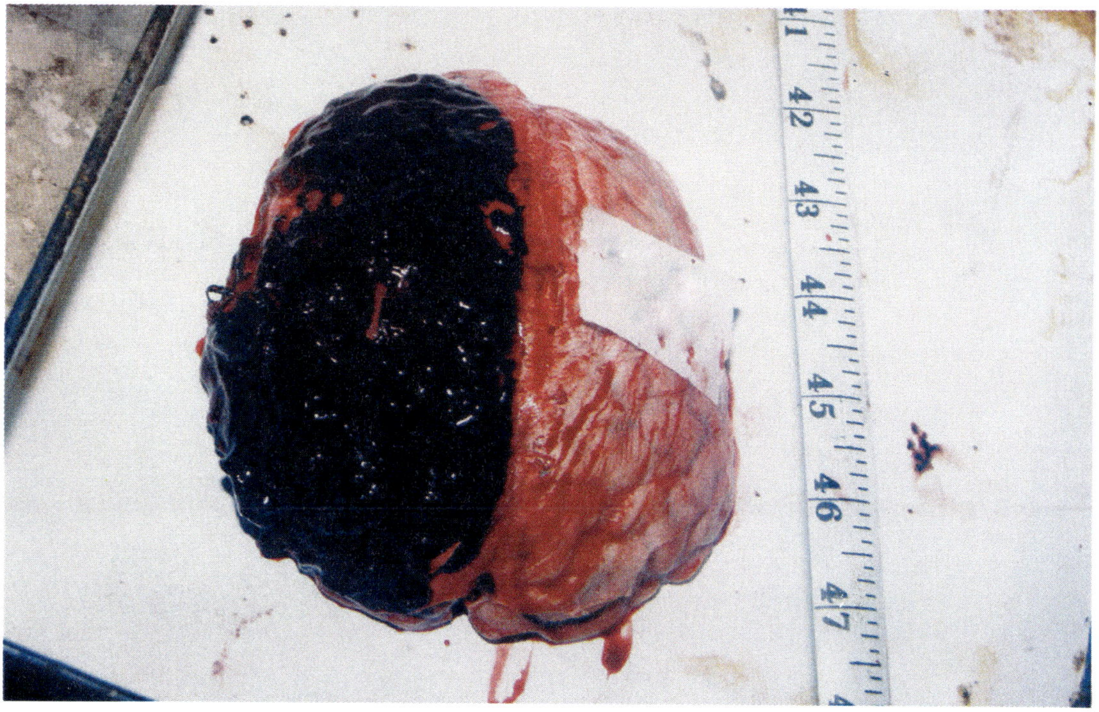

Haematoma of scalp

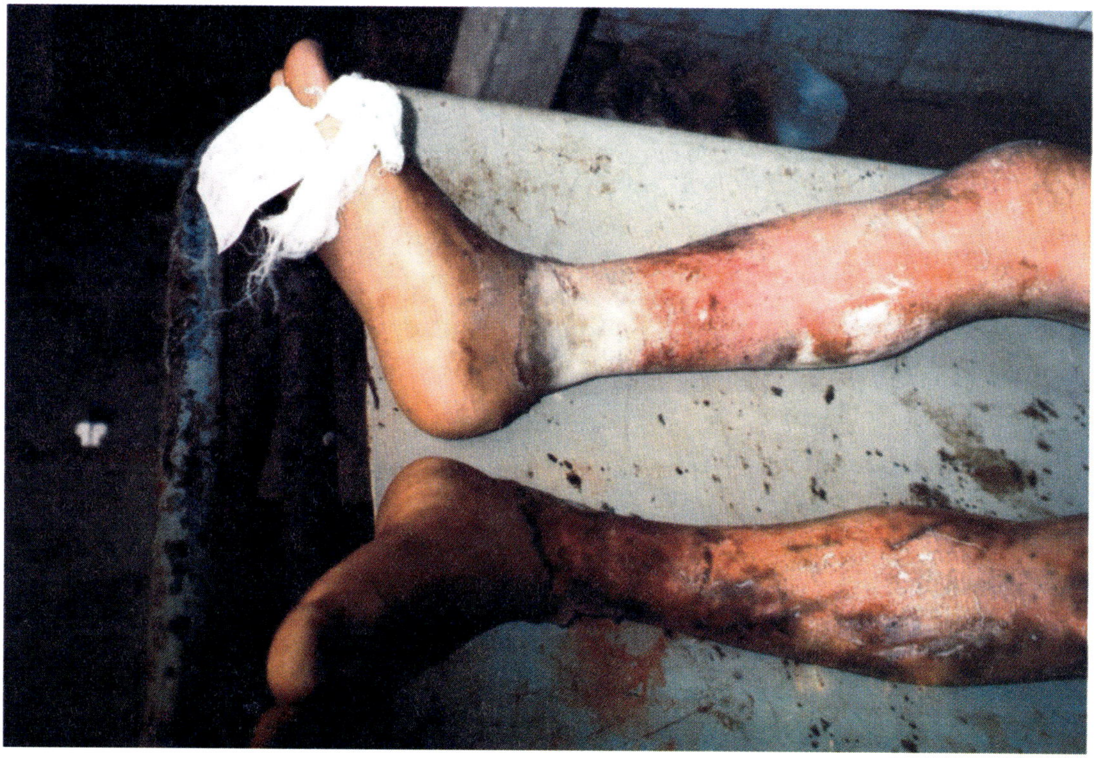

Note the left leg and foot contused and abraded injury

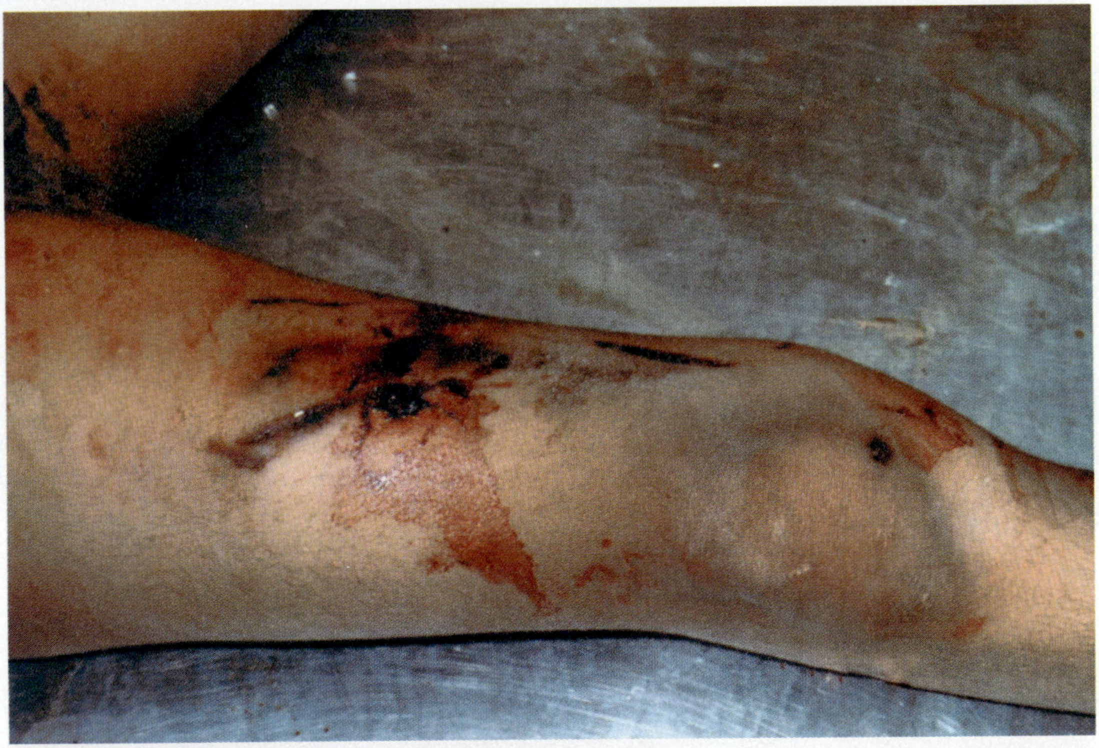

Abraded contused wound

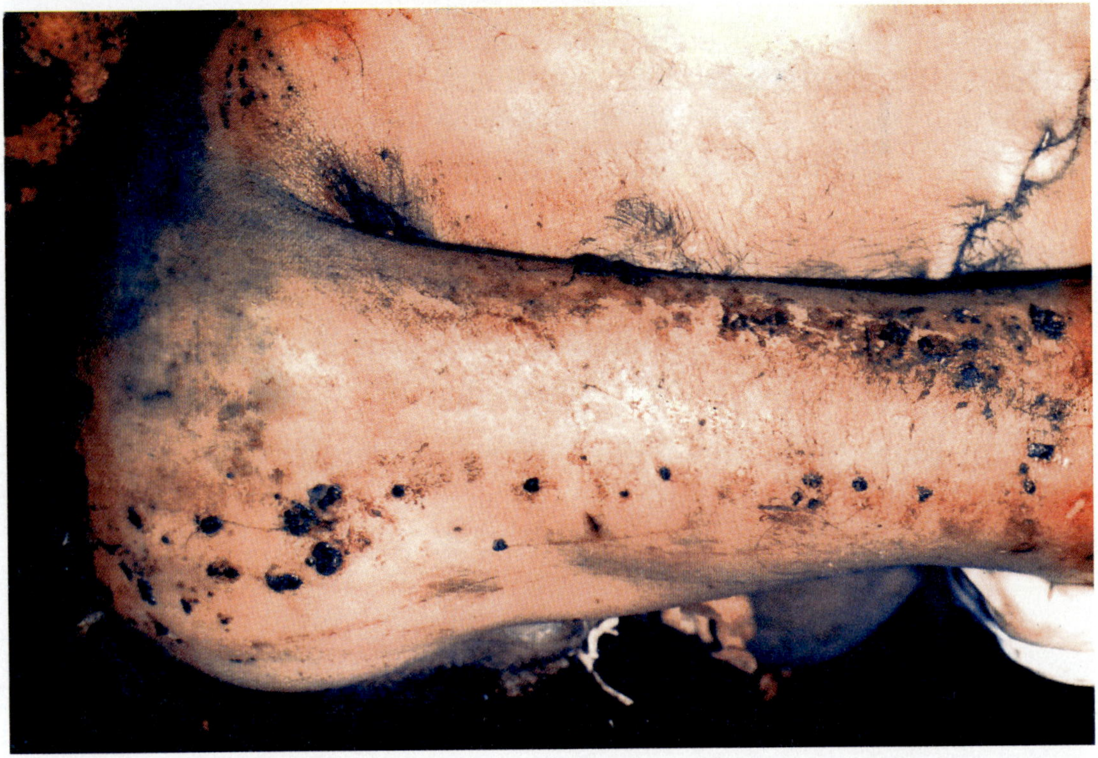

Firearm injury wound of entry. *Note* multiple scattered pallet marks

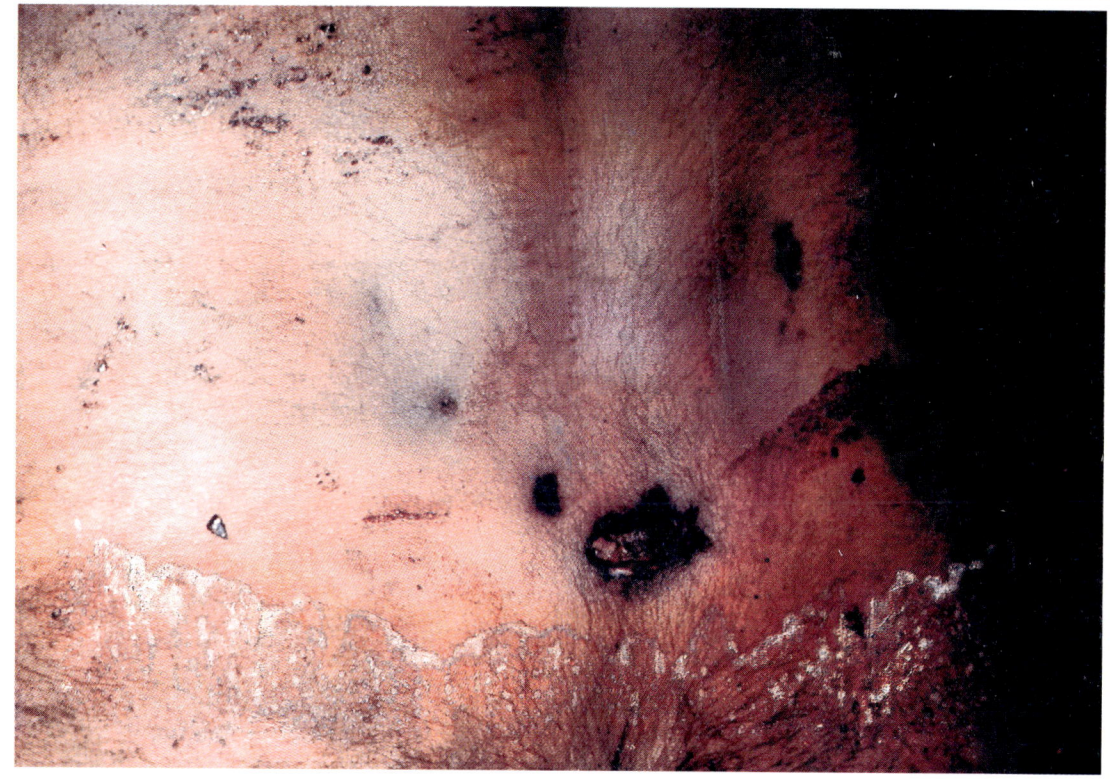

Firearm injury wound of entry

CHAPTER 6

Anoxia due to Mechanical Violence

INTRODUCTION

Anoxia begets anoxia—CK Drinker

- Violent mechanical deaths due to anoxia are very commonly seen in medicolegal practice.
- They are being known as asphyxial deaths. Asphyxia means lack of oxygen and excess of carbon dioxide.
- This does not occur in deaths due to mechanical violence.
- In these cases, death is brought about by different ways of privation of oxygen to the brain.

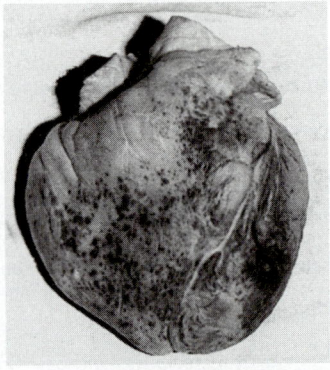

Fig. 6.1: Multiple petechial haemorrhages over surface of heart in asphyxial death

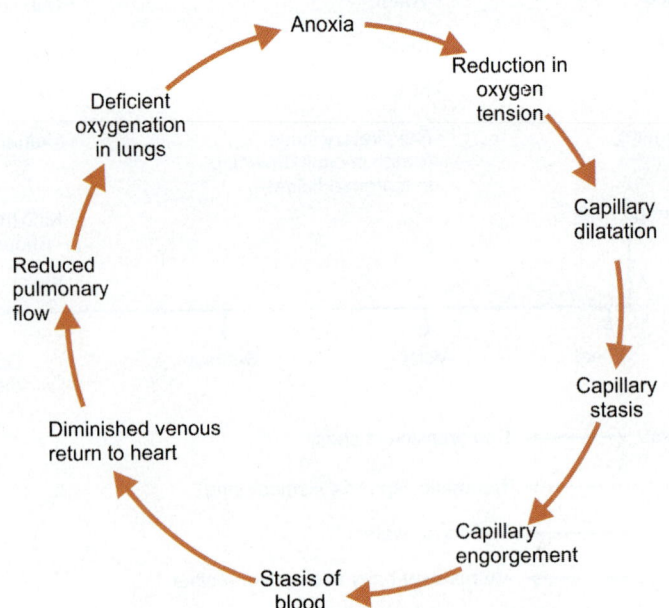

Fig. 6.2: Vicious cycle of anoxia, i.e. anoxia begets anoxia

Common Causes

- Obstruction of air passage from outside, e.g. hanging, strangulation, throttling, etc.
- Occlusion of air passages from inside as in case of choking with solid object or in drowning or in spasm of larynx.
- Closing of external respiratory orifices, i.e. nostrils (and mouth) as in smothering.
- Compression of chest as in traumatic asphyxia.

General Features of Anoxia Deaths due to Mechanical Violence

- Cyanosis
- Capillary dilatation
- Capillary stasis

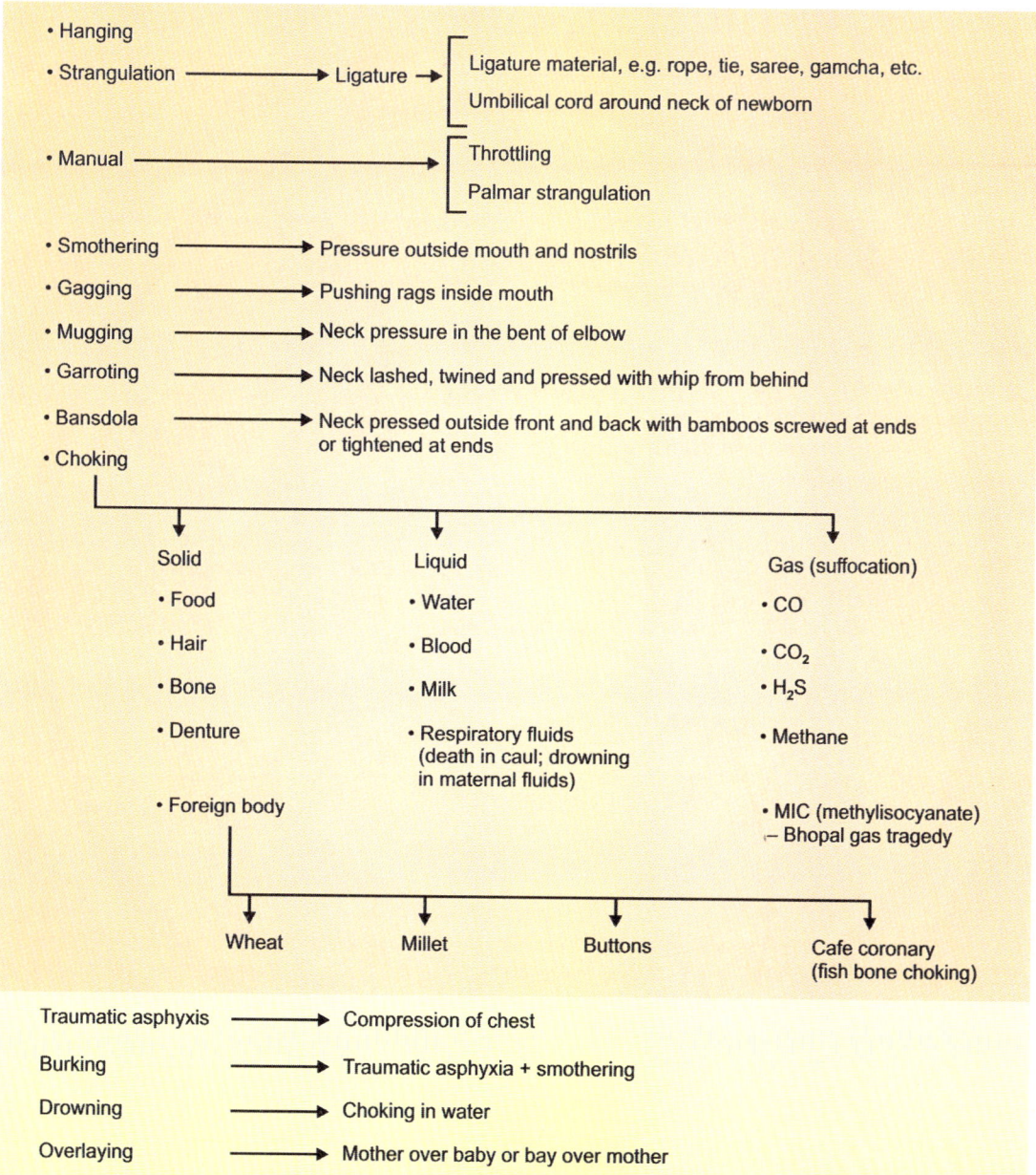

Fig. 6.3: Anoxic deaths due to mechanical violence

- Increase in capillary pressure.
- Increased capillary permeability.
- Petechial haemorrhages (Tardieu's spots)
- Fibrinolysis (fluidity of blood)
- Relaxation of sphincters.

Autopsy Findings (Postmortem Features)

External

Blue face, prominent eyeballs due to congestion; subconjunctival petechial haemorrhages (Tardieu spots), prominent neck veins, dilated pupil, protruded and often bitten tongue, cyanosis of lips and fingernails.

- Turgid penis; semen at the tip.
- Purple postmortem staining.

Internal

- Blood is fluid and purple due to decreased oxygen tension and increased reduced haemoglobin.
- Lungs are congested, distended and sometimes emphysematous.
- Associated pulmonary oedema present.
- Subpleural petechial haemorrhages seen.
- On cutting the lungs, frothy, bloodstained fluid comes out.
- The mucosa of the respiratory passage is congested.

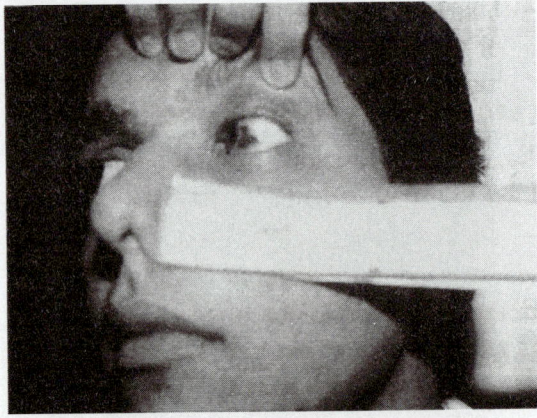

Fig. 6.5: Subconjunctival petechial haemorrhage

- Abdominal organs show congestion.
- Congestion of brain with scattered petechial haemorrhages seen.

These general features are common to all the following types of violent anoxic (asphyxial) deaths.

Exceptions and additional features are described in individual cases.

HANGING

- Hanging is a type of violent, mechanical, anoxic (asphyxial) death brought about by constriction of neck due to suspension.

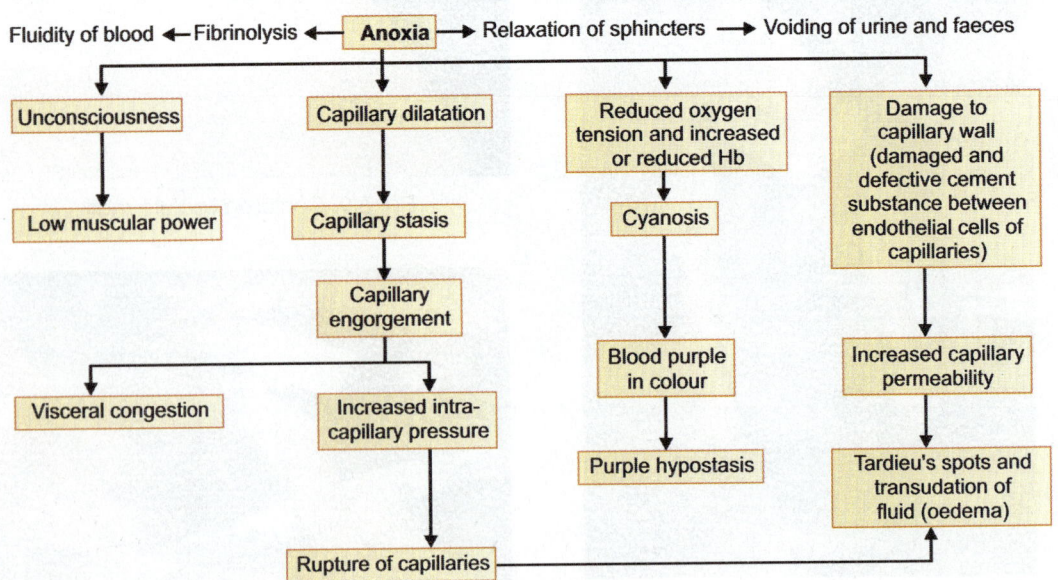

Fig. 6.4: Pathology of anoxia

• The suspending force is generally the weight of the body and sometimes only the head.

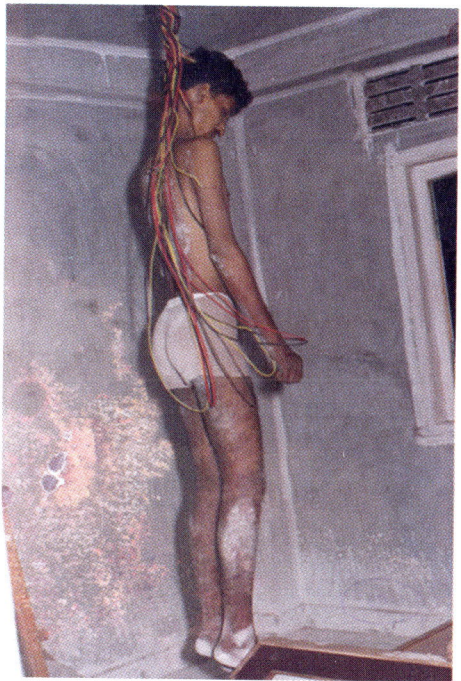

Fig. 6.6: Hanging using cable wires to show feet *in situ*

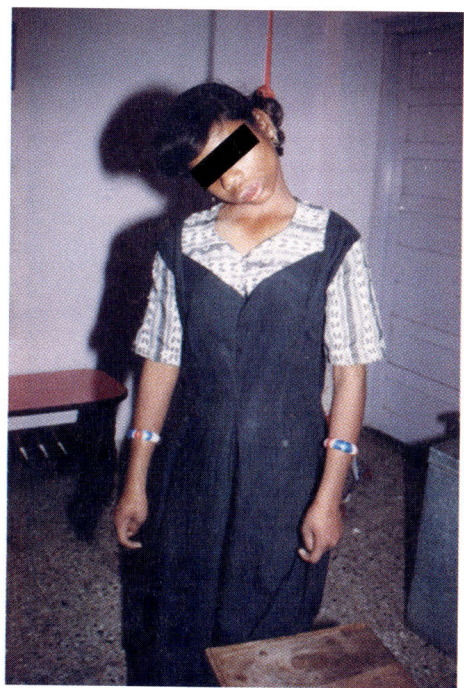

Fig. 6.7: Hanging using nylon rope

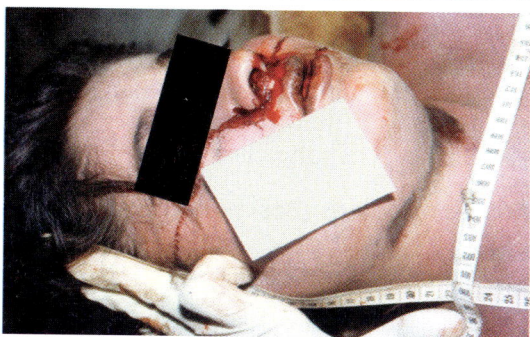

Fig. 6.8: Parchmentized ligature mark

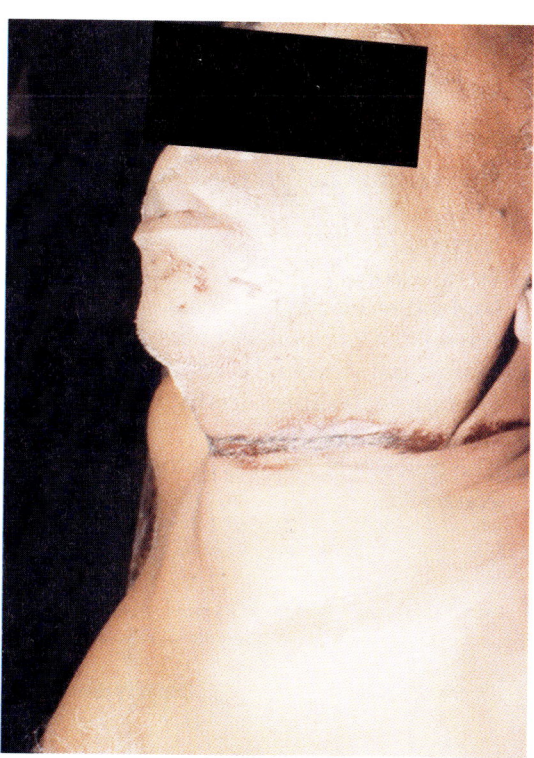

Fig. 6.9: Contused ligature mark

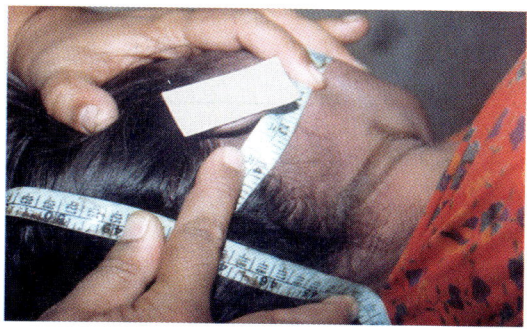

Fig. 6.10: Slipping noose marks

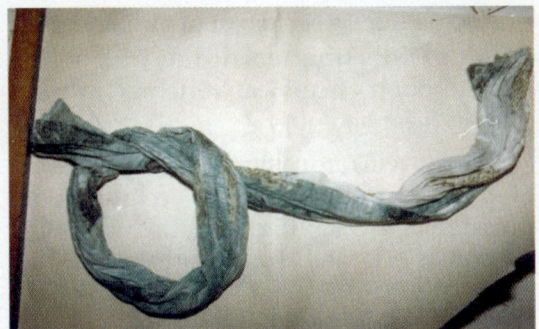

Fig. 6.11: Ligature

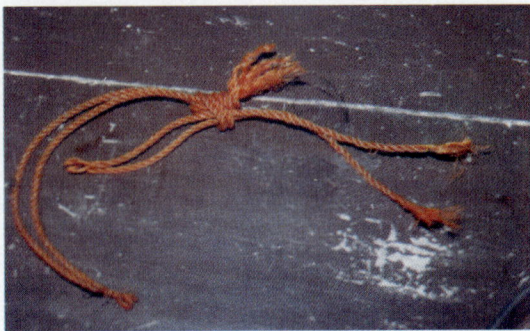

Fig. 6.12: Demonstrating how to preserve ligature

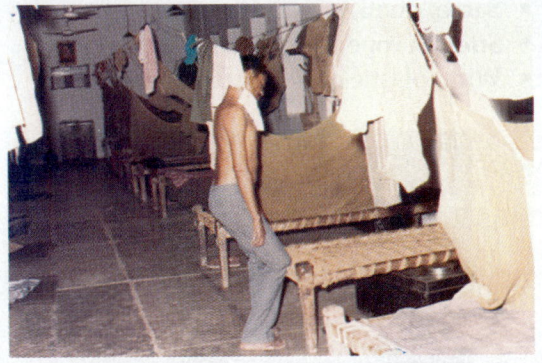

Fig. 6.13: Suicidal partial hanging

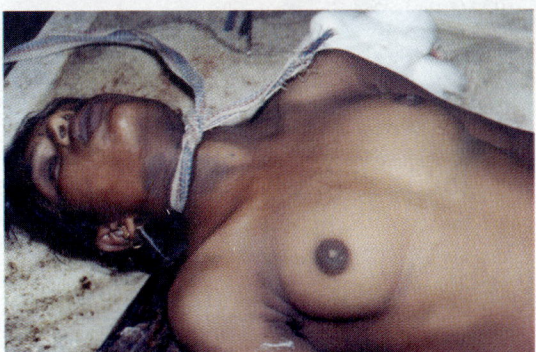

Fig. 6.14: Ligature *in situ*

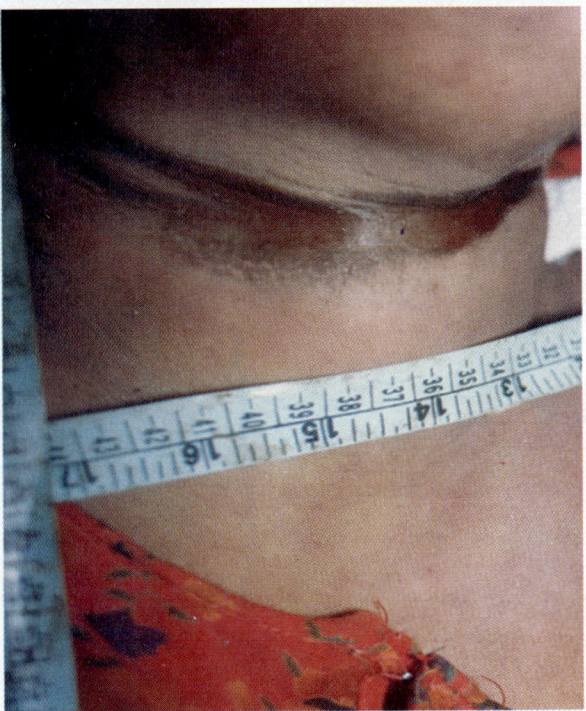

Fig. 6.15: Abraded parchmentized ligature mark

Typical Hanging

In a case of typical hanging, the pressure on the neck is caused by weight of the body, pulling on the ligature around the neck, it presses the tongue upwards and backwards against the posterior wall of pharynx causing occlusion of air passages.

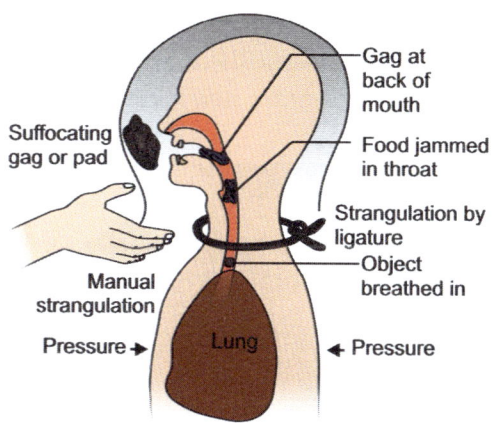

Fig. 6.16: Mechanism of violent mechanical anoxic deaths

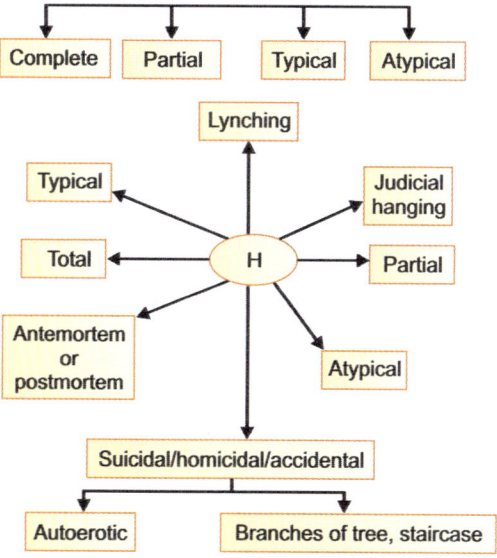

Fig. 6.17: Types of hanging

Causes of Death in Hanging Cases

- Cerebral anoxia due to pressure on carotid arteries and jugular veins.
- Reflex cardiac inhibition due to pressure on vagus (trigger area).
- Anoxia due to occlusion of air passage. Injury to spinal cord due to fracture dislocation of cervical vertebrae in cases of judicial hanging.

Jugular veins are compressed with pressure of 2 kg; carotid arteries are occluded with pressure of 4–5 kg; trachea is occluded with pressure of 15 kg and vertebral arteries by 30 kg.

Types of Ligature Material used

The common types of ligature material used are:

- Saree, dhoti, gamcha
- Smooth rope, twisted rope, coir rope.
- Wire, plastic cable, electric wires.

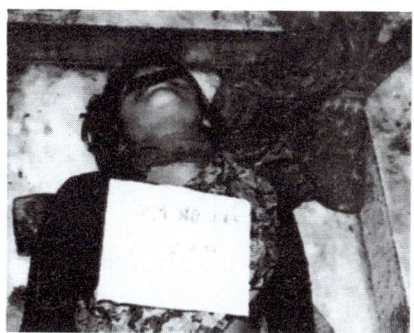

Fig. 6.18: Hanging with saree—ligature material *in situ*

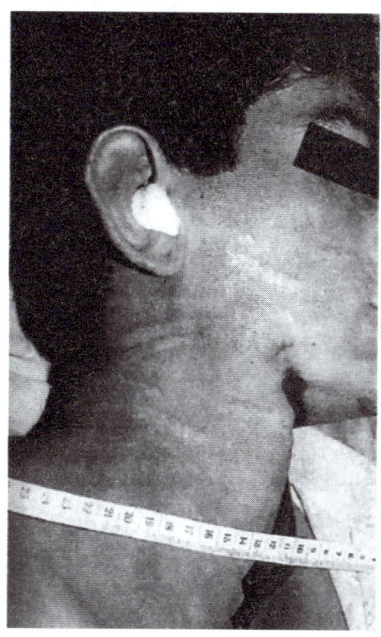

Fig. 6.19: Patterned (rope) ligature mark in hanging

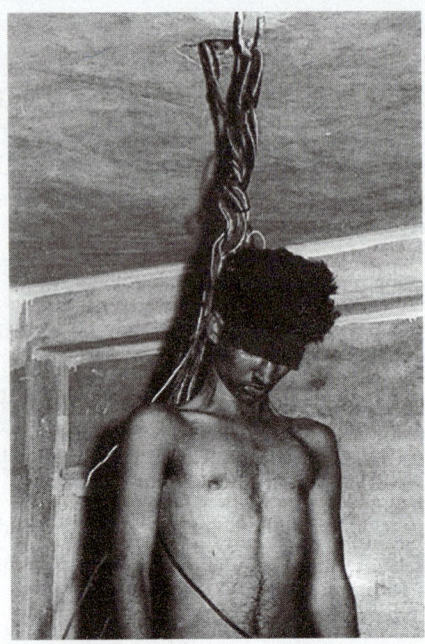

Fig. 6.20: Hanging—suspension with electrical wires

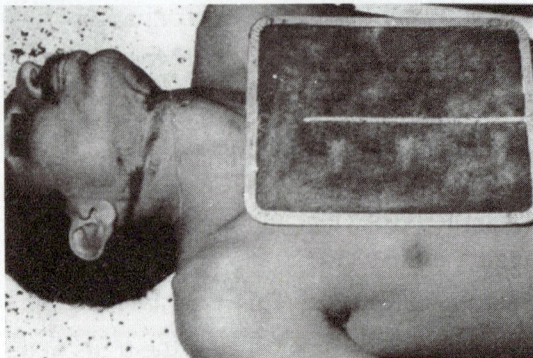

Fig. 6.21: Ligature mark

Features of Hanging
General Features
- The head is away from the knot. Face becomes pale.
- Drooling of saliva along the angles of mouth seen due to ligature mark pressing upon the salivary glands. This is considered as **surest sign of typical antemortem** hanging because salivation is a vital process.
- Hypostasis is seen in lower limbs below knees and in upper limbs below elbow.
- Emission of semen at the tip of penis or on the floor of scene or on the underwear.

Ligature Mark
- The ligature mark is oblique around the neck, above Adam's apple with dry parchmentised leathery base.
- The edges show abrasions or petechial haemorrhages.
- The ligature resembles the shape of material used.
- When many rounds of ligature are present skin between ligature marks is abraded and bruised.

- **Internally** beneath the ligature mark subcutaneous tissues of neck show extravasation of blood.
- Vertical fracture of thyroid cartilage is sometimes seen.
- The platysma and sternomastoid muscles show tears.
- Hyoid bone fracture is rare. When present, it is due to anteroposterior compression.
- The greater cornu shows outward divergence.
- The fragments of bone show outward angulation.
- Internal rupture carotid artery may be seen.
- Haemorrhage in the lymph node above and below the ligature is seen.
- Suicidal hanging is more common.
- Incomplete or partial hanging suggests suicide.
- Accidental hanging may occur in children during play.
- In adolescents, accidental hanging may occur as a sexual misadventure (in such cases pornographic literature may be seen by the side of victim).
- Hanging or suspension of a person after death is done sometimes to camouflage or divert the attention of investigating officers.
- Therefore, it is advisable that in all cases of hanging other causes of death should not be ruled out including poisoning.

- The author has seen a case of hanging of a Malaysian citizen of Indian origin on the outskirts of Tirupathi during 1971.
- At autopsy the viscera were preserved and sent for chemical analysis.
- The chemical analyser detected pethidine in that case.
- This case was one out of a number of murder carried out by a gang operating in Tamil Nadu.
- A special court conducted the trails of all these cases and the accused were awarded death sentence or life imprisonment.

Atypical Hanging

- In atypical hanging, the ligature knot may be seen on the front below the jaw, or on sides right or left.
- Accordingly at the site of the knot, the deficiency in the ligature mark is seen.

Partial Hanging

- It is a type of atypical hanging where feet of the person are found touching the ground and the individual is seen standing or sitting or kneeling with head bent.
- The bent head acts as the suspension force.
- Ordinarily, partial hanging suggests antemortem hanging and suicide.

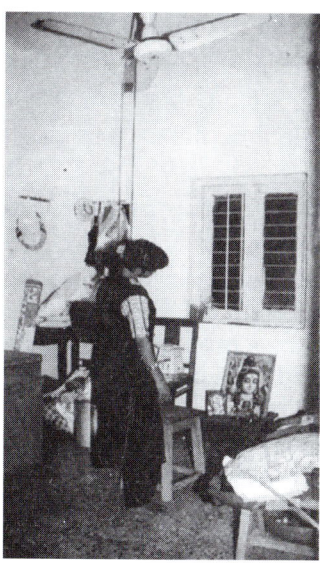

Fig. 6.22: Partial hanging—suspension by plastic rope with feet touching the ground

Lynching

- This type of hanging is done by mass of people after overpowering an individual, e.g. black men raping a white woman.
- Lynching is named after captain William Lynch who used to order on-the-spot hanging without trial in USA.

Judicial Hanging

- Execution of death sentence by judicial hanging exists in India.
- The face of condemned person is covered with dark mask.
- The noose is put around neck with knot under chin or behind the ears.
- The victim is asked to stand on a **trap door** when the trap door is drawn drops the person into the pit below.
- The **drop** is calculated by noting the length and weight.
- Usual drop is about 7 feet.
- The person dies due to fracture or dislocation at C2–C3 cervical vertebrae with injury to spinal cord.
- Death is claimed to be instantaneous and painless.

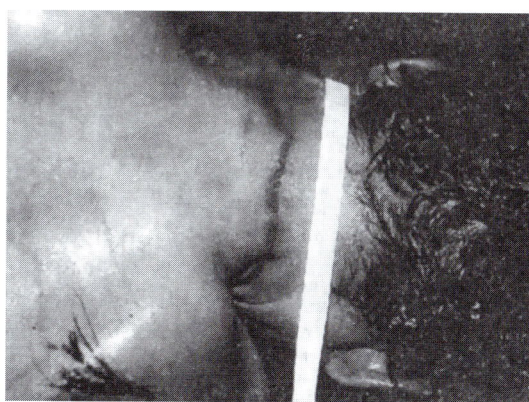

Fig. 6.23: Horizontal ligature mark over back of neck

Postmortem Hanging

- People resort to postmortem hanging of their victims to divert the attention of the doctors and police.
- The doctors examining, the ligature mark on neck must note the presence of bruises and abrasions along the edges of ligature

mark, look for the seminal stains at the tip of penis or undergarments, look for salivary stains, subconjunctival petechial haemorrhages, etc. to differentiate post-mortem hanging from antemortem hanging.

Autoerotic Hanging

- Autoerotic sadomasochistic exercises accidentally terminate in violent anoxic death.
- Generally adolescent or young adult males (in lonely environment) after indulging himself in pornography, sex literature and blue films may masturbate and use a soft cloth to apply pressure on the neck, thus making a noose with a loose knot and slipping into it.
- In 1982, a case was brought about by IG, CID Crime Mr. Vaishnav, from a place called Dehgam near Ahmedabad.
- In this case a young adult male was autopsied by the medical officer who found bleeding from the penile urethra, with ligature around the neck and death due to mechanical violent anoxia.
- A visit to the scene of crime 10 months after, the autopsy could bring of crime out

a 6 inches long screw on the beam from which this person is said to have been hanged.
- The screw revealed the presence of blood.
- The deceased was watching a young couple having sexual act inside the room, got emotionally motivated, inserted the screw into his urethra and hanged himself—a unique case of autoerotic hanging presented as homicide at first instance.

STRANGULATION

- In strangulation, there is pressure on the neck, or constriction of the neck, caused by a violent mechanical force other than the body weight, leading to death.
- When a ligature is used to constrict the neck, it is called ligature strangulation and while manual pressure is applied, it is called manual strangulation or throttling.
- In ligature strangulation, the common materials used as ligature are scarf, saree, belt, rope, wire cable, coir rope, lungi, gumcha, umbilical cord in newborn sometimes twist around the neck.

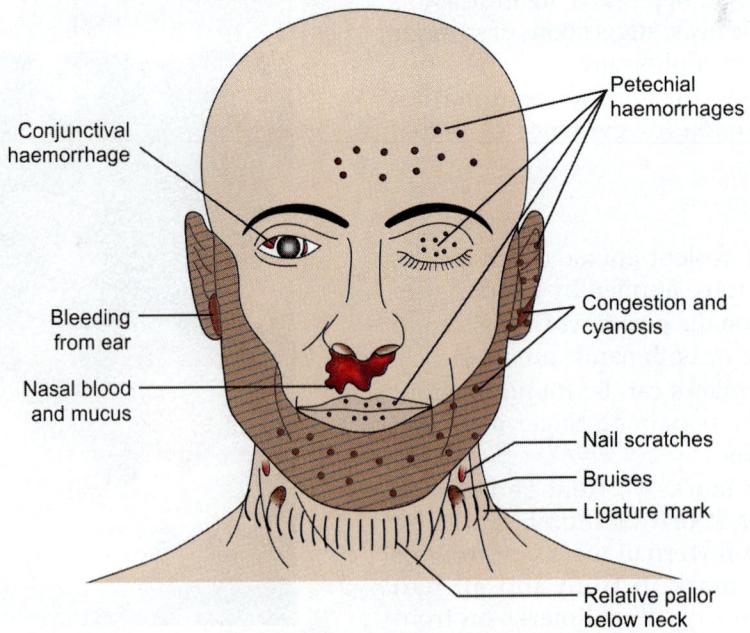

Fig. 6.24: Appearance of pressure mark upon the neck

The Autopsy Appearances

Externally

- Protruding tongue, bleeding ears due to rupture of tympanic blood vessels, congested face and eyes, petechial haemorrhages, cyanosis.
- Ligature mark is usually all around the neck, at the level of Adam's apple, runs horizontal, encircles the neck, one or more rounds may be seen.
- The ligature mark looks like a depressed mark.
- The edges are contused and abraded, the pattern corresponds to the type of ligature material.
- At the place of the knot, there is a wider skin impression.

Internally

- Under the ligature mark, extravasation of blood is seen.
- Neck muscles, larynegal cartilages, intima of carotids are injured.
- Hyoid bone fracture may occur at greater cornu or at the junction of body and greater cornu.
- Ligature strangulation is generally homicidal in nature.
- Gagged mouth, tied limbs, ligature knots on back of the neck, suggestions of struggle indicate homicidal nature.
- In female victim genital examination should be made for evidence of sexual assault.

THROTTLING

- It is type of violent anoxic death due to mechanical force applied by hands.
- Depending on the position of accused and whether one or both hands are used.
- The thumb marks can be found on front and back, the remaining finger marks on opposite side.
- Two thumb marks on front and all nail marks on back or two thumb marks on back and all fingernail marks on front or one thumb mark in front and all nail marks on back or all nail marks on front and one thumb mark on back can be seen.

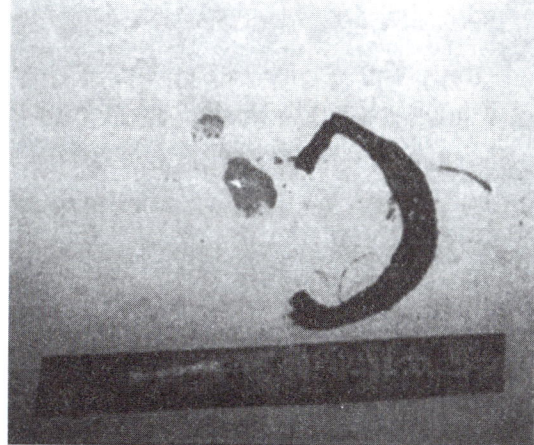

Fig. 6.25: Inward compression fracture of cornua of hyoid bone in strangulation

- On dissection, under the nail marks contused areas are seen.
- Crescentric abrasions or bruises or both can be seen.
- If there is a movement of the victim, scratches may also be seen.
- Internally, fracture of the hyoid bone due to inward compression or due to squeezing pressure of cornu of the bone, the broken fragments move freely inwards.
- The periosteum is torn on outer aspect of the fracture.

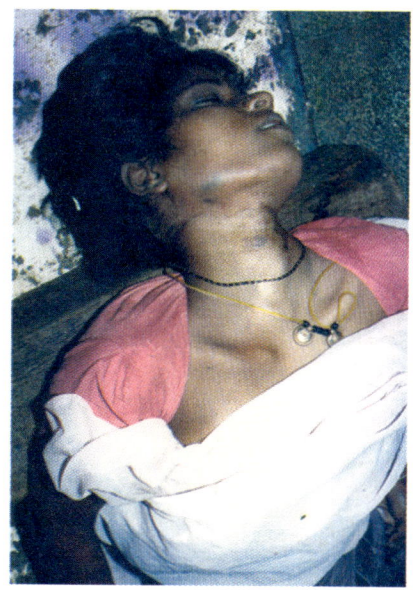

Fig. 6.26: Diffuse faint interrupted ligature mark

Medicolegal Importance

- Throttling is homicidal in nature.
- In females, evidence of sexual assault must be considered.

Palmar Strangulation

- When manual strangulation is achieved by applying pressure of palm or palms instead of fingers to cause violent mechanical

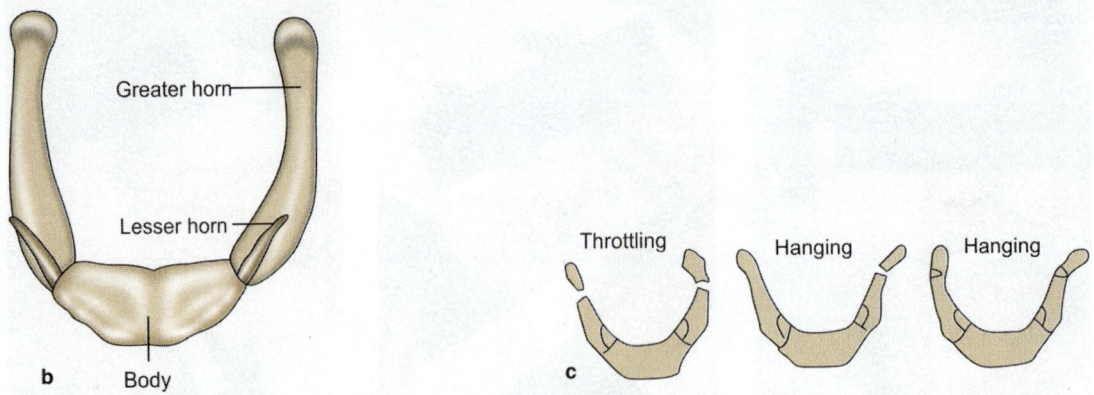

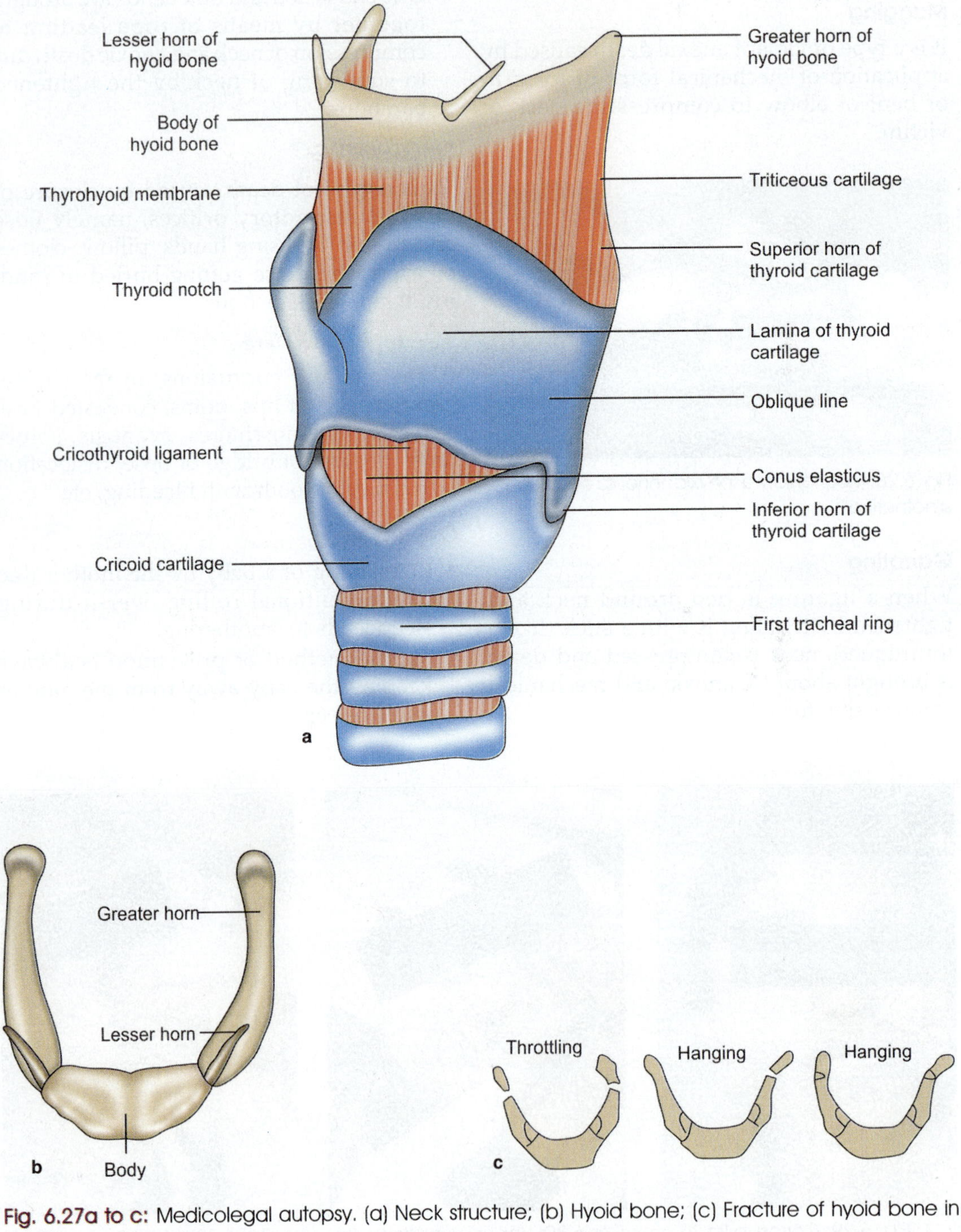

Fig. 6.27a to c: Medicolegal autopsy. (a) Neck structure; (b) Hyoid bone; (c) Fracture of hyoid bone in throttling and hanging

force, anoxic death occurs due to compression of neck.

- Diffuse bruising with underneath fracture of thyroid cartilage suggests palmar strangulation.

Mugging

It is a type of violent anoxic death caused by application of mechanical force of forearm or bent of elbow to compress the neck of victim.

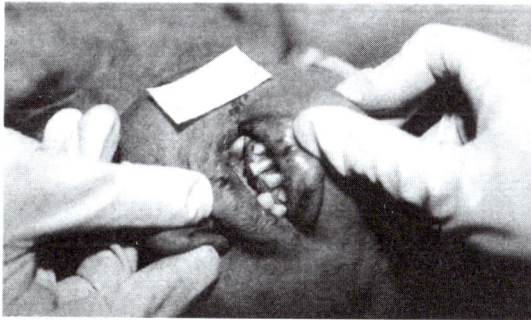

Fig. 6.28: Mechanical asphyxia: Inner lip contusion—smothering

Garroting

When a ligature is tied around neck and tightened by twisting it with a stick (like a tourniquet), neck is compressed and death is brought about by anoxia and mechanical compressive force.

Bansdola

- Bans means bamboo.
- In Assam and some Northern states of India, bamboo sticks are used, one in front and other behind.
- One end is tied and other ends are brought together by means of rope leading to compression of neck and anoxic death due to squeezing of neck by the tightened bamboos.

SMOTHERING

"It is a type of death caused by closure of external respiratory orifices, namely nose and mouth by using hands, pillow, clothes or even when face getting buried in sand, mud, hay-stack or flour".

The appearances are

Abrasions and contusions on face, nose, inner aspects of lips, gums, congested face, petechial haemorrhages, cyanosis, sometimes fracture of bridge of nose, dislocation or fracture of tooth with bleeding, etc.

Overlaying

- Overlaying of a baby by the mother due to unintentional rolling over it during sleep leads to smothering.
- Simple method of prevention is always keeping the baby away from the mother while asleep.

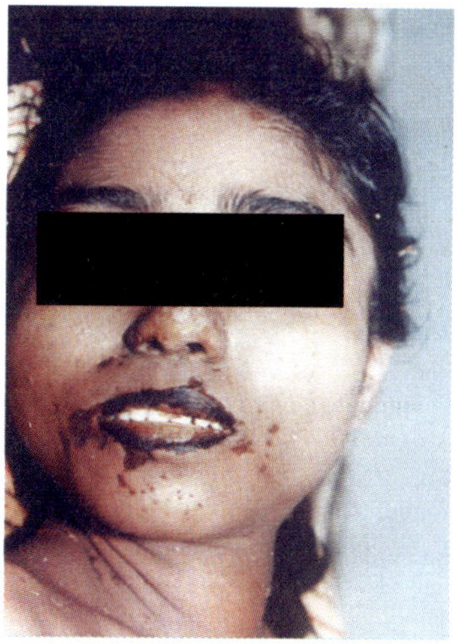

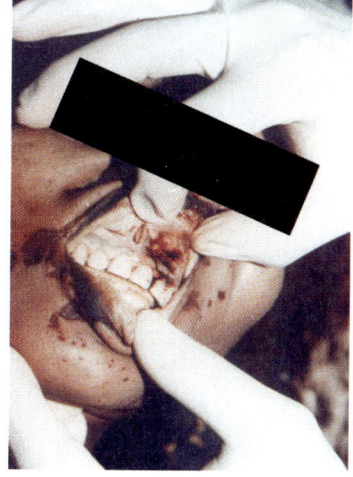

Fig. 6.29: Corrosive lip

Fig. 6.30: Upper lip inside bruise

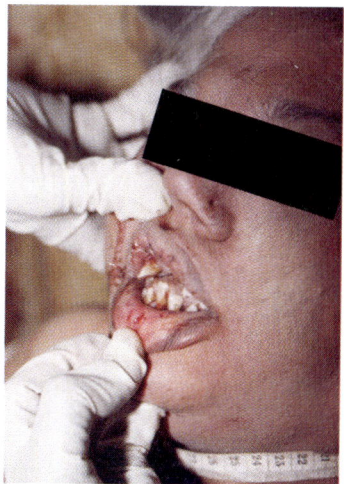

Fig. 6.31: Smothering case

- Homicidal smothering is more common among infants and children.
- When the victim is over powered by assailant or assailants, only then overlaying is possible in adults.

Gagging

- It is a type of choking caused by obstruction of mouth and throat.
- The material used for gagging is cloth or any soft material like scarf, tie, socks, handkerchief, etc. Gagging is homicidal in nature.
- The victim of gagging is generally a small baby or a helpless woman or an old sick woman or man.

CHOKING

- Choking is a form of death caused by occlusion of the air passage from inside by solid objects, e.g. coins, dentures, fish bone, marbles, worms, vomitus, food particles, blood in cut-throat injury, etc.
- Sometimes irrespirable gases and thick material like mud can also cause choking.
- The blocking need not be total or complete.
- Even a cotton wisp or a small hair can trigger laryngeal spasm and leads to death from choking.

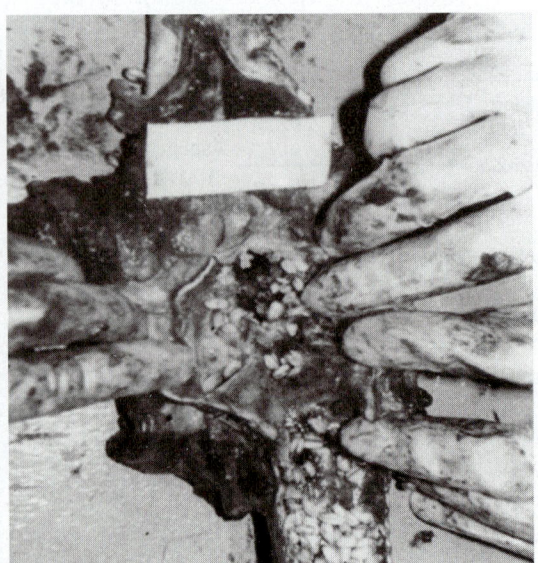

Fig. 6.32: Choking by *sucked in* wheat

- The autopsy findings are those of anoxic death—petechial haemorrhage, cyanosis and recovery of the object choking the respiratory passage.
- Sometimes, a bullet may be the object choking the respiratory passage.

Cafe Coronary

- This term is applied to sudden death of a person in a café or restaurant at the time of munching food or fish bone or steak that suddenly causes spasm in the respiratory passages and death due to choking.
- During autopsy, a lump food may be found obstructing the glottis.

TRAUMATIC ASPHYXIA

- When there is a compression of chest or chest and abdomen preventing the respiratory excursions of chest wall, death results.
- This is commonly know as traumatic asphyxia.
- Continued compression of the chest obstructs the venous return from head and arms.
- Stasis pools up deoxygenated blood causing intense cyanosis.
- Below the level of compression the skin is pale. Fracture of ribs, contusion of lungs, rupture of liver, spleen, kidney and stomach are commonly seen.
- For example, getting caught between two shunting bogies of train, sandwiched as a result of wall collapse, room collapse, mass disasters like earthquake, tree fall and trampled down in stampede, *Kumbh Mela, Tirupathi Temple Mela, Jagannath Ratha Yatra, Puri*, etc.

Burking

- Burking is a combination of homicidal smothering and traumatic asphyxia.
- It is named after Burke and Hare who used to kill people and supply dead bodies to Edinburgh Medical School in UK.
- A case of burking due to sexual jealousy in Banaras was noticed.
- A big ladle was forcibly thrusted into the private parts of a middle-aged woman

before she was killed by smothering and traumatic asphyxia.

DROWNING

- Drowning is a type of violent mechanical anoxic death brought about by exclusion of air in respiratory passages due to presence of fluid medium, medium can be water, milk, etc.
- Suicidal drowning is more common.
- Postmortem drowning and disposal of dead bodies in water (as a tradition) are also known.
- The human body has a specific gravity (1.080) which is a little more than that of water (1.000).
- A little beating movements can keep the body afloat.
- When a person falls in water, he starts gulping more and more of water while trying to breath air.

- This stimulates a vicious cycle of water entering the respiratory passages, coughing, gulping more water.
- Churning of water in the lungs produces fine, foamy, lathery, copious froth under pressure.
- In fresh water, ventricular fibrillation and in salt water severe pulmonary oedema occurs leading to death.

Death in cases of drowning can be due to

- Laryngeal spasm
- Vagal inhibition
- Head injury
- Exhaustion
- If the person survives, delayed death can occur due to septic aspiration pneumonia.
- The person struggling in water before death inhales diatoms in the water.

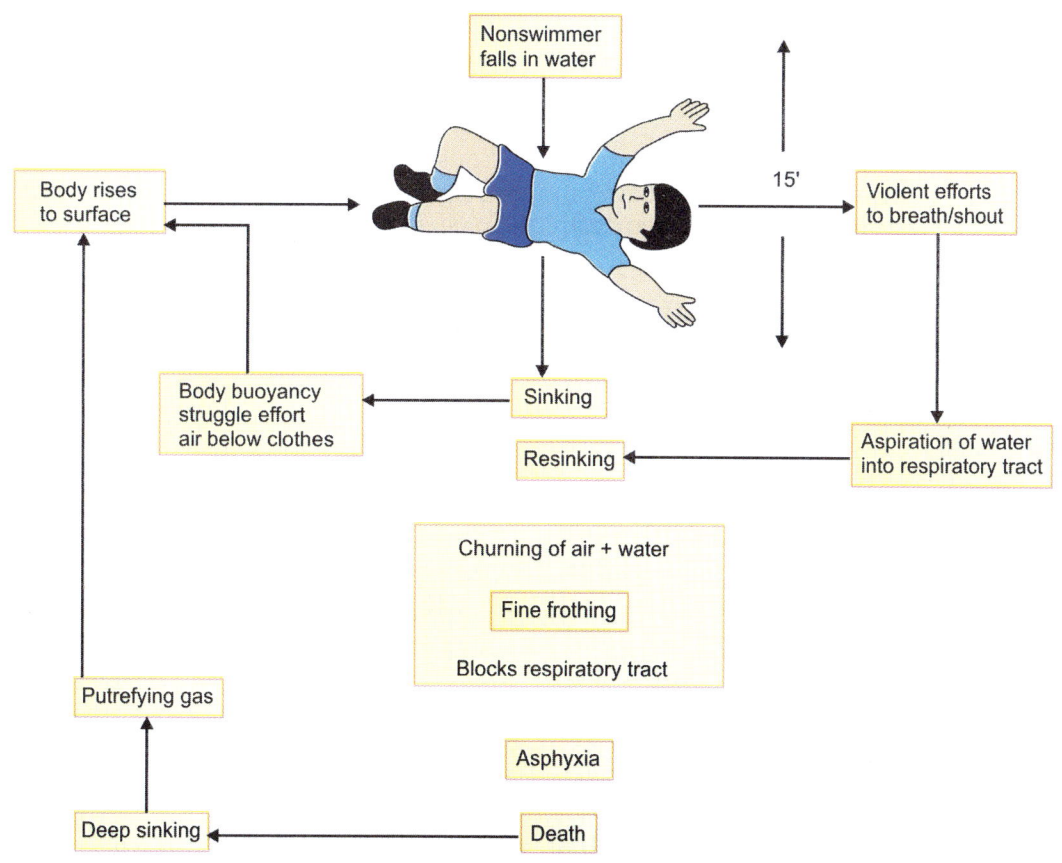

Fig. 6.33: How one struggles to breath before drowning death

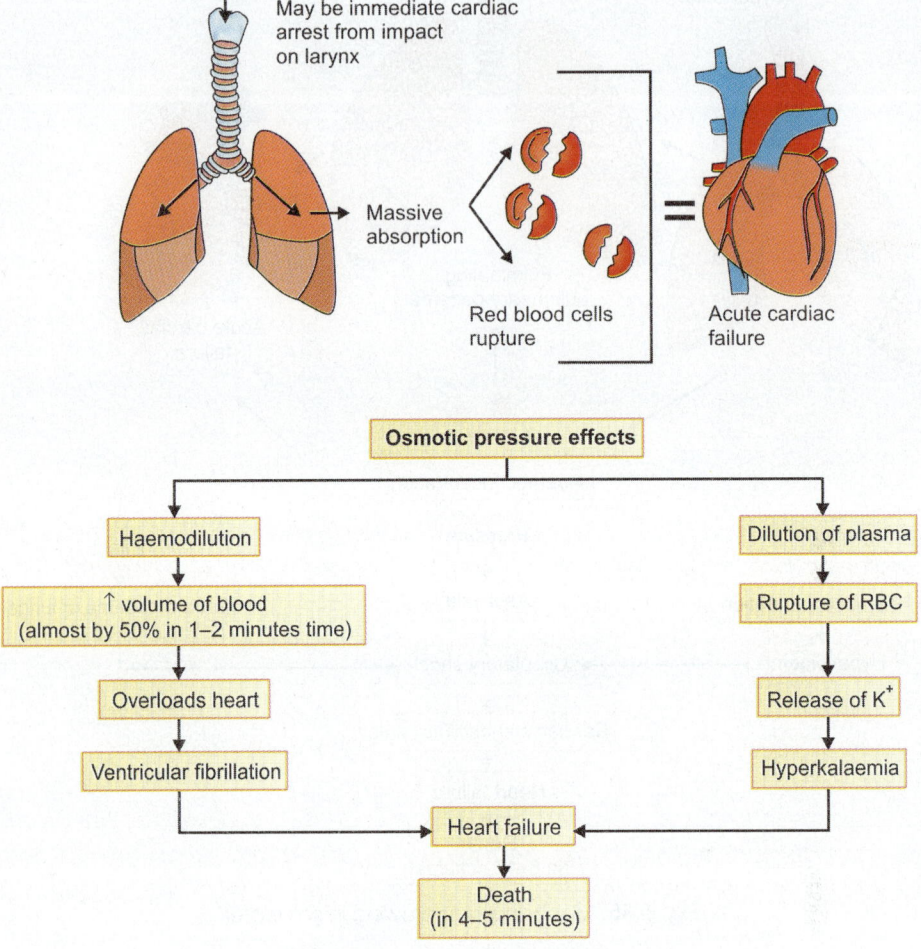

Fig. 6.34: Drowing mechanism in fresh water

- These diatoms pass through the lungs, liver and get stored in bone marrow of long bones.
- Diatoms are double-layered transversely striated, unicellular microscopic planktons or algae.
- The skeleton of diatoms resists acid digestion, so they can be demonstrated in acid digested tissue from drowning death cases.
- Their refractory walls shine under the microscope.
- They have different shapes like wheels, spindles, etc.
- However, persons in polluted humid environments during normal process of breathing are likely to inhale diatoms.

Postmortem Appearances (Typical Case of Drowning)

- In typical drowning, the face is pale, eyes may be half open, tongue swollen and protruded–bruised or bitten (during submersion of epileptics).
- Postmortem lividity on face, neck, front of upper chest and both hands.
- Fine white foamy leathery froth found in mouth and nostrils which reappears on wiping (due to the emphysema aquosum or **hydraemia of the lung**).
- The skin of extremities shows goose skin or goose flesh appearance because of contraction of erectorum pilae muscles.
- The water wrinkled appearance on hands and feet look like that of a washerwoman.

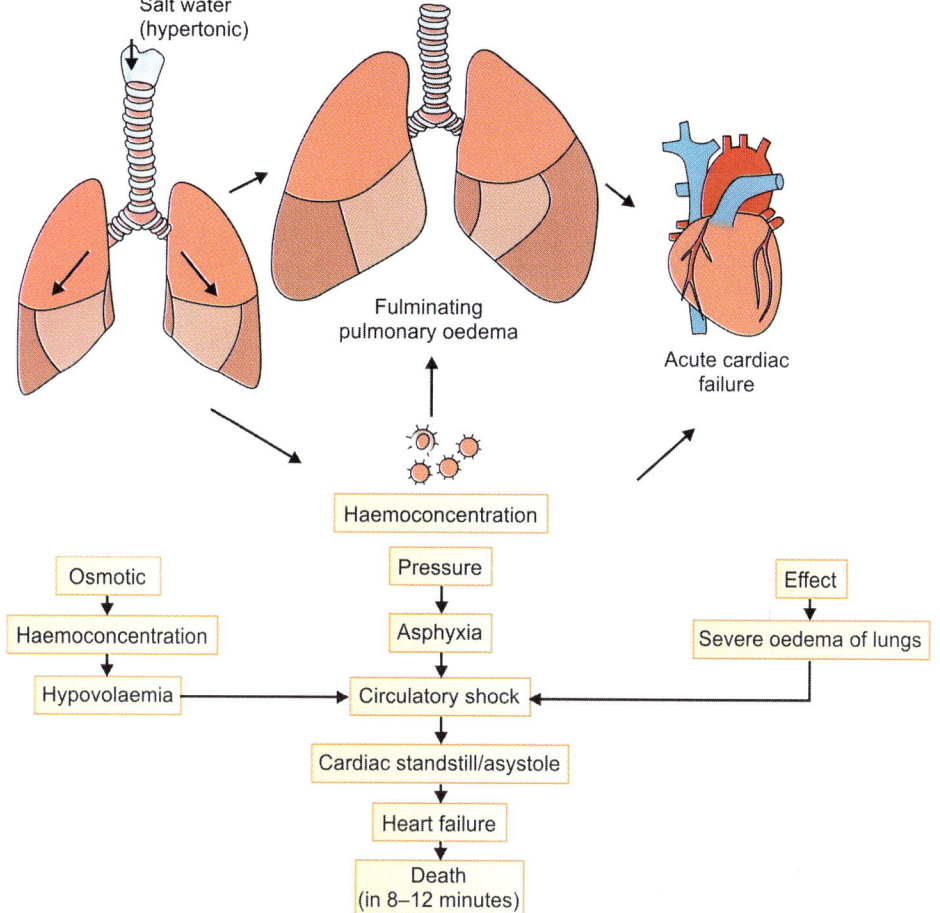

Fig. 6.35: Mechanism of drowing in salt water

- The person may be holding in his hands gravel, sand and weeds due to cadaveric spasm.
- Rigor mortis appears early in drowning.

Internally

- The lungs are volumnious, distended and are ballooned out.
- The distended surface of lungs shows rib marks.
- The lungs are doughy, boggy and heavy.
- They show pit on finger pressure.
- Mottled red and grey areas of alveoli also known as Paltauf's haemorrhages occur due to the blood effusion on the alveolar walls.

- On cut section the lungs exude copious quantities of frothy blood, when lung is filled with airless water.
- It is called oedema acquosum, when lung is filled with frothy air mixed fluid (water).
- In fresh water drowning, emphysema acquosum is seen but because of the air, cut section shows crepitus.

GETTLER'S TEST

- In salt water drowning, left side of the heart shows more chloride and magnesium than the right side.
- In fresh water drowning the chloride content on left side is less than on the right side because of dilution by water.

- So, determination of chloride content of blood helps in differentiation of fresh and salt water drowning.
- Stomach and intestines are also filled with water in typical cases of drowning.
- Diatoms are present in liver and bone marrow in typical cases of drowning.

Manifestations of Atypical Cases of Drowning

- In atypical cases, the death may be due to reflex cardiac arrest due to stimulation of vagal nerve endings.
- When cold water suddenly enters larynx or when a person dives into cold water and the water hits the pit of the stomach, death may occur due to laryngeal spasm.
- When the person is submersed in water, logging of water is absent in lungs. Foamy forth is not seen around mouth and nostrils.
- When a person drowns in a state of unconsciousness as in the cases of head injury, epilepsy, cerebral haemorrhage, intoxication, inebriation or a coronary attack/associated findings are seen.

Floating of the body: A dead body floats in water by 36–48 hours. The floatation depends upon male or female, fatty or thin, heavily built or lightly built, young or child, clothed or unclothed, fresh or decomposed. In advanced decomposition cases, the body floats with belly upwards.

Nonfloating of the body: The body may not float if it is entangled in weeds, when soft parts of the body are eaten by aquatic animals, when the body is tied and fixed to a fixed object in water, or when a heavy weight is tied to the body.

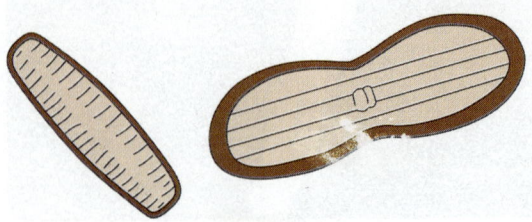

Fig. 6.36: Diatoms

Secondary Drowning

- When delayed death occurs due to causes other than drowning, it is called secondary drowning.
- Death occurs due to inhalation pneumonia, pulmonary oedema, chemical pneumonitis, metabolic acidosis and electrolyte imbalance.

Medicolegal Issues

- In dry drowning water is prevented from entering lungs due to severe laryngeal spasm.
- The dead body shows cyanosis, congestion of organs, fluidity of blood, petechial haemorrhages, but not water laden lungs.
- When cold water stimulates nerve endings on body surface like pit of stomach, tympanic drum, death occurs from cardiac arrests due to vagal inhibition.
- This is called **hydrocution** or **immersion syndrome.**
- A case presenting all typical manifestations is called **wet drowning.**
- When only face falls in water or fluid and leads to submersion, internal findings of drowning are seen but not external.
- In suicidal drowning cases by women, the women secure their clothing such a way that clothes continue to cover the body.
- In homicidal drowning, the limbs may be found tied or smell may be associated head injury or blunt force injuries.
- In all drowning cases, chemical analysis of the viscera helps in knowing whether the person consumed any poison before drowning or was given poison prior to drowning.
- Postmortem drowning cases do not show froth and Paltauf's haemorrhages.
- These cases show evidence of injuries and for poisoning.
- In all female bodies, evidence for sexual violence and pregnancy should be looked for.

Time Since Death

- *As per the Casper's dictum, the postmortem appearances take double the time to appear in water compared to when the body is outside.*

  - The body temperature falls rapidly after drowning.
  - Rigor mortis sets in early but lasts longer.
  - The destocking in summer takes 2–3 days.
  - In winter, the time roughly doubles.
  - Adipocere formation may occur in about three weeks time, washerwoman hands are seen in about 18 hours.

  - Floatation of the body is seen by 1–2 days in summer and 2–4 days in winter.

Inhalation of Irrespirable Gases (Suffocation)

- Inhalation of irrespirable gases or suffocation causes death due to interference with respiration.
- Gases like hydrogen sulphide, carbon monoxide, carbon dioxide, sulphur dioxide, chlorine, iodine, etc. are considered toxic.
- Seen in sewage workers (sewer gas) entering man holes (H_2S, CH_4, CO_2, etc.)
- Seen in people entering deep unused wells (CO_2).

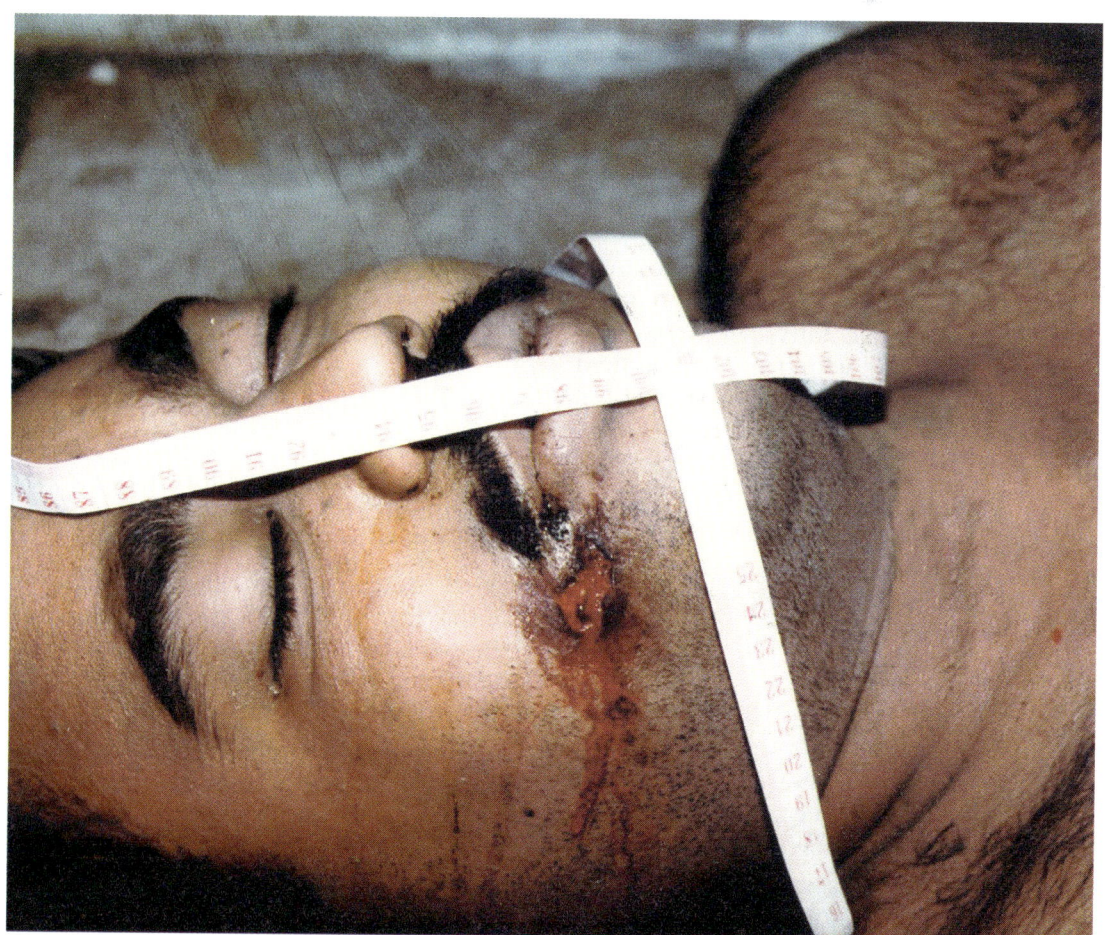

Note the drooling of stained saliva

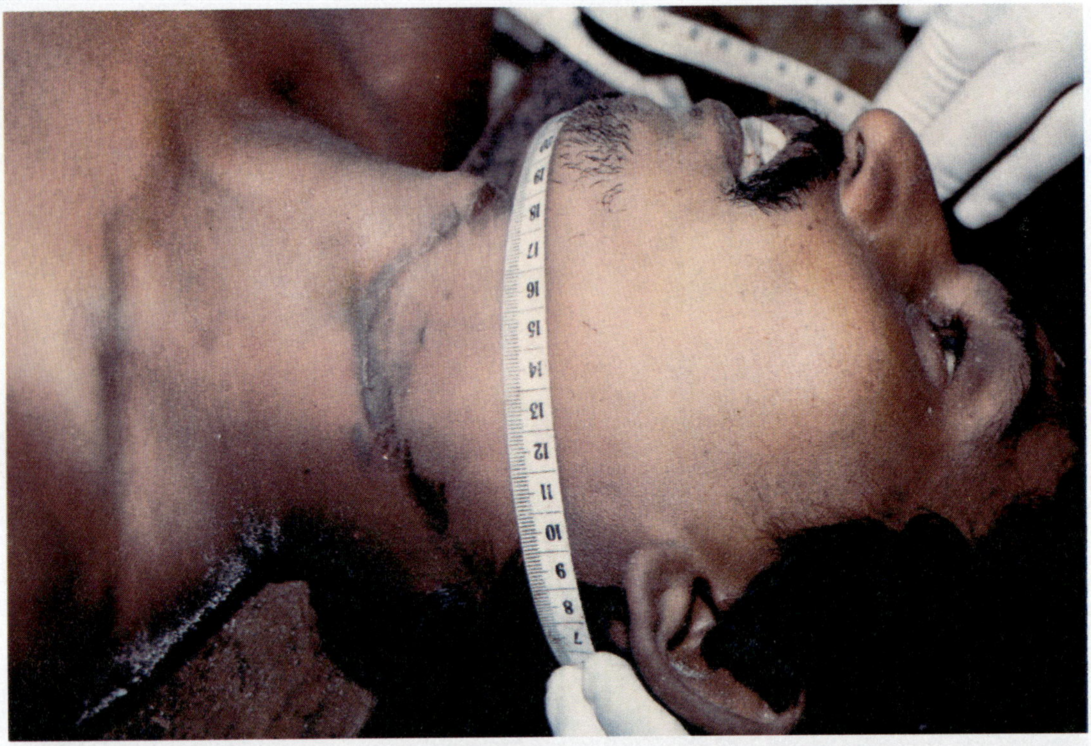

Strangulation mark patterned

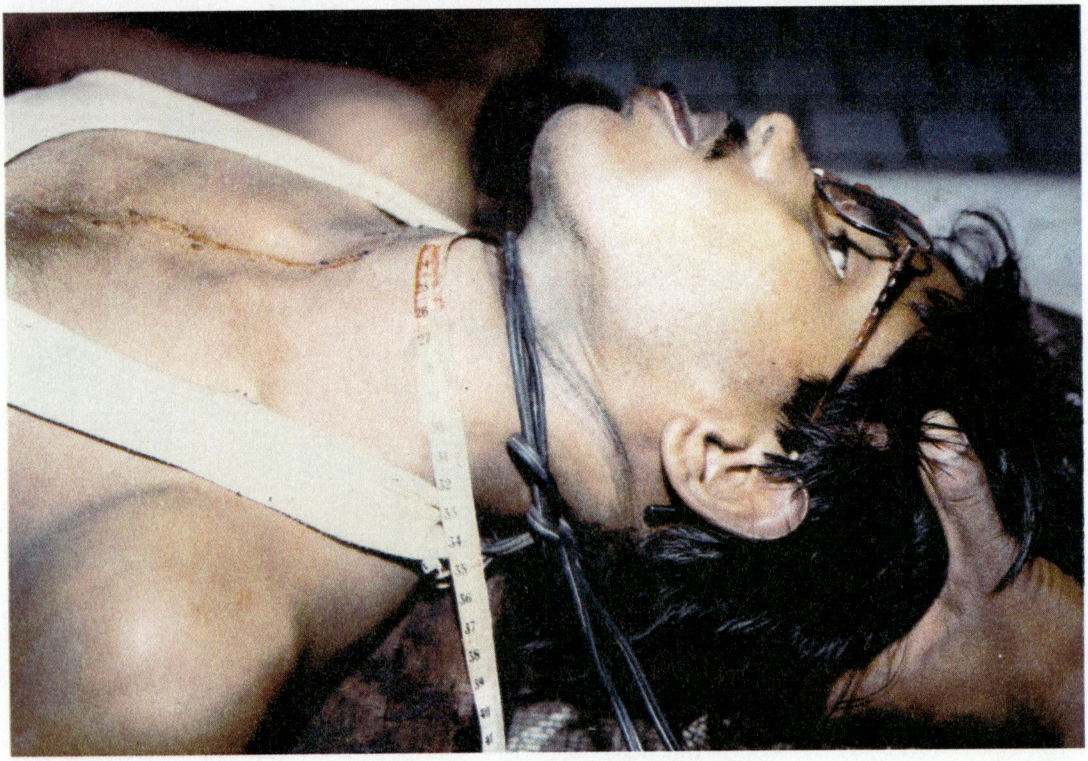

Note ligature mark and slipped ligature

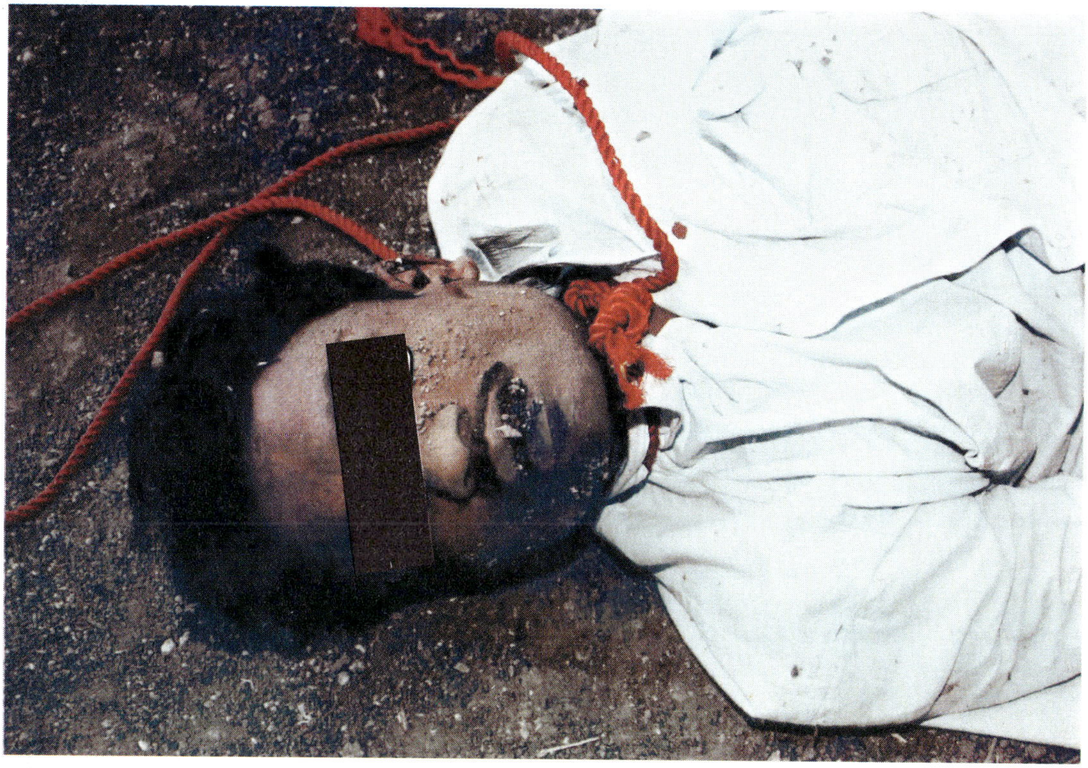

Ligature *in situ* case of strangulation

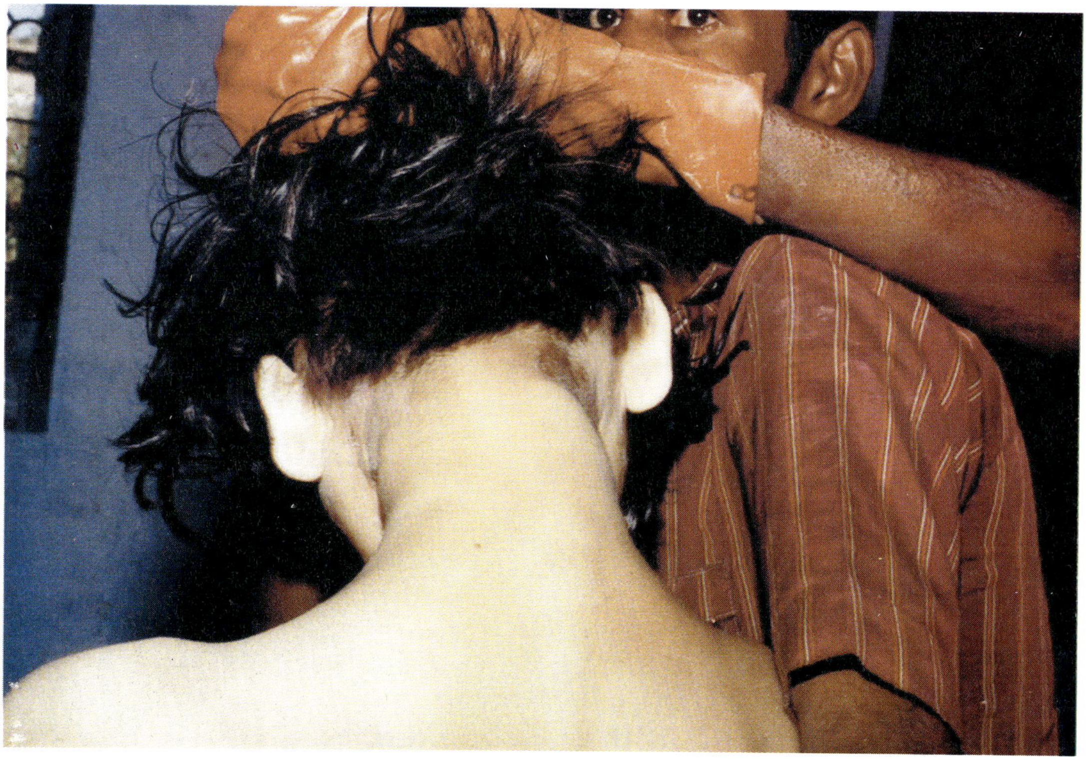

Ligature at the hanging—gap in the nape of the neck

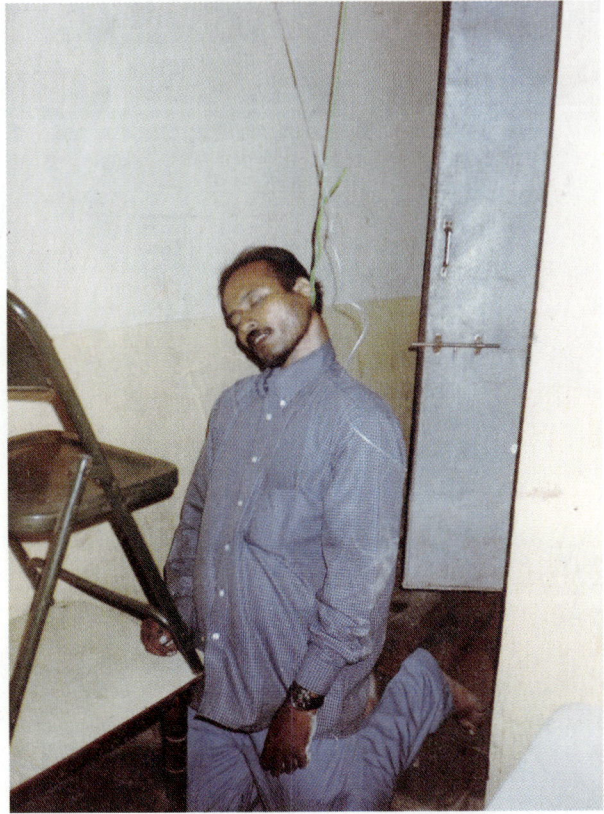

Antemortem suicidal partial hanging

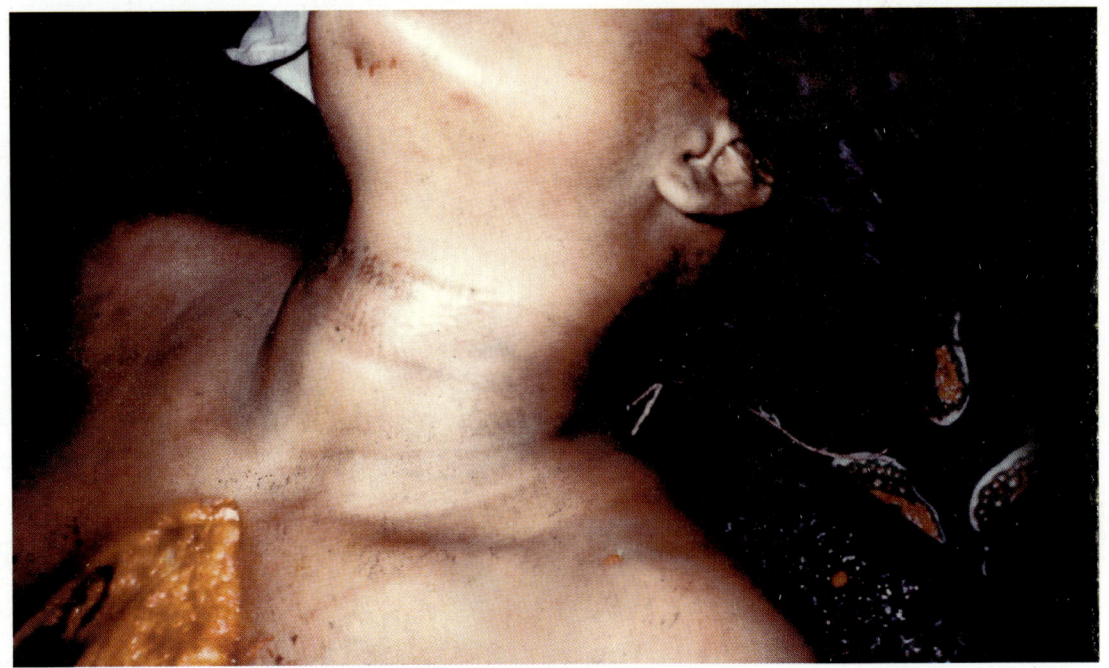

Strangulation

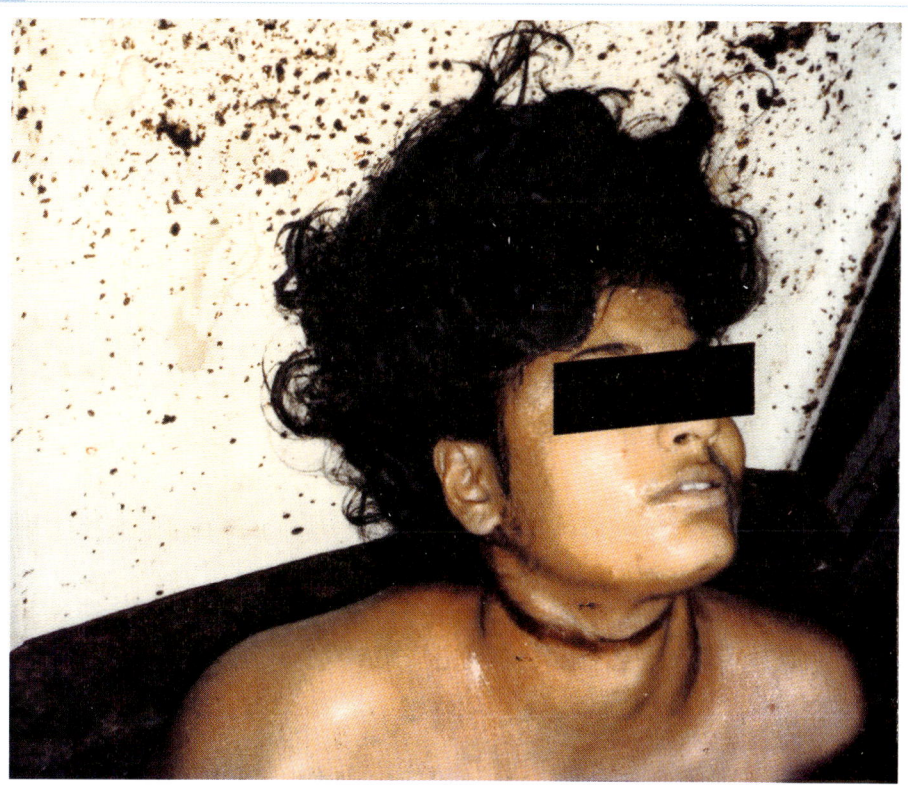

Ligature mark in case of hanging. *Courtesy*: Dr PH Barai

of traumatic intracranial
...rachnoid haemorrhage is

...d contusions of brain.
...rry aneurysms.
...surface vessels of cerebral
...e.
...vertebral artery.
...matic subarachnoid haemorrhage
...rupture of blood vessels caused by
...ertension, e.g. brain stroke.

When the subarachnoid haemorrhage becomes older, it causes yellow discolouration of the meninges. When the subarachnoid haemorrhage spreads into the basal cisterns, the ventricles show bleeding haemorrhage in the fourth ventricle is an indicator of subarachnoid haemorrhage.

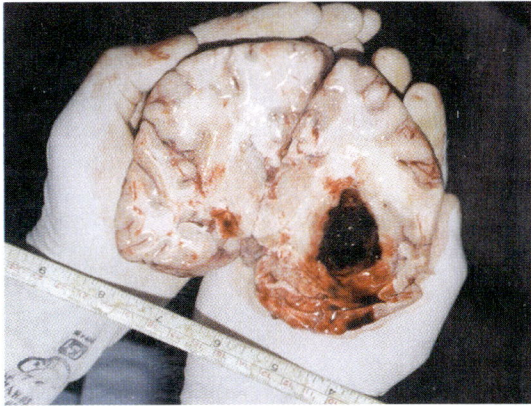

Fig. 5.71: Intracerebral haemorrhage

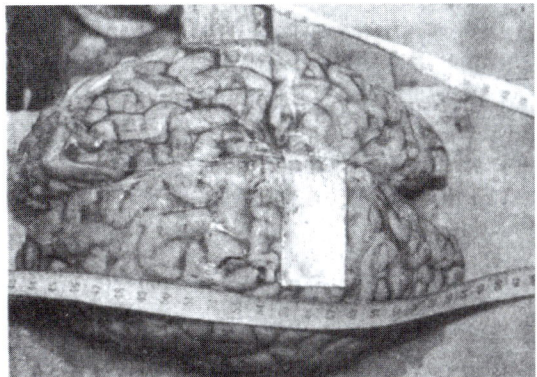

Fig. 5.70: Subarachnoid haemorrhage (seen below meninges on right side and through cut open meninges on left side)

Intracerebral Haemorrhage

Cortical contusions are common due to trauma. Blow on the head, with or without fracture of the skull can cause intracerebral haemorrhage. Severe blow on the vertex pushes the brain towards the base of the skull. This causes haemorrhage inside the brain nearer to the caudate nucleus.

Intraventricular Haemorrhage

It generally arises from the extension of nontraumatic intracerebral haemorrhage through the ventricle. In the absence of history of trauma, disease must be looked for.

Internal Capsule Haemorrhage

It is due to the verticulostriate branch of the anterior thalamic artery. Atherosclerosis and hypertension are common causes. Trauma to internal capsule occurs during crush injuries of head.

Pontine Haemorrhage

Haemorrhage into pons occurs due to pull, push or rotation of the brain stem, during trauma. Localized visible pontine haemorrhages are traumatic in nature. Diffuse petechial type pontine haemorrhages are usually no traumatic in nature.

Post-traumatic manifestations
- Amnesia or loss of memory
- Post-traumatic automatism
- Epilepsy or convulsions
- Post-traumatic headache
- Confusion
- Localizing and focal signs

Neck
Cut-throat Injuries

Cut-throat injuries are generally suicidal in nature. Hesitation cuts are seen, before the final sweep of cut-throat is made by the suicide. Hesitation cuts are multiple, superficial, tentative, generally parallel or criss-cross near the beginning of the cut-

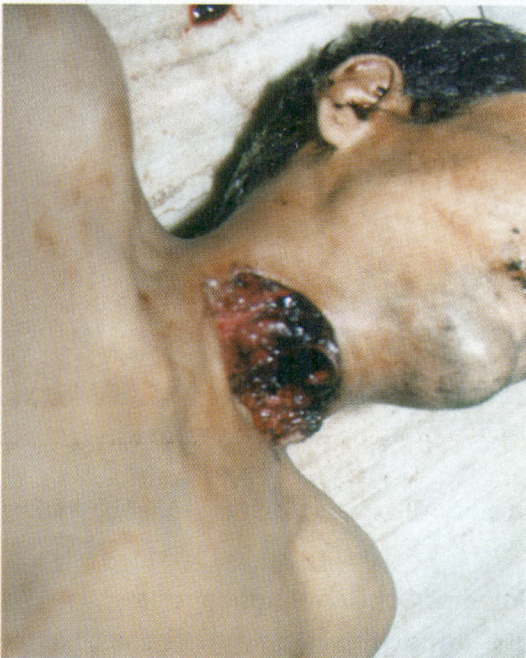

Fig. 5.72: Homicidal cut-throat

throat wound. Once the initial hesitation is overcome, a deep cut-throat wound is made, beginning of which is deeper than the end. The end may show tapering. Generally, it is above the level of Adam's apple. The various structures that may be cut in cut-throat wounds are trachea, oesophagus, vagus nerve, sometimes recurrent laryngeal nerve, carotid arteries, jugular veins.

In homicidal cut-throat wounds, hesitation cuts are not seen. The cut is deep even involving vertebral bodies or even spinal cord. The wound is generally directed backwards. Injury to subclavian vessels, pleura and even lung may be seen in the case of homicidal stabs, oesophagus may be cut.

Death occurs commonly due to blood entering the respiratory passages. Injury to the carotid vessels, injury to the spinal cord, jugular veins also cause death. Suction of air into cervical veins may cause death from pulmonary embolism also.

Fracture of Vertebral Bodies

When a person falls from height and lands on his feet, fracture of one or both calcanea

occurs. The force is transmi
gradual compression of v
wedge compression of ve
can cause spinal concussio
laceration or crushing of the
4th cervical vertebra fractures
nerves and may cause immed

Whiplash Injury

This injury is usually caused in the
of the front seat of the vehicle. Whe
comes to a sudden halt, a forward i
force causes acute hyperflexion. Spinal cord
suffers fatal contusion or laceration without
a fracture.

Railway Spine

Concussion of the spinal cord commonly occurs in railway and motor car collisions. It goes by the name of railway spine. It can also occur due to severe blows on the back due to compression or fracture dislocation of vertebrae, due to effusion of blood, due to fall from height or bullet injury.

It produces temporary paralysis of arm, bladder, rectum or lower extremities. Recovery occurs in about two days.

HANGMAN'S FRACTURE

Fracture of the neuronal arch of axis (2nd cervical vertebra between superior and inferior articular processes) is called Hangman's fracture, as it is associated with judicial execution.

Chest Injuries

They are of two types
- Penetrating or open
- Nonpenetrating or closed

Penetrating Injuries

They are caused due to stab injuries, broken ribs, firearm injuries, arrow injuries. They can cause open pneumothorax, pleural effusion, emphysaema, haemothorax, haemopneumothorax. Blunt force trauma to the chest can cause chest wall abrasions, contusions, lacerations, fractures of ribs, injury to large blood vessels. Death can occur due to concussion of chest and shock.

Commotio cordis: This is due to a sudden jolt received by an individual by a Karate kick or a hit by a ball on the chest.

He may collapse instantaneously or immediately and lead to sudden death due to primary ventricular dysrhythmia. This is induced by a sudden blunt, precordial blow at the peak of the T wave of ventricular excitability of a normal cardiac electrical flow even though the heart is normal and not associated with any structural injury. This is called commotio cordis because there is a commotio of the heart due to a jolt and sudden death occurs following sudden nonpenetrating blunt force jolt. This can cause sudden death from cardiac arrest without any visible trauma. The impact in many cases may be on left ventricle.

Buckled Sternum

It is a typical steering wheel impact on the sternum of the driver of the vehicle, when the chest hits the steering wheel as the vehicle comes to a sudden halt. The sternum yields and breaks and buckles inside with a confusion in front and behind. Under the buckled sternum, cardiac contusions can also be seen. Sometimes haemopericardium may also be seen.

Contrecoup Contusion on the Lungs

Sudden compression of the chest sometimes cause contrecoup contusions as a result of forceful displacement of air into the lungs, near the angles of the ribs on the posterior surfaces of the lungs.

Complications of Chest Injuries

Cardiac tamponade: When rapid accumulation of 300–400 ml of blood occurs in pericardial sac, there is mechanical hindrance for pumping of heart. It leads to death.

Arterial air embolism: Through a punctured or lacerated pulmonary vein, air emboli become arterial and gets lodged in cerebral arterial terminal segment.

Interstitial emphysema: Lung injury forces air into the disrupted alveoli, produces large subpleural blebs. They may rupture and even cause pneumothorax.

Haemothorax: Usually associated with pneumothorax. Generally from heart, lungs or large blood vessels.

Pneumothorax: It can be open or closed pneumothorax. When air enters lungs through an open wound of lungs are pleura, it causes open pneumothorax. Where air passes into pleural cavity through a wound in lung and visceral pleura, closed pneumothorax occurs.

Chylothorax: When there is injury to thoracic duct, chylothorax occurs.

Abdominal Trauma

Injuries are

- Nonpenetrating or closed
- Penetrating or open

Open types of abdominal injuries are generally stab injuries or firearm injuries or due to bullous (injuries by horns of animals, e.g. buffalo, cow, goat, deer, etc.) injuries.

Blunt force injuries of abdomen cause abrasion, contusion or lacerations on front, back and sides. Tyre treated marks are commonly seen in heavy vehicles running over the abdomen.

Penetrating injuries of hollow organs like stomach, intestines cause peritonitis. **Perforating injuries** are caused when the stabbing instrument cause entry and exit in hollow viscera.

Liver

Liver injuries are due to blunt force and also due to stab injuries. The **lacerations of liver** are on:

- Convex surface of the liver transcapsular laceration, i.e. rupture of capsule.
- Convex surface of the liver subcapsular laceration, i.e. without rupturing the capsule.
- Noncommunicating or central lacerations in liver substance.
- Superior surface of coronal laceration.
- Inferior surface of laceration (undersurface)
- Contrecoup laceration of the back surface.

Liver injuries cause bleeding sufficient to lead to death. Mild trauma may cause rupture of diseased liver, e.g. fatty liver, malaria, abscess, etc.

Spleen

Spleen has protection of the ribs better than liver. Blunt force trauma to spleen is more common. Compression produces lacerations, pulling or traction causes tears from its pedicle. Hilar surface causes more ruptures. Splenic bleeding is fast and profuse. Enlarged spleens rupture with minor trauma, e.g. malaria, kala-azar.

Rupture of Urinary Bladder

Extraperitoneal rupture: Extraperitoneal rupture causes extravasation of urine up to kidneys and downwards up to scrotum.

Intraperitoneal rupture: Intraperitoneal rupture of the bladder occurs, when the bladder is distended and receives a fall or kick or blow. The peritoneum over the upper surface tears causing the urine to enter the peritoneal cavity.

Rupture of Urethra

Male urethra ruptures under the pubic arch, when there is a kick on perineum, fracture of pubic bone, foreign body, fall on projecting object, etc.

Trauma to Major Vessels

- Stab injuries to femoral artery and profunda femoris branch, popliteal vessels.

- Penetrating or nonpenetrating injury to the aorta.

- Penetrating or nonpenetrating injury to common iliac or iliac vessels.

- Penetrating or nonpenetrating injury to renal vessels.

- Penetrating injury to brachial, subclavian and carotid vessels.

Injuries to the above vessels due to blunt trauma or stab injuries without any other injuries can cause death.

FALL FROM HEIGHT

In simple fall from a high building the body is nearer to the foot of the building when the person falls on the head, both vault and base can fracture.

When a person falls on feet, the following injuries can occur:

- Fracture of tibia and femur
- Fracture of femoral neck
- Dislocation of hip joint
- Fracture—dislocation of sacroiliac joint
- Fracture of vertebral body
- Ring fracture of skull

When a person falls on the side of the body, this can be:

- Fractures of multiple ribs
- Fracture of shoulder blades
- Contusions and lacerations of back, buttocks, limbs
- Severe abdominal and thoracic injuries.

Boxing Injuries

Boxing is one of the dangerous games. Professional boxers end up with **punch-drunk syndrome,** e.g. Mohammed Ali. Boxers suffer acute and chronic injuries.

Acute boxing injuries are

- Subdural haematoma (fatal)
- Retinal detachment
- Black eyes
- Extradural haemorrhage
- Fracture of nasal bones
- Lip bruises
- Dental breaks and dislocations, etc.

Punch-drunk Syndrome

Slurred speech, defective memory, slow thought, stiff limbs, ataxia, broad based gait, Parkinson facies, dementia, violent outbursts.

Intracranial findings

- Subdural, subarachnoid and intracerebral haemorrhages, cortical atrophy, contusions of brain, focal ischaemic lesions, etc.
- Repeated punches on the head cause small haemorrhages and degenerative changes in cortices, thalamus, deep central grey matter and central pathways.

Aircraft Injuries

- Commonly aircraft accidents occur at the time of landing. During 'take off' accidents are less common.

CHAPTER 7

Thermal Deaths

HEAT

- When the environmental heat increases, the body temperature may go up if thermoregulatory mechanism does not cope up.
- Heat stroke occurs when the body is unable to compensate the environmental heat.

Factors Influencing Heat Stroke

- Alcoholism
- Cerebral or cardiac artherosclerosis
- Tranquillizers
- Antidepressants
- Obesity
- Old age
- In younger individuals due to extreme exertion like long distance runners, football players, etc. manifestations of heat stroke like hot dry skin, nausea, vomiting, breathlessness, muscle cramps, circulatory collapse, cardiac failure are seen.
- If the person lives for sometimes, conditions like pneumonia, supra-renal haemorrhage, chronic renal failure, liver necrosis or DIC (disseminated intravascular coagulation) may occur.
- When the person suffers minor attack of heat, heat cramps can occur.
- During vigorous exercise leg muscle cramps are common.
- Skin is moist, body is cool and body temperature is normal.

- Intake of salt tablets relieves the cramps. When both salt and water are lost, the person suffers from heat exhaustion, headache, nausea, vomiting, weakness and cramps and treatment includes salt and water replenishment.

HYPOTHERMIA

- As the temperature goes down, the body exhibits changes below 95°F or 35°C.
- Severe hypothermia is seen below 30°C, moderate is seen between 30°–34°C and above 34°C, it is mild hypothermia.

Susceptibility to Cold Depends Upon

- Newborns are most susceptible followed by infants and children.
- Lean and thin are more susceptible than fat persons.
- Men are more susceptible than women.

The Effects of Cold

- At 32°C → Shivering is lost, hallucinations, slow reflexes, analgesia occur.
- At 30°C → Cold nercosis appears.
- Below 30°C → Atrial fibrillation.
- Between 28–25°C → Ventricular fibrillation, loss of pupillary reflex.
- Below 25°C → Very low heartbeats. Flat ECG
- At 10°C → No heart activity.

Postmortem Findings

Postmortem staining is bright red or pinkish colour due to under utilization of oxyhaemoglobin (cherry red staining is also seen in refrigerated bodies, HCN and CO poisoning).

Other Manifestations

Haemorrhagic pancreatitis, pneumonia, acute tubular necrosis of kidney, cardiac muscle necrosis, etc.

BURNS

Burns due to heat are very common in India. Primus stove bursting in kitchen causes burns among many young cooking women.

Classification of Burns

Dupuytren's Classification of Burns

Six degrees

- First degree—erythema.
- Second degree—erythema and blister formation.
- Third degree—partial destruction of true skin.

- Fourth degree—total involvement of skin.
- Fifth degree—skin, subcutaneous tissue, deep fascia and muscles.
- Sixth degree—blood vessels, nerves and bones.

Wilson's Classification

- Epidemral → 1st and 2nd of Dupuytren.
- Dermoepidermal → 3rd and 4th of Dupuytren.
- Deep → 5th and 6th of Dupuytren.

Calculation of the Area/Body Surface Involved

- The area involved is calculated by using the burns chart which facilitates more accurate calculation.
- The percentage of total body surface area (TBSA) is taken into account, and the areas are divided into half of head (A), half of one thigh (B) and half of lower leg (C).
- These areas show different percentages depending on various age groups.

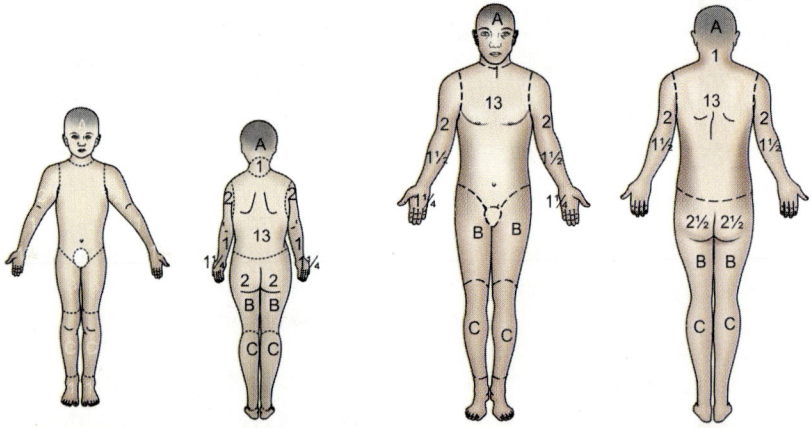

Percentage (%) of TBSA					Percentage (%) of TBSA			
	Age					Age		
	0	1	5			10	15	Adult
A= half of head	9½	8½	6½	A= half of head		5½	4½	3½
B= half of thigh	2¾	3¼	4	B= half of one thigh		4¼	4½	4¾
C= half of one lower leg	2½	2½	2¾	C= half of one lower leg		3	3½	3½

TBSA= Total body surface area

Fig. 7.1: Percentage of total body surface area

Table 7.1: Estimation of percentage of body surface area burnt in adults and children

Area of the body	Percentage (%)		
	Infant	Child	Adult
Head and neck	20	15	09
Anterior chest	20	20	18
Back	20	20	18
Upper extremity			
Right	10	10	09
Left	10	10	09
Lower extremity			
Right	10	15	18
Left	10	15	18
Genitalia and perineum	0	0–1	01
Total	**100**	**100**	**100**

PEADIATRIC BURNS

5 years child with flames burns over face, chest and abdomen, both upper limbs

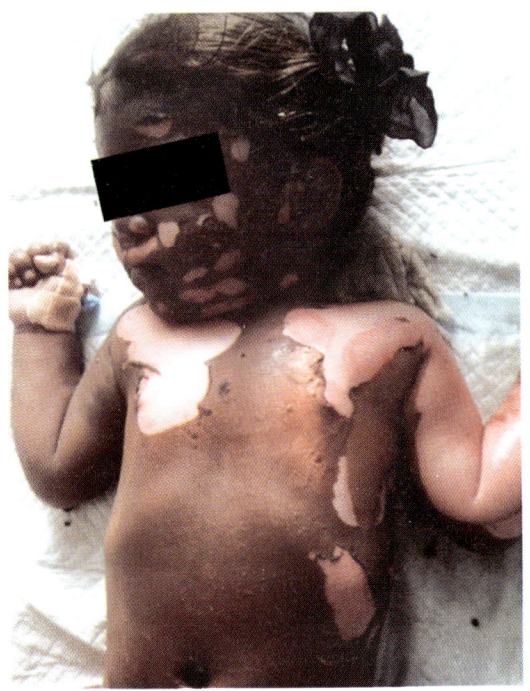

Fig. 7.2: Preoperative

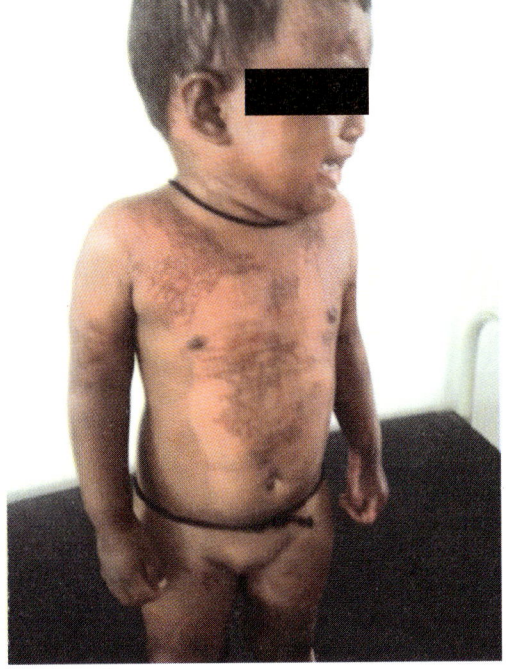

Fig. 7.3: Postoperative

- The remaining parts of the body are given same percentage irrespective of the age.
- Age
- Sex

The Factors Affecting Burns

- Intensity of heat
- Duration of exposure
- Nature of clothes on body

Types of Burns

- Flame burns
- Contact burns
- Radiant burns

- Scalding burns
- Chemical burns
- Microwave burns
  - Flame burns occur due to direct contact with flame.
  - Contact burns occur when hot object comes in contact with skin (e.g. hot iron, hot iron rod).
  - Radiant burns occur when skin is exposed to heat waves.
  - Scalding occur when skin comes in contact with hot fluids at boiling point (exposure to steam, splashing or spilling of hot liquid or immersion in hot fluid).

Causes of Death due to Burns

a. Immediate Causes

- Neurogenic shock
- Thermal shock—shock, hypovolaemia and acute renal failure.

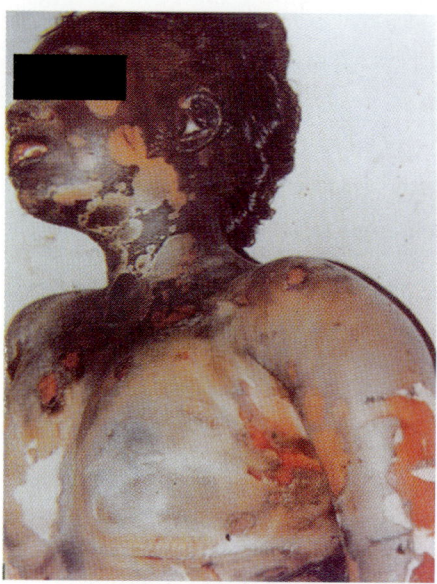

Fig. 7.4: Corrosive burns

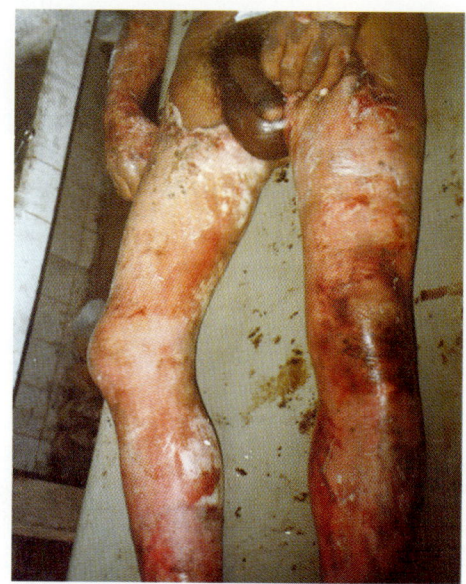

Fig. 7.5: Corrosive burns

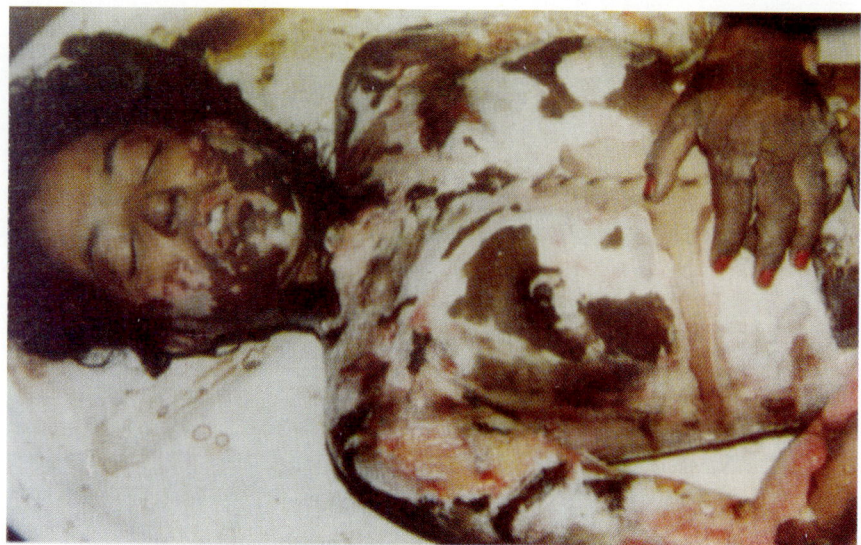

Fig. 7.6: Corrosive burns. *Courtesy:* Prof. Amar Raghu Narain, Burns (Plastic Surgery) NMCHS, Nellore

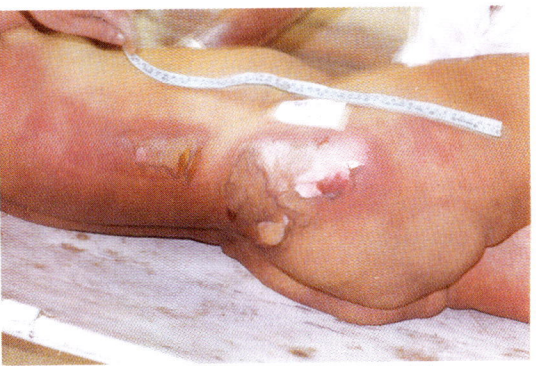

Fig. 7.7: Blebs

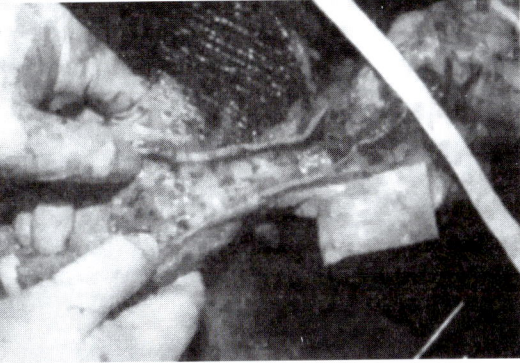

Fig. 7.8: Soot in trachea suggests antemortem burns due to hydrocarbon

- Inhalation of smoke—CO and other noxious gases.

b. Delayed Causes
- Renal failure
- Respiratory failure due to acute respiratory distress syndrome
- Septicaemia
- Pneumonia
- Pulmonary embolism.

Postmortem Manifestations
- Presence of black carbonaceous matter, i.e. soot in the upper and lower respiratory passages is considered as a reliable sign of life before catching fire, i.e. it is antemortem burns.
- If the burns patient goes into carbon monoxide poisoning and death, soot deposition may or may not be found in respiratory passages.
- Rim or redness at blister margins is considered in favour of antemortem burns.
- Blister fluid rich in albumin and chlorides is again antemortem indicator of burns.
- Postmortem blisters do not show red margin, albumin, chlorides.
- Under the microscope, the antemortem burns show elongated and flat epithelial cells.
- When kerosene is used for burns, kerosene smell is found on the body and chemical analysis can detect the kerosene.
- Haemoconcentration and carboxyhaemoglobin in blood are seen.

- Cerebral congestion and oedema are present.
- The skull bones may burst and show fractures.
- If the burns victim lives for a week or 10 days, stomach and duodenum may show **Curling's ulcers.**
- These ulcers are caused by release of histamine and protein breakdown products, capillary endothelial damage and thrombosis.
- Changes in skin, muscles, bones look like lacerations and fractures, but they can be differentiated from the absence of bleeding and clotting. The ruptured organs and heat haematomas show chocolate brown colour due to heat coagulation of proteins.

Pugilistic Attitude
With flexion of upper limbs like a boxer holding is hands in front of face, is due to coagulation of muscle proteins.

Preternatural Combustibility
- Preternatural means unnatural and combustibility means ability to catch fire.
- In the alimentary tract, due to bacterial fermentation and digestive processes, sometimes inflammable gases like hydrogen, methane and hydrogen sulphide are formed.
- They may come out by belching or flatus during that time if there is any flame

nearby gases catch fire and create terror in the person.

- Sometimes during operations when diathermy is used in the large intestine, mild explosions can occur due to same phenomenon.

Medicolegal Importance

- Conflagrations can cause mass burns. In such mass disasters, identification becomes a problem.
- By subjecting bodies to X-ray, age and sex determination becomes easy.
- Dental data helps in identification.
- Suicidal burns are very common in India especially among the young married women in their husband's home.
- These cases are known as bride burning cases.
- In a married woman up to 7 years of marriage or completion of 30 years when death occurs in *sasural* (mother-in-law's place), the autopsy should be conducted by panel of two doctors.
- The inquest is carried out by magistrate.
- Homicidal burns are sometimes seen.
- The homicide victims may be drugged or tied down with ropes or some other material before they are burnt. Sometimes burns are associated with other injuries like head injuries, neck injuries and strangulation.
- In women, sexual violation should be looked for.
- Many times women are pregnant and how pregnancy may become the cause of bringing end of life.

Postmortem Burns

- Such as the cause of death is other than burns, poisoning, head injuries, rape followed by murder are the possible causes.
- Postmortem burns can be identified by absence of carboxyhaemoglobin.
- In antemortem burns, if death had occurred before carboxyhaemoglobin levels could raise, evidence of carbon monoxide may not be found.

Contact Burns

When an object like red hot iron from blacksmith's fire comes into contact with human body, the burns caused, present the shape of object touching the body.

Radiant Burns

When the skin is exposed to heat waves, the burns are due to radiation.

Scalding Burns (Scald)

Scalding can occur due to steam generated by boiling fluid, by spilling or splashing of hot liquid like the transformers oil or when the person is immersed in hot fluids either accidentally or homicidally. It is an accidental in nature.

Chemical Burns

- Chemical burns are caused by strong acids like nitric and sulphuric acids. Substances like phosphorus and carbolic acid also cause chemical burns.
- Alkalies like sodium hydroxide and potassium hydroxide can also cause chemical burns.
- Alkalies—coagulation and liquefaction necrosis. Acid burns are superficial erosion with redness. Alkali burns are pale, slippery and leather-like.
- Acids—precipitate proteins. The extent of burns depends on concentration of the chemical and the time duration of contact.

Microwave Burns

- Microwave gadgets are very popular and common in India also.
- Microwave burns are accidental. The microwave causes burns by reflection, absorption or passing through the target. Muscles are affected more than the body fat in the microwave burns.
- Microwaves are electromagnetic waves. Their wavelength varies from 1 mm to 30 cm.

Scene of Burns

- A careful look at the scene of burns gives clues about the nature of burns.

- Bursting of primus stove; spilling of hot fluids like transformer oil; using of fuel like kerosene, petrol, diesel; slowly burning coal *chulha* (stove) should be looked for; whether the walls are showing these materials or smoke, whether room is closed or an open space and whether other materials in the room are burnt or not, should be looked for. More disturbed scene suggests homicide or accident.

ELECTRICAL INJURIES

- Electrical injuries occur due to high tension wires falling on the ground or the person; short circuit of electricity; faulty electrical appliances like iron, heater, etc. can cause accidental electrocution.
- The human skin provides greatest resistance to electrocution.
- Dry thick skin can offer resistance up to one million ohms. Thin and moist skin offers resistance up to 100 ohms.
- When a person wears insulated materials like rubber, gloves and boots, he is protected. The least resistant tissues are blood and body fluids.
- When electricity flows through the body, it tries to take the shortest path.

An 11-year-old boy with high voltage electric burns, involving face, neck and left ear.

The common paths are

- Hand to foot
- Head to foot
- Hand to hand with chest in between
- When the current passes through heart or brain, death results faster.

Effects of Electricity on Body

- Tingling, muscle tremors, muscular contractions, loss of consciousness, ventricular fibrillation, ventricular arrest occur as the intensity of current increases from one milliampere to two milliamperes.
- Generally, electricity causes entry and exit wounds. Concealed electrical burns may be seen inside the mouth of small children playing with defective electrical gadgets and unknowingly putting into mouth.
- Entry sites are fingertips or palms, top of the head, back of the chest. Exit sites are soles of feet, hands, etc. A typical electrical burn is chalky white or yellowish with a raised pale border and central crater. Blackening may be seen sometimes.
- The size is from 1–2 mm to 1–2 cm.
- Fresh electrical burns may give a burnt odour. High voltage electricity can cause many small pit like burns due to the arc of current striking the body.
- The heat generated can cause explosive trauma like shattering of limbs or rupture of internal organs like liver, spleen. The

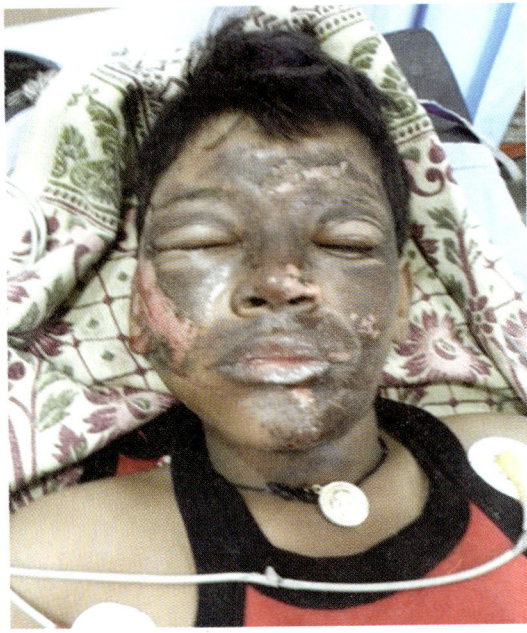

Fig. 7.9: High voltage electric burns

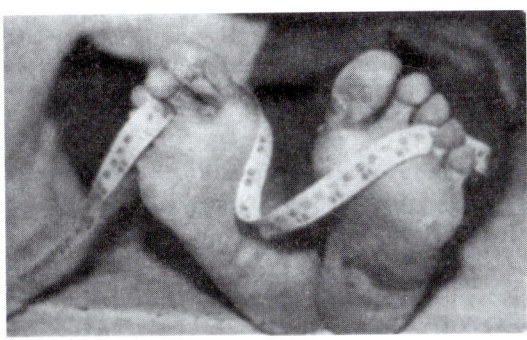

Fig. 7.10: Electrical exit wounds. *Courtesy*: Dr BD Gupta, Jam Nagar

person may die of secondary injuries when he is thrown away by high voltage electricity.

- The victim may suffer from head injury or fracture of bones.

Joule's Burns

- Joule's burn is heat generated in the body as a result of electricity entering, so it is called **endogenous thermal burn.**
- The burn may appear in shape and size like the object causing electrocution.
- The entry burn shows metallization.
- The exit burn does not show metallization.

Causes of Death in Electrical Burns

- Ventricular fibrillation, when current passes through the heart.
- Medullary paralysis when current passes through brain (medulla oblongata).
- Cerebral anoxia.

JUDICIAL ELECTROCUTION

- The condemned person is comfortably seated in a wooden chair. His head is shaven, a conducting paste is applied, one electrode is attached to head, the other electrode is attached to right leg in the lower part.
- An alternating current of 7 ampere and 1700 volts is passed through for a minute, which is repeated for another minute after a brief gap to make sure that he is dead.
- Judicial electrocution for capital punishment as death sentence was introduced in New York.
- Autopsies revealed burning of body tissues and burns of skin.
- USA, Albania, Virginia, Ohio and other states follow this method.

Medicolegal Importance

- Accidents are common. Torture by electricity is on increase.
- In one case brought to author from Valsad, South Gujarat, an adolescent boy was given repeated shocks of electricity on thighs.
- He was brought with impotence.

FLASH BURNS

- These are exogenous thermal burns.
- These are extensive and severe burns with gross destruction of soft tissues and charred bones underneath.
- These are caused when a very high voltage electricity passes on the body producing a lot of intense heat, causing burns.

LIGHTNING

- The upper surface of clouds are positively charged.
- The lower surfaces are negatively charged.
- When there is accumulation of negative charge at lower surface of a cloud, it crosses the insulating barries of the atmosphere and creates an electrical field on reaching near the earth.
- The earth has a positive charge so the earth's positive discharge touching the cloud's negative discharge creates a return stroke, thus the lightning is released as a flash with a tremendous amount of energy.
- There is an agitation of air in the path of lightning.
- The electricity generated is a direct current of 20,000 ampere and 1,000 mV.
- When it directly strikes a person, it causes death.
- The victim sustains blast-like injuries, contusions, lacerations and even fractures.
- The clothes may be torn and thrown out of him.
- The heat of lightning melts the metal like keys or buttons.
- There may be magnetization of metallic objects.
- Burns like branches of a tree are seen on the front of the chest.
- They are called *arborescent markings (filigree burns), Lichtenberg's flowers.*
- When the electrical discharge exits through the feet, skin of the sole at exit point is ruptured.
- Victim's shoes may be torn. These arborescent marks are greenish in colour due to the copper deposition.
- Surface burns and linear burns are also seen on the skin.

- Tympanic membrane may be ruptured. Internally organ congestion and pulmonary oedema are seen.
- Scattered petechial haemorrhages in brain and spinal cord are seen.

Medicolegal Issues

- Majority of human loss occurs because of cloud to ground lightening strikes.
- It is one of the natural disasters, during thunderstorms.
- Singeing of the body hairs is also seen
- Death is due to immediate irreversible cardiopulmonary arrest.

- The injuries may create a false impression of homicide.
- So, one should carefully look for metallization, magnetization, arborescent marks and exit wound.

Primary Blast Injury (Shock Wave)

- It results from the dramatic change in barometric pressure which spreads concentrically from the site of explosion at about the speed of sound.
- A wave of very high pressure (shock wave) is followed by a weak wave of negative pressure (below atmosphere),

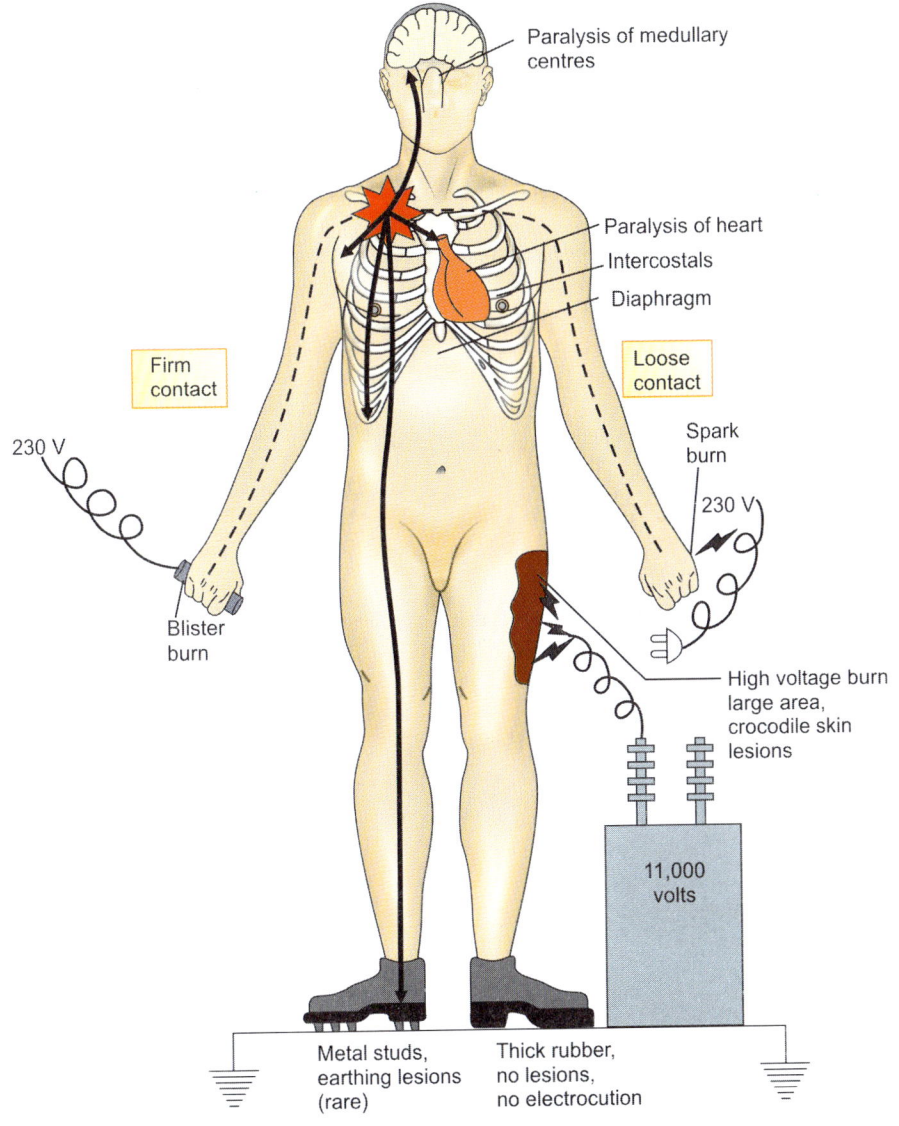

Fig. 7.11: Effects of electrocution

a suction which lasts about 5 times as long.

- A shock wave >700 kilo Pascals (100 lb/ sq. inch) pressure is necessary to cause serious damage to body.
- Lung shows subpleural patchy haemorrhages (in line of ribs), rupture of alveolar septa, intrapulmonary haemorrhage, bullae at margins, reactive pulmonary oedema, blood-stained froth and bronchopneumonia later.
- This injury of air blast is called blast lung. This is the commonest organ involved in primary blast injury.

Type of Blast Injuries

Blast injury type	Mechanism of injury	Health impact
Primary	Rapid, crushing over pressure	Damage to hollow organs such as ears, eyes, lungs, gastrointestinal tract
Secondary	Flying debris	Penetrating and blunt trauma injuries
Tertiary	Blast wind	Fracture and blunt trauma
Quarternary	Any complicating factor not in the other three categories	Burns, crush injuries, respiratory problem

a. Air blast (explosion in air)
  - Barotrauma to air filled hollow organs
  - Tympanic membrane (eardrum) is most sensitive and most commonly injured.
  - Lung is 2nd most sensitive and commonly injures hollow organs but lung injury is the most common cause of life-threatening injury. Death may occur from systemic air embolism.
  - Middle ear and cochlea
  - Eyes
  - Bowels mesentery and omentum
  - Brain
  - Homogenous solid tissues, e.g. liver and muscle are usually not affected.
b. Under water blast (explosion under water)
  - Gastrointestinal tract (most common)
  - Lungs due to pressure transmitted from abdomen through diaphragm)
  - No injury due to secondary impact so very little external but massive internal damage.
c. Solid blast (explosion energy spreads through rigid structure, e.g. tank or warship)
  - Skeleton (most common).
d. Moltov cocktail is an incendiary bomb (a bottle filled with gasoline and a rag to serve as a wick) that is thrown by hand.

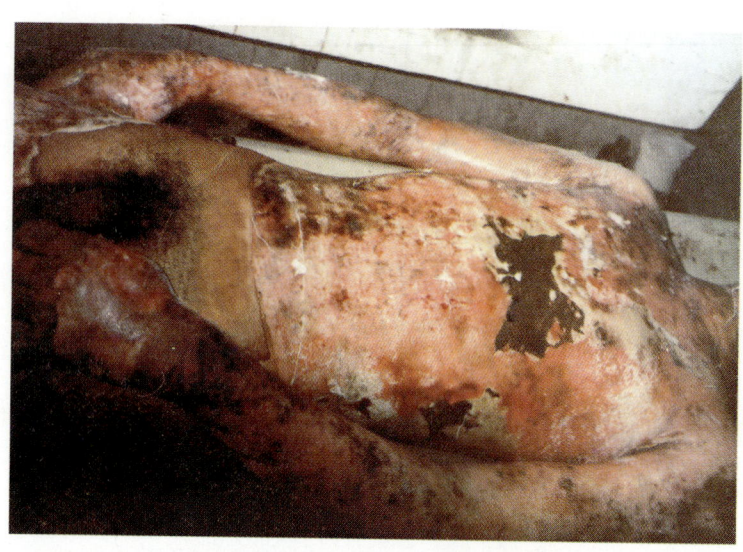

Burns in varying stages of healing

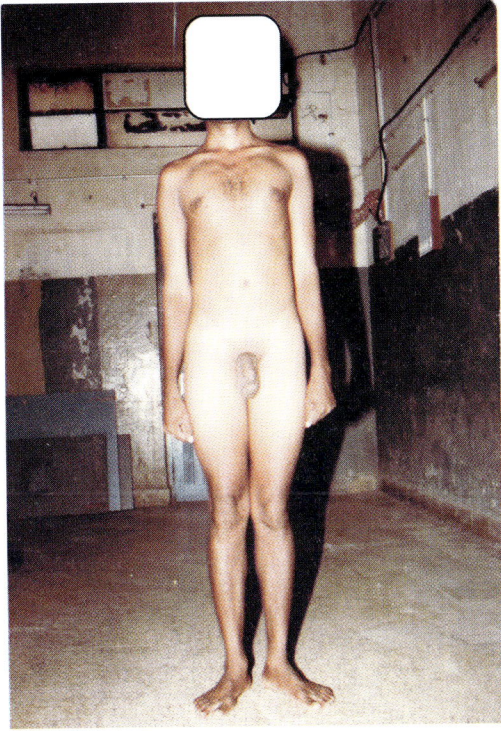

Case of impotence due to electric current
applied at the scrotal region

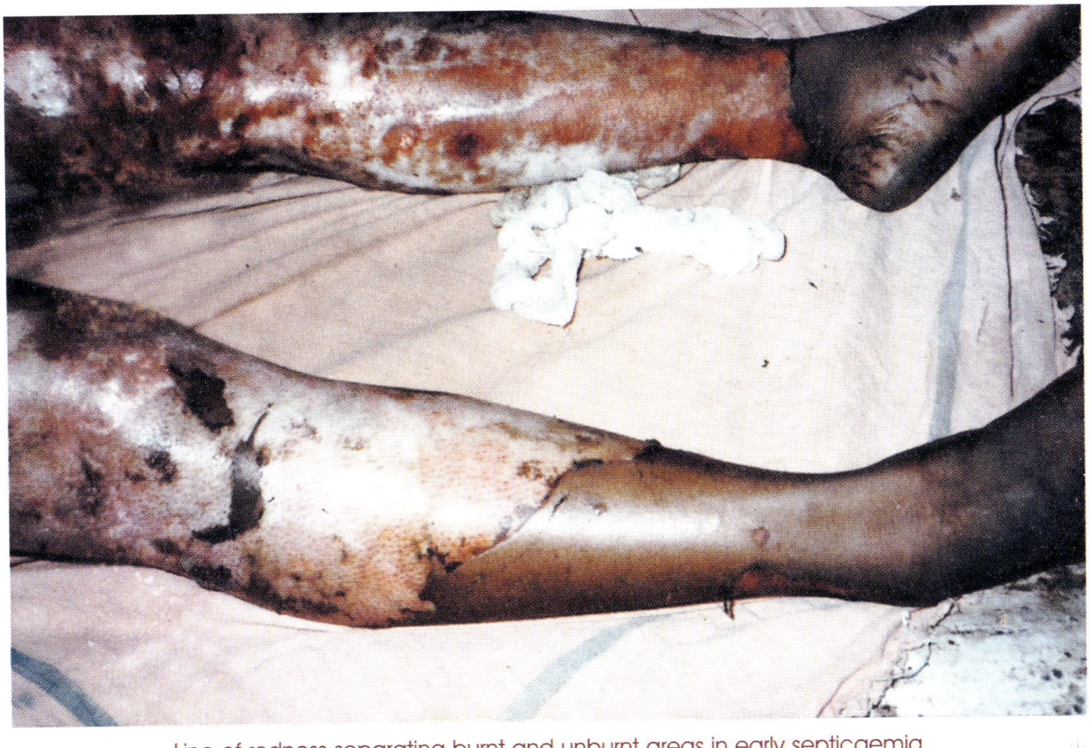

Line of redness separating burnt and unburnt areas in early septicaemia

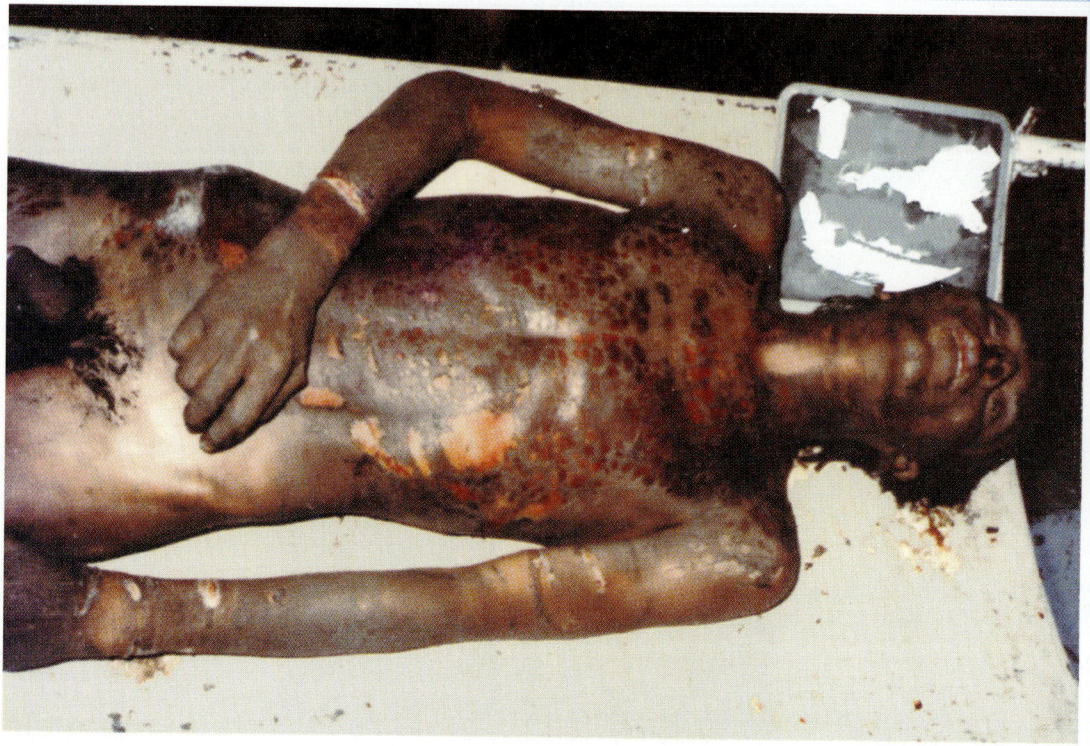

Crocodiling of skin electrocution

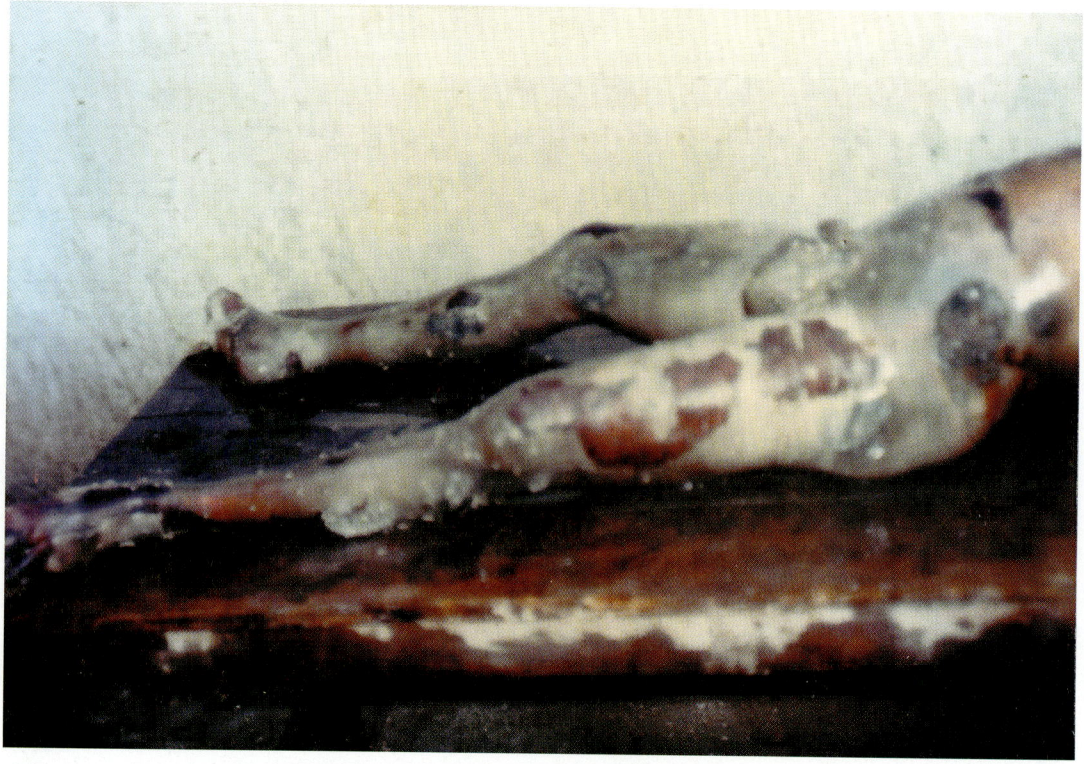

Septicaemia in case of burns. *Courtesy*: Dr PH Barai

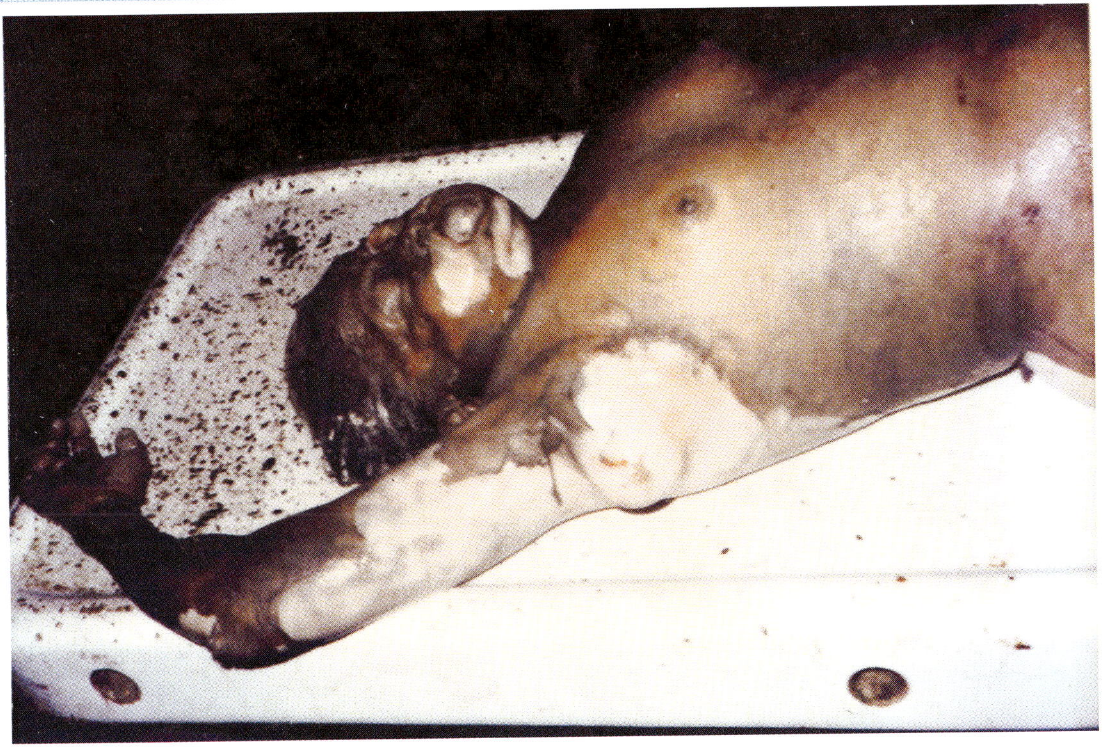

Burns—septicaemic. *Courtesy*: Dr PH Barai

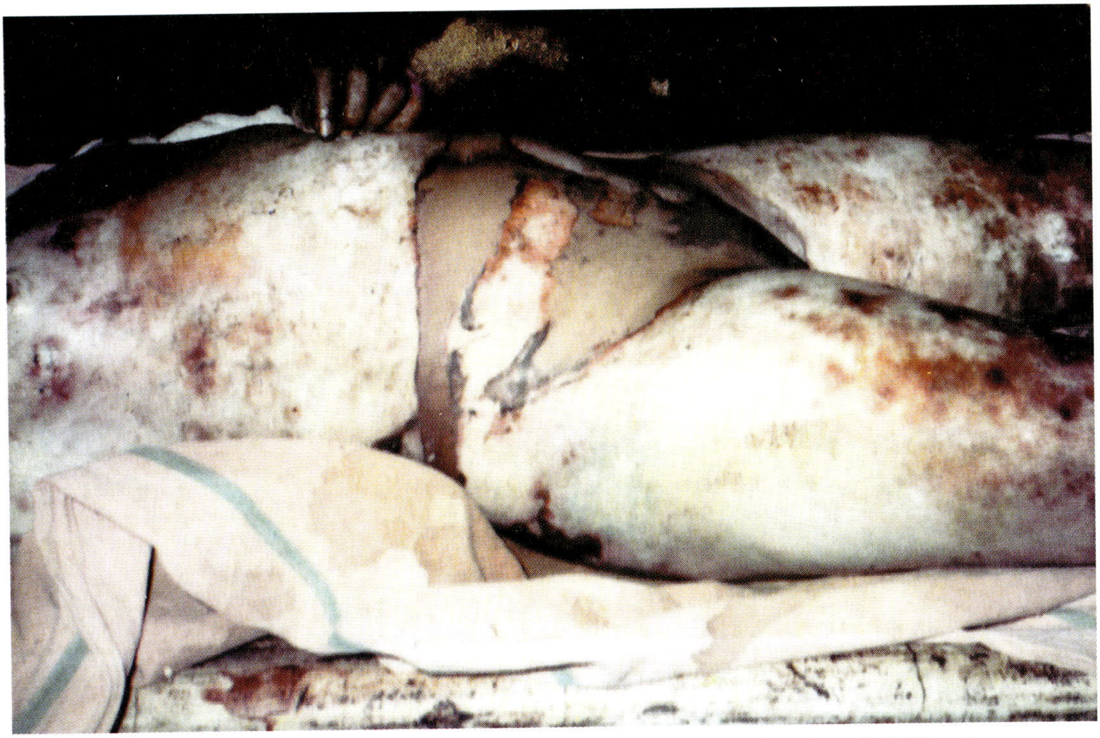

Burnt and unburnt area line of demarcation septicaemia. *Courtesy*: Dr PH Barai

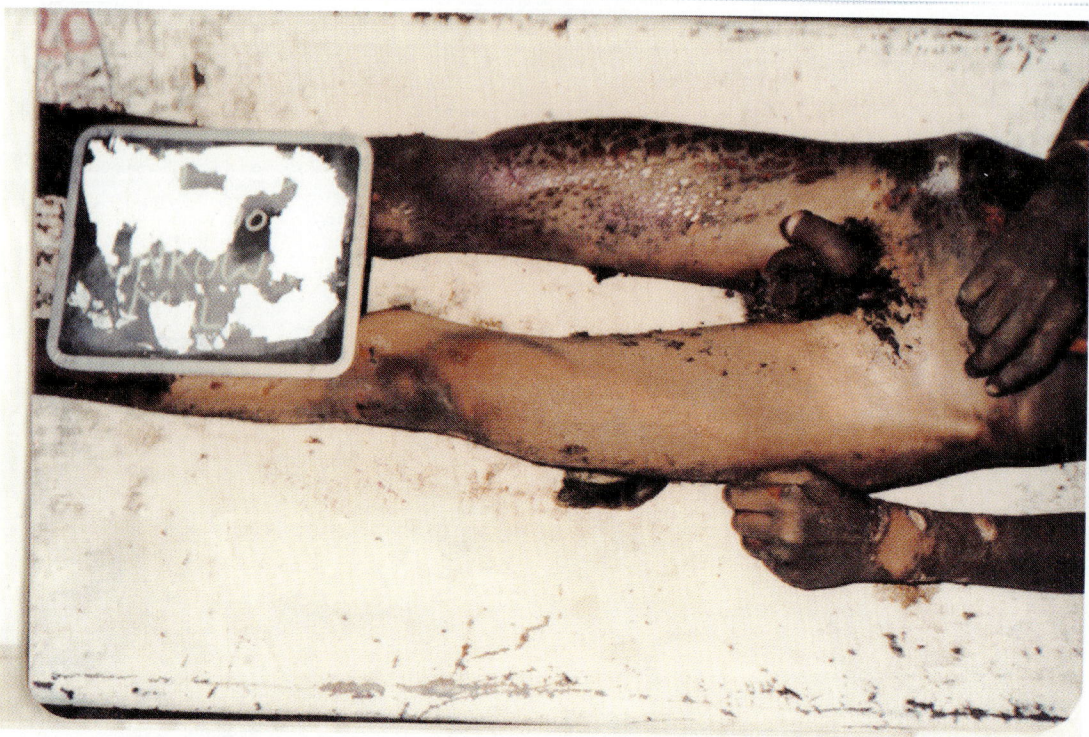

Crocodiling of skin electrocution over railway line 11,000 watts. *Courtesy*: Dr PH Barai

CHAPTER 8

Sexual Offences

Crimes connected with sexual activity are sexual offences. Rape is considered as a natural sexual offence sodomy is concerned as unnatural sexual offence. Bestiality is also unnatural sexual offence.

RAPE (UNDER SECTION 375 OF IPC)

A man is guilty of rape if he has coitus with a woman:

- Without consent
- Against her will
- With her consent when consent is obtained by putting her in fear of death or hurt.
- With her consent, when consent is obtained under intoxication or when woman is of unsound mind and unable to understand the act for which she has consented.
- With her consent, when she believes him to be the person lawfully married to and the person knows that he is not her husband.
- With or without consent, when she is less than 16 years of age.
  - To constitute rape, coitus must be unlawful because lawful intercourse is in between legal wedlock couple.
  - Coitus by a man with his own wife is rape if she is less then 15 years of age.
  - Coitus means genital intercourse between male and female or union of male and female genitalia.
  - The term sexual intercourse is inappropriate as it does not convey a clear meaning.

- Full penile penetration into vagina is not necessary to constitute coitus.
- Partial penetration even up to vulva is sufficient.
- Proof of hymenal rupture is also not necessary.
- Similarly ejaculation of semen is also not necessary to constitute coitus.

Consent means voluntary permission

- It must be either expressed, implied and legally valid.
- A woman above 16 years of age can give valid consent.
- Consent and will are not the same.
- A person may consent though not willing for intercourse and vice versa.
- Consent should be obtained before the Act is commenced and in full senses (not under intoxication).
- Consent must have been freely and voluntarily given and must not have extorted by force, fraud, undue influence or intoxication. Just because she has submitted herself to coitus, it does not mean that she has given consent.
- Consent must be obtained even in the case of prostitutes.

Statutory Rape

- Statutory rape is the rape committed by a man on a girl who is below the age of 18 years even with her consent (with his wife when she is below 15 years of age).

161

Gang Rape

When more than one person commit rape on a woman it is called gang rape.

Custody Rape

When rape is committed on a woman by a person in whose custody she is presumed to be kept safe, e.g. police officer, management or staff of hospital, superintendent of jail or remand home, etc.

Sexual Offences not Considered as Rape

When a person has coitus with a woman with her consent, it does not amount to rape when she is above 18 years (or age of consent). However, if the accused has custody, guardianship or control of the woman and with her consent such coitus is considered as natural sexual offence not amounting to rape and is punished.

Examination of Rape Victim

- No age is safe from rape.
- Rape of children is common in our country because of false belief that venereal diseases are cured by coitus with virgins.

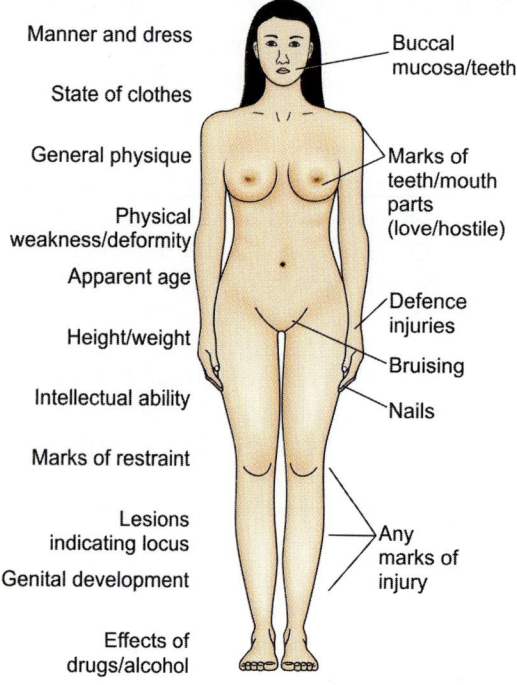

Manner and dress

State of clothes

General physique

Physical weakness/deformity

Apparent age

Height/weight

Intellectual ability

Marks of restraint

Lesions indicating locus

Genital development

Effects of drugs/alcohol

Buccal mucosa/teeth

Marks of teeth/mouth parts (love/hostile)

Defence injuries

Bruising

Nails

Any marks of injury

Fig. 8.1: Examination of rape victim

Because of genital disproportion, extensive genital injuries are seen and even death may result.

- It is normally impossible to rape a healthy, robust female in full possession of her senses.
- When older women are raped, extra-genital injuries are less as they do not resist like young and healthy women.

Usually sent by police officers/magistrate. Careful and thorough examination is required and must be conducted without any delay as follows:

Name: ....

Parent/Guardian's Name: ....

Sex: ....

Age: ....

(Confirmed by physical and radiological examinations)

Height

Weight   } to assess the age

Dental formula

Build: ....
Important for reasons of offering resistance. A labour class sturdy woman can resist the assault and so it is difficult to rape her. Similarly, physique of the accused must also be noted.

Consent: ....
Written consent of the victim if she is above 12 years and of parent/guardian if below 12 years.

Name of female attendant in the presence of whom victim is examined: ....

Identification Marks

Marital status: In case of married woman it is difficult to prove rape as she is already used to coitus.

History of incident: ....
Detailed history with date and time of incident, place and circumstances when offence was committed.

Position of both persons during the offence; resistance offered, etc.

Gait of the victim: ....
Due to genital pain, gait is painful and broadbased.

Clothing: ....
Look for tears, loss of buttons, stains like blood, mud, grass, saliva, semen.

Hair on the clothes: ....
The stains must be preserved for grouping. Presence of seminal stains on clothes of victim is insignificant but on the body is significant.

General Examination

Breasts: ....
Examined for their development, presence of bite marks, suction marks, salivary stains, etc.

Extragenital injuries: ....
Like abrasions, contusions, etc.

Genital Examination

Done in lithotomy position in good light (Fig. 8.2).

Pubic hair: .... Look for matting (due to semen); loose hair (victim's hair).

Vulva: .... Look for injuries, blood/seminal stains.

Vagina: .... Look for injuries, 10–20 ml of saline is put into posterior fornix and aspirated back and sample examined for motile sperms. Sperms live in vagina for only two hours and in uterus/cervix for up to 72 hours.

Presence of sperms is a definite proof of rape in a child but not in adult. Absence of sperm, does not rule out rape. If vaginal smear shows *Mycobacterium smegmatis*, it indicates coitus.

Presence of spermatozoa in female genital tract

Spermatozoa	Detected for about
Motile sperms in vagina	6–8 hours and occasionally about 12 hours
Nonmotile sperms in vagina	24 hours, occasionally up to 48–72 hours and rarely 96 hours
Motile sperms in uterine cavity	3–5 days
Nonmotile form in female genital tract	Week to months after death

Smear should also be examined for presence of gonococci. If chancre is present exudate should be examined for *Treponema pallidum*. If venereal disease is present, look for:

- The disease in the accused.
- The disease appeared in victim after the alleged act of coitus.
- Victim was healthy before coitus.
- Hymen may be intact (elastic) or torn. If ruptured, note number of tears, position, edges, tenderness, etc.

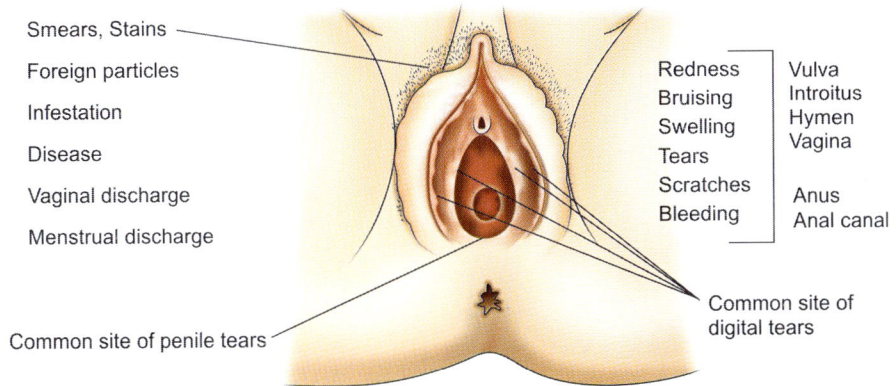

Fig. 8.2: Examination of external genitals of victim of rape

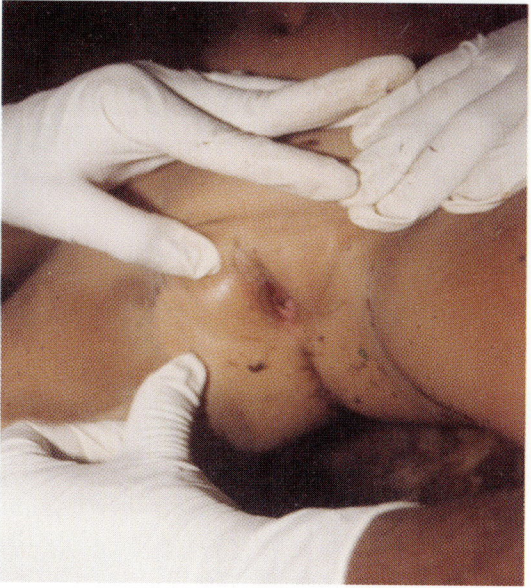

Fig. 8.3: Hymen—tear

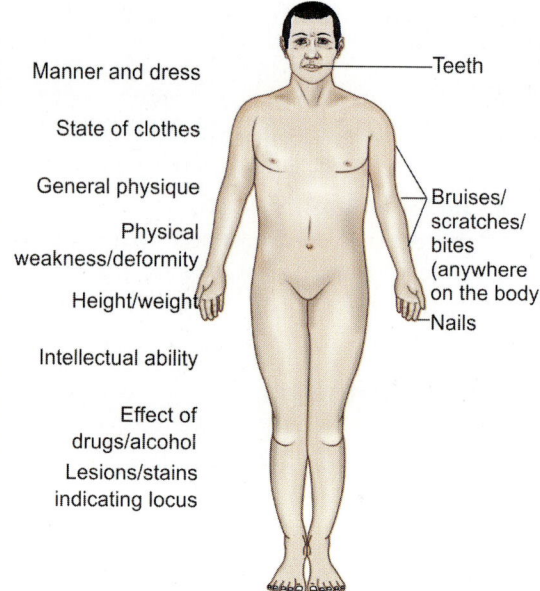

Fig. 8.5: Examination of rape accused

- Frenulum injured when great force is used.
- Perineum—perineal tear may be present if there is gross genital disproportion.

Examination of Accused

The accused is also examined in the same manner:

- He should also be examined for impotence.
- Penis should be examined for presence of frenum tears and vaginal epithelial cells.

Penis is wiped with clean filter paper and then paper is exposed to vapours of Lugol's iodine. Brownish discolouration due to presence of glycogen indicates presence of vaginal epithelial cells.

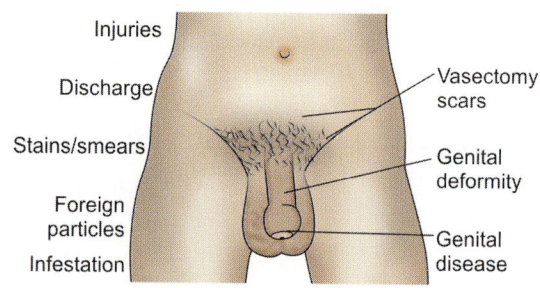

Fig. 8.6: Examination of genitals of accused of rape

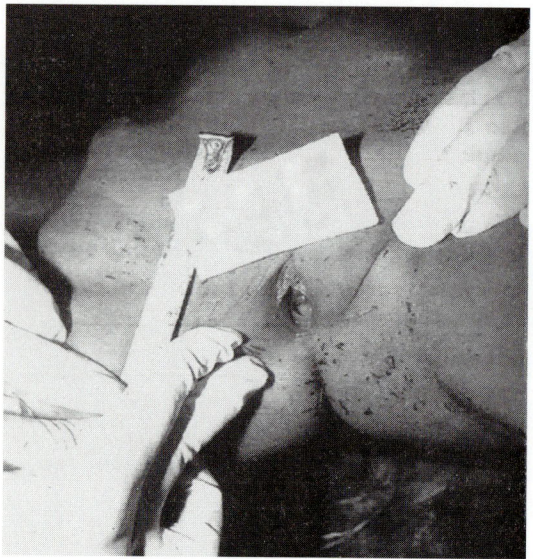

Fig. 8.4: Demonstration of hymen

SEXUAL DEVIATIONS

- Both law and customs permit only heterosexual intercourse between man and wife with the sexual organs intended for the purpose.
- Anything which departs from this is abnormal and is called **sexual** deviation.
- A person who indulges in sexual deviation is called **deviate.**

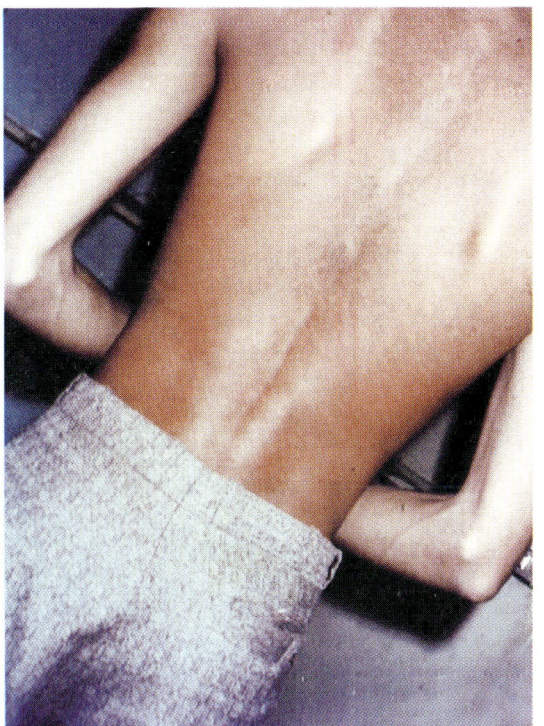

Fig. 8.7: Parallel bruise mark (fresh) accused of rape. *Courtesy*: Dr PH Barai

• These are usually the result of sexual starvation. When natural outlet of coitus is denied to a man, he indulges in abnormal sexual practices.

Sodomy (Buggery)

• A man is said to commit sodomy if he has anal intercourse and is called **active agent** and the victim of intercourse is another man or woman.

• The victim is **passive agent.** If passive agent is a child, it is called **paederasty** and the child is called **catamite.**

• In sodomy, both the persons can act as active or passive agents alternatively. Usually practiced among inmates of jail, hostel, etc.

• If Act is committed with consent, both are punished; if without the consent, only assailant is punished.

• An adult cannot commit sodomy on a sleeping child without waking him up. The catamite is generally murdered after the Act.

• False allegations are quite common. While investigating, both active and passive agents are to be examined.

Findings of Active Agent

• Usually adult male
• Presence of signs of struggle

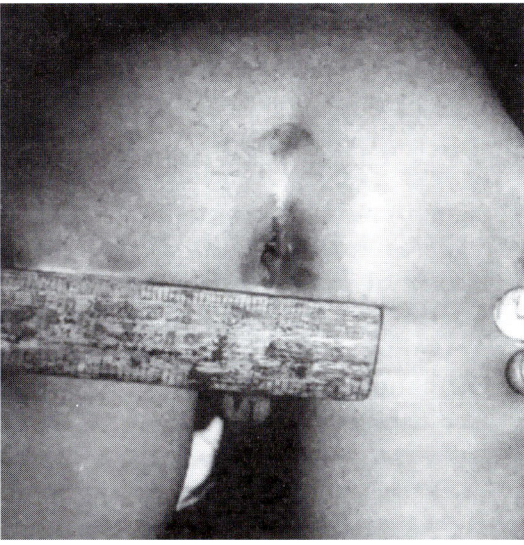

Fig. 8.8: Fresh tear in a passive agent of sodomy

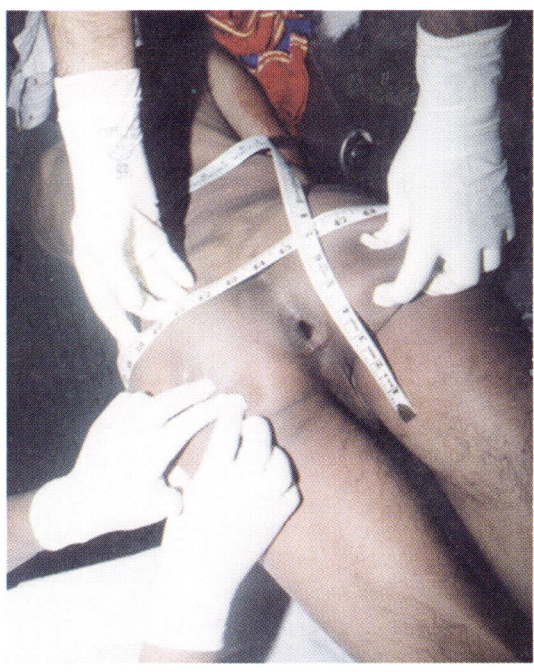

Fig. 8.9: External anal examination in sodomy case

- Presence of mud, seminal fluid, blood or faecal stains on clothes of person.
- Genital findings:
  - Shaved pubic hairs.
  - Faecal stains on penis.
  - Evidence of lubrication on penis.
  - Torn frenum.
  - Occasionally constriction near tip of penis due to anal sphincter in case of repeated sodomy.

Findings of Catamite

- Usually a young boy
- Painful gait
- Signs of struggle on clothes of person
- Signs of faecal, blood, seminal stains on clothes of person
- Anal hair may be shaven or matted
- Anus may be lubricated
- Defecation painful
- In a habitual, anal skin may be thickened and keratinized
- Evidence of recent injury (tear) or venereal disease
- Loss of anal rugosity, infundibulum type anus and laxity of anal sphincter.

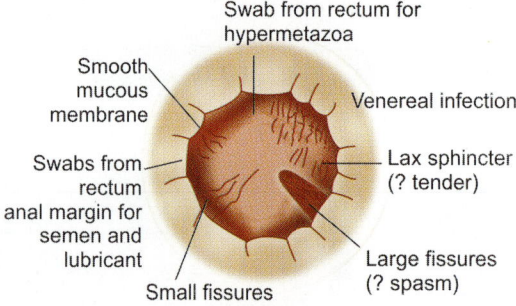

Fig. 8.10: Sodomy: Examination of victim

Hijrah and Zenana (Male Prostitutes)

- Hijrahs are the people who earn livelihood by prostituting themselves as catamites of sodomy.
- They are habitual catamites.
- Because their genitals are cut, they are safe from mischief.
- Hijrahs however perpetuate their tribe by recruiting boys to their tribe and cutting off their genitals.

- This is performed by their own barber; opium is used as a dose and hot oil is used to dress the operated area when the wound heals.
- On cursory examination, the genitals resemble female ones.
- If castration is done before puberty, these boys develop feminine characteristics.
- They dress like women and are a source of pleasure for vulgar youth.
- Zenanas are people who serve the same purpose, but their genitals are intact.

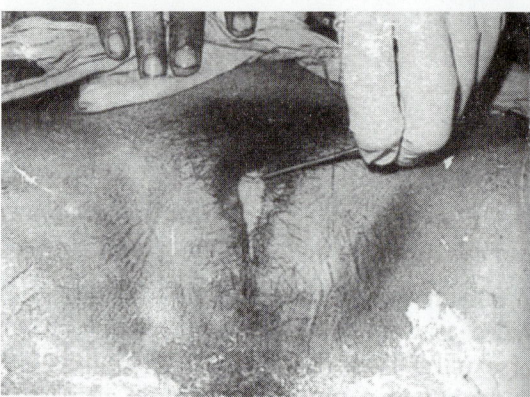

Fig. 8.11: External genitals of a Hijrah (the iron nail tied with thread around waist is kept inserted in urethra to prevent urethral stricture)

Bestiality

- It is sexual intercourse by a man or woman with a lower animal.
- May be committed by both man and woman.
- Any animal may be used, e.g. sheep, cat, dog, buffalo, etc.
- Sexual intercourse may be effected through any orifice of the animal, e.g. anus, vagina, mouth, nostril.
  - Generally because of the result of sexual starvation and also due to a belief that venereal diseases are cured by having coitus with animal.
  - Difficult to prove without a thorough examination of accused and animal.

Findings on Accused

- Usually a young adult
- Injuries due to bites or kicks

- Animal hairs or blood on person
- Blood or faecal stains on penis
- Injuries over penis.

Findings on Animal

- Presence of human hairs
- Presence of sperms in animal orifice.

Exhibitionism (Indecent Exposure)

- It is a sexual offence wherein sexual pleasure is obtained by indecently exposing genitals to members of opposite sex in public (*exhibere*—to display).
  - More common in males
  - Usually seen in public lavatories and may be followed by masturbation.

Tribadism

- A sexual deviation wherein women derive sexual pleasure by mutual friction of genitals. Also called female homosexuality.
- In Greek mythology, woman of Isles of Lesbos practised this deviation, hence called **lesbianism**.
- Usually seen in women suffering from nymphomania (excessive sexual desire) or who have repulsion for men.
- It is not punishable in law.

Transvestism

- A deviation where sexual pleasure is obtained by wearing clothes of opposite sex (*trans*—opposite; *vest*—cloth).
- The person is called **transvestite.**

Sadism

- Type of sexual deviation where sexual pleasure is obtained by beating, whipping, biting or torturing the sexual partner.
- May be practised by both sexes, but more common in males.
- The deviate is called the **sadist** (named after Marquis De Sade, a French man, a sexual pervert).
- Rarely a sadist may murder his partner which is called **lust murder.**

Necrophagia

It is the extreme form of sadism where sadist drives sexual pleasure by tearing out genitals of corpse and eating them (*necros*—corpse; *phagia*—to eat).

Necrophilia

- The sadist derives pleasure by having coitus with dead body.
- Common in young males (*necros*—corpse; *philia*—to defile).

Masochism

- Type of sexual deviation where sexual pleasure is obtained by being tortured by one's sexual partner.
- It is opposite of sadism named after Leopold Masoch who has described this deviation in the characters in his books.

Bondage

Condition where both sadism and masochism are present.

Incest

- Refers to coitus between persons who are within forbidden degrees of marital relationships, i.e. blood relatives.
- If a man is so related with woman that he is prohibited to marry her, has coitus with her, then he commits incest, e.g. father and daughter, brother and sister, etc.

Buccal Coitus

- Refers to sexual intercourse through mouth and is usually practised by adult males on young children.
- This practice was prevalent in a town by name of Gomorrah.

Fetichism

- Refers to sexual deviation wherein sexual pleasure is obtained by contact or sight of clothes of opposite sex.
- To the person, also called fetichist, the object serves as a symbol of real sex.
- The very sight or touch of the object arouses him and he may masturbate on it.

Masturbation

- Refers to a condition wherein sexual pleasure is derived by self stimulation of genitals.
- Seen in both men and women.
- In males, pleasure is obtained by rubbing the penis or moving the penis against bed or any other object.
- In females, genitalia may be rubbed by hand or against pillow or bed or by insertion of fingers, bananas, test tubes, etc. into the vagina.
- It is an offence when practised in public.

Voyeurism

- It is opposite of exhibitionism.
- Sexual pleasure is obtained by seeing at sexual organs of opposite sex or sexual intercourse of any couple.
- The person is called voyer or **Peeping Tom.**
- The person may masturbate afterwards. In India, voyeurism is crime as per the recent criminal law amendment.

Undinism

Sexual pleasure is obtained by seeing someone else urinate or by urinating on person of opposite sex or by getting urinated upon by person of opposite sex.

Trolism

Refers to a condition where a person gets sexual pleasure by inducing his wife to have sexual intercourse with another man and observing the same.

Satyriasis

Excessive sexual desire in man is called satyriasis.

Nymphomania

Excessive sexual desire in females is called nymphomania.

Frotteurism

- Here sexual pleasure is obtained by rubbing one's private parts with others in public.
- Section 377 of IPC lays down the punishment for such unnatural sexual offences.

SEMENOLOGY (STUDY OF SEMINAL STAINS)

- Detection of seminal stains arises in cases of rape and other sexual offences.
- Stains may be found on accused or victim, clothes, bed clothes, place of offence, etc.
- Routine examination of seminal stains is carried out by chemical examiner.
- When clothing bears seminal stains, it is dried in shade, to prevent putrefaction and then sealed and sent.

Semen

- It consists of fluid portion and a cellular portion.
- The fluid portion is formed in seminal vesicles and prostate.
- Cellular portion is formed in testes.

Contents

Fluid portion

- Choline and lecithin—seminal vesicles.
- Acid phosphatase, phosphorus and spermin—prostate.
- Lipoglycoprotein, deoxyriboglycoprotein, hyaluronidase.

Cellular portion

- Spermatozoa and epithelial cells—testes.
- Tests for semen depend upon detection of these substances from it.

Examination

Naked Eye Examination

- Quantity—single ejaculation is usually 2–5 ml.
- Colour—yellowish white opalescent.
- Odour—typical seminal odour.
- Consistency—viscous and sticky when fresh and becomes fluid later.
- Reaction—slightly alkaline pH 7.5.
- Miscellaneous—when semen dries on cloth, it stiffens the cloth and gives starchy feel.

When semen is examined under ultraviolet light, it glows with bluish fluorescence. This is however nonspecific as other albuminous materials like urine and faeces are also positive.

Chemical Examination

- Stains on clothing are extracted as follows:
  - Part of the stained cloth is cut out and soaked in a petridish containing acidulated water (1 drop of H_2SO_4 in 30 ml of water) for one hour and the extract is used for the test.
  - If dry stains are present on body they are gently scraped out with scalpel and mixed with normal saline in petridish.

Acid Phosphatase Test

- Introduced by F. Lundquist in 1945, based on the fact that semen contains a very high quantity of acid phosphatase 25 KA units or more. Other body fluids also contain acid phosphatase but in less amount.
- The great advantage of this test lies in its value in detecting seminal origin of stains as in aspermia.

The following tests are not specific for semen. Also called primary sorting tests

- *Alizarin test*: 0.01% aqueous solution of alizarin sodium sulphate when added to extract turns violet in colour.
- *Ammonium molybdate test*: Ammonium molybdate when dissolved in nitric acid renders the extract a deep yellow colour due to phosphorus.
- *Creatine phosphokinase test*: CPK is in high concentration in seminal fluid. It is detected up to 6 months. More than 400 units means presence of sperms.
- p30 semen specific glycoprotein of prostatic origin is detected up to 27–47 hours (detected in aspermic or normal).

Microchemical Tests

- **Barberio's test** (named after Michele Barberio, a physician of Naples): When Barberio reagent (saturated aqueous solution of picric acid) is added to the extract on glass slide, rhomboid needle shaped crystals of spermin picrate are formed. Detects spermine and the crystals resemble charcoal layden crystals.
- **Florence test** (named after Albert Florence, a French physician): When few drops of Florence's reagent (iodine + potassium iodide + distilled water) is added to the extract on the glass slide, dark brown rhombic crystals of choline periodide are formed. Detects choline; neither specific nor sensitive. May be negative if stain is decomposed or when choline is low. Other body fluids may be positive too.
- **On adding:** A few drops of dilute sulphuric acid to extract of seminal stain, a white crystalline precipitate of calcium sulphide is formed.
- **Seminal:** Stains when treated with 2% aqueous solution of eosin yields lanceolate crystals.

Microscopic Examination

- Consists of looking for sperms in an unstained preparation or stained slide.
- In a healthy adult, total number of sperms in one ejaculate is about 500 millions of which at least 80% must be actively motile. Sperm count can be done by using haemocytometer pipette and counting chamber and a suitable diluting fluid, just like blood cell counts are made.
- Examination of fresh specimen from vagina is done by aspirating vaginal contents with pipette.
- Spermatozoa remain motile in vagina for only 2 hours. So, if motile sperms are seen it means coitus has been indulged within that period. Care must be taken not to mistake *Trichomonas vaginalis* with sperms. Absence of sperms does not rule out coitus.
- For staining, haemotoxylin and eosin or Ziehl-Neelsen staining methods are used. In haemotoxylin and eosin stain, tail, body and proximal part of the head appears red and rest of the head appears blue.
- A sperm atazoan has an oval flattened head measuring 5 μm in length and 3 μm in breadth, a short body and a long filamentous tail. Total sperm length is 50–55 μm.
- If entire sperm or fragment is seen, it is an absolute proof that the stain is seminal. Positive acid phosphatase and other tests indicate stain to be of seminal origin. In case of azoospermia, immuno-electrophoretic determination of specific

protein components of semen helps in identification.

DNA analysis: This can be performed on any tissue or substance that contains nucleated cells. The two most common tissues examined are blood and semen.

Serological examination: Based on precipitin test. This helps in finding out whether seminal stain is human or not, also acid phosphatase test like blood, seminal grouping can also be done.

Other Stains which Resemble Seminal Stains

• **Starch stains**—show starch granules in microscope and do not show fluorescence.

• **Pus stains**—show presence of large number of pus cells and microorganisms.

• **Leucorrheal stains**—show epithelial cells as well as microorganisms.

• **Egg white stains**—all the tests for semen are negative.

RAPE: ADDITIONAL READING

DEFINITION

Rape has been defined as the Act of taking anything by force. Most statutes in the United States define rape as carnal knowledge of a person against the will of the person. Two elements are necessary to constitute the crime:

1. Sexual intercourse, and
2. Failure to seek or to obtain the consent of the victim. Neither complete penetration of the vagina by the penis nor emission of seminal fluid is necessary. Most rapes include force or violence applied to the victim in order to accomplish the Act, but acquiescence can be obtained by verbal threat or other circumstances indicating lack of consent.

In group rape there is evidently a higher frequency of both alcohol intake and prior criminal records, especially of sexual offences. The assault is usually planned and is more brutal in terms of beatings and subjecting the victim to sexually humiliating practices in addition to the rape.

When the complaint reaches trail, there are three major elements of the legal defense in a rape case:

1. Lack of identification—that the man accused is not the perpetrator of the crime.
2. Lack of penetration—that a sexual act did not take place.

3. Consent—that the intercourse was consented to or voluntary on the part of the woman.

Gates and Wood recommend a redefinition of rape to include oral and anal intercourse and a delineation of varieties of rape to be contingent on the degree of force or violence used. They suggest that the resistance standard be dependent on "reasonable fear" and whether victim resistance was reasonable to expect under the circumstances of the assault. Reduced or graded penalties as with a system of degrees for rape, line with comparable violent crimes, would increase the likelihood of convictions.

RAPE TRAUMA SYNDROME

Rape is an ultimate violation of self short of homicide, with invasion of one's inner and most private space, as well as the loss of autonomy and control. Thus, it is irrelevant to differentiate vaginal, anal, or oral intercourse when it is the self and not an orifice that has been invaded. The core meaning of rape would be the same, whether the victim were a virgin, a prostitute, a housewife, or a lesbian.

Descriptions of stress reactions generally define **four stages** which vary in intensity and duration. These responses are also found in rape victims.

An anticipatory or threat phase in which some anxiety facilitates perception of potentially dangerous situations so that they can be avoided. Most people protect themselves with a combination of internal psychological mechanisms which enable them to maintain an illusion of invulnerability, with enough reality perception to be protected from real danger. Thus, in situations where a potential stress is planned (i.e. elective surgery), individuals can protect themselves by strengthening those mechanisms which will ward off feelings of helplessness.

An impact phase in which varying degrees of disintegration may occur in a previously well-adapted person, depending on the degree of trauma and the adaptive capacity of the individual. During this phase, major physiologic reactions, including cardiovascular and sensorial shifts, may occur. The responses of people vary, from those who remain calm to those who respond with confusion, anxiety, and even hysterical outburst. Most victims show variable but less extreme responses. They demonstrate restricted attention span and automatic or stereotyped behaviour. This clinical picture is seen in rape victims as well as in other crisis victims.

A post-traumatic or "recoil" phase in which emotional expression, self-awareness, memory, and behaviour control are gradually regained. Nevertheless, perspective may remain limited and dependency feeling may increase. Individuals perceive adaptive and maladaptive responses in themselves and may question their own reactions. A positive or negative view of one's ability to cope may affect the course of resolution of the particular trauma and future capacity to respond to stress. Self-esteem may be enhanced or damaged during this phase.

Self-awareness, memory and behavioural control are gradually regained. Nevertheless, perspective may remain limited and dependency feelings may increase. Individuals perceive adaptive and maladaptive responses in themselves and may question their own reactions. A positive or negative view of one's ability to cope may affect the course of resolution of the particular trauma and future capacity to respond to stress. Self-esteem may be enhanced or damaged during this phase.

Post-traumatic, reconstitution phase in which victims try to put their lives back together again. At this time, the loss of self-reassuring mechanisms which had fostered a sense of invulnerability may result in a decrease in self-esteem. The victim then blames herself for lack of perception or attention to danger. When individuals begin to question themselves, and then the ability of the group or of society to be protective, a resulting traumatic neurosis may develop which is designed to protect the individual against further exposure to trauma, but which is psychologically costly, especially since it results in loss of self-esteem and of ability to take risks or to be innovative in other situations.

Rape trauma syndrome is sometimes described in **two stages. An immediate or acute response** in which the victim's lifestyle is disrupted by the rape, and a **long-term process** in which the victim reorganizes herself. In addition, they comment on **two types of acute response: The expressed style** in which the victim is emotional and visibly upset, in contrast with the **controlled style** in which the victim may appear to be calm to the casual observer.

Long-term consequences of rape: There are no systematic data currently available about the long-term consequences of rape. In addition, it is difficult to predict all the long-term needs of the rape victim, since individual response patterns and circumstances differ so much of the reactions which do appear clinically, often at a later date, area as follows:

• Mistrust of men with consequent avoidance or hesitation to form relationships.
• A variety of sexual disturbances, often presenting as sexual dysfunctions and marital conflicts.
• Persistent phobic reactions.
• Anxiety and depression which may be precipitated by seemingly unrelated events which in some way bring back the original trauma.

- Persistent anxiety and avoidance of gynaecologic examinations or procedures.
- Suicide or suicide attempts: Preliminary studies of female suicide attempters suggest the possibility of a relationship between an earlier rape experience and suicide attempts.

Rape crisis centres have the following goals:

1. To provide supportive services to victims.
2. To reform the institutions which deal with victims.
3. To educate themselves and the public on rape-related issues.
4. To reform the law.

Medical Concerns

Medical concerns include the quality of the victim's treatment in the hospital; interactions with medical and nursing staff; extent and type of physical injury; the possibilities of pregnancy and venereal disease; and the pelvic examination. The pelvic examination is a frequent focus for the victim's anger. Because many victims experience the pelvic examination as another rape, adequate preparation is important. Victims also are fearful that their bodies are irrevocably damaged.

Medicolegal Considerations

The physician treating the rape victim has several tasks including immediate care of physical injuries, prevention of venereal disease, prevention of pregnancy, proper medicolegal examination with documentation by evidence collection for law-enforcement purpose, and prevention or alleviation of permanent psychological damage.

As lady doctors must examine the victims, every lady doctor should know all aspects about this crime. If lady doctor is not available a male doctor examines in the presence of female nurse.

Rape: Incidence in India. According to a study done by WHO, every 54 minutes a woman is raped in India. According to the centre for development of women's studies

42 women are raped, everyday in India (i.e.) one every 35 minutes. Only ten out of 100 cases are reported, this is a serious issue for a medicolegal man/woman.

- Presence of sperms is a definite proof of rape in a child, but not in adult. Absence of sperms does not rule out rape.
- If vaginal smear shows smegma bacilli, it indicates coitus.
- Smear should also be examined for presence of gonococci. If venereal diseases are present, look for:
- Disease in the accused.
- Disease appeared in victim after the alleged Act of coitus.
- Victim was healthy before coitus.
- Hymen may be intacat or torn. If ruptured, note number of tears, position, edges, tenderness.
- Frenulum injured when great force is used.
- Perineal tear may be present if there is gross genital disproportion.

SEX-RELATED DEATHS

Deaths during Sexual Activity

Men die not infrequently during sexual intercourse and almost invariably as the result of pre-existing cardiovascular disease, although an occasional death may occur as the result of a ruptured berry aneurysm with intracerebral and subarachnoid haemorrhage. Studies have shown that during sexual intercourse there is an increase in blood pressure, tachycardia, and hyperventilation due to emotional response and muscular exertion. In the presence of a significant degree of cardiovascular disease and an insufficient cardiac reserve, the increased demand on the cardiovascular system cannot be met, and the subject may die.

An autopsy is absolutely mandatory, not only to document the cardiovascular disease but also to rule out the remote possibility of foul play. In addition to any natural disease, one should examine the gastric contents obtain blood for alcohol analysis, and be sure to note lipstick marks on the body surfaces or clothing, as well as any clumsy attempts that have been made to dress the body after death, such as clothing worn backwards or inside out.

Trauma and Mutilation of the Genitals

The male genitalia, by virtue of their pendulant condition and easy vulnerability, are frequently traumatized, and such trauma may result in death. Self-mutilation of the genitalia is not unknown, and the circumstances surrounding such cases often show common features. In another case, a genitals and threw them on the fire in the fireplace. In another case, a subject upset by his homosexuality amputated his genitals after applying a tourniquet. Unfortunately, the tourniquet slipped from the amputation stump and the victim bled to death. In a third case, the subject became contrite after consorting with a prostitute, cut off his genitals and threw them on the kitchen table.

Female Death Related to Sexual Activity

Women almost never suffer a natural death during normal sexual intercourse. Perhaps they have greater control of tendencies to overexcitement, perhaps they take a more passive role, or perhaps they are less susceptible to cardiovascular disease, but for whatever reason, they tend not to die. An unnatural death of female during sexual activity may occur under a variety of circumstances. For instance, death may result from aspiration of semen or impaction of the penis in the hypopharynx. With the increase of interest in oral sex within recent years, we will no doubt see more of these cases. The diagnosis is made by finding where the circumstances so indicate. Because ejaculate loses its opaque, gelatinous consistency with rapidly, the seminal fluid may look no different at autopsy than the normal secretions seen in the trachea and larynx.

A type of death which presents great difficulty for the investigator is the accidental strangulation or suffocation of a female during sexual intercourse. If intercourse is performed in a relatively confined space, such as the back seat of a car, it is possible for the male, during intercourse in the missionary position, to apply undue pressure to the thorax, neck, or face of his partner either with the weight of the body or by application of the forearm to the upper chest and neck. Under these circumstances, the female partner may be asphyxiated and her struggles go unnoticed in the heat of passion.

Sperm survival and prostatic acid phosphatase activity in the vagina of a dead woman are subject to a great deal of variation. Both sperm and prostatic acid phosphatase are extremely resistant to autolytic and decomposition changes and can persist under unsterile conditions for years. In the live female who has sexual intercourse and thereafter assumes an upright position, sperm and acid phospatase are diluted with the natural secretions and drain from the vagina in a matter of hours. In the Christie murders in London in 1953, the bodies of three young women who had been strangled and asphyxiated were found secreted in a kitchen cupboard. Two of them had been dead for approximately 8 weeks. Not only identifiable sperm were so well preserved that the prosector always regretted that he had stained the preparations instead of examining wet mounts, for the felt that the sperm were in such good condition that they might have still been viable.

Simultaneous Sex-related Deaths

A student nurse and her boyfriend were seen to park in front of the nurse's dormitory 5 minutes before the 12 o'clock curfew. At midnight while locking the dormitory doors, the custodian noted the couple still seated in the front seat of the car. Upon investigation he found them both dead in the car through the passenger's window which was rolled down only about 4 inches. In 5 minutes, enough carbon monoxide had entered through this small opening to asphyxiate both occupants. Small wonder then that we see this type of death so frequently where two people are engaged in sexual activity, whose minds are many miles away from the possibility of a defective exhaust system and carbon monoxide intoxication.

The sex murder is understood to involve the killing of an adult female by an adult male. A few of these crimes are premeditated in the sense that the assailant deliberately sets out to find a victim, then sexually assaults and kills her. The usual objective of an assailant is rape or sexual abuse, often with an element of sadism involved. The victim is generally unknown to the assailant and is selected at random from among women who happen to be easily accessible, not uncommonly a waitress, a bar girl, or a prostitute.

In the sadistic killing, infliction of pain upon the victim is a direct source of sexual stimulation and gratification to the assailant. When the sadistic aspect of the crime is emphasized, one often finds mutilation, evisceration, or even evidence of cannibalism. The absence of sperm or acid phosphatase in or on the victim in no way detracts form the sexual nature of the crime, for the sadistic criminal obtains his gratification from the inflicting of pain, not necessarily from sexual contact with the victim. If the body has been mutilated, the disfigurement usually involves the breasts and genital area. If dismemberment is the only form of mutilation present, this does not mean that the crime was committed by a sadistic killer, or in the majority of cases, dismemberment by itself is a method of concealing the crime and preventing identification of the victim, or for allowing for easy disposal of the body.

Occasionally, the victim has a foreign object inserted in her vagina or rectum. This foreign object may be a bottle, table leg, broom handle, or stick, and there may or may not be injury to the genital organs. Death will occur as a result of manual or ligature strangulation, bearing witness once again to the spontaneity of the crime. In such a case, the assailant was usually known by deceased. By this is meant that the subject has had some type of social contact or relationship with the deceased prior to the time of death, not simply a rapist-victim type of relationship. The situation which results in death and the insertion of a foreign object into the vagina follows a pattern. The assailant and victim have sexual relations, usually after a considerable amount of drinking. At the end of the intercourse, the victim may desire to continue the activity or may berate the assailant for his lack of stamina or the quality of his performance. At this point, an argument ensues and the assailant ends by strangling the victim and inserting the foreign object into the vagina. The thought behind this action is that since the assailant cannot fill the victim's vagina with what she desired, he will leave her with a substitute instead. This was graphically demonstrated in a case which occurred in Cleveland, in which an assailant got a sausage from the refrigerator and inserted it into the victim's vagina after she had been strangled.

Child Molestation Deaths

The deliberate killing of a child that does not involve the battered child syndrome may be considered to have an underlying sexual motive, whether or not there is physical evidence of rape or sexual molestation. The male assailant will kill male or female children, depending upon his particular aberration.

Death at the hands of such an assailant is as the result of manual or ligature strangulation, blunt trauma to the head, or stabbing. One does not ordinarily encounter mutilation of the male or female genitalia, any sustained injury being associated with forcible rape, sodomy, or vigorous fondling or rubbing. Traumatic injury may be slight, and tears in the vaginal or rectal mucosa are not always easy to identify. A careful dissection must be carried out after removal of these structures.

Homosexually Related Deaths

Homosexuality is a sexual perversion, not an alternate life style. Many homosexuals are desperately unhappy, and they commit suicide for a number of reasons. The homosexual may be consumed by feelings of guilt about his way of life. He may be threatened with exposure, blackmail, or disgrace before family or friends. He may commit suicide because of unrequited love or a blighted romance.

Sudden death may occur during fellatio as the result of aspiration of ejaculate with subsequent asphyxiation, or as the result of asphyxiation due to impaction of the penis in the hypopharynx.

It is not unusual for the anal inserter to grasp the passive partner's neck in his hands, or to twist a towel or pillowcase around the neck, or to cover the head or upper part of the body with pillows or a mattress during the sex act.

One cannot make the diagnosis of homosexuality solely on the basis of physical findings at autopsy, although, in the confirmed sodomite, one may see epithelialization of the rectal mucosa.

A male homosexual will sometimes become attached to, and often marry a wealthy older woman. She provides money, social status, and makes no sexual demands; he provides companionship and, quite often, care and genuine affection.

Autoerotic Asphyxia

Basically, the death involves asphyxiation by constriction of the neck in the course of a sexual fantasy or masturbation. In most cases, a rope or ligature is placed around the neck, and the free end of the rope is secured to a fixed object (hanging) or to one of the extremities of the body. Anoxia is produced by placing tension on the rope with resultant constriction of the veins of the neck and decreased blood flow to the brain. Death occurs when the anoxia is carried too far and the subject blacks out, at which time the weight of the body or the weight or tension of the extremity causes the ligature around the neck to tighten and the subject dies. It is thought that the production of partial anoxia during sexual activity heightens the feeling of sexual pleasure.

In addition, constriction of the neck, there may be binding of the head with a gag, mask, or blindfold; binding of the trunk and extremities with ropes. Ligatures, tape, or chains; pinioning of the extremities with handcuffs, shackles, leg irons, belts, or leather thongs; binding of the genitals or suspension of heavy weights from the genitals; or insertion of foreign objects into the rectum.

In the early adolescent stage, we find the individual suspended with the body fully clad, but with the penis or genitals exposed and frank evidence of masturbation. In this type of case, if the body is first discovered by the family, the clothing may be disturbed before the authorities are called.

In the sex hanging we see manifestations of sadism, masochism, transvestism, fetishism, and narcissism.

THE PROTECTION OF CHILDREN FROM SEXUAL OFFENCES ACT, 2012

1. Short Title, Extent and Commencement

1. This Act may be called the **Protection of Children from Sexual Offences Act, 2012**.
2. It extends to the **whole of India**, except the state of Jammu and Kashmir.
3. It shall come into force on such date as the Central Government may, by notification in the Official Gazette, appoint.

2. Definitions

1. In this Act, unless the context otherwise requires:
   a. "Aggravated penetrative sexual assault" has the same meaning as assigned to it in Section 5.
   b. "Aggravated sexual assault" has the same meaning as assigned to it in Section 9.
   c. "Armed forces or security forces" means armed forces of the Union or security forces or police forces, as specified in the Schedule.
   d. **"Child" means any person below the age of eighteen years.**
   e. "Domestic relationship" shall have the same meaning as assigned to it in clause (f) of Section 2 of the Protection of Women from Domestic Violence Act, 2005 (43 of 2005).
   f. "Penetrative sexual assault" has the same meaning as assigned to it in Section 3.

g. Prescribed means prescribed by rules made under this Act.

h. Religious institution shall have the same meaning as assigned to it in the Religious Institutions (Prevention of Misuse) Act, 1988 (41 of 1988)

i. "Sexual assault" has the same meaning as assigned to it in Section 7.

j. "Sexual harassment" has the same meaning as assigned to it in Section 11.

k. "Shared household" means a household where the person charged with the offence lives or has lived at any time in a domestic relationship with the child.

l. "Special Court" means a court designated as such under Section 28.

m. "Special Public Prosecutor" means a Public Prosecutor appointed under Section 32.

2. The words and expressions used herein and not defined but defined in the Indian.

Penal Code (45 of 1860), the Code of Criminal Procedure, 1973 (2 of 1974), the Juvenile Justice (Care and Protection of Children) Act, 2000 (56 of 2000) and the Information Technology Act, 2000 (21 of 2000) shall have the meanings respectively assigned to them in the said Codes or the Acts.

SEXUAL OFFENCES AGAINST CHILDREN

A. PENETRATIVE SEXUAL ASSAULT AND PUNISHMENT THEREFOR

3. Penetrative Sexual Assault

A person is said to commit "penetrative sexual assault" if

a. He penetrates his penis, to any extent, into the vagina, mouth, urethra or anus of a child or makes the child to do so with him or any other person; or

b. He inserts, to any extent, any object or a part of the body, not being the penis, into the vagina, the urethra or anus of the child or makes the child to do so with him or any other person; or

c. He manipulates any part of the body of the child so as to cause penetration into the vagina, urethra, anus or any part of body of the child or makes the child to do so with him or any other person; or

d. He applies his mouth to the penis, vagina, anus, urethra of the child or makes the child to do so to such person or any other person.

4. Punishment for Penetrative Sexual Assault

Whoever commits penetrative sexual assault shall be punished with imprisonment of either description for a term which shall not be less than seven years but which may extend to imprisonment for life, and shall also be liable to fine.

B. AGGRAVATED PENETRATIVE SEXUAL ASSAULT AND PUNISHMENT THEREFOR

5. Aggravated Penetrative Sexual Assault

a. Whoever, being a police officer, commits penetrative sexual assault on a child

   i. Within the limits of the police station or premises at which he is appointed; or

   ii. In the premises of any station house, whether or not situated in the police station, to which he is appointed; or

   iii. In the course of his duties or otherwise; or

   iv. Where he is known as, or identified as, a police officer; or

b. Whoever being a member of the armed forces or security forces commits penetrative sexual assault on a child

   i. Within the limits of the area to which the person is deployed; or

   ii. In any areas under the command of the forces or armed forces; or

   iii. In the course of his duties or otherwise; or

   iv. Where the said person is known or identified as a member of the security or armed forces; or

c. Whoever being a public servant commits penetrative sexual assault on a child; or

d. Whoever being on the management or on the staff of a jail, remand home, protection home, observation home, or other place of custody or care and protection established by or under any law for the time being in force, commits penetrative sexual assault on a child, being inmate of such jail, remand home, protection home, observation home, or other place of custody or care and protection; or

e. Whoever being on the management or staff of a hospital, whether government or private, commits penetrative sexual assault on a child in that hospital; or

f. Whoever being on the management or staff of an educational institution or religious institution, commits penetrative sexual assault on a child in that institution; or

g. Whoever commits gang penetrative sexual assault on a child. Explanation. When a child is subjected to sexual assault by one or more persons of a group in furtherance of their common intention, each of such persons shall be deemed to have committed gang penetrative sexual assault within the meaning of this clause and each of such person shall be liable for that act in the same manner as if it were done by him alone; or

h. Whoever commits penetrative sexual assault on a child using deadly weapons, fire, heated substance or corrosive substance; or

i. Whoever commits penetrative sexual assault causing grievous hurt or causing bodily harm and injury or injury to the sexual organs of the child; or

j. Whoever commits penetrative sexual assault on a child, which

   i. Physically incapacitates the child or causes the child to become mentally ill as defined under clause (b) of Section 2 of the Mental Health Act, 1987 (14 of 1987) or causes impairment of any kind so as to render the child unable to perform regular tasks, temporarily or permanently; or

   ii. In the case of female child, makes the child pregnant as a consequence of sexual assault.

   iii. Inflicts the child with human immunodeficiency virus or any other life-threatening disease or infection which may either temporarily or permanently impair the child by rendering him physically incapacitated, or mentally ill to perform regular tasks; or

k. Whoever, taking advantage of a child's mental or physical disability, commits penetrative sexual assault on the child; or

l. Whoever commits penetrative sexual assault on the child more than once or repeatedly; or

m. Whoever commits penetrative sexual assault on a child below twelve years; or

n. Whoever being a relative of the child through blood or adoption or marriage or guardianship or in foster care or having a domestic relationship with a parent of the child or who is living in the same or shared household with the child, commits penetrative sexual assault on such child; or

o. Whoever being, in the ownership, or management, or staff, of any institution providing services to the child, commits penetrative sexual assault on the child; or

p. Whoever being in a position of trust or authority of a child commits penetrative sexual assault on the child in an institution or home of the child or anywhere else; or

q. Whoever commits penetrative sexual assault on a child knowing the child is pregnant; or

r. Whoever commits penetrative sexual assault on a child and attempts to murder the child; or

s. Whoever commits penetrative sexual assault on a child in the course of communal or sectarian violence; or

t. Whoever commits penetrative sexual assault on a child and who has been previously convicted of having committed any offence under this Act or any sexual offence punishable under any other law for the time being in force; or

u. Whoever commits penetrative sexual assault on a child and makes the child to strip or parade naked in public, is said to commit aggravated penetrative sexual assault.

6. Punishment for Aggravated Penetrative Sexual Assault

Whoever, commits aggravated penetrative sexual assault, shall be punished with rigorous imprisonment for a term which shall not be less than ten years but which may extend to imprisonment for life and shall also be liable to fine.

C. SEXUAL ASSAULT AND PUNISHMENT THEREFOR

7. Sexual Assault

Whoever, with sexual intent touches the vagina, penis, anus or breast of the child or makes the child touch the vagina, penis, anus or breast of such person or any other person, or does any other act with sexual intent which involves physical contact without penetration is said to commit sexual assault.

8. Punishment for Sexual Assault

Whoever, commits sexual assault, shall be punished with imprisonment of either description for a term which shall not be less than three years but which may extend to five years, and shall also be liable to fine.

D. AGGRAVATED SEXUAL ASSAULT AND PUNISHMENT THEREFOR

9. Aggravated Sexual Assault

a. Whoever, being a police officer, commits sexual assault on a child
  i. Within the limits of the police station or premises where he is appointed; or
  ii. In the premises of any station house whether or not situated in the police station to which he is appointed; or
  iii. In the course of his duties or otherwise; or

  iv. Where he is known as, or identified as a police officer; or
b. Whoever, being a member of the armed forces or security forces, commits sexual assault on a child
  i. Within the limits of the area to which the person is deployed; or
  ii. In any areas under the command of the security or armed forces; or
  iii. In the course of his duties or otherwise; or
  iv. Where he is known or identified as a member of the security or armed forces; or
c. Whoever being a public servant commits sexual assault on a child; or
d. Whoever being on the management or on the staff of a jail, or remand home or protection home or observation home, or other place of custody or care and protection established by or under any law for the time being in force commits sexual assault on a child being inmate of such jail or remand home or protection home or observation home or other place of custody or care and protection; or
e. Whoever being on the management or staff of a hospital, whether government or private, commits sexual assault on a child in that hospital; or
f. Whoever being on the management or staff of an educational institution or religious institution, commits sexual assault on a child in that institution; or
g. Whoever commits gang sexual assault on a child.

  Explanation: When a child is subjected to sexual assault by one or more persons of a group in furtherance of their common intention, each of such persons shall be deemed to have committed gang sexual assault within the meaning of this clause and each of such person shall be liable for that act in the same manner as if it were done by him alone; or

h. Whoever commits sexual assault on a child using deadly weapons, fire, heated substance or corrosive substance; or

i. Whoever commits sexual assault causing grievous hurt or causing bodily harm and injury or injury to the sexual organs of the child; or

j. Whoever commits sexual assault on a child, which

  i. Physically incapacitates the child or causes the child to become mentally ill as defined under clause (l) of section 2 of the Mental Health Act, 1987 (14 of 1987) or causes impairment of any kind so as to render the child unable to perform regular tasks, temporarily or permanently; or

  ii. Inflicts the child with human immunodeficiency virus or any other life-threatening disease or infection which may either temporarily or permanently impair the child by rendering him physically incapacitated, or mentally ill to perform regular tasks; or

k. Whoever, taking advantage of a childs mental or physical disability, commits sexual assault on the child; or

l. Whoever commits sexual assault on the child more than once or repeatedly; or

m. Whoever commits sexual assault on a child below twelve years; or

n. Whoever, being a relative of the child through blood or adoption or marriage or guardianship or in foster care, or having domestic relationship with a parent of the child, or who is living in the same or shared household with the child, commits sexual assault on such child; or

o. Whoever, being in the ownership or management or staff, of any institution providing services to the child, commits sexual assault on the child in such institution; or

p. Whoever, being in a position of trust or authority of a child, commits sexual assault on the child in an institution or home of the child or anywhere else; or

q. Whoever commits sexual assault on a child knowing the child is pregnant; or

r. Whoever commits sexual assault on a child and attempts to murder the child; or

s. Whoever commits sexual assault on a child in the course of communal or sectarian violence; or

t. Whoever commits sexual assault on a child and who has been previously convicted of having committed any offence under this Act or any sexual offence punishable under any other law for the time being in force; or

u. Whoever commits sexual assault on a child and makes the child to strip or parade naked in public, is said to commit aggravated sexual assault.

10. Punishment for Aggravated Sexual Assault

Whoever, commits aggravated sexual assault shall be punished with imprisonment of either description for a term which shall not be less than five years but which may extend to seven years, and shall also be liable to fine.

E. SEXUAL HARASSMENT AND PUNISHMENT THEREFOR

11. Sexual Harassment

A person is said to commit sexual harassment upon a child when such person with sexual intent:

  i. Utters any word or makes any sound, or makes any gesture or exhibits any object or part of body with the intention that such word or sound shall be heard, or such gesture or object or part of body shall be seen by the child; or

  ii. Makes a child exhibit his body or any part of his body so as it is seen by such person or any other person; or

  iii. Shows any object to a child in any form or media for pornographic purposes; or

  iv. Repeatedly or constantly follows or watches or contacts a child either directly or through electronic, digital or any other means; or

v. Threatens to use, in any form of media, a real or fabricated depiction through electronic, film or digital or any other mode, of any part of the body of the child or the involvement of the child in a sexual act; or

vi. Entices a child for pornographic purposes or gives gratification therefor. Explanation. Any question which involves sexual intent shall be a question of fact.

12. Punishment for Sexual Harassment

Whoever, commits sexual harassment upon a child shall be punished with imprisonment of either description for a term which may extend to three years and shall also be liable to fine.

USING CHILD FOR PORNOGRAPHIC PURPOSES AND PUNISHMENT THEREFOR

13. Use of Child for Pornographic Purposes

Whoever, uses a child in any form of media (including programme or advertisement telecast by television channels or internet or any other electronic form or printed form, whether or not such programme or advertisement is intended for personal use or for distribution), for the purposes of sexual gratification, which includes:

a. Representation of the sexual organs of a child;

b. Usage of a child engaged in real or simulated sexual acts (with or without penetration);

c. The indecent or obscene representation of a child, shall be guilty of the offence of using a child for pornographic purposes. Explanation. For the purposes of this section, the expression "use a child" shall include involving a child through any medium like print, electronic, computer or any other technology for preparation, production, offering, transmitting, publishing, facilitation and distribution of the pornographic material.

14. Punishment for Using Child for Pornographic Purposes

1. Whoever, uses a child or children for pornographic purposes shall be punished with imprisonment of either description which may extend to five years and shall also be liable to fine and in the event of second or subsequent conviction with imprisonment of either description for a term which may extend to seven years and also be liable to fine.

2. If the person using the child for pornographic purposes commits an offence referred to in Section 3, by directly participating in pornographic acts, he shall be punished with imprisonment of either description for a term which shall not be less than ten years but which may extend to imprisonment for life, and shall also be liable to fine.

3. If the person using the child for pornographic purposes commits an offence referred to in Section 5, by directly participating in pornographic acts, he shall be punished with rigorous imprisonment for life and shall also be liable to fine.

4. If the person using the child for pornographic purposes commits an offence referred to in Section 7, by directly participating in pornographic acts, he shall be punished with imprisonment of either description for a term which shall not be less than six years but which may extend to eight years, and shall also be liable to fine.

5. If the person using the child for pornographic purposes commits an offence referred to in Section 9, by directly participating in pornographic acts, he shall be punished with imprisonment of either description for a term which shall not be less than eight years but which may extend to ten years, and shall also be liable to fine.

15. Punishment for Storage of Pornographic Material Involving Child

Any person, who stores, for commercial purposes any pornographic material in any form involving a child shall be punished with imprisonment of either description which may extend to three years or with fine or with both.

ABETMENT OF AND ATTEMPT TO COMMIT AN OFFENCE

16. Abetment of an Offence

A person abets an offence, who first, instigates any person to do that offence; or secondly, engages with one or more other person or persons in any conspiracy for the doing of that offence, if an act or illegal omission takes place in pursuance of that conspiracy, and in order to the doing of that offence; or thirdly, intentionally aids, by any act or illegal omission, the doing of that offence.

Explanation I: A person who, by willful misrepresentation, or by willful concealment of a material fact, which he is bound to disclose, voluntarily causes or procures, or attempts to cause or procure a thing to be done, is said to instigate the doing of that offence.

Explanation II: Whoever, either prior to or at the time of commission of an act, does anything in order to facilitate the commission of that act, and thereby facilitates the commission thereof, is said to aid the doing of that act.

Explanation III: Whoever employ, harbours, receives or transports a child, by means of threat or use of force or other forms of coercion, abduction, fraud, deception, abuse of power or of a position, vulnerability or the giving or receiving of payments or benefits to achieve the consent of a person having control over another person, for the purpose of any offence under this Act, is said to aid the doing of that act.

17. Punishment for Abetment

Whoever abets any offence under this Act, if the act abetted is committed in consequence of the abetment, shall be punished with punishment provided for that offence.

Explanation: An act or offence is said to be committed in consequence of abetment, when it is committed in consequence of the instigation, or in pursuance of the conspiracy or with the aid, which constitutes the abetment.

18. Punishment for Attempt to Commit an Offence

Whoever attempts to commit any offence punishable under this Act or to cause such an offence to be committed, and in such attempt, does any act towards the commission of the offence, shall be punished with imprisonment of any description provided for the offence, for a term which may extend to one-half of the imprisonment for life or, as the case may be, one-half of the longest term of imprisonment provided for that offence or with fine or with both.

PROCEDURE FOR REPORTING OF CASES

19. Reporting of Offences

1. Notwithstanding anything contained in the Code of Criminal Procedure, 1973 (2 of 1974), any person (including the child), who has apprehension that an offence under this Act is likely to be committed or has knowledge that such an offence has been committed, he shall provide such information to:
   a. The Special Juvenile Police Unit; or
   b. The local police.

2. Every report given under sub-section (1) shall be:
   a. Ascribed an entry number and recorded in writing;
   b. Be read over to the informant;
   c. Shall be entered in a book to be kept by the Police Unit.
3. Where the report under sub-section (1) is given by a child, the same shall be recorded under sub-section (2) in a simple language so that the child understands contents being recorded.
4. In case contents are being recorded in the language not understood by the child or wherever it is deemed necessary, a translator or an interpreter, having such qualifications, experience and on payment of such fees as may be prescribed, shall be provided to the child if he fails to understand the same.
5. Where the Special Juvenile Police Unit or local police is satisfied that the child against whom an offence has been committed is in need of care and protection, then, it shall, after recording the reasons in writing, make immediate arrangement to give him such care and protection (including admitting the child into shelter home or to the nearest hospital) within twenty-four hours of the report, as may be prescribed.
6. The Special Juvenile Police Unit or local police shall, without unnecessary delay but within a period of twenty-four hours, report the matter to the Child Welfare Committee and the Special Court or where no Special Court has been designated, to the Court of Session, including need of the child for care and protection and steps taken in this regard.
7. No person shall incur any liability, whether civil or criminal, for giving the information in good faith for the purpose of sub-section (1).

20. Obligation of Media, Studio and Photographic Facilities to Report Cases

Any personnel of the media or hotel or lodge or hospital or club or studio or photographic facilities, by whatever name called, irrespective of the number of persons employed therein, shall, on coming across any material or object which is sexually exploitative of the child (including pornographic, sexually-related or making obscene representation of a child or children) through the use of any medium, shall provide such information to the Special Juvenile Police Unit, or to the local police, as the case may be.

21. Punishment for Failure to Report or Record a Case

1. Any person, who fails to report the commission of an offence under sub-section (1) of Section 19 or Section 20 or who fails to record such offence under sub-section (2) of Section 19 shall be punished with imprisonment of either description which may extend to six months or with fine or with both.
2. Any person, being in-charge of any company or an institution (by whatever name called) who fails to report the commission of an offence under sub-section (1) of Section 19 in respect of a subordinate under his control, shall be punished with imprisonment for a term which may extend to one year and with fine.
3. The provisions of sub-section (1) shall not apply to a child under this Act.

22. Punishment for False Complaint or False Information

1. Any person, who makes false complaint or provides false information against any person, in respect of an offence committed under Sections 3, 5, 7 and 9, solely with the intention to humiliate, extort or threaten or defame him, shall be punished with imprisonment for a term which may extend to six months or with fine or with both.
2. Where a false complaint has been made or false information has been provided by a child, no punishment shall be imposed on such child.
3. Whoever, not being a child, makes a false complaint or provides false information

against a child, knowing it to be false, thereby victimising such child in any of the offences under this Act, shall be punished with imprisonment which may extend to one year or with fine or with both.

23. Procedure for Media

1. No person shall make any report or present comments on any child from any form of media or studio or photographic facilities without having complete and authentic information, which may have the effect of lowering his reputation or infringing upon his privacy.

2. No reports in any media shall disclose, the identity of a child including his name, address, photograph, family details, school, neighbourhood or any other particulars which may lead to disclosure of identity of the child: Provided that for reasons to be recorded in writing, the Special Court, competent to try the case under the Act, may permit such disclosure, if in its opinion such disclosure is in the interest of the child.

3. The publisher or owner of the media or studio or photographic facilities shall be jointly and severally liable for the acts and omissions of his employee.

4. Any person who contravenes the provisions of sub-section (1) or sub-section (2) shall be liable to be punished with imprisonment of either description for a period which shall not be less than six months but which may extend to one year or with fine or with both.

PROCEDURES FOR RECORDING STATEMENT OF THE CHILD

24. Recording of Statement of a Child

1. The statement of the child shall be recorded at the residence of the child or at a place where he usually resides or at the place of his choice and as far as practicable by a woman police officer not below the rank of sub-inspector.

2. The police officer while recording the statement of the child shall not be in uniform.

3. The police officer making the investigation, shall, while examining the child, ensure that at no point of time the child come in the contact in any way with the accused.

4. No child shall be detained in the police station in the night for any reason.

5. The police officer shall ensure that the identity of the child is protected from the public media, unless otherwise directed by the Special Court in the interest of the child.

25. Recording of Statement of a Child by Magistrate

1. If the statement of the child is being recorded under Section 164 of the Code of Criminal Procedure, 1973 (2 of 1974) (herein referred to as the Code), the Magistrate recording such statement shall, notwithstanding anything contained therein, record the statement as spoken by the child: Provided that the provisions contained in the first proviso to sub-section (1) of Section 164 of the Code shall, so far it permits the presence of the advocate of the accused shall not apply in this case.

2. The Magistrate shall provide to the child and his parents or his representative, a copy of the document specified under Section 207 of the Code, upon the final report being filed by the police under Section 173 of that Code.

26. Additional Provisions Regarding Statement to be Recorded

1. The Magistrate or the police officer, as the case may be, shall record the statement as spoken by the child in the presence of the parents of the child or any other person in whom the child has trust or confidence.

2. Wherever necessary, the Magistrate or the police officer, as the case may be, may take the assistance of a translator

or an interpreter, having such qualifications, experience and on payment of such fees as may be prescribed, while recording the statement of the child.

3. The Magistrate or the police officer, as the case may be, may, in the case of a child having a mental or physical disability, seek the assistance of a special educator or any person familiar with the manner of communication of the child or an expert in that field, having such qualifications, experience and on payment of such fees as may be prescribed, to record the statement of the child.

4. Wherever possible, the Magistrate or the police officer, as the case may be, shall ensure that the statement of the child is also recorded by audio-video electronic means.

27. Medical Examination of a Child

1. The medical examination of a child in respect of whom any offence has been committed under this Act, shall, notwithstanding that a First Information Report or complaint has not been registered for the offences under this Act, be conducted in accordance with Section 164A of the Code of Criminal Procedure, 1973 (2 of 1974).

2. In case the victim is a girl child, the medical examination shall be conducted by a woman doctor.

3. The medical examination shall be conducted in the presence of the parent of the child or any other person in whom the child reposes trust or confidence.

4. Where, in case the parent of the child or other person referred to in sub-section (3) cannot be present, for any reason, during the medical examination of the child, the medical examination shall be conducted in the presence of a woman nominated by the head of the medical institution.

SPECIAL COURTS

28. Designation of Special Courts

1. For the purposes of providing a speedy trial, the State Government shall in consultation with the Chief Justice of the High Court, by notification in the Official Gazette, designate for each district, a Court of Session to be a Special Court to try the offences under the Act: Provided that if a Court of Session is notified as a children's court under the Commissions for Protection of Child Rights Act, 2005 (4 of 2006) or a Special Court designated for similar purposes under any other law for the time being in force, then, such court shall be deemed to be a Special Court under this section.

2. While trying an offence under this Act, a Special Court shall also try an offence [other than the offence referred to in sub-section (1)], with which the accused may, under the Code of Criminal Procedure, 1973 (2 of 1974), be charged at the same trial.

3. The Special Court constituted under this Act, notwithstanding anything in the Information Technology Act, 2000 (21 of 2000), shall have jurisdiction to try offences under Section 67B of that Act in so far as it relates to publication or transmission of sexually explicit material depicting children in any Act, or conduct or manner or facilitates abuse of children online.

29. Presumption as to Certain Offences

Where a person is prosecuted for committing or abetting or attempting to commit any offence under Sections 3, 5, 7 and 9 of this Act, the Special Court shall presume, that such person has committed or abetted or attempted to commit the offence, as the case may be unless the contrary is proved.

30. Presumption of Culpable Mental State

1. In any prosecution for any offence under this Act which requires a culpable mental state on the part of the accused, the Special Court shall presume the existence of such mental state but it shall be a defence for the accused to prove the fact that he had no such mental state with respect to the Act charged as an offence in that prosecution.

2. For the purposes of this section, a fact is said to be proved only when the Special Court believes it to exist beyond reasonable doubt and not merely when its existence is established by a preponderance of probability.

Explanation: In this section, "culpable mental state" includes intention, motive, knowledge of a fact and the belief in, or reason to believe, a fact.

31. Application of Code of Criminal Procedure, 1973 to Proceedings Before a Special Court

Save as otherwise provided in this Act, the provisions of the Code of Criminal Procedure, 1973 (2 of 1974) (including the provisions as to bail and bonds) shall apply to the proceedings before a Special Court and for the purposes of the said provisions, the Special Court shall be deemed to be a Court of Sessions and the person conducting a prosecution before a Special Court, shall be deemed to be a Public Prosecutor.

32. Special Public Prosecutors

1. The State Government shall, by notification in the Official Gazette, appoint a Special Public Prosecutor for every Special Court for conducting cases only under the provisions of this Act.

2. A person shall be eligible to be appointed as a Special Public Prosecutor under sub-section (1) only if he had been in practice for not less than seven years as an advocate.

3. Every person appointed as a Special Public Prosecutor under this section shall be deemed to be a Public Prosecutor within the meaning of clause (u) of Section 2 of the Code of Criminal Procedure, 1973 (2 of 1974) and provision of that Code shall have effect accordingly.

PROCEDURE AND POWERS OF SPECIAL COURTS AND RECORDING OF EVIDENCE

33. Procedure and Powers of Special Court

1. A Special Court may take cognizance of any offence, without the accused being committed to it for trial, upon receiving a complaint of facts which constitute such offence, or upon a police report of such facts.

2. The Special Public Prosecutor, or as the case may be, the counsel appearing for the accused shall, while recording the examination-in-chief, cross-examination or re-examination of the child, communicate the questions to be put to the child to the Special Court which shall in turn put those questions to the child.

3. The Special Court may, if it considers necessary, permit frequent breaks for the child during the trial.

4. The Special Court shall create a child-friendly atmosphere by allowing a family member, a guardian, a friend or a relative, in whom the child has trust or confidence, to be present in the court.

5. The Special Court shall ensure that the child is not called repeatedly to testify in the court.

6. The Special Court shall not permit aggressive questioning or character assassination of the child and ensure that dignity of the child is maintained at all times during the trial.

7. The Special Court shall ensure that the identity of the child is not disclosed at any time during the course of investigation or trial: Provided that for reasons to be recorded in writing, the Special Court may permit such disclosure, if in its opinion such disclosure is in the interest of the child.

Explanation: For the purposes of this sub-section, the identity of the child shall include the identity of the child's family, school, relatives, neighbourhood or any other information by which the identity of the child may be revealed.

8. In appropriate cases, the Special Court may, in addition to the punishment, direct payment of such compensation as may be prescribed to the child for any physical or mental trauma caused to him or for immediate rehabilitation of such child.

9. Subject to the provisions of this Act, a Special Court shall, for the purpose of the trial of any offence under this Act, have all the powers of a Court of Session and shall try such offence as if it were a Court of Session, and as far as may be, in accordance with the procedure specified in the Code of Criminal Procedure, 1973 (2 of 1974) for trial before a Court of Session.

34. Procedure in Case of Commission of Offence by Child and Determination of Age by Special Court

1. Where any offence under this Act is committed by a child, such child shall be dealt with under the provisions of the Juvenile Justice (Care and Protection of Children) Act, 2000 (56 of 2000).

2. If any question arises in any proceeding before the Special Court whether a person is a child or not, such question shall be determined by the Special Court after satisfying itself about the age of such person and it shall record in writing its reasons for such determination.

3. No order made by the Special Court shall be deemed to be invalid merely by any subsequent proof that the age of a person as determined by it under sub-section (2) was not the correct age of that person.

35. Period for Recording of Evidence of Child and Disposal of Case

1. The evidence of the child shall be recorded within a period of thirty days of the Special Court taking cognizance of the offence and reasons for delay, if any, shall be recorded by the Special Court.

2. The Special Court shall complete the trial, as far as possible, within a period of one year from the date of taking cognizance of the offence.

36. Child not to see Accused at the Time of Testifying

1. The Special Court shall ensure that the child is not exposed in any way to the accused at the time of recording of the evidence, while at the same time ensuring that the accused is in a position to hear the statement of the child and communicate with his advocate.

2. For the purposes of sub-section (1), the Special Court may record the statement of a child through videoconferencing or by utilising single visibility mirrors or curtains or any other device.

37. Trials to be Conducted in Camera

The Special Court shall try cases in camera and in the presence of the parents of the child or any other person in whom the child has trust or confidence: Provided that where the Special Court is of the opinion that the child needs to be examined at a place other than the court, it shall proceed to issue a commission in accordance with the provisions of Section 284 of the Code of Criminal Procedure, 1973 (2 of 1974).

38. Assistance of an Interpreter or Expert while Recording Evidence of Child

1. Wherever necessary, the court may take the assistance of a translator or interpreter having such qualifications,

experience and on payment of such fees as may be prescribed, while recording the evidence of the child.

2. If a child has a mental or physical disability, the Special Court may take the assistance of a special educator or any person familiar with the manner of communication of the child or an expert in that field, having such qualifications, experience and on payment of such fees as may be prescribed to record the evidence of the child.

MISCELLANEOUS

39. Guidelines for Child to Take Assistance of Experts, etc.

Subject to such rules as may be made in this behalf, the State Government shall prepare guidelines for use of non-governmental organisations, professionals and experts or persons having knowledge of psychology, social work, physical health, mental health and child development to be associated with the pre-trial and trial stage to assist the child.

40. Right of Child to Take Assistance of Legal Practitioner

Subject to the proviso to Section 301 of the Code of Criminal Procedure, 1973 (2 of 1974), the family or the guardian of the child shall be entitled to the assistance of a legal counsel of their choice for any offence under this Act: Provided that if the family or the guardian of the child are unable to afford a legal counsel, the Legal Services Authority shall provide a lawyer to them.

41. Provisions of Sections 3 to 13 not to Apply in Certain Cases

The provisions of Sections 3 to 13 (both inclusive) shall not apply in case of medical examination or medical treatment of a child when such medical examination or medical treatment is undertaken with the consent of his parents or guardian.

42. Alternative Punishment

Where an act or omission constitute an offence punishable under this Act and also under any other law for the time being in force, then, notwithstanding anything contained in any law for the time being in force, the offender found guilty of such offence shall be liable to punishment only under such law or this Act as provides for punishment which is greater in degree.

43. Public Awareness About Act

The Central Government and every State Government, shall take all measures to ensure that

a. The provisions of this Act are given wide publicity through media including the television, radio and the print media at regular intervals to make the general public, children as well as their parents and guardians aware of the provisions of this Act;

b. The officers of the Central Government and the State Governments and other concerned persons (including the police officers) are imparted periodic training on the matters relating to the implementation of the provisions of the Act.

44. Monitoring of Implementation of Act

1. The National Commission for Protection of Child Rights constituted under Section 3, or as the case may be, the State Commission for Protection of Child Rights constituted under Section 17, of the Commissions for Protection of Child Rights Act, 2005 (4 of 2006), shall, in addition to the functions assigned to them under that Act, also monitor the implementation of the provisions of this Act in such manner as may be prescribed.

2. The National Commission or, as the case may be, the State Commission, referred to in sub-section (1), shall, while inquiring into any matter relating to any offence under this Act, have the

same powers as are vested in it under the Commissions for Protection of Child Rights Act, 2005 (4 of 2006).

3. The National Commission or, as the case may be, the State Commission, referred to in sub-section (1), shall, also include, its activities under this section, in the annual report referred to in Section 16 of the Commissions for Protection of Child Rights Act, 2005 (4 of 2006).

45. Power to Make Rules

1. The Central Government may, by notification in the Official Gazette, make rules for carrying out the purposes of this Act.
2. In particular, and without prejudice to the generality of the foregoing powers, such rules may provide for all or any of the following matters, namely:
   a. The qualifications and experience of, and the fees payable to, a translator or an interpreter, a special educator or any person familiar with the manner of communication of the child or an expert in that field, under sub-section (4) of Section 19; sub-sections (2) and (3) of Section 26 and Section 38.
   b. Care and protection and emergency medical treatment of the child under sub-section (5) of Section 19.
   c. The payment of compensation under sub-section (8) of Section 33.
   d. The manner of periodic monitoring of the provisions of the Act under sub-section (1) of Section 44.

3. Every rule made under this section shall be laid, as soon as may be after it is made, before each House of Parliament, while it is in session, for a total period of thirty days which may be comprised in one session or in two or more successive sessions, and if, before the expiry of the session immediately following the session or the successive sessions aforesaid, both Houses agree in making any modification in the rule or both Houses agree that the rule should not be made, the rule shall thereafter have effect only in such modified form or be of no effect, as the case may be; so, however, that any such modification or annulment shall be without prejudice to the validity of anything previously done under that rule.

THE CRIMINAL LAW (AMENDMENT) BILL, 2013

NEW OFFENCES

This new Act has expressly recognised certain acts as offences which were dealt under related laws. These new offences like acid attack, sexual harassment, voyeurism, stalking have been incorporated into the Indian Penal Code:

Section	Offence	Punishment	Notes
326A	Acid attack	Imprisonment not less than ten years but which may extend to imprisonment for life and with fine which shall be just and reasonable to meet the medial expenses and it shall be paid to the victim	Gender neutral
326B	Attempt to acid attack	Imprisonment not less than five years but which may extend to seven years, and shall also be liable to fine	Gender neutral

(Contd.)

(Contd.)

Section	Offence	Punishment	Notes
354A	Sexual harassment	Rigorous imprisonment up to five years, or with fine, or with both in case of offence described in clauses (i) and (ii) Imprisonment up to one year, or with fine, or with both in other cases	Gender neutral i. Physical contact and advances involving unwelcome and explicit sexual overtures; or ii. A demand or request for sexual favours; or iii. Making sexually coloured remarks; or iv. Forcibly showing pornography; or v. Any other unwelcome physical, verbal or non-verbal conduct of sexual nature
354B	Public disrobing of woman	Imprisonment not less than three years but which may extend to seven years and with fine	Assaults or uses criminal force to any woman or abets such act with the intention of disrobing or compelling her to be naked in any public place
354C	Voyeurism	In case of first conviction, imprisonment not less than one year, but which may extend to three years, and shall also be liable to fine, and be punished on a second or subsequent conviction, with imprisonment of either description for a term which shall not be less than three years, but which may extend to seven years, and shall also be liable to fine	Watching or capturing a woman in "private act", which includes an act of watching carried out in a place which, in the circumstances, would reasonably be expected to provide privacy, and where the victim's genitals, buttocks or breasts are exposed or covered only in underwear; or the victim is using a lavatory; or the person is doing a sexual act that is not of a kind ordinarily done in public
354D	Stalking	Imprisonment not less than one year but which may extend to three years, and shall also be liable to fine	Only for women. To follow a woman and contact, or attempt to contact such woman to foster personal interaction repeatedly despite a clear indication of disinterest by such woman; or monitor the use by a woman of the internet, email or any other form of electronic communication. There are exceptions to this section which include such act being in course of preventing or detecting a crime authorised by state or in compliance of certain law or was reasonable and justified

Changes in Law

Section 370 of Indian Penal Code (IPC) has been substituted with new Sections 370 and 370A which deals with trafficking of person for exploitation. If a person (a) recruits, (b) transports, (c) harbours, (d) transfers, or (e) receives, a person or persons, by using threats, or force, or coercion, or abduction, or fraud, or deception, or by abuse of power, or inducement for exploitation including prostitution, slavery, forced organ removal, etc. will be punished with imprisonment ranging from at least 7 years to imprisonment for the remainder of that person's natural life depending on the number or category of persons trafficked. Employment of a trafficked person will attract penal provision as well.

The most important change that has been made is the change in definition of rape under IPC. The word rape has been replaced with sexual assault in Section 375, and have added penetrations other than penile penetration an offence. The definition is broadly worded and gender neutral in some aspect, with acts like penetration of penis, or any object or any part of body to any extent, into the vagina, mouth, urethra or anus of another person or making another person do so, apply of mouth or touching private parts constitutes the offence of sexual assault. The section has also clarified that penetration means "penetration to any extent", and lack of physical resistance is immaterial for constituting an offence. Except in certain aggravated situation the punishment will be imprisonment not less than seven years but which may extend to imprisonment for life, and shall also be liable to fine. In aggravated situations, punishment will be rigorous imprisonment for a term which shall not be less than ten years but which may extend to imprisonment for life, and shall also be liable to fine. A new Section 376A has been added which states that if a person committing the offence of sexual assault, inflicts an injury which causes the death of the person or causes the person to be in a persistent vegetative state, shall be punished with rigorous imprisonment for a term which shall not be less than twenty years, but which may extend to imprisonment for life, which shall mean the remainder of that person's natural life, or with death. In case of "gang rape", persons involved regardless of their gender shall be punished with rigorous imprisonment for a term which shall not be less than twenty years, but which may extend to life and shall pay compensation to the victim which shall be reasonable to meet the medical expenses and rehabilitation of the victim. The age of consent in India has been increased to 18 years, which means any sexual activity irrespective of presence of consent with a woman below the age of 18 will constitute statutory rape.

Certain changes have been introduced in the CrPC and Evidence Act, like the recording of statement of the victim, more friendly and easy, character of the victim is irrelevant, presumption of no consent where sexual intercourse is proved and the victim states in the court that there has been no consent, etc.

The Criminal Law (Amendment) Act, 2013

Offence	Changes in ordinance
Acid attack	Fine shall be just and reasonable to meet medical expenses for treatment of victim, while in the ordinance it was fine up to rupees 10 lakhs
Sexual harassment	"Clause (v) any other unwelcome physical, verbal or nonverbal conduct of sexual nature" has been removed. Punishment for offence under clause (i) and (ii) has been reduced from five years of imprisonment to three years. The offence is no longer gender-neutral, only a man can commit the offence on a woman
Voyeurism	The offence is no longer gender-neutral, only a man can commit the offence on a woman
Stalking	The offence is no longer gender-neutral, only a man can commit the offence on a woman. The definition has been reworded and broken down into clauses. The exclusion clause and the following sentence has been removed "or watches or spies on a person in a manner that results in a fear of violence or serious alarm or distress in the mind of such person, or interferes with the mental peace of such person, commits the offence of stalking". Punishment for the offence has been changed; A man committing the offence of stalking would be liable for imprisonment up to three years for the first offence, and shall also be liable to fine and for any subsequent conviction would be liable for imprisonment up to five years and with fine

(Contd.)

(Contd.)

Offence	Changes in ordinance
Trafficking of person	"Prostitution" has been removed from the explanation clause
Rape	The word sexual assault has been replaced back to rape. The offence is no longer gender-neutral, only a man can commit the offence on a woman. The clause related to touching of private parts has been removed

a. After the entries relating to Section 166, the following entries shall be inserted, namely:

1	2	3	4	5	6
"166A	Public servant disobeying direction underlaw	Imprisonment for one year or fine or with both	Noncognizable	Bailable	Magistrate of the first class"

b. After the entries relating to Section 326, the following entries shall be inserted, namely:

1	2	3	4	5	6
"326A	Voluntarily causing grievous hurt by use of acid, etc.	Imprisonment for not less than 10 years but which may extend to imprisonment for life and fine of 10 lakh rupees	Cognizable	Nonbailable	Court of Session
326B	Voluntarily throwing or attempting to throw acid.	Imprisonment for five years but which may extend to seven years and fine	Cognizable	Nonbailable	Court of Session"

c. For the entries relating to Section 354, the following entries shall be substituted, namely:

1	2	3	4	5	6
"354	Assault or use of criminal force to woman with intent to outrage her modesty	Imprisonment of 1 year which may extend to 5 years, and with fine	Cognizable	Nonbailable	Any Magistrate.
354A	1. Sexual harassment of the nature of unwelcome physical contact and advances or a demand or request for sexual favours	Imprisonment which may extend to 5 years or with fine or with both	Cognizable	Nonbailable	Any Magistrate

(Contd.)

(Contd.)

1	2	3	4	5	6
	2. Sexual harassment of the nature of making sexually coloured remark or showing pornography or any other unwelcome physical, verbal or nonverbal conduct of sexual nature	Imprisonment which may extend to 1 year or with fine or with both	Noncognizable	Bailable	Any Magistrate
354B	Assault or use of criminal force to woman with intent to disrobe	Imprisonment of not less than 3 years but which may extend to 7 years and with fine	Cognizable	Nonbailable	Any Magistrate
354C	Voyeurism	Imprisonment of not less than 1 year but which may extend to 3 years and with fine for first conviction	Noncognizable	Bailable	Any Magistrate
		Imprisonment of not less than 3 years but which may extend to 7 years and with fine for second or subsequent conviction	Cognizable	Nonbailable	Any Magistrate
354D	Stalking	Imprisonment of not less than 1 year but which may extend to 3 years and with fine	Cognizable	Nonbailable	Any Magistrate"

d. For the entries relating to Section 370, the following entries shall be substituted, namely:

1	2	3	4	5	6
"370	1. Trafficking of person	Imprisonment of not less than 7 years but which may extend to 10 years and with fine	Cognizable	Nonbailable	Court of Session
	2. Trafficking of more than one person	Imprisonment of not less than 10 years but which may extend to imprisonment for life and with fine	Cognizable	Nonbailable	Court of Session

(Contd.)

1	2	3	4	5	6
	3. Trafficking of a minor	Imprisonment of not less than 10 years but which may extend to imprisonment for life	Cognizable	Nonbailable	Court of Session
	4. Trafficking of more than one minor	Imprisonment of not less than 14 years but which may extend to imprisonment for life	Cognizable	Nonbailable	Court of Session
	5. Public servant or a police officer involved in trafficking of minor	Imprisonment for life which shall mean the remainder of that person's natural life	Cognizable	Nonbailable	Court of Session
	6. Person convicted of offence of trafficking of minor on more than one occasion	Imprisonment for life which shall mean the remainder of that person's natural life	Cognizable	Nonbailable	Court of Session
370A	1. Employing of a trafficked child	Imprisonment of not less than 5 years but which may extend to 7 years and with fine	Cognizable	Nonbailable	Court of Session
	2. Employing of a trafficked adult person	Imprisonment of not less than 3 years but which may extend to 7 years and with fine	Cognizable	Nonbailable	Court of Session"

e. For the entries relating to Sections 376, 376A, 376B, 376C and 376D, the following entries shall be substituted, namely:

1	2	3	4	5	6
376	1. Sexual assault	Rigorous imprisonment of not less than 7 years but which may extend to imprisonment for life and with fine	Cognizable	Nonbailable	Court of Session

(Contd.)

(Contd.)

1	2	3	4	5	6
	2. Sexual assault by a police officer or a public servant or member of armed forces or a person being on the management or on the staff of a jail, remand home or other place of custody or women's or children's institution or by a person on the management or on the staff of a hospital, and sexual assault committed by a person in a position of trust or authority towards the person assaulted or by a near relative of the person assaulted	Rigorous imprisonment of not less than 10 years but which may extend to imprisonment for life and with fine	Cognizable	Nonbailable	Court of Session
376A	Person committing an offence of sexual assault and inflicting injury which causes death or causes the person to be in a persistent vegetative state	Rigorous imprisonment of not less than 20 years but which may extend to imprisonment for life which shall mean the remainder of that person's natural life or with death	Cognizable	Nonbailable	Court of Session
376B	Sexual assault by the husband upon his wife during separation	Imprisonment for not less than 2 years but which may extend to 7 years and with fine	Cognizable (but only on the complaint of the victim)	Nonbailable	Court of Session
376C	Sexual intercourse by a person in authority	Rigorous imprisonment for not less than 5 years but which may extend to 10 years and with fine	Cognizable	Nonbailable	Court of Session

(Contd.)

(Contd.)

1	2	3	4	5	6
376D	Sexual assault by gang.	Rigorous imprisonment for not less than 20 years but which may extend to imprisonment for life which shall mean the remainder of that person's natural life and com pensation to the victim	Cognizable	Nonbailable	Court of Session
376E	Repeat offenders.	Imprisonment for life which shall mean the remainder of that person's natural life or with death	Cognizable	Nonbailable	Court of Session

f. Entry relating to Section 509, in column 3, for the words "Simple imprisonment for one year, or fine, or both," the words "Simple imprisonment for 3 years and with fine" shall be substituted. In case the victim is below 12 years, punishment of full life imprisonment and even death sentence is recommended.

CHAPTER 9

Autopsy in Females

VIRGINITY

- A virgin is a girl/a woman who has never experienced sexual intercourse or coitus.
- The question of virginity may arise in relation to true or false allegations of rape, defamation, or character assassination, nullity of marriage due to noncon-summation.
- The opposite of virginity is defloration.
- The status of a woman who has experienced sexual intercourse is called defloration.

The data used to establish virginity

- Areola is pink in colour, nipples are small and pink.
- Breasts are firm and hemispherical.
- The labia majora are firm and lie in apposition. They cover labia minora.
- The labia minora are pink in color, soft and sensitive to touch.
- Clitoris is small, the vagina is narrow, the mucosa is rugose.
- The hymen is intact; doest not allow the entry of tip of little finger without pain unless the hymen is elastic.

In a woman who has experienced sexual intercourse

- The labia majora are separated.
- Labia minora are visible through labia majora.
- The hymen is torn and easily admits two fingers without pain.
- Breasts are not firm and hemispherical.
- The nipples are prominent and enlarged.

Various types of hymen

- Semilunar—moon shaped.
- Annular—ring shaped.
- Cribriform—seived.
- Infundibuliform—funnel shaped.
- Septate—partitioned.
  - All the above descriptions pertain to nature of opening in the hymen.
  - When there is no opening it is called imperforate hymen.
- Hymen is a circular fold of connective tissue about 1 mm thick. It may be thin elastic and yielding or thick elastic and unyielding.
- After parturition or birth of a child, the hymen is left out as small remnants called carunculae hymenalis/carunculae myrtiformis.

Medicolegal issues

- 'Virgo intacta is a *rara avis*' remarked a learned judge.
- Presence of intact hymen is useful only if it is thin, nonyielding and allows the tip of little finger with pain.
- In case of elastic fleshy hymen, intact hymen is not of significance.
- Rupture of hymen due to sexual intercourse is the 5 o' clock, 6 o' clock, 7 o' clock positions when viewed in lithotomy positions.
- Anterior tears are more in favour of trauma of nonsexual nature.
- Sometime threadworms also can cause erosions which are mistaken for tears.

- Similarly diphtheritic ulcers may destroy the hymen causing scar formation.
- False virginity is the status of woman who presents intact hymen though she has experiences acts of sexual intercourse.
- In these cases, labia majora are not in apposition, labia minora may be cutaneous. Though the hymen is intact it allows two fingers.

PREGNANCY

Pregnancy is the status of a woman who is carrying a baby in her womb. The question of pregnancy may arise in relation to:

- In an expecting couple or in a couple who do not want a child or couple who want to delay pregnancy but failed in the attempt.
- Following rape or alleged rape.
- Suspected infidelity.
- For the postponement of death sentence or rigorous imprisonment.

- Postponement of trial of the case.
- In cases of abortion, concealment of birth.
- In cases of nullity of marriage.
- Inheritance of property.
- Divorce.

Diagnosis of Pregnancy

- Positive signs of pregnancy.
- Probable signs of pregnancy.
- Presumptive sings of pregnancy.

Positive Signs of Pregnancy

Ultrasonography

- By sonography we can diagnose pregnancy.
- By 6 weeks→gestational ring is made out.
- By 8 weeks→distinct echoes from the embryo within the gestational ring.

At this stage, if pregnancy is not progressing further, we call it *blighted ovum*. This is made out in the sonography by loss of

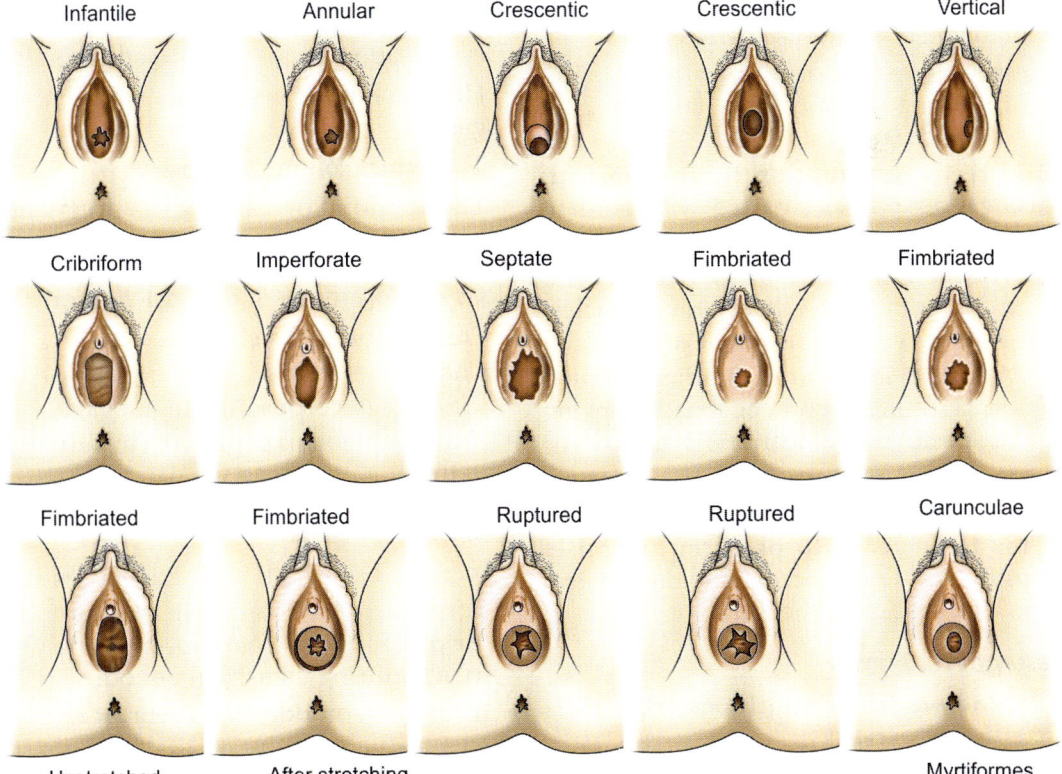

Fig. 9.1: Types of hymen

gestational ring and loss of foetal echoes after 8 weeks of pregnancy.

- By 12 weeks → foetal heartbeats made out.
- By 14 weeks → foetal head and thorax are made out.

X-ray examination

By 16th weeks, X-ray examination shows ossification centres. A circular outline of skull, beaded shadow of spine, ladder shadow of ribs.

Foetal movements

- By 16–20 weeks, the foetal movements are seen as well as felt.
- By 24 weeks, the foetal parts can be felt by bi-manual examination per vaginum.

Foetal heart sounds

- By 18–20 weeks, foetal heart sounds are heard like muffled ticks of a watch.
- The rate at this stage is 120–160/min.

Probable Signs of Pregnancy

- Softening of cervix: 6–8 weeks.
- Enlargement of uterus: 8 weeks.
- Test for human chorionic gonadotrophin in the urine becomes detectable by 2nd week of pregnancy.
- **Indirect agglutination inhibition test** using latex particles coated with human chorionic gonadotrophin.
  - The morning urine is first treated with hCG antibodies—then latex particles coated with hCG hormone are added.
  - Agglutination occurs if the urine does not contain human chorionic gonadotrophin. So, positive test means no pregnancy.
  - If there is no agglutination, it means that the woman is pregnant.
- This test is easy to perform but false positive result can occur in hydatidiform mole or chorionepithelioma.

Presumptive Signs

- **By 2nd week:** Amenorrhoea (absence/missing of period).
- **By 6–10 weeks:** Morning sickness (vomiting on getting up from bed).

- **By 3–4 weeks:** Breast changes.
- **By 6 weeks:** Vaginal discolouration.
- **By 18–20 weeks:** Quickening (feeling of movement of baby by the mother).

Duration of pregnancy

Normal gestation period is 10 lunar months or 280 days.

Death of Foetus *in utero*

Sonography

- Blighted ovum is detected after 8 weeks of gestation.
- Instead of increasing in size, foetus decreases in size. This is the indicator during early months.
- In later half of pregnancy, foetal movements disappear, uterus size and pregnancy duration do not tally, size of uterus becomes smaller than during earlier observation.

Radiology

- Due to liquefaction of brain, there is gross overlapping of skull bones on X-ray examination. This is called **Spadling's sign.**
- Heart and great vessels show presence of gas.
- The spinal column collapses.
- The immunological test for pregnancy becomes negative.

Signs of Pregnancy in a Dead Women

- Presence of foetus or ovum.
- Changes in uterus.
- Presence of corpus luteum in ovary.
- Presence of foetus or placenta in the uterus in the womb of dead woman.

Changes in Uterus

- Increased size both in length and width.
- Corpus luteum is formed in the ovary after the escape of ova from rupture of graafian follicle during menstrual period.
- If fertilization does not occur, it ends as an avascualr scar by 10–12 days.
- If pregnancy occurs, corpus luteum grows in size up to 16 weeks and continues to be

present up to delivery and 1–2 months even after delivery.

- It is not a positive sign of pregnancy. False positives are seen in fibroids, in non-pregnant and menstruating woman also.

DELIVERY

The question of delivery arises in cases of

- Concealment of birth
- Suppositious child
- Abortion
- Infanticide
- Contested legitimacy
- Disputed chastety

Signs of Delivery

- Up to few hours after delivery, the uterus is felt as a flabby mass extending up to umbilicus.
- Involution (return to its normal size) of uterus starts immediately after delivery.
  - The size reduces by 1 cm per day. By third day, it is felt like a cricket ball at level of umbilicus above symphysis pubis.
  - By fourteen days, it is just palpable at or above symphysis pubis.

Vagina

- There is tenderness of labia, bruising or laceration may be seen, vagina is smooth, relaxed; shows recent tears that heal by 7 days.
- In caesarean deliveries, these findings are not seen.

Cervix

- The internal **os** begins to close within 24 hours.
- The external **os** admits two fingers for a few days.
- At the end of 7 days, it admits one finger.
- By two weeks, it returns to normal size.
- These changes are not seen in caesarean deliveries.

Lochia

- It is discharge from womb with a peculiar, disagreeable odour (labour room smell).

- The discharge is bright red up to 5 days consisting of blood clots, so it is called **lochia rubra.**
- In the next four days, it is pallor in colour and serous, so it is called **lochia serosa.**
- After 9 days, it becomes slightly yellowish grey, is called **lochia alba.** It disappears by two weeks.
- The breast is bulky and contains milk. The woman looks tired for 2–3 days after delivery.
- Intermittent contractions of uterus may be seen for 3–5 days.

Signs of Delivery in Dead

The findings found in living person are also seen in dead, namely changes in uterus, vagina, cervix, lochia and breasts.

During of Autopsy

- The size of the uterus can be measured.
- The corpus luteum of pregnancy in the ovaries can be seen.
- The weight of uterus soon after delivery is 840 gm.
- End of 1 week → 360 gm
- End of 1 month → 90 gm
- The length of uterus.

Table 9.1: Period of gestation and length of uterus

Period of gestation	Length of uterus
Nonpregnant uterus	7 cm
By end of 3rd month	12.5 cm
By end of 6th month	15 cm
By end of 7th month	20 cm
By end of 8th month	24 cm
By end of 9th month	26 cm

Remote Signs of Delivery in Living

- **These are not reliable**
  - Breasts—areola dark, nipples prominent with linea albicantes.
  - Abdomen—striae gravidarum.
  - Vagina—rugae absent.
  - Carunculae myrtiformis present.

Cervix shows transverse cleft with irregular margins.

Signs of Remote Delivery in the Dead

- Uterus, larger thicker and heavier.
- Uterine walls concave from inside.
- Top of fundus convex.
- Cervix is irregular.
- Old scars seen on edges of cervix.
- External **os** patulous.

Above findings can be observed at autopsy.

Causes of Death in Pregnancy

1. Direct
- Haemorrhage
- Toxaemia of pregnancy
- Sepsis
- Other complications
  - Pulmonary embolism
  - Amniotic fluid embolism
  - Cortical venous thrombosis

2. Indirect
- Anaemia
- Jaundice
- Heart disease

3. Unrelated—causes of maternal deaths due to haemorrhage
- Post-partum haemorrhage (PPH)
- Ante-partum haemorrhage (APH)
  - Placenta previa
  - Accidental haemorrhage
- Ruptured uterus
- Retained placenta
- Abortion
- Ruptured ectopic pregnancy
- Hydatidiform mole.

ABORTION

"Abortion is defined as the premature expulsion of products of conception from the womb at any time before the completion of period of gestation" (*aboriri*—to detach from the proper site).

The average period of gestation is 280 days. The product of conception is called **ovum** up to 2 weeks, **embryo** from 3rd to 5th weeks, foetus after 5 weeks, till birth.

Abortion may be
- Threatened abortion
- Natural abortion (spontaneous abortion)
- Therapeutic abortion
- Justifiable abortion
- Criminal abortion.

Threatened Abortion

In a pregnant woman, bleeding may appear but it is controlled if pregnancy continued until delivery. This is threatened abortion. Here abortion is only threatened, it is not real and complete.

Natural Abortion

It can be spontaneous or accidental. In up to 15% of cases of normal pregnancies, abortion may occur in 2nd or 3rd month. In later months, foetal delivery occurs first, followed by amniotic sac, placenta and decidual tissues.

Accidental abortion occurs due to trauma or drug toxicity, accidental consumption of arsenic, lead or some vegetable poison.

Abortions when induced are not natural and are called **induced** or **unnatural abortions.**

Therapeutic Abortions

Those abortions carried out to save the life of the mother or to extrude the retained products of conception.

Justifiable abortion: Therapeutic abortions done in good faith are justifiable abortions. These abortions are also permitted under Medical Termination of Pregnancy Act.

Under the Medical Termination of Pregnancy Act, termination of pregnancy is allowed under the following conditions:
- Qualified and authorized doctor
- Recognized or authorized centre
- Length of pregnancy not beyond 20 weeks
- Consent.
- Punishment for not following the rules to doctor:
  - Doctors who are MBBS with experience of carrying out MTPs, at least 25 cases at recognized centre.
  - Gynaecologists with MD/DGO.

- Centre should be recognized by the authorized government office or board.
- Up to 12 weeks of pregnancy, a single doctor can decided about MTP. Between 12–20 weeks, a second doctor's opinion is required.
- Above 20 weeks, only if the mother's life is in danger, even a single doctor can perform the operation, irrespective of whether the centre is recognized or not.

Indications

1. **Therapeutic:** When there is danger to life or serious injury to physical and mental health of mother.
2. **Eugenic:** If the pregnancy is allowed to continue, the child is likely to be born with physical and mental abnormalities.
3. **Humanitarian:** Pregnancy following rape.
4. **Social:** When a married couple used contraceptive methods and there is failure of contraceptive method, it causes mental anguish, so MTP is allowed.

Consent

Consent of the pregnant woman must be obtained. If she is not eligible to give valid consent, i.e. below 18 years or mentally unsound, then consent of guardian is required. If the doctor fails to follow MTP rules, a private doctor is liable for fine up to Rs 1000. A government doctor is liable for dismissal from service.

Methods of MTP

- Vacuum suction and curettage
- If pregnancy is above three months, then
  - Induction by prostaglandins
  - Aminocentesis
  - Abdominal hysterotomy
  - By the MTP Act, abortions are only liberalised but not legalised.

Criminal Abortion

Any abortion which does not come under the purview of MTP Act, becomes a criminal abortion, even if it is carried out by qualified doctors in recognized centres.

This category of abortions is described and punishable under Sections 312–318 of IPC.

Criminal abortion is an abortion done with criminal intent. It is the unlawful and deliberate destruction of products of conception. Both the woman and person doing the abortion are punishable.

Attempted abortion is also a punishable offence.

Criminal abortion is induced by

- Drugs
- Mechanical trauma
- Mechanical trauma like repture of membranes by catheter, needle or uterine sound, injection of hot irritant fluids like soap and water, dilation of cervix using bougies, application of galvanic current on uterine region of abdomen, use of abortion stick. Abortion stick is used by professional abortionists (*dai*). The abortion stick is 12–18 cm long cotton wool is wrapped at one end, it is soaked in substances like madar juice (calotropis), marking nut juice (*Semicarpus anacardium*), arsenic paste, etc.
- Ecbolics like ergot, emenagogues like borax, urinary irritants like cantharides, systemic poisons like arsenic.

Causes of Death in Cases of Criminal Abortion

- Reflex vagal inhibition
- Shock and haemorrhage
- Peritonitis
- Air embolism
- Fat embolism
- Electrocution

Duties of doctor in cases of criminal abortion: The patient's history should be kept secret (professional secrecy). If the suspects criminal abortion and there is danger of death, he should get the dying declaration recorded. If she dies, he should not issue death certificate and report the matter to police.

Examination of Victim of Criminal Abortion

This consists of:

- Examination of woman
- Products of conception
  - The woman presents signs of recent delivery.
  - She also presents evidence of interference with pregnancy.
  - The products of conception consist of ovum/embryo/foetus, placental tissue, membranes and amniotic fluid.
  - The doctor has to identify products of conception and opine about age of products (i.e. foetus).
- In the case of a dead person, uterus and appendages are subjected for histopathology and chemical analysis.
- If drugs are the cause of criminal abortion, viscera should be sent for chemical analysis.
- If stick or some other material is found, it should be subjected for chemical analysis.

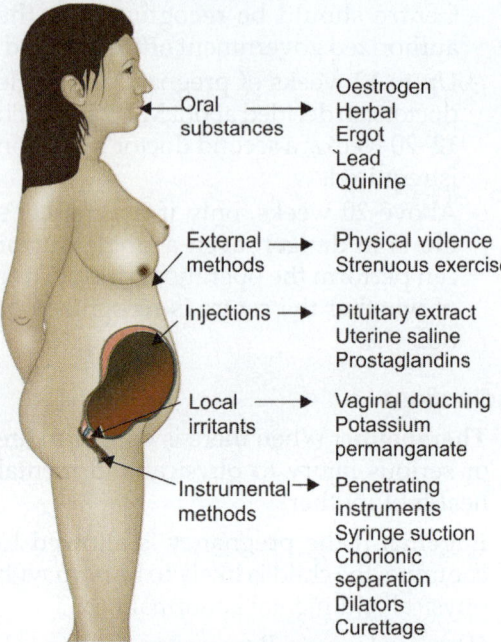

Fig. 9.2: Methods of criminal abortion

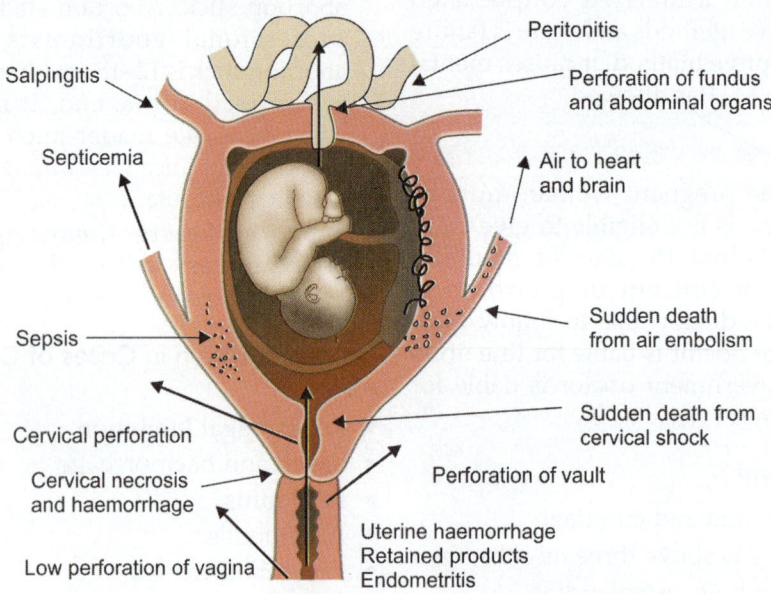

Fig. 9.3: Complications of criminal abortion

CHAPTER 10

Assisted Reproduction

IMPOTENCE

- Impotence is inability of a man to perform sexual intercourse.
- The presumption is in favour of potency.
- Functional causes are more common than organic causes in impotence.
- 95% cases are of psychological origin.
- In women, frigidity (equivalent of male impotency) occurs due to vaginismus.

Vaginismus

It is a severe spasm of vaginal muscle because of which the woman cannot allow penetration of male organ.

Sterility

It is the inability to conceive in woman. The problem of infertility and impotence arises under the following circumstances:

- Nullity of marriage
- Divorce
- Legitimacy
- Disputed paternity
- Rape
- Other sexual offences
- Adultery
- Blackmailing
- Defamation, etc.

Causes of Impotence

- Very young and very old age.
- Drug dependence (alcohol, opium, cannabis, arsenic, lead, etc.)

- Psychological causes
  - Worry, depression, fear.
  - Timidity, guilt, complex.
- Impotence 'Quoad Hanc'
  - Condition where a man is unable to perform sexual intercourse with particular woman but is potent with others (e.g. impotent with wife but potent with others).
- **Diseases**
  - Acute fever, hypopituitarism.
  - Sexual infantilism.
  - Tabes dorsalis, spinal cord injury involving **nervi erigentes of Wrisburg** (genital branch of genitourinary nerves).
- Congenital abnormalities
  - Maldevelopment of penis, vagina.
- Acquired conditions
  - Hydrocele, elephantiasis of penis and scrotum.
  - While issuing an impotence certificate, the medical officer will use double negative form. The patient is well developed physically and genetically.
  - The sexual organs are well developed. There are no visible causes for impotence. After a complete physical and general examination, there is nothing to suggest that the person is incapable of performing sexual intercourse.
  - A sterile man may not be potent.
  - An impotent man need not be sterile.
  - Impotence and sterility may coexist.

Sterilization

- Sterilization is different from sterility. It should not be confused with sterility. Sterility or infertility means that person is incapable of procreation.
- "Sterilization is a process by which a person is made sterile by medical or surgical intervention".
- In India, surgical sterilization is voluntary.
- There are temporary and permanent methods.
- The indications for sterilizations are:
  - Contraceptive
  - Therapeutic
  - Eugenic
  - Socioeconomic
  - Convenience
- Sterilization practiced for restricting number of children as family planning measure is known as **contraceptive sterilization.**
- When sterilization is carried out in the interest of health of the mother, it is called **therapeutic sterilization.**
- When sterilization is carried out to prevent children with birth defects, it is called **eugenic sterilization.**
- In male, surgical sterilization is carried out by vasectomy, in female by ligation of fallopian tubes.

Precautions

- Consent of both husband and wife is required for sterilization of either spouse.
- After vasectomy, patient is advised contraception for two months.

Laparoscopic sterilization in women is the method of choice nowadays. Sometimes death occurs in laparoscopic sterilization due to:
- Vagal inhibition.
- Air embolism.
- Rupture of major vessels.

Sometimes this laparoscopic sterilization fails.

The causes of failure are
- Misidentification of tube.
- Spontaneous rejoining.

- Absence of band on one side.
- Superficial application.

Failure of vasectomy can be due to
- Spontaneous recanalization
- Unrecognized double vas
- Failure to divide each vas
- Temporary appearance of sperms
- Failure to empty pre-existing sperms
- Delayed onset of sterility.

DEFINITIONS CONNECTED TO ASSISTED REPRODUCTION

Artificial Insemination (AI)

AI is the procedure of artificially transferring semen into the reproductive system of a woman. This technique comprises artificial insemination with husband's (AIH) or with donori's (AID) sperm.

Aspiration Cycle

Initiated ART cycle in which more follicles are punctured and aspirated irrespective of whether or not oocytes are retrieved.

Assisted Hatching

Assisted hatching allows easier release of the embryo from its shell (zona pellucida), helping implantation and increasing the pregnancy rate.

Assisted Reproductive Technology (ART)

For the purpose of these guidelines. ART would be taken to encompass all techniques that attempt to obtain a pregnancy by manipulating the sperm and/or oocyte outside the body, and transferring the gamete or embryo into the uterus.

Blastocyst

An embryo with a fluid-filled blastocele cavity (usually developing by five or six days after fertilization).

Controlled Ovarian Hyperstimulation (COH)

Medical treatment to induce the development of multiple ovarian follicles to obtain multiple oocytes at follicular aspiration.

Cryopreservation

Freezing and storage of gametes, zygotes or embryos.

Donation of Gametes

Donation of gametes is a process by which a person voluntarily offers his or her gametes for the process of procreation.

Ectopic Pregnancy

A pregnancy in which implantation takes place outside the uterine cavity.

Embryo

Embryo is defined as the fertilized ovum that has begun cellular division and continued development up to the blastocyst stage till the end of eight weeks.

Embryo Donation

The transfer of an embryo resulting from gametes that did not originate from the recipient and/or her partner.

Embryo Transfer (ET)

Procedure in which embryo(s) are placed in the uterus or fallopian tube.

Fertilization

The penetration of the ovum by the spermatozoon and fusion of genetic materials resulting in the development of a zygote.

Foetus

The product of conception starting from completion of embryonic development (at eight completed weeks after fertilization) until birth or abortion.

Foetal Reduction

Foetal reduction is an invasive/interventional process, by which a higher order multiple pregnancy is reduced to a single or twin pregnancy in order to improve the perinatal outcome.

Gamete

Oocytes and sperm are called gametes.

Hatching

It is the process that precedes implantation by which an embryo at the blastocyst stage separates from the zona pellucida.

Intracytoplasmic Sperm Injection (ICSI)

In intracytoplasmic sperm injection (ICSI) is a single sperm injected into the cytoplasm of the ovum to effect fertilization before the fertilized ovum is transferred to the uterus of the woman.

Implantation

The attachment and subsequent penetration by the zona-free blastocyst (usually in the endometrium) which starts five to seven days following fertilization.

Infertility

Failure to conceive after at least one year of unprotected coitus.

Intrauterine Insemination (IUI)

Intrauterine insemination involves the introduction of sperm into the uterus of the woman. In IUI, specially prepared sperm are injected into the uterine cavity via a fine cannula passed through the cervix. At this site, the sperm are near the uterine entrance of each of the two fallopian tubes and thus have a shorter distance to swim in order to reach the oocyte(s) released at the time of ovulation.

IVF-ET (in vitro Fertilization—Embryo Transfer)

In vitro fertilization—embryo transfer (IVF-ET) is the fertilization of an ovum outside the body and the transfer of the fertilized ovum to the uterus of a woman.

IVMTS and IVMO (in vitro maturation of testicular sperm and in vitro maturation of oocytes).

In vitro maturation of testicular sperm (IVMTS) involves keeping the testicular sperm in a culture medium under optimal conditions where they can attain physiological maturity and acquire motility.

In vitro maturation of immature oocytes involves keeping the immature oocytes in an appropriate culture medium under optimal conditions where they can attain physiological maturity.

Oocyte Donation

An ART procedure performed with third party oocytes.

Ovum/Oocyte

Ovum/oocyte is the female gamete produced in the ovary.

PESA (Percutaneous Epididymal Sperm Aspiration) and TESA/TESE (Testicular Sperm Aspiration/Extraction)

Percutaneous epididymal sperm aspiration (PESA) and testicular sperm aspiration (TESA) are simplified, minimally invasive outpatient procedures that allow the physician to recover the sperm for fertilization in patients with obstructive azoospermia (lack of sperm in semen).

PESA requires a needle to be introduced into the epididymis and the contents aspirated. The aspirate is observed under the microscope to determine if motile sperm are present.

In TESA, the needle is introduced into the testicle itself.

Pre-implantation Genetic Diagnosis (PGD)

Pre-implantation genetic diagnosis is a technique in which an embryo formed through IVF is tested for specific genetic disorders (e.g. cystic fibrosis) or other characteristics prior to implantation.

Preterm Birth

A birth which takes place after at least 20, But less than 37, completed weeks of gestation. This includes both live births and stillbirths. Births are counted as birth events (e.g. a twin or triplet live birth is counted as one birth event).

Semen

A thick, whitish fluid discharged through the penis during ejaculation containing spermatozoa, secretions from the testes, seminal vesicles, prostate gland, bulbourethral and other glands associated with the male reproductive system.

Semen Donor

Semen obtained from third party for purpose of inseminating the wife in cases where husband is unable to produce healthy semen.

Sperm

Sperm are the male gametes produced in the testicles.

Spontaneous Abortion

Spontaneous loss of a clinical pregnancy before 20 completed weeks of gestation or, if gestational age is unknown, a weight of 500 gm or less.

Surrogacy

Surrogacy is an arrangement in which a woman agrees to carry a pregnancy that is genetically unrelated to her and her husband, with the intention to carry it to term and handover the child to the genetic parents for whom she is acting as a surrogate.

Surrogacy with Oocyte Donation

Surrogacy with oocyte donation is a process in which a woman allows insemination by the sperm/semen of the male partner of a couple with a view to carry the pregnancy to term and handover the child to the couple.

Zygote

Fertilized oocyte prior to first cell division is called zygote.

Artificial Insemination with Donor (AID) Semen Indications

  a. Nonobstructive azoospermia
  b. The husband has a hereditary genetic defect; or
  c. When the couples have Rh incompatibility.

Indications

- Husband has non-obstructive azoospermia.
- Husband has a hereditary genetic defect.

- The couple has Rh incompatibility.
- The woman is isoimmunized and has lost previous pregnancies and intrauterine transfusion is not possible.
- Husband has severe oligozoospermia and the couple does not wish to undergo any of the sophisticated ART such as ICSI.

Intrauterine Insemination with Either Husband's or Donor's (IUI-H or IUI-D) Semen

Pure, activated sperm, directly placed into the uterus.

Indications

- Hostile uterine cervix that does not respond to medication
- Husband's sperm cannot be used.
  - Success rate of IYF: One in every 4–5 women.
- Irreversible pathology of the fallopian tubes.
- Infertility due to a subnormal male factor.
- Idiopathic infertility
- Endometriosis
- Infertility of immunological origin.

IVF-ASSOCIATED TECHNIQUES

Gamete intrafallopian tube transfer (GIFT) and tubal embryo transfer (TET) are recommended for patients with fallopian tubes in good condition. Access to the tube is gained by laparoscopy or by retrograde catheterization through the uterine cervix. GIFT is associated with higher levels of pregnancy than IVE.

A sizeable number of couples is not suitable for IVF because their sperm count is far below 10 million/ml with less then 30% sperm being motile and more than 30% having abnormal morphology.

Partial zona dissection (PZD), subzonal insemination (SUZI) and intracytoplasmic sperm injection (ICSI) are done in such case.

ICSI is the most widely accepted choice of treatment for male factor infertility. ICSI is carried out with fresh or frozen thawed ejaculated or epididymal/testicular motile or live spermatozoa.

Indications

- Severe male-factor infertility.
- Fertilization failure after standard IVF treatment.
- Number of spermatozoa in the ejaculate too low for IVF.

Indications of ICSI with Epididymal Spermatozoa Obtained by Microsurgical/ Percutaneous Epididymal Sperm Aspiration (MESA/PESA)

- Congenital bilateral absence of the vas deferens (CBAVD).
- Failed vasoepididymal anastomosis.
- Failed vasovasal anastomosis.
- Obstruction of both ejaculatory ducts. An ejaculation because of spinal cord injury.
- Retrograde ejaculation.

Indications of ICSI with Testicular Spermatozoa (TESA)

- Extensive scarring rendering MESA/ PESA impossible
- Germ cell hypoplasia (hypospermato-genesis).
- Germ cell aplasia with focal sperma-togenesis.
- Sertoli cell-only syndrome with focal spermatogenesis.

Indications for Oocyte or Embryo Donation

- Gonadal dysgenesis
- Premature ovarian failure
- Iatrogenic (due to ovarian surgery or radiation or chemical castration) ovarian failure.
- Women who have resistant ovary syndrome, or who are poor responders to ovulation induction.
- Women who are carriers of recessive autosomal disorders.
- Women who have attained menopause.

Cryopreservation

Freezing semen: Men, suffering from psychological stress at the time of ovum pick-up and those who cannot be present at the time of ovum pick-up can get their semen frozen for use at the appropriate time. Donor semen is quarantined for six months. The safety of using frozen sperm is proved by experimental work and the actual human results. Donors who are infected with venereal diseases, hepatitis B or C, or HIV are not included sperm freezing causes 20% loss of motility after thawing. Donors are asked to report to the semen bank six months after donation to be checked for HIV, HBV or HCV infection/disease status.

Freezing embryos: Embryos are cryo-preserved to store supernumerary embryos, as up to a maximum of only three embryos are allowed for transfer to avoid the risk of multiple pregnancies. Embryo freezing is a widespread routine procedure to increase cumulative pregnancy rates.

Human embryos can be successfully cryopreserved at any stage from zygote to blastocyst, using one or two propanediol (PROH) or dimethylsulphoxide (DMSO) for zygotes and cleaved embryos and glycerol for blastocysts.

Consent is obtained concerning the agreement for embryo freezing as well as for the future use of the embryos.

ARTIFICIAL INSEMINATION

Artificial insemination is insemination of woman for purpose of impregnation by means other than sexual intercourse. It is of two types:

1. Artificial insemination homologus (AIH), husband's semen.
2. Artificial insemination donor (AID), donor's semen.

Indications for Donor Insemination

- Sterility of husband.
- Rh incompatibility between husband and wife.
- Genetic defects in husband.
- Husband has non-obstructive azoospermia.
- Husband has a hereditary genetic defect.
- The couple has Rh incompatibility.
- The woman is isoimmunized and has lost previous pregnancies and intrauterine transfusion is not possible.
- Husband has severe oligozoospermia and the couple do not wish to undergo any of the sophisticated ART such as ICSI.

Donor Selection

- The donor must be below 40 years of age.
- There should be no Rh incompatibility between donor and recipient.

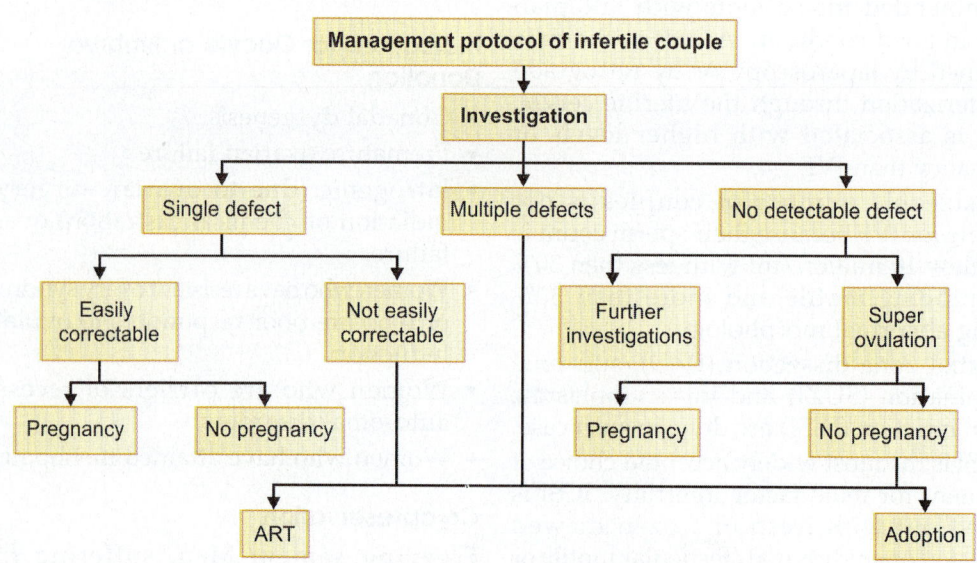

Fig. 10.1: Infertility protocol

- The donor must be in sound health.
- No history of hereditary or familial diseases.
- The consent of wife of donor is required.
- The identity of donor is kept confidential.
- The donor should have resemblance to the recipient and her husband.

Medicolegal Problems

- The law presumes that child produced during the period of legal marriage is legal child, unless it is consented.
- In AIH, the problem is still less as husband is treated as father of the child.
- Artificial insemination cannot be a ground for divorce/nullity of marriage.

Surrogate Mother

- A surrogate mother is one who offers her womb for carrying out the pregnancy of another woman.
- The pregnancy may be the result of artificial insemination or ovum fertilized *in vitro*.
- A surrogate mother has no claim on the baby delivered by her.
- The methods of assisted reproduction have very much advanced.

- A spermatozoa may be taken out form the testes and introduced into the ovum obtained from the woman desirous of begetting child from that person.
- Fertilization is carried out under laboratory conditions and embryo is transferred either to biological or surrogate mother.

Medicolegal Issues

- The baby in the womb may not be the product of the woman carrying out the pregnancy.
- The baby in the womb may be the product of the woman bearing the pregnancy but not with her husband.

The problems faced by the baby by assisted reproduction are:

- Who is the father?
- Who is the mother?
- Who is his/her legal guardian?
- Who is the biological parent?
- Can he/she inherit the property?

All these questions have to be answered in individual cases depending on their own merits and on legal questions that arise.

CHAPTER 11

Legitimacy and Paternity

INTRODUCTION

The question of legitimacy of a child arises in cases of affiliation, inheritance and supposititious children.

Affiliation cases: In these cases the maintenance of a child is handed over to the biological father of the child, irrespective of whether the woman is married to him or not.

Inheritance: Only a legitimate child has a right to inherit the property of his father.

Supposititious child: A supposititious child is a child supposed to be the child of a woman but infact he is not the child of that woman. In this case woman assumes pregnancy, pretends delivery and presents the supposititious child as her own.

Such a child is not the valid offspring of father or mother.

Establishment of Legitimacy of a Child

To establish the legitimacy, i.e. the status of a child born in lawful wedlock, the following criteria have to be taken into consideration.

- Whether the woman was pregnant?
- What was the duration of pregnancy?
- Whether the woman delivered child (male/female)?
- Whether the husband is not impotent and not infertile?
- Paternity status of the child?

If the woman was pregnant and carried pregnancy for 280 days and then she delivered the full term child.

- If the woman shows signs of recent delivery then her status as a delivered woman is confirmed.
- Examination of the husband for semen status and possibilities of impotence confirm his capacity to impregnate.
- Paternity of the child is decided by examination of the blood of the child, mother and father.
- If the father dies with the woman being pregnant but before the delivery of the child, the child born is legitimate child and is called **posthumous child.**
- If a child is born during the legal continuation of a marriage, it is considered to be a **legitimate child.**
- Even if there is a separation or divorce between husband and wife, if the child is born within 280 days of separation or divorce, the child is presumed to be legitimate.
- When a man and woman are not married and at that time woman becomes pregnant but they get married before the child is delivered, then also the child born is treated as legitimate child.

PATERNITY

- The question of paternity may arise due to disputes in relation to property, guardianship, maintenance, etc.
- Paternity means fatherhood. However, in practice paternity means parenthood/parentage, i.e. whether the child C is born

to a husband H and wife W during their accessibility to each other.

Paternity is determined by the following data

Resemblance to parents

Features

• Facial features
  – Gestures
  – Gait
  – Colour of iris
  – Complexion
  – Hair
  – Mannerisms
  – Personal peculiarities
  – DNA profile of parents and child.

Table 11.1: Blood group in establishing paternity and nonpaternity

Blood groups of parents	Possible groups of children	Blood groups of children not possible
O, O	O	A, B, AB
O, A	O, A	B, AB
O, B	O, B	A, AB
O, AB	A, B	O, AB
A, A	O, A	B, AB
A, B	A, B, AB, O	–
A, AB	A, AB, B	O
B, B	B, O	A, AB
AB, AB	A, B, AB	O

DNA profile also helps in paternity testing. **Mitochondrial DNA from mother shows link with mother**

• Sometimes, the child may not resemble the parents it may resemble the grandfather/grandmother (atavism).
• Atavism is the state of a child when it resembles the grandparents and not the parents (atavism grandfather).
• If the alleged father is impotent and infertile, if he did not have access to the woman, if the child's blood group is not possible with that couple, if the parents belong to one race and the child belongs to another race, then it is easy to say that the child does not belong to the couple.

Superfoetation

In this case, fertilization of two ova of different ovulatory periods by different acts of coitus lead to double pregnancy. The resulting twins are of different ages.

Superfecundation

• When the fertilization of two ova of same ovulatory period occurs by two different acts of coitus, leading to double pregnancy; the twins delivered are equality developed and are of same age.
• In one case reported, the woman gave birth to one dark skinned and other fair skinned child of equal uterine development and age.

CHAPTER 12

Infant Deaths

INFANTICIDE

- Infanticide is defined as deliberate and unlawful killing of an infant by an Act of omission or Act of commission.

- *Is it punishable?* It is regarded as murder in the court of law. It is punishable under Section 302 of IPC.

Infant: An infant is any live born child up to the age of one year after birth.

Acts of Omission and Infanticide

Any willful omission or failure in taking are of the infant to preserve or maintain the infant life is an act of omission.

Examples

- As soon as the baby is born, the umbilical cord must be ligated before it is cut.

- If this is not done it is an Act of omission.

- The newborn baby is given bath and kept warm.

- Before that the fluids from nose and mouth need to be sucked to facilitate proper breathing. Failure to do any of these Acts become an Act of omission.

Acts of Commission

- Acts of commission are those Acts which are intentionally done to take the life of an infant like poisoning, strangulation, drowning, abandoning the child in cold unprotected place and so on.

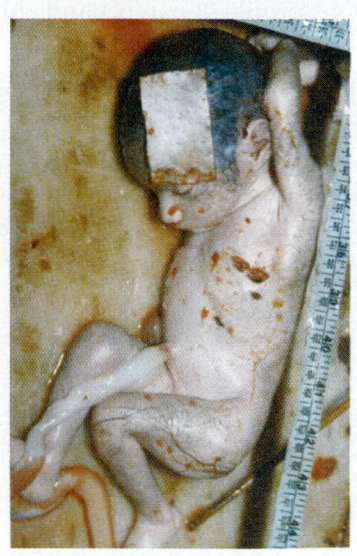

Fig. 12.1: Mother stabbed causing multiple stabs to the baby in side

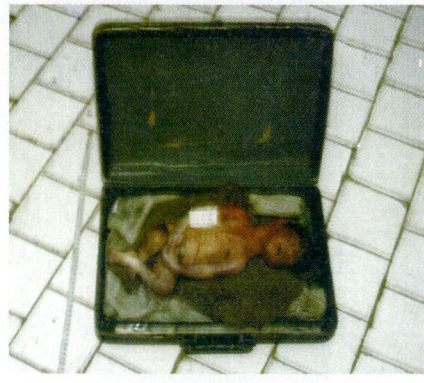

Fig. 12.2: Newborn disposed via briefcase, creased a "Bomb-scare" on Surat railway station platform bomb squad called for defusing

Some Questions Arise when a Dead Body is brought for Examination

- Whether the child is dead born/still born?
- Whether the child was born alive?
- If the child was born alive, how long did the child live?
- What was the cause of death?
- When did the child die?
- How did the child die homicidal or accidental?
- Where did the child die in the house or anywhere else?

Still Born Child

A still born child is one who did not breathe at all or show any other sign of life like breathing/swallowing or heart-beats after it is delivered.

Dead Born Child

- A dead born child has died in the uterus. It shows maceration (or) aseptic autolysis.
  - The foetus is softened. The body is soft and pliable, flattens out on table (it does not retain shape when kept on the table).
  - The skin is sodden and coppery red in colour. It shows blisters. Abdomen is distended. Umbilical cord is thick.
  - The joints are unduly mobile.
  - The tissues are oedematous. Body cavities contain reddish serum. Organs are soft and oedematous. Skull bones are loose.
  - No gases are formed.
  - Maceration takes about 7 days.
  - A child who has died a week before delivery shows signs of maceration.
  - There is a rancid odour from foetus. Sometimes **adipocere** may be formed in place of maceration.

Live Born Child

A child born alive shows signs of live birth. The signs of live birth are seen in:

- External appearances
- Examination of ear
- Examination of chest
- Examination of umbilicus

- Examination of lungs
- Examination of heart
- Examination of gastrointestinal tract.

External appearances

- A well clothed body suggests live birth. If the body is washed well, the vernix caseosa disappears.
- Body is washed well and vernix caseosa disappears.
- *Vernix caseosa* is a dirty, whitish, cheesy substance present on the skin consisting of sebaceous secretions and epithelial cells. It protects foetal skin from amniotic fluid. When the body is washed, it disappears which indicates postnatal care.

Examination of ear

- The middle ear contains gelatinous embryonic tissue during foetal life. After birth this is replaced by air when respiration starts.
- *Wredin's test* is positive when middle ear contains air. It indicates breathing and live birth.

Examination of chest

- The chest flat before respiration.
- After respiration, the chest expands.
- Its circumference is greater than abdominal circumference.

Examination of umbilicus

- After the umbilical cord is cut, the stump attached to the abdomen starts getting dried from cut end by 1st day.
- The base of stump shows redness by 2nd day.
- The stump shows mummification by 3rd day.
- It falls off within a week.
- The healing of umbilicus occurs by about 10 days.
- The umbilical arteries are obliterated by 3rd day and umbilical veins by 5th day. All these are evidences of life activity in umbilicus.

Examination of lungs

- After the baby starts breathing, the lungs get inflated.

- The unrespired lung is liver like dry, no blood escapes on section.
- They are bluish red in colour, do not fill the thoracic cavity, lie behind close to the spine.
- The margins are sharp. The surface is smooth, consistency is solid. The weight is 30–40 gm.

Fodere's test or static test

- The respired lung occupy the chest cavity, mottled in appearance, blood oozes from cut sections, the margins are rounded, surface is uneven, spongy in consistency and crepitant.
- The weight is doubled, i.e. 60–70 gm. The doubling of weight of respired lung is called "Fodere's test or static test".

Plouquete test

The ratio of weight of lung and of the body is 1:70 before respiration and 1:35 after respiration. This is called *Plouquete test.*

The respired lung is lighter than water so it floats on water. This test of *floatation or Raygat's hydrostatic test* is based on testing the floatation of bits of lungs until the pieces are compressed under strong pressure to remove even the tidal air. Even these pieces of respired air float because the residual air still remians. **It is also know as the first life test.**

Fallacies of hydrostatic test

- The unrespired lungs float after decomposition.
  - Because of gases decomposition in the lungs. When artificial respiration is given to the lungs of newborn, some areas of lung float.
  - Respired lungs sink in case of collapse or atelectasis of lung, consolidation or pneumonitis.
- The unrespired alveoli appear hollow, and look like glands lined by cuboidal/columnar epithelium. The alveoli of respired lung are covered by flattened epithelium.
- The presence of alveolar duct membrane lining the alveolar ducts indicate live birth.

It is made up of fat, can be seen by colouring with fat stains.

Examination of heart

- The ductus arteriosus closes in 4–10 days time, foramen ovale closes in about 2 months after birth.
- Closure of these live births and time of survival.

Examination of GI tract

- Presence of milk in **stomach bowl test:** It is based on presence of air in stomach which is gulped during respiration.
- The stomach is ligated at pyloric and cardiac ends and opened under water. Bubbles of air escape. The same is repeated with intestine.
- **Fallacies of Breslau's test:** If the child did not swallow air it may be negative even if the child was born alive.
- Decomposition gases give positive test even if the child is not born alive.
- Artificial respiration can show air in stomach. However, small intestines do not show air in artificial respiration.

Presence of Meconium

- **Meconium** is a greenish inspissated bile found in upper part of large intestines of foetus.
- Within the first two days, meconium is voided by the baby.
- Absence of meconium suggests live birth except in breech delivery where it may be passed during delivery.

Survival Time

It is estimated from the changes in heart, umbilical cord, gastrointestinal tract. Caput succedaneum, changes in blood, changes in urinary system.

Caput Succedaneum

- During the process of delivery, the presenting part (head) is pressed.
- The tissues become engorged and oedematous.
- The presenting part is generally head so there is caput haematoma. When

there is greater extravasation, it is called **cephalohaematoma.**
- It is observed from 24 hours onwards and the caput disappears by about one week after birth.
- Caput succedaneum is seen in any presenting part other than buttocks to a variable extent.

Changes in Blood

- The newborn presents nucleated cells in peripheral blood up to 24 hours after birth, after which they disappear.
- Foetal haemoglobin is seen up to 6 months after birth.

Changes in Urinary System

Uri acid crystals are seen in pyramids of kidneys up to two days. After this they disappear.

Causes of Death

- Natural causes
- Accidental causes
- Criminal causes

Natural Causes

- Erythroblastosis foetalis
- Immaturity
  - A child whose weight is 2000 gm is immature baby.
  - A child born before full term is premature child.

Accidental Causes

- Prolonged labour
- Prolapse of cord
- Twisting of cord around neck
- Precipitate labour
  - Precipitate labour is the labour that occurs in multiparous woman with lax and roomy passages, small child without any forewarning.
  - There is telescoping of all the 3 stages of labour. Placenta delivered along with baby.
  - Caput succedaneum and cephalohaematoma absent.

- If the woman is standing, child may sustain head injuries. If the baby is born in comode, he/she may be asphyxiated.
- Umbilical cord may be torn in precipitate labour.

Criminal Causes

- Acts of omission
- Acts of commission.
  - Exposure to cold; failure to ligate umbilical cord; failing to feed.
  - Drowning, strangulation, throttling, head injury, poisoning.

Foetal Autopsy

- Skull is opened along the four directions from the middle of anterior frontanelle.
- Ossification centres are examined in foot, at knee and in sternum.
- Abdomen is opened before chest to note the level of diaphragm levels.
- Weight of organs taken; viscera subjected to histopathology and chemical analysis.

Age of the Foetus

- The products of conception are called ovum up to age of 2nd week of pregnancy, from third to fifth weeks, it is called embryo and after fifth week, it is called foetus.
- **After first month:** Length is 4 cm, eyes seen as two dark spots, mouth as cleft and limbs as bud-like processes.
- **After second month:** Length is 4 cm, anus seen as dark spot; umblical cord begins to develop; limbs are webbed; ossification centre in mandible and clavicle.
- **After third month:** Length is 9 cm; pupillary membrane appears; nails appear; placenta is formed.
- **After fourth month:** Length is 16 cm; sex distinguishable; lanugo present; meconium present in duodenum.
- **After fifth month:** Length is 25 cm; vernix caseosa present; meconium reaches large intestine; ossification centre in calcaneum.
- **After sixth month:** Length is 30 cm; scalp hairs; eyelashes and eyebrows formed; testes lie with kidneys; ossification in 4 divisions of sternum.

- **After seventh month:** Length is 35 cm; pupillary membrane disappears; eyelids open; testicles up to external inguinal ring; ossification centre in talus, child becomes viable.
- **After eighth month:** Length is 40 cm; weight in 2 kg; nails extend beyond finger-tips; left testicle in scrotum.
- **After ninth month:** Length is 45 cm; weight in 2.5–3 kg. Dense scalp hair; both testicles descended; ossification centres in cuboid, lower end femur, upper end tibia; meconium in entire large intestine.

Full Term Features

- Length: 50 cm
- Weight: 2.5–3 kg
- Dark scalp hair: 4 cm long
- Umbilicus midway between xiphoid and symphysis pubis.
- Umbilical cord: 50 cm long
- Placenta: 500 gm; 22 cm in diameter, 1.5 cm thick at centre.

SUDDEN INFANT DEATH SYNDROME (SIDS)

Sometimes an infant sleeping in a cot or crib is found lying dead causing alarm, wonder and shock in the minds of parents. As it is possible due to more than one cause. This type of sudden death of infant is also called as sudden infant death syndrome.

Predisposing Causes

- Season (rainy and winter)
- Prematurity
- Male sex
- Age of middle infancy
- Social status of lower and middle class
- Late night time of death.

Precipitating Causes

The commonest cause is prolonged state of apnoea during sleep.

Others

- Viral infection of respiratory tract.
- Hypersensitivity to cow's/buffalo's milk when baby is fed on such milk causing inhalation of milk and laryngeal spasm to death.

- The sleeping/intoxicated mother causes death of the baby due to overlaying.
- Bed clothes smothering the baby.

Medicolegal Issues

- Generally, cot deaths are natural.
- Sometimes sudden death is represented as Criminal Act to deviate the attention of investigating agencies.

BATTERED BABY SYNDROME/CAFFEY'S SYNDROME

- Majority of the victims are <2 years.
- Common in male children.
- Illigitimate or unwanted child is battered one.
- Victim is usually the single child in the family.
- Both parents are busy with their own work.
- Young, wreckless in lifestyle with low tolerance threshold, aggressive personalities.
- Battering is done frequently to punish the child for real or imaginary disobedience.
- The parents present the case to the doctor with a history inconsistent with time of incident, nature of injuries.

Findings

- Multiple injuries of varying ages.
- The injuries simple to serious.
- Frequently rib fractures of different ages can seen in X-ray examination. These fractures were first noticed by Caffey on X-ray examination, so this syndrome is called Caffey's syndrome.
- Bruises, abrasions, fractures of skull, limbs, etc. are seen.
- The baby may be kept in hot water tub; burnt by cigarette butts; thrashed against a wall.

Medicolegal Issues

- Battered baby syndrome is a marital and social problem.
- Punishments are given based on the crime and also depend upon nature of injuries.
- Parents need counselling.

MUNCHAUSEN SYNDROME BY PROXY (GENTLE HOMICIDE)

- In this case, the mother inflicts repeated minor injuries to the child. The child is admitted frequently in the hospital, he/she may be unconsciousness and treated for resuscitation leading to unnecessary investigations.
- It may be serious health problem including death of child.

Shaken Baby Syndrome

- It is an alleged condition characterized by intracranial bleeding and retinal haemorrhage.
- When a young child is violently shaken with resultant whiplash movement of head, bridging veins are torn causing subdural/subarachnoid haemorrhage.

Munchausen Syndrome

- These individuals feign physical and psychological symptoms and their basic motive seems to get hospitalized.
- They may even inflict injury on themselves or may take drugs which produce symptoms.
- They usually do not have any external motive which differentiates them from malingerers.

The Following is Required for Firm Diagnosis

- The individual feigns physical/psychological symptoms consistently.

- There is no evidence of any physical or psychological disease.
- History of repeated hospitalisation.
- Repeated investigation and treatment.
- No external motivating factors.

SOME IMPORTANT POINTS

- False negative Raygat's hydrostatic test is seen in atelectasis in live born foetus.
- Adipocere formation is not seen in a dead born foetus.
- Rigor mortis develops in a foetus of 7 months intrauterine life.
- Mummification is seen in late intrauterine death.
- Spalding's sign is diagnostic of foetal death.
- Gas in great vessels of foetus suggests foetal death. If the ossification centre of lower end of femur is present, the foetus is viable one. In cases, where the foetal heart rate is 160/minute in fifth month and 120 per minute in ninth month.
- Under PNDT Act, prenatal test is not permitted. After delivery the uterus walls are concave from inside and the top of the fundus convex.
- Cervical canal shows mucosal folds (arbor vitae).
- Karyotyping of the foetus can be done from lymphocyte, fibroblast, and amniocyte, but not monocyte.

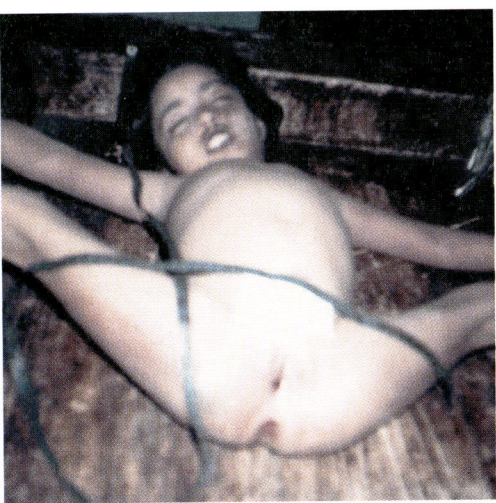

Injury to vulva in a small child

CHAPTER 13

Trace Evidence

INTRODUCTION

- When any crime is committed, the accused, the victim and the scene of offence are involved.
- According to the **Locard's principle of exchange,** whenever and wherever two individuals come across each other there is an exchange of material.
- Accordingly in a reported crime, material exchanged from the accused can be found on the victim, material exchanged from the victim can be found on accused; material from the scene can be found on accused or victim, mateiral from the accused can be found at the scene of crime.
- This material gives the connection between accused, victim and the scene of offence.
- This is a very valuable trace evidences, helpful in the establishment of chain of evidences or corpus delicti.
- Therefore, the doctor doing autopsy examination, examination of sex offences, examination of injured persons in accidents and in all cases requiring examination and reporting should look for trace evidence like blood stains, seminal stains, hair, saliva, bite marks, nails, spent cartridges, latent fingerprints, bullets or pellets or unused cartridges, paints, greasy materials, condoms, etc.

Examination of Hair

The following questions arise during examination of hair:

- Identification of hair?
- If hair, human or animal?
- If human hair, which part of the body it belongs to?
- How it is removed from the body? Cut or crushed or pulled?
- Is it of natural colour or dyed?
- Is there any poison in the hair?
- What is the sex of the person?
- Can the cause of death be given from hair?
- Can the identity be told from hair to DNA typing?

1. **Identification of hair?**
   - Hair differs from other fibres. It has an outer layer of cuticle, middle layer of cortex and inner layer of medulla.
   - The cuticular pattern of human hair is irregularly annular. This pattern can be examined by taking the impression of cleaned hair on a gelatin smeared slide and lifting the hair.
   - The cuticular scale pattern is printed on the smear which can be examined under low power and high power compound microscope.
   - Any fibre other than hair can thus be differentiated.

2. **Whether animal or human hair?**
   - The human hair differs from animal hair. Medulla is very thin in diameter in human hair, cortex is many times more in diameter. In animal hair, cortex and medulla are nearly equal in diameter.

- Some indices of the hair help in identification like medullary index, scale count index.
- The number of cuticular scales in a given area for a given person is constant and varies from person to person.

3. **Which part of the body does the human hair belong?**
- Beard hair are triangular in cross section, scalp hair are long, soft with tapering tip.
- Due to combing, there is fraying of the hair nearer to the ends.
- When the hair naturally falls, the root of the hair is atrophied, shrunken and distorted. The hair bulb has round end, smooth surface. The hair root cells help in sex determination by sex chromatin.
- Hair of eyelashes, eyebrows and nostrils are stiff, thick and tapering.
- The axillary or pubic hair are oval or oblong in cross section.

- Body hairs are less pigmented, fine and soft. The hair of the newborn lack pigment cells.
- They are fine and dawny. The Europeans have wavy hairs with light, dark, brown or red pigment.
- Chinese and other Asians have long straight black coarse hair.
- Negroes have highly curled wire like hair, black in colour.
- When examined under the microscope, the dyed hair can be differentiated.
- The dye is found superficially nearer the growing end and absent towards the root.
- The cut hair is clean at the end.
- The crushed end is irregular.
- As the time passes the cut end smoothens and becomes rounded.
- When the hair is exposed to heat, it gets singed.

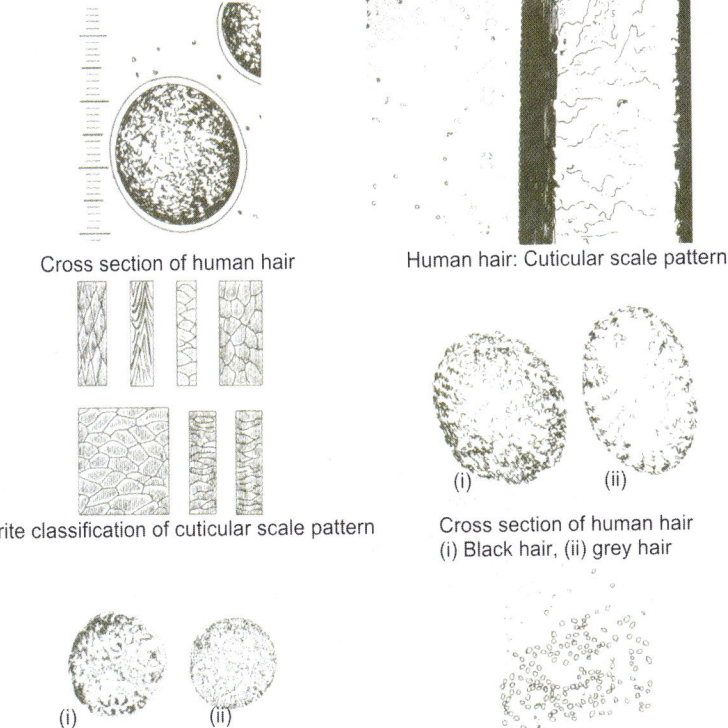

Cross section of human hair

Human hair: Cuticular scale pattern

Morite classification of cuticular scale pattern

Cross section of human hair
(i) Black hair, (ii) grey hair

Cross section of human hair
(i) Pigmented medullated, (ii) nonmedullated

Cross section of bunch of human hair

Fig. 13.1: Examination of human hair

- ABO blood group can be determined from hair by modified absorption elution method.
- Certain poisons are deposited in the hair like arsenic, mercury, thallium, copper, antimony, etc.
- Neutron activation analysis of the hair for trace elements helps in individualization.
- **DNA profiling,** the latest tool available for biometric profiling and individualisation is possible from the hair bulb.
- Hair cannot grow after death. From the hair length on the beard, the time of last shave can be determined as hair grows at the rate of 0.4 mm/day.
- So, from the examination of hair, clues are available and evidences traced in rape, sodomy, bestiality, hit and run accidents, poisoning cases, nature of weapon, rape of the person and identification of the person.
- Hair may be found on the weapon.

Blood

Blood stains are found in relation to crime on the body of victim, on the weapon and scene of crime.

The following questions arise in relation to blood stains:

- Whether the stain in question is blood or not?
- If it is blood, whether it is human or animal?
- If human, male or female blood?
- Whether it is menstrual blood?
- Is it haematemesis?
- Is it from an abscess?
- What is the age of blood stain?
- What is the approximate age?
- Is it from living or dead person?
- Is it from accused or victim?
- Human blood has biconcave disc-like red blood cells which are non-nucleated in nature.
- Whether it is blood or not, is also decided by physical examination, chemical examination, microscope studies, microchemical tests?

- The camel blood is oval, biconvex and non-nucleated. The blood of reptiles and birds is oval, biconvex and nucleated.
- Spectroscopic examination studies are haemoglobin bands.
- Various bands that are studied are carboxyhaemoglobin, haemochromogen, cyanhaemochromogen, methaemoglobin, sulphmethaemoglobin, haematoporphyrin, cyanmethaemoglobin, etc.
- Microchemical tests are also used to study haemoglobin, haemin and haemochromogen crystals.
- Haemin crystals are faint yellow or dark crystals are pink, rhomboidal crystals in cluster.
- Among the serological tests for the species origin, the precipitin test is conducted to detect human species.
- It is done as ring or capillary tube test.
- Antihuman sera in dilutions up to 1 in 50,000 can react and detect human serum.
- From the blood, sex can be known by examination of polymorph leucocytes or by studying Davidson bodies.
- Menstrual blood is acidic, contaminated with vaginal epithelial and endometrial cells.
- Haematemesis blood is acidic, contaminated with regurgitated food material.
- Haemoptysis blood is frothy and bright red, contains mucosal shreds.
- If animal bite or crushing of the insect is in the blood, the crushed parts of mosquito, bed-bugs, etc. can be seen under microscope.
- Biochemical analysis of blood helps in estimation of time since death.
- Ageing of the blood is estimated from dissolution of blood pigments to some extent.
- Blood group determination helps in identification.
- Cause of death from blood examination is detected in many poisoning cases. DNA profiling of blood helps in the identification of the person.

The Various Types of Blood Group Systems

- ABO system
- MN system

- Rh system
- Ss group
- P group
- Kell system
- Lutheran system
- Duffy system
- Kidd system
- Gm groups
- Haptoglobin
- As groups.
- Red cell enzyme groups
- Serum lipoprotein groups
- G6PD
- Bombay blood group
- Even after taking help of all blood group systems we cannot fix paternity in all cases.

- However, with the advent of DNA profiling, the results are more specific nowadays.
- DNA profiling is useful because both maternal and paternal components are seen in the child.
- At the scene of crime from the nature of blood stains certain inferences can be made.
- The spurting or splashing of blood causes stains on the walls, first in upward direction followed by downward trickling.
- The tailing of the blood stain suggests the direction of bleeding.
- When the blood oozes from dead body, stains are found settled on floor, bed or clothes with diffusion due to oozing.
- For DNA profile, *refer* to Chapter 3.

CHAPTER 14

Artefacts

- According to McMillan's dictionary, an artefact is an object made by man.
- However, in medicolegal parlance, artefacts are anything intentionally or inadvertently introduced in a human body for diagnostic or therapeutic interventions by the doctor before the death of the person and also by any means introduced after. Careful death handling and protection from animals or insects during postmortem examination by the doctors or the mortuary staff is necessary. Any negligence or mishandling can produce artifacts.

DISADVANTAGES OF ARTEFACTS

- Artefacts interfere with natural events in the human body so they may create confusion in the mind of the person, examining the body. It may cause misinterpretation of the observations leading to wrong inferences.
- Artefacts can lead to wrong cause of death, wrong manner of death, and miscarriage of justice.

Antemortem artefacts are caused by

- Cardiac massage.
- Interference in pre-existing injuries for surgical purpose.
- Regurgitation of fluids into mouth and respiratory passages.

Postmortem artefacts are caused by

- Embalming
- Changes like rigor mortis, hypostasis, decomposition.

- Animal and insect bites
- Refrigeration
- Toxicology

Artefacts due to cardiac massage

- External cardiac massage can lead to fracture of ribs along mid-axillary line or sternum in middle of body or manubriosternal joint.
- Fat or bone marrow embolism may follow sometimes.

Interference in pre-existing injuries for surgical purpose

- Positive pressure ventilation may cause acute emphysaema, tension, pneumothorax.
- Carotid angiography may cause bruising of neck, muscles, surgeons excise, extend, explore, repair and alter the wounds.

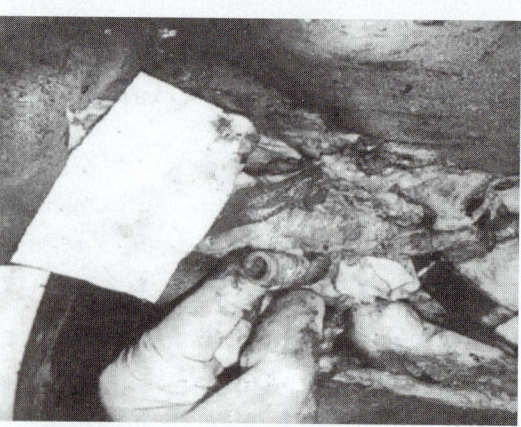

Fig. 14.1: Endotracheal tube in stomach

Regurgitation

Agonal regurgitation, i.e. the leakage of fluids into respiratory passage or stomach and their re-entry or presence in the mouth, trachea, oesophagus create agonal artefacts.

POSTMORTEM ARTEFACTS

- Embalming artefacts: Embalming fluid is pushed through a trocar passed through subclavian area of neck, axilla, abdomen, femoral region.
- The trocar wounds resemble as stab wounds or firearm wounds.
- Embalming fluid may cause effusion of blood in and around injured areas.
- Embalming may alter the pre-existing or other injuries.

Rigor Mortis, Decomposition and Lividity

- Rough handling can break the rigor mortis.
- Heat, cold and gases of decomposition interfere with rigor mortis.
- Hypostasis and decomposition cause colour change and distortion of the organs externally and internally.
- These changes often confuse the observer or examiner.

Animal and Insect Bites

- Rats, cats, dogs, jackals, vultures, ants, cockroaches, flies damage the body after death.

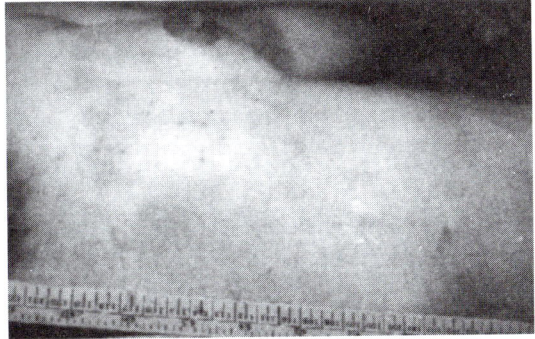

Fig. 14.2: Multiple needle punctures during resuscitation

- These lesions can resemble similar to abrasions, lacerations, firearm wounds, etc.
- They also can change the character of pre-existing wounds.

Refrigeration Artefacts

- The refrigerated bodies show bright-coloured blood and bright tissues inside.
- It prolongs rigor mortis, hypostasis and retards decomposition.

Autopsy-related Artefacts

During autopsy, while dissecting and examining the dead body, the detailed analysis of the following points can be made.

- Air in blood vessels
- Skull fractures damage the organ
  - Tears of midbrain
  - Diaphragm tears
  - Injury to neck structures
- Extravasation of blood
- Fracture of hyoid bone
- Injury to blood vessels
- Toxicological artefacts like:
  - Contaminaiton of stomach contents
  - Mistake while collection of samples
  - Wrong usage of preservatives
- Faulty technique in collection of sample can give false results.
- While collecting blood from heart with needle it may get contaminated with stomach contents and regurgitated material.
- If sample is contaminated with cavity fluids, false results may be obtained.
- Anticoagulants used for blood, e.g. EDTA, formalin, heparin, etc. may give false positive result for alcohol.
- Bacterial decomposition itself produces ethyl as well as higher alcohols.
- Decomposition itself causes increase in concentration of CO in blood.
- Cyanide in significant quantities is produced in blood after death and also in death due to burns.

- Many substituted phenols are formed in decomposing bodies.
- In buried bodies, arsenic may be imbibed from surrounding tissues (keratin tissues absorb arsenic more, so concentration in hair and nail is much greater than concentration of arsenic in contaminating fluid).

CONCLUSION

- The medical officer must be aware of possibility of artefacts whenever he conducts postmortem examination.
- Once he keeps in mind these possibilities and proceeds with examination, changes of error are minimized and even eliminated.

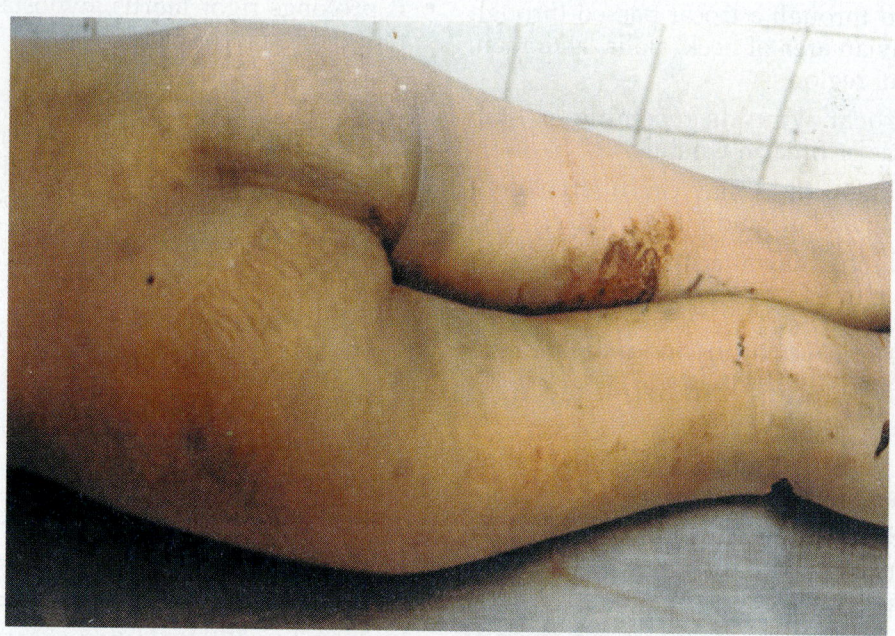

Artefact elastic underwear parallel marks: Contusion abrasion

CHAPTER 15

Tripped Forensic Issues

Five categories of medicolegal cases

1. Violent deaths, i.e. unnatural deaths (accidents, suicides and homicides).
2. Suspicious deaths, i.e. those that may be due to violence.
3. Sudden and unexpected deaths.
4. Unattended deaths, i.e. those in which a physician was not present at the time of death.
5. Deaths in custody.

Individual jurisdiction may modify these categories, either by expanding or by contracting them.

Cause, mechanism and manner of death

The manner of death is how the death occurrred.

- Natural
- Accidental
- Suicide
- Homicide
- Undetermined
- Unclassified

Handling of bodies from a hospital

a. If the deceased did not die immediately and was transported to a hospital, a number of surgical and medical procedures may have been carried out. This is why:
  - The complete medical records of the deceased from the time of admission to the time of death should be obtained.
  - In addition, EMS and ambulance transport records should also be obtained.

b. All hospitals in the area served by the medicolegal system should be informed about the cases.
  - Life saving additional tubes should not be removed from the body after death, e.g. endotracheal tubes, intravenous lines and Foley catheters.
  - Injection sites should be circled with ink by the hospital staff to indicate that they are of therapeutic origin and did not antedate hospitalization.
  - Surgical stab wounds should be labelled or described in the medical records.
  - If an injury is incorporated into a thoracotomy or laparotomy incision, this should be noted.
  - If death occurs within a few hours after hospitalization, paper bags should be placed on the hands, just as if the death had occurred at the scene.
  - Any clothing worn by the deceased should be transferred to the medical examiner's office.
  - All medical records having details of the procedures performed should accompany the body.
  - Any blood withdrawn on admission in the hospital should be sent for toxicology.
  - Blood obtained for transfusion purposes in trauma cases is often reserved for one to two weeks in the hospital blood bank.
  - The blood bank should be queried for retained initial blood samples.

DNA ANALYSIS

- DNA analysis can be performed on any tissue or substance that contains nucleated cells.
- The two most common tissues examined are blood and semen.
- The analysis is also performed on hair and saliva.

1. a. If the DNA profile of evidence from crime scene or victim is different from that of the suspected source, then that evidence absolutely did not come from the suspected individual.

   b. If the DNA profile of the evidence matches to that of an individual, then the individual is not excluded as the source of the evidence.
      - One then makes a statistical evaluation as to ascertain the suspect is the source of the evidence.

2. Whenever, a DNA analysis is performed there are three possible results:

   a. The specimen is inadequate in size, degraded, or contaminated, thus resulting in an insufficient amount of DNA for analysis.

   b. The DNA profiles are different and one has an exclusion.

   c. The DNA profiles match. If this last situation occurs, the match can be due to:
      - The samples come from the same person.
      - The samples come from different people but an error was made in either the collection of the material or in the laboratory, or
      - Two individuals have the same DNA profile.
      - This could because they are identical twins or because an insufficient number of tests has been performed so as to differentiate between the two.

3. While it is true that one's total DNA pattern is unique (except for an identical twin), the DNA testing currently being performed involves examination of a very minute portion of one's genetic blueprint.
   - The reason that one concludes that two samples came from the same source (i.e.

the same individual) is not same because one perform a complete analysis of the genetic structure of an individual, but other one performs a number of tests in which the DNA profiles from the individual tests are identical.

- Then, on the basis of probability calculation (i.e. statistics) we say that an individual is the source of the specimen.

4. There are two methods of DNA analysis in common use today, these are:
   - RFLP (restriction fragment length polymorphism), and
   - PCR (polymerase chain reaction) based methods of analysis. The nucleus of all cells in the body, excluding sperm and eggs, contains 23 pairs of chromosomes.

- Each of the 46 chromosomes consists of thread of deoxyribonucleic acid (DNA).
- This DNA thread is made up of two strands of bases held together by a sugar phosphate backbone arranged in a double helix (Fig. 15.1).

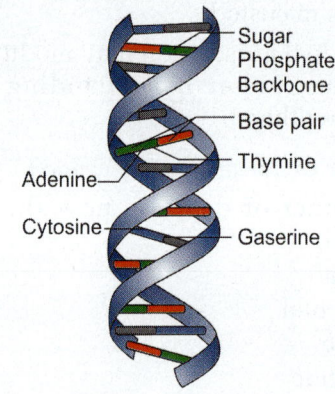

Fig. 15.1: Double helix

- The double helix has the configuration of a twisted ladder whose steps are formed by the four bases—adenine, thymine, guanine and cytosine.
- Adenine (a purine) always binds to thymine (a pyrimidine) and guanine (a purine) always binds to cytosine (a pyrimidine).
- Gene is a portion of this DNA thread (chromosome) that produces a specific product.

- The length of this gene can range from a few thousand to ten thousands of base pairs.
- The order of the four bases on the double helix determines the functions of the gene.
- Genes, however, constitute only a small fraction of the total length of the chromosome. The purpose of the test the chromosome is unknown.
- There are usually more one form of a gene for each location or locus on the chromosome.
- The alternate forms are called alleles.
- Most of the length of a chromosome serves no known function. In these areas, there are regions consisting of multiple copies of identical base sequences arranged in tandem, one behind the other. The repeated sequences are known as tandem repeats and the areas as variable number of tandem repeats (VNTR).
  - A VNTR region consists of any where from 500 to 10,000 of the base pairs arranged in these tandems repeated units of from 50 to 60 base pair lengths.
  - These VNTR loci are used in DNA typing because of the large number of alleles of these tandem repeats.
  - A VNTR loci may have a hundred or more alleles, although only 15–25 can be distinguished.
  - VNTR loci are used to full advantage in RFLP analysis.

Restriction Fragment Length Polymorphism (RFLP)

Analysis was the first method of DNA profiling widely used. In this method of analysis:

1. The DNA is cut into VNTR fragments by restriction enzymes.
2. These fragments are then detected and identified using electrophoresis and radioactive DNA probes.
3. A probe is a piece of single-stranded DNA, usually about 50 base pairs in length, which recognizes a specific region or locus in the DNA by virtue of complementary base pairing.

4. The single strand probe binds with a single strand DNA to produce a stable double strand molecule (thread).
5. This binding takes place on nylon membrane which is placed next to a X-ray film. Beta emissions from the probe expose the film.
6. After exposure for several hours to several days, the X-ray film is developed and the resulting film is called an autoradiograph or autorad. Where the probe has adhered to the VNTR fragment, bars appear on the X-ray film.
7. The autorad is then interpreted.
   - After the interpretation is complete, the probe is stripped by heating or by chemical action from the membrane and a new probe is applied.
   - This can be done for up to several probes.
8. Initial interpretation of the autorad is usually by visual inspection to see whether the samples have the same general pattern.
   - This eliminates obvious mismatches.
   - The autorad is then subjected to a more objective method of analysis to determine the fragment size present. This is accomplished with a computer.
   - If an exclusion has occurred, then one is finished. If not, then one has to determine the relative probabilities (frequencies).

The frequency of occurrence of a DNA profile is calculated using a standard population genetic equation with appropriate databases.

Polymerase Chain Reaction (PCR)

The second method of analysis involves PCR based systems.

1. The polymerase chain reaction (PCR) is a method for amplifying or copying a short sequence of DNA repeatedly, thus going from a small amount of DNA to a very large amount.
2. In the PCR methodology, polymerase enzymes are used to copy specific regions of DNA in order to obtain numerous copies of these areas to perform typing.

3. PCR based typing system allow alleles to be identified as discrete entities thus avoiding the statistical issues in matching and binning of the VNTR alleles.

4. The PCR process has advantages over the RFLP in that:
   - It is relatively simple and easily carried out in the laboratory.
   - The results are obtained in a short time (within a matter of a few days), and
   - Because of the unlimited capacity to reproduce the DNA segments, the PCR based methods permits analysis of extremly tiny amount of DNA.

5. The advantages of this method are:
   - It is susceptible to contamination.
   - Most PCR loci have fewer alleles than the VNTR areas utilized in RFLP, and
   - In addition, unlike RFLP which uses areas that have no functions, some natural selection leading to greater differences among population subgroups.

6. Instead of adding probes to a membrane in which DNA has been separated by electrophoresis, the probes are already bound to the membrane. Detection of the DNA is by a colour change to a dot on a membrane.

Short Tandem Repeats (STR)

STR is a PCR technique that will probably replace RFLP and presently used PCR methods in forensic labs in future.

1. The repeat unit in this system is much smaller than VNTR loci, being normally 2 to 6 base pairs.

2. STR loci occur throughout the genome at an estimated frequency of one STR every 300,000 to 500,000 base pairs.

3. While most STR loci have only 6–12 alleles, there are a large number of such systems that can be exploited for identification purposes.

4. In combination, they can produce a high power of discrimination.

5. As a general rule, in RFLP, a battery of four VNTR loci produces the power of exclusion of greater than 99% used of 8–9 STR loci gives at least the same percentage of exclusion.

6. STR technology has several advantages over conventional RFLP technology:
   - It is more rapid and can be done in two to three days; and
   - It can be performed on very small quantities of DNA (from one-tenth to one-hundredth the amount of DNA used in RFLP).

7. STR can be performed on wiping from full metal jacketed bottles that have perforated the body even if no tissue is visible.

8. While STR fragments from different STR loci differ in size, they are still small. Thus, it is possible to run the products from several STR loci simultaneously on one as long as the fragment sizes do not overlap.

9. STR analyses are performed by:
   - Isolating the DNA
   - Replicating the STR fragments by PCR
   - Performing gel electrophoresis, and
   - Identifying the fragments using stains, chemiluminescene or laser techniques.

10. The use of PCR robotics, an automated electrophoresis and analysis technology, allows automation of the STR typing.

Eruption of Deciduous Teeth (Subadult)

Tooth	Maxillary	Mandibular
Central incisor	7–8 months	6–7 months
Lateral incisor	8–1 months	8–11 months
Cuspid	17–20 months	16–20 months
First molar	12–16 months	12–16 months
Second molar	20–30 months	20–30 months

Eruption of Permanent Teeth (Adult)

Tooth	Maxillary	Mandibular
Central incisor	7–8 years	6–7 years
Lateral incisor	8–9 years	7–8 years
Cuspid	11–12 years	9½–11 years
First bicuspid	10–12 years	10–11 years
Second bicuspid	10–12 years	6–7 years
First molar	6–7 years	11½–13 years
Third molar	17–24 years	17–24 years

BRONCHIAL ASTHMA

Chronic bronchial asthma is associated with sudden death in a small percentage (–5%) of all cases of chronic asthma.

1. Sudden death can occur without a prolonged attack (acute asthmatic parozysm).
2. The frequency of sudden death in these cases appears to be increased at night or in the early morning.
3. There are several known triggers of asthmatic attacks are:
   - Allergens, both airborne and food (house dust, mites, peanuts)
   - Infections (viral or bacterial)
   - Occupational exposure to allergens
   - Certain drugs (e.g. aspirin)
   - Certain gases (such as sulphur dioxide, ozone)
   - Psychological stress
   - Exertion/exercise
   - Cold air.
4. Death results due to reduction of flow with ventilation perfusion mismatches which lead to decreased oxygenation of the blood, an elevation in the pCO_2 and right ventricular overload.
5. Decreased airflow occurs as a result of allergic release of histamine and other vasoactive compounds from inflammatory cells (eosinophils and mast cells), which in turn cause bronchial smooth muscle contraction, and intrabronchial mucous secretion.
6. In non-resuscitated individuals, autopsy usually shows hyperexpanded, puffy, pale lungs, with abundant mucous plugging of the bronchi (central and peripheral). In cases where cardiopulmonary resuscitation is done typical picture may not be seen (Table 15.1).

Microscopic examination: The lungs show characteristic changes of chronic asthma, with increased numbers of eosinophils present in the bronchial mucosa, submucosa, and/or peribronchiolar tissue. Representative section should be taken from all areas of the bronchial tree (central, mid, and peripheral).

Table 15.1: Samples/items collected before release of unidentified body

	Non-decomposed body	Decomposed body	Burned body	Skeletal
Colour photo of face, with ID number frontal and profile views	X	X	X	–
Colour photos of identifying marks (totterus, scars piercing, etc.)	X	X	–	–
Complete sets of classifiable fingerprints and palm prints in selected cases	X	If possible	–	–
Dental chart and X-ray of upper and lower jaw	X	X	X	X
X-ray, total body (especially skull with sinus views) 10–20 cc whole blood in EDTA	X	If available	X	–
Hair with root bulb	–	X	–	If present
Clothing, jewellery, personal effects, such as eyeglasses, dentures, hearings, aids, pacemaker	X	X	X	X

SUDDEN INFANT DEATH SYNDROME (SIDS)

SIDS is also referred to as cot or crib death:

a. SIDS was originally defined in 1969 at the Second International Conference on causes of sudden deaths in infants, as "the sudden death of any infant or young child, which is unexpected by history, and in which a thorough postmortem examination fails to demonstrate an adequate cause for death".

b. The definition was revised in 1989 by United States National Institute of Child
   • Health and Human Development Group, as "the sudden death of an infant under one year of age which remains unexplained after a thorough case investigation, including performance of a complete autopsy, examination of the death scene, and review of the clinical history".

c. **Incidence:** Estimated as approximately 2 per 1,000 live births in the United States. In Western countries, most common cause of death of infants in-between one week to one year of age.

d. Large number of deaths occur between first two days of child birth to few months of age.

e. Male predominance.

f. Higher occurrence in winter months of the year, and in countries with colder climates.

g. Premature infants are at a higher risk, but in the majority of cases the infant is full term.

h. Maternal risk factors include:
   • Low socioeconomic status.
   • Age less than 20 years at first pregnancy.
   • Cigarette smoking during and after pregnancy.
   • Use of illicit drug (cocaine, heroin) during pregnancy.

i. No apparent association between maternal caffeine or alcohol consumption during pregnancy and subsequent SIDS has been demonstrated.

j. Can occur at any time of the day, but the peak time is between midnight and the early morning hours.

Diseases which may result in sudden natural death in pediatric population

Cardiac
• Defections (myocarditis, endocarditis, rheumatic fever) of congenital cardiac defects.
• Cardiomyopathies
• Valvular abnormalities (aortic stenosis, mitral valve prolapse)
• Subaortic stenosis
• Tumour (rhabdomyoma, fibroma, myxoma)
• Conduction system disorders
• Endocardial fibroclastosis
• Emotional stress

Vascular
• Bronchial asthma
• Upper airway obstruction (congenital deformities, infections)
• Bronchopulmonary dysplasia
• Acute bronchopneumonia
• Massive pulmonary haemorrhage
• Idiopathic pulmonary haemosiderosis
• Tension pneumothorax.

Respiratory
• Bronchial asthma
• Upper airway obstruction (congenital deformities, infections)
• Bronchopulmonary dysplasia
• Acute bronchopneumonia
• Massive pulmonary haemorrhage
• Idiopathic pulmonary haemosiderosis
• Tension pneumothorax

Central nervous system
• Tumors (primary, metastatic)
• Epilepsy
• Infections (meningitis, encephalitis)
• Bleeding diathesis
• Tuberous sclerosis

Haematological
• Haemoglobinopathies (sickle cell disease)
• Lymphoma, leukaemia
• Coagulation disorders (inherited and acquired, bleeding diathesis and hypercoagulable syndromes)

- Congenital asplenia
- Splenic rupture (Western countries infectious mononucleosis, leukaemia).

Gastrointestinal

- Gastroenteritis with electrolyte abnormalities.
- Intestinal obstruction (intussusception or volvulus with associated blood infarction, sepsis).
- Late-presenting congenital diaphragmatic hernia.
- Anorexia nervosa or malnutrition.

Genitourinary

- Primary renal disease (pyelonephritis, glomerulonephritis).
- Ovarian torsion.

Metabolic/endocrine

- Fatty and oxidation disorders (MCAD, LCAD).
- Carbohydrate disorders (galactosaemia, glycogen storage disease).
- Amino acid disorders
- Newly onset diabetes mellitus
- Adrenal hypoplais
- Reye's syndrome

Miscellaneous

- Chromosomal disorders (Down, fragile, X-Turner syndrome).
- Anaphylaxis (food related—nuts, eggs, milk).

k. In many cases, there is a history of minor respiratory or gastrointestinal illness in the day's prior to death.

l. Sleeping position may play a role in the causation of SIDS, recently a marked reduction in the incidence of SIDS followed advertising campaign in some countries, which publicized possible link between SIDS and prone sleeping position.

m. Death usually occurs during sleep without evidence of distress or a struggle.

n. May occur anywhere, including cribs, or beds, automobiles, daycare centres, strollers, even in the arms of an adult.

o. Diagnosis of SIDS is one of exclusion and cannot, therefore, be made without a complete autopsy, including microscopic and toxicologic testing. In approximately 15% of cases where the initial impression is that of SIDS, another cause of death is found at autopsy.

p. Nonspecific gross findings which may be present include:
- Blood-tinged oedema fluid at the nostrils or between the lips.
- Hands clenched with fingers curled to palms, occasionally fibres from the bedding may be found in the hand.

q. Nonspecific autopsy findings may include:
- Thymic, pleural, and epicardial petechiae, present in 70–95% of cases.
- Congested or oedematous lungs with oedema, froth in the tracheobronchial tree.
- Sparse or foetal submucosal chronic inflammation of the airways.
- Gliosis of the brain stem.

r. Scene investigation should be conducted in all cases of suspected SIDS. The investigation should include questions regarding:
- Age of the infant, prior birth and medical history, including immunization history.
- The last time the infant was seen alive, and the time found deceased or unresponsive.
- The last time the infant was fed, amount and matter, and by whom.
- How as the infant was put down (position and bed covering), and how was the infant found?
- Was the infant sleeping alone?
- The type and condition of bed and mattress.
- Temperature of the room.
- Was resuscitation attempted?
- The recent health of the infant (sniffles, cold, etc.).
- Was the infant currently taking any medications, on prescription or not on prescription?

- Had any other family members been sick?
- History of any other SIDS deaths in the family.

s. The occurrence of repeat SIDS in the same family may be due to undetected or undiagnosed or undiagnosed inherited metabolic disorders, but may also be due to homicidal asphyxia.

t. The exact cause of sudden infant death syndrome is unknown, despite many theories which have been proved through the years. Multiple factors are probably involved. Some of the popular theories are:

- Older theory of status thymolymphaticus—death due to enlarged thymus gland, in association with arterial and adrenal hypoplasia. This theory became obsolete. When it was documented that the thymus is normally enlarged in healthy infants.
- More recent theories.
  - Related to diphtheria, pertussis, tetanus, DPT inoculations. Recent studies have disproved this theory,
  - Idiopathic apnoea—most cases subsequently proven to be due to repeated smothering episodes (Munchausen's syndrome by proxy).
  - Mechanical upper airway obstruction due to anatomical abnormalities such as narrow nasal passages, short mandibular rami, etc.
  - Defective or immature brain stem respiratory or cardiac control centres.
  - Activation of the "diving" reflex
  - Anaphylaxis
  - Adrenal insufficiency
  - Hyperthermia
  - Vitamin or trace metal deficiency
  - Gastro-oesophageal reflux leading to bradycardia and apnoea.

BLUNT FORCE INJURY

Stages in the Healing

First stage—scab formation: If fibrin, serum, and red blood cells accumulate on the surface of the abrasion, this is usually interpreted as "survival" following the injury.

- From 2 to 6 hours after the injury, polymorphonuclear cells may infiltrate in a perivascular fashion.
- By 8 hours, a zone of infiltrating polymorphonuclear cells is seen underlying the area of epithelial injury.
- At 12 hours, collagen in the area of injury may stain abnormally.
- From 12–18 hours postinjury, the wound is progressively infiltrated by polymorphonuclear cells.

Second stage—epithelial regeneration: Arises in hair follicles, and at the edges of the abrasion.

- May appear as early as 30 hours postinjury in superficial scrape abrasions.
- Clearly visible by 72 hours postinjury in most abrasions.

Third stage—subepidermal granulation: Becomes prominent within 5–8 days.

- Occurs only after epithelial covering of an abrasion.
- Perivascular infiltration and chronic inflammation is prominent.
- Overlying epithelium becomes more and more thick with new keratin.
- Most prominent at 9–12 days postinjury.

Fourth stage—regression: Begins at about 12 days postinjury. Epithelium becomes thinner and occasionally atrophic. New collagen fibres are now prominent. Definite basement membrane is present, and vascularity of the dermis decreases.

Blunt Force Injury to the Chest (Thorax)

Rib Injuries

Four classes or types of rib fractures exist.

1. Spontaneous, or pathologic, rib fractures may occur with primary or metastatic tumour of the bone.
2. Therapeutic iatrogenic rib fractures may be caused by cardiopulmonary resuscitation, especially in elderly individuals.
   - May be accompanied by sternal fractures, mediasternal and substernal haemorrhages, and pneumothorax.
   - Tend to be more left-sided than right, but can be bilateral or only right-sided.

- If present, the pathologist should be certain that CPR was administered before determining the fractures were due to resuscitation.
3. Rib fractures due to direct, localized trauma:
   - May be simple, displaced, or compounded with projection through the pleura.
   - Usually lie immediately beneath the point of impact.
   - If compounded, may puncture underlying organs, leading to hemo- or pneumothoraces.
   - Fracture of ribs 1–3 is frequently associated with severe injuries of the trachea, and great vessels of the upper chest (aorta, vena cava, subclavian veins).
   - Fracture of ribs 10–12 may be associated with injuries of the spleen, liver and diaphragm.
4. Rib fractures due to indirect trauma: Compression or squeezing of the chest can cause rib fractures.
   - If compression is front to back (anteroposterior), lateral rib fractures may result.
   - If compression is back to front, the ribs tend to fracture near the spine.
   - If compression is side to side, the ribs may fracture near the spine and sternum.

Blunt Force Injury to the Genitalia (Internal and External)

a. Male Genitalia

- Forceful blows to the male external generation can cause total or subtotal amputation. Blows of less force cause abrasions and lacerations penile or scrotal, and contusions with or without scrotal haematomas.
- A wide range of injuries can occur to the male internal genitalia.
  - Injury produced depends upon the severity of the blow and the structure injured.
  - Injuries include contusion, laceration of ductal structure and parenchyma, testicular haematomas, interstitial haemorrhage.
- In rare cases, a **kick or blow** to the scrotal region can cause immediate or instantaneous death, due to cardiac asystole.
  - Blow to the testicles imitates simultaneous stimulation of vagi
  - Hypervagal stimulation is presumed to cause cardiac standstill.

b. Female Genitalia

- Injuries to the external female genitalia, due to blunt force, if present, are usually due to sexual assault.
  - Injuries include contusions, lacerations or abrasions.
  - If present and possibly related to sexual assault, the injuries should be extensively photographed (with and without comparison scale) before proceeding with collection of trace evidence which may be present, or internal amputation.
- Blunt force injury of the internal genitalia in a non-pregnant female, can occur, but is rare.
- Blunt force injury to the pregnant uterus or foetus occurs more often, especially as a result of vehicular accidents, and less commonly due to falls or assaults.
  - Mechanism of foetal death is placental separation with rapid or delayed intrauterine death.
  - Following intrauterine death, lobour usually begins within 48 hours but may be delayed for as long as a few weeks.
  - If pelvic fractures result from the blunt trauma, direct fetal injury is possible.

Skeletal Fractures due to Blunt Force Trauma

a. Bone fractures are caused by direct trauma and indirect trauma.

   Direct trauma is subdivided into three types, depending on the amount of force applied and the size of the area impacted.
   - Focal (tapping frame produced by small force striking a small area).
     - Usually transverse.
     - In regions where two bones lie adjacent to each other, usually only one bone is fractured.

- Crush fracture produced by a great force striking a large area:
  - Usually comminuted
  - Usually accompanied by soft tissue injury.
- Penetrating fracture—produced by a great force striking a small area (i.e. gunshot wound).

Indirect trauma is produced by a force acting at a location remote from the fracture site. It is subdivided into **six categories:**

1. Traction fracture—bone pulled apart.
2. Angulation fracture—bone is bent until it snaps, usually a transverse fracture is produced.
3. Relational fracture—bone is twisted, producing a spiral fracture.
4. Vertical compression fracture—produces oblique fracture of the body of long bones, in the femur, it produces a T-shaped fracture at the distal end of the bone.
5. Angulation and compression fractures are usually curved, not transverse.
6. Angulation, rotation and compression fractures.

b. Vertebral column fractures are usually indirect, except for those produced by gunshot wounds, which are direct.
  - Vertebral column mobility is greatest in the cervical region, least in the thoracic region, and intermediate in the lumbar region.
  - Most common spinal fracture is anterior compression fracture of the vertebral body at or near the thoracic lumbar junction, this fracture is most common in individuals of middle age or older, and can follow minor trauma in older individual with osteoporosis.

c. Pelvic fractures are caused by direct or indirect (through force applied to lower extremities) trauma.
  - Usually require great force to be produced.
  - Can be subdivided into three major types:
    - **Open book fracture:** Produced by anterior posterior compression with fracture separation of symphysis pubis.
    - **Lateral compression fractures**
      - If lateral force is applied to the iliac crest, usually the ipsilateral pubic rami are fractured and the ipsilateral sacroiliac joint is impacted, less frequently, there may be fracture of the contralateral pubic rami, or fracture of all four pubic rami.
      - If the force is to the femoral head such that it drives into the acetabulum, then usually acetabular fracture results as well as fractures of the ipsilateral pelvic rami and disruption or impaction of the sacroiliac joints.
    - **Vertical shear fractures** are produced by an extremely severe force vertically displacing one hemipelvis in relation to the other:
      - Anterior disruption of symphysis or pubic rami.
      - Posterior gross disruption of the sacroiliac joints or fractures of adjacent sacrum or ilium.
      - Usually accompanied by massive haemorrhage.
- In order to evaluate pelvic fractures at autopsy, soft tissue should be scraped away in the area if suspected fracture so direct visualization of the fracture is possible.
- Most frequent complication of pelvic fracture is haemorrhage, and in severe fractures, severe haemorrhage almost always occurs.
  - The fatality rate from haemorrhage associated with fracture, with current management techniques, ranges from 5 to 20%.
  - In case of severe pelvic fracture, it is not uncommon to see two to three little haemorrhages from small vessels.
  - Massive intraperitoneal and retroperitoneal haemorrhages resulting from severe pelvic fracture may be the only finding, and therefore, the cause of death in some traumatic deaths.

- Occasionally, the presence of the extremities will be discussed. Fractures may provide a clue as to the mechanism of injury. Some examples include.
  - A fall on the outstretched hand can cause a fracture of the distal radius (i.e. colles fracture).
  - Fractures of the metacarpal bones occur most commonly by striking the closed hand against a firm surface (boxer's fracture).
  - Fractures of the heels (calcaneal fracture) can occur in falls from a great height, when landing on the feet in a relatively upright position.

Fat Embolization may Result in the Fat Embolization Syndrome

- Classically, the syndrome of fat embolization has three main symptoms and signs:
  - Pulmonary distress—present in 75% of cases
  - Cerebral signs—occur in 86% of cases, vary from confusion, lethargy, convulsions to coma.
  - Petechial rash—50% of cases. Rash is on mucous membranes and/or skin of the anterior chest and neck in-between shoulder blades.
- The symptoms manifest within 24–48 hours after injury.
- The incidence of the syndrome increases as the number of fractures increases.
- The syndrome is more likely to occur after pelvic or lower limb fractures and is seldom seen with isolated fracture of an upper limb.
- The syndrome is rare in children.
- At autopsy, gross evidence of cerebral fat embolization may appear as multiple punctate haemorrhage (petechiae) on the cut surface of the brain, mostly within the white matter.
- At autopsy, the diagnosis of fat embolization may be made by demonstration of fat globules in capillaries of the lung, brain, kidney, and skin, usually through a fat stain of fat embolization is suspected, frozen portions of lung, brain, and kidney should be retained for fat stain such as oil red.
- In some cases, small fragments of bone and bone marrow will be readily apparent in pulmonary vessels with routine stains. These emboli can also be seen following aggressive resuscitation, which may make differentiation as to their source difficult.
- Infection—more common in open wounds than in crushing injuries with infected skin.

Cerebral Laceration

- May result from a displaced skull fracture, or occur in the absence of any skull fracture.
- When severe cerebral laceration is present, usually and massive skull trauma is also present.
- Cerebral lacerations are usually bloodless, despite antemortem infliction.
- In young infants (5 months or less), blunt head trauma results more frequently in cerebral laceration than contusion.
  - Grossly visible lacerations may occur in the white matter of the frontal and temporal lobes, while microscopic examination lacerations may occur in the superficial cortex.
  - While evaluating suspected lacerations in brain of infants, it is important to remember that artificial linear defects can occur in these brains as a result of removal, due to their extremely soft, gelatinous nature. Microscopic examination may not help in the determination of significance, as cellular reaction to the injury may not be evident until 36 hours post-injury.
  - Unlike cerebral contusions, the location of a cerebral laceration, in relation to the point of impact, is not indicative of the mode or mechanism of injury (fall versus blow).

Cerebral Swelling

Cerebral swelling can occur as a complication of blunt head trauma. The swelling may be diffuse, focal, adjacent to a specific area of brain injury (such as a contusion or laceration), or one sided, following removal of a subdural or epidural haematoma.

- The swelling may be due to:
  - An increase in the cerebral intravascular blood volume due to vasodilation, or
  - An absolute increase in the water content of the brain tissue is termed cerebral oedema.
- Significant delayed brain swelling is rare:
  - Usually associated with less severe forms of brain trauma.
  - Usually diffuse
  - The most severe form of delayed brain swelling occurs more commonly in children (4–10 years of age).
- Brain swelling can cause symmetrical or asymmetrical herniation of the brain.

Wounds Produced by Pointed, Sharp-edged and Chopping Implements

Stab wounds: By definition, these are wounds produced by a pointed instrument (i.e. knife, ice pick) in which the depth of penetration into the body is greater than the length of the wound on the skin, stab wounds, therefore, consist of an outer, visible skin wound (external component) and deeper, inner wound (internal component).

a. A distinguishing characteristic of stab wounds is the absence of **bridging tissue** in the depth of the wound. If connecting tissue strands are present in the base of the wound, it is more likely the wound was produced by, a blow with a blunt object, and not a stab with a sharp-edged implement, as the later would cut through, not tear, the tissue. Therefore, the terms laceration and stab wound (or cut) should never be used interchangeably (Table 15.2).

b. The force needed to penetrate the body, when stabbed, is dependent on
   - The configuration of the tip of the weapon (sharp *vs* dull)
   - The amount and composition of clothing covering the body on the area stabbed.

Time period followed injury	States of clot	Side of membrane facing dura	Side of membrane between clot and arachnoid
24 hours	Fresh red blood cells	Thin layer of fibrin between dura and clot	–
48–72 hours	Fresh red blood cells	Rare fibroblast	Fibrin only
4–5 days	RBC begin to break down	2–5 cell thick layer of fibroblasts	Occasional spindle cell within fibrin
5–10 days	RBCs are staked, fibroblasts may extend into clot, early capillary formation	3–14 cell thick layer of fibroblast, occasional small capillaries may be present, pigment/laden macro-phages present	Layer still mostly with some fibroblasts
10–20 days	A few RBC remain, capillary formation continues	Fibroblast layer 1/3 to 1/2 as thick as dura, capillaries and pigment laden macro-phages present	Early fibroblastic membrane is evident
3–4 weeks	Nearly liquefied	Membrane equal to dura in thickness, pigment laden macrophages present	Fibroblastic membrane about 1/2 as thick as dura, occasional pigment laden macrophages
5 weeks	Large capillaries present	Membrane well-formed	Membrane well-formed
1–3 months	Large capillaries present	Membrane well-formed	Membrane well-formed
3–6 months	–	Hyalinized membrane	Hyalinized membrane

Table 15.2: Stages in organisation of subdural haematoma

For example, clothing items made from leather (jacket, material such as a nylon nightgown).

- The toughness or thickness of the skin in the area stabbed, skin within the same individual varies in thickness depending upon the body location. Other factors that affect the skin thickness or toughness include pre-existing medical conditions which affect the skin, age, and sun exposure.

c. Stab wounds may be homicidal, suicidal, or accidental.

- *In suicidal stabbings*
  - The wounds are usually multiple and to the mid or left anterior chest, with most of the wounds superficial or barely breaking the skin ("hesitation wounds").
  - The stab wounds do not usually go through the clothing, consistent with the individual pushing aside or pulling up the clothing prior to stabbing him or herself.
  - Stab wounds to the neck or head do occur occasionally, but these are much less common than those to the chest, suicidal stab wounds to the abdomen are very rare.
- *In homicidal stabbings*
  - Multiple wounds are usually present, with scar penetrating deep into the body.
  - Most fatal chest wounds involve injury to the heart or aorta. A stab wound to the heart that sever the left anterior descending artery can cause rapid death.
  - The abdominal organs may be injured by stab wounds to the abdomen or lower chest. Fatal stab wounds of the abdomen usually involve the liver and major blood vessels, abdominal stab wounds may cause delayed death due to peritonitis and sepsis.
  - Wounds of the head and neck are less common than wounds of the chest or abdomen.
- Stab wounds of the neck cause death acutely by exanguination, air embolism, or asphyxia by compression of the neck organs if massive soft tissue haemorrhage is present.
  - Delayed death may occur from cellulitis, or arterial thrombosis leading to cerebral infarction.
  - If stab wounds are present in the neck, a postmortem radiograph of the chest should be made prior to autopsy, as an aid in demonstrating an air embolus.
- Fatal stab wounds of the head are uncommon. When present, they may cause injury of the skull or brain.
  - The thinner areas of the skull are more likely to be penetrated (orbit, temporal bones).
  - Intracranial haemorrhage resulting from a stab wound may be sub-arachnoid, subdural, intracerebral, or a combination of these.
- *Accidental stabbings*
  - Can occur, but are very rare.
  - Usually involve an individual being in placed after an accidental fall onto a sharp or pointed object, or by a moving sharp object striking the individual.

Postmortem stab wounds are usually yellow to tan in colour, due to the absence of tissue perfusion. Stab wounds inflicted shortly before, or at the time of death (antemortem or perimortem) may also appear relatively bloodless, if significant blood loss has already occurred and lowered the blood pressure. If several bloodless, yellow stab wounds are present, in addition to the obvious lethal wound, this is a clearer indication that some wounds were inflicted after death, and therefore, after the victim had ceased to struggle, or "put up a fight".

Chop wounds are caused by heavy instruments, or weapons, which have at least one sharp cutting edge. Examples of such weapons include axes, hatchet, meat cleavers, and matchet.

a. A chop wound consists of an incised wound with an associated groove or cut in the underlying bone.

b. If the chopping is tangential then a disk-shaped portion of bone or skin and soft tissue may be cut away.

c. Dull-edged chopping weapons (such as heavy shovel), may cause more crushing than incision of the tissue, and may, therefore, result in a wound more consistent with a laceration than an incised wound.

d. Moving propellant (boat or aeroplane) may cause severe chop like wounds.

e. The pressure of soft tissue haemorrhage associated with a chop or incised wound is generally considered good evidence, the wound occurred prior to death prolonged immersion of a body in water can cause haemorrhage initially present in the wound to be leached out, giving the wound a postmortem appearance, and making the determination of its true nature difficult.

FIREARM INJURIES

Gunshot

Rifling is a series of parallel spiral grooves and cut caused by the bore of barrel.

- The metal left between the grooves is the land.
- The number of grooves can vary from 2 to 20 with the direction of the rifling either clockwise (right) or counterclockwise (left).
  - Virtually all handguns have 5 or 6 grooves with a right hand twist. Colt has a left hand twist.
  - In centrefire rifles, virtually all weapons have a right hand twist with the number of grooves varying from 4 to 6.
  - 0.22 reinfine weapons generally have a right hand twist with 4, 6 or more than 6 grooves.
- Rifling imparts a rotational spin on the bullet as it travels down the barrel. The spin imparted to the bullet stabilizes its flight through the air, preventing it from tumbling.

Caliber

The caliber of a rifled weapon is supposed to be the diameter of the bore measured from land to land. This practice is not strictly followed and some of the caliber designations are essentially arbitrary.

- In the metric system used in Europe, the caliber identifies the bullet diameter and the cartridge case length in millimetres. Thus, a 7.62 × 39 mm cartridge fires a bullet 7.62 mm long.

Ammunition

a. Ammunition for rifled weapons is divided into two categories, centrefire and rimfire, depending on the location of the primer.
  - In rimfire cartridges the primer composition is in the rim of the cartridge case with the propellant in contact with the primer.
    - On firing, the firing pin crushes the rim of the cartridge case, detonating the primer composition, igniting the powder.
    - Current reinfine ammunition is limited to three calibers—22 short rifle, 22 long rifle and 22 magnum.
    - Reinfine ammunition may be fired in either handguns or rifles.

b. Cartridge case is usually made of brass, though sometimes aluminium and steal cases are also made.
  - On firing, the cartridge case contains the gases from the ignition of the powder.
  - Most handgun cartridges have a straight design, while rifle cartridges are bottlenecked.
  - In commercial ammunition, the caliber and the name of the manufacturer are stamped on the base of the cartridge.
  - In military ammunition the plant that manufactured the ammunition (either by letter or by code number) and year of manufacture are stamped on the base of the cartridge.
  - The powder used in the cartridge case is smokeless powder, a nitrocellulose compound, to which nitroglycerin may or may not be added. The physical forms of the powder in the United States are generally.
    - Disk (flake) or ball in handguns and shotguns.

– Either cylindrical or ball powder in rifles.

The barrel is the part of the cartridge that leaves the muzzle on filling the weapon.

- Because of their high velocities, centrefire rifle bullets have to be either a full or partial metal jacket.
    – This jacket is usually copper or copper alloy or may be of steel sometimes.
    – The cone is usually lead but in the case of military bullets mild steel or a combination of steel and lead are seen. The configuration of the bullet is variable.
    – Handgun ammunition tends to be:
        ▪ Round nose
        ▪ Semi-wad cutter
        ▪ Hollow point, or
        ▪ Wad cutter (cylindrical shaped)
    – Centrefire rifle ammunition is either:
        ▪ Full metal jacketed, or
        ▪ Semi jacketed
        ▪ With a spitzer point or round nose.

Gunshot wounds: Whenever a gun is fired, the exiting barrel is accompanied by:

- A jet of flame, one to two inches in length, having temperature of approximately 1400°F.
- A cloud of gas.
- Burning and unburnt grains of gunpowder.
- Carbon, or soot, from burnt gunpowder.
- Vapourized metal from the bullet, cartridge case and primer.

Based on their appearence, and thus their range, gunshot wounds can be divided into four broad categories:

- Contact
- Near contact
- Intermediate range
- Distant range.

In contact wounds, the muzzle of the gun is against the skin at the time of discharge.

- If the gun is pushed "hard" against the skin, indenting it, and thus guaranteeing a complete seal between the muzzle and skin on discharge, the wound is called a hard contact.

– In hard contact wounds, all the material exiting the muzzle of the gun goes beneath the skin.
– The edges of the wound will be seared burnt and blackened by a combination of burning from the flame exiting the muzzle, as well as impregnation of soot in the area of burning.

The picture is completely different in contact wounds of the head where a thick layer of scalp, is stretched over bone.

- In contact wounds of the head from handguns, one can have:
    – A round entrance with blackened and burnt margin.
    – An entrance wound with a muzzle imprint around it.
    – A stellate entrance.
    – The latter two pictures are due to the gas coming out of the muzzle of the weapon and collecting between the scalp and bone. This may cause hallowing outward of the scalp with the scalp impacting the muzzle producing a muzzle imprint, or the hallowed out skin tearing at the entrance producing a stellate entrance.
    – Careful examination of the edges of the stellate entrance will reveal the original circular defect with blackened and seared margin, from which the tears radiate.
    – The appearance and extent of the injury depends to a degree on the caliber of the weapon.
- With 0.22 reinfine bullets, the entrance wound tends to be round with blackened and seared margins.
- With a 0.357 magnum, one gets the typical stellate wound with ejection of brain tissue. In loose contact wounds, the muzzle is against the skin, but for a shortime following discharge of the weapon, a gap opens up between the muzzle and skin so that a ring of soot is deposited around the extreme hole. This can be washed away.

In near-contact wounds, the muzzle is held at a short distance from the skin such that there is a bullet hole surrounded by a band of blackened and seared skin. This band is significantly wider than one sees in a contact wound. With handguns, near-contact wounds occur at ranges of less than 10 mm.

Intermediate range: Gunshot wounds are characterized by the presence of powder tattooing around the wound of entrance.

- Powder tattooing occurs when the muzzle of the weapon is held away from the body at the time of fixing, yet is sufficiently close so that the powder grains emerging from the muzzle with the bullet strike the skin, producing punctate abrasions on the skin. These are called powder tattoo marks.
- Powder tattooing consists of multiple reddish-brown to orange-red punctate lesions of the skin surrounding the entrance wounds.
- Powder tattoo marks are punctate abrasions.
  - They cannot be wiped away
  - They are not burns
  - The term powder burn should not be used in describing powder tattooing or the searing or blackening of the skin by the flame and/or soot.
- Distant gunshot wound.
- Distant gunshot wounds have entrances that tend to be round to oval with sharp punched out margins. Typically, the edges are surrounded by an abrasion ring.
- The abrasion ring is caused by the bullet scraping the edges of the skin as it indents and perforates it. It is not due to the heat of the bullet or its rotary movement.
- Irregular abrasion rings can be due to:
  - The bullet impacting the skin at an angle.
  - Irregularities of the skin at the point of entrance.
  - A deformed bullet.
  - Destabilization of the bullet in flight.

Ricochet bullets are relatively rare. Most bullets on striking break up a hard surface or punctate the surface. There is, however, a critical angle of imput below which a bullet striking a surface will ricochet.

- For water, this angle ranges from 3° to 8°. Bullets ricocheting off water will ricochet off at angles greater than the input angle.

- The critical angle of impact for ricochet for hard surface is much more variable. It may vary from 10° to 30°. When the bullet is on the ricochet surface, it ricochet at an angle smaller than the impact angle.
- The entrance wounds produced by ricochet bullets tend to be larger and more irregular in shape with very large irregular areas of abrasion around the entrance wound.
- Bullets that ricochet off a hard surface have one side typically flattened with a mirror like surface. This is true for both jack lid and lead bullets.
- Shotguns are designed to fire multiple pellets down the barrel. The size of the pattern thrown by a shotgun depends to a great degree on the choke of the barrel:
  - The choke is a partial constriction of the bore of the gun at the muzzle end that controls the size of the shot pattern.
  - There are four levels of choke:
    - Full
    - Modified
    - Improved
    - Cylinder
  - Different degrees of choke give different spreads.
  - Excluding the 0.410, shotguns of 12, 16 and 20 gauges of the same choke should throw the same size pattern at the same range. The only difference is that there will be more pellet holes in the pattern produced by the 12 than the 16 and 20.

Wounds of Bone

- The entrance is round to oval with sharp punched out margins.
- Fragments of bone show broken edges of the exiting surface and is propelled forward due to bullet on its path. Thus, the exit is bevelled out in a cone-like fashion.
- When one is dealing with very thin bone, such as the orbital plates or in some distance temporal bone, this bevelling appearance may not be present.
- If the bullet strikes the skull at a very shallow angle, a gutter wound may occur. The most superficial such wound involves

only the outer table while the most severe involves the complete thickness of bone.

- In a key hole wound of the skull, the bullet striking at a very shallow angle produces a combined entrance/exit type effect. At the point the bullet impacts, there will be a punched out sharp edge entrance defect. The distal end of thin hole will have a beveled out appearance, typically seen in an exit. This is usually due to the bullet striking at a very shallow angle and breaking into two pieces with one entering the skull and the outer exiting.
- Contact wounds of the head from shotguns tend to be explosive, resembling centrefire rifle wounds, X-rays will usually reveal at least a few pellets.
- Contact wounds of the chest and abdomen are circular in configuration with blackened and seared margins. A muzzle imprint may be present.
- From contact to two feet, birdshot fired from a shotgun produces a single round entrance anywhere from three-fourths inch to one inch in diameter.
- By **three feet,** the wound has widened and will have scalloped margins due to the separating pellets.
- By **four feet,** one will have an entrance hole approximately one inch (rat hole appearance) in diameter surrounded by **scattered satellite pellet holes**.
- As the range increases, the number of surrounding pellet holes increases.
- By approximately 10 feet, there tends to be a ragged central hole surrounded by numerous pellet holes.
- Beyond **10 feet,** the pattern changes dramatically depending upon the choke, so that one will often get just a pattern of multiple pellet holes.
- The size of the shotgun pattern should always be measured and recorded for subsequent range determinations. At that time, the shotgun and identical ammunition are fired at known ranges in an attempt to reproduce the same sized pattern found on the body.

- The wadding fired from the shotgun tends to go into the entrance for the first 5 to 6 feet of range. After that, it tends to drift to the side and may make a separate impact abrasion on the adjacent skin.
- Winchester birdshot wadding consists of cylindrical discs of cardboard. If they impact the skin adjacent to the entrance, there will be a circular mark produced. They will mark the skin generally out to 15 feet.
- In Remington and Federal ammunition, birdshot pellets are enclosed in a cup with four petals. With plastic wadding in 12, 16 and 20 gauge, it takes at least one foot of travel for the cup to open up.
- At less than 1 foot of range, one tends to get a circular hole.
- Between one and two feet, the wadding has opened up so that the four petals stick out. One gets a circular entrance wound with a maltase cross pattern of abrasions encircling it.
- As the wadding goes through the air, resistance folds back the petals so that by 3 feet, one will again have a single hole of entrance and not the open petal pattern.
- 0.410 shotgun ammunition, no matter the manufacturer, uses plastic cups with three petals. The petal marks appear at about 6 inches and are gone by about 3 feet.

SIGNS OF POISONING

This section describes how to examine a patient for some common signs of poisoning (Table 15.3):

- Unconsciousness
- Changes in the skin, breathing, pulse, temperature and diarrhoea
- Dehydration
- Not passing urine
- Fits
- Signs of liver damage.

Some Poisons Make the Patient Restless, Overactive or Aggressive

- This can also happen when people suddenly stop use of drugs or drinking alcohol after doing so for a long time.

- Some poisons may cause overactivity, restlessness or irritability.
- **Medicines:** Aminophylline, atropine-like substances, chlorpromazine and other phenothiazines, ephedrine.
- **Drugs of abuse:** Amphetamines, cocaine.

Some Substances that may Affect the Eyes

a. Very small " pinpoint" pupils
   Medicines: Opiates
   Pesticides: Organophosphorus and carbamate insecticides.
b. Large pupils
   - Medicines: Amitriptyline and other tricyclic antidepressants, antihistamines, atropine like medicines, carbamazepine, ephedrine, isocarboxazide and other monoamine oxidase inhibitors, quinine.
   - Drugs of abuse: Amphetamines.
   - Other substance: Methanol.
c. Blurred vision
   - Medicines: Atropine like medicines, ephedrine, pseudoephedrine.
   - Other substances: Ethanol, methanol.
d. Loss of sight or complete blindness
   - Medicines: Chloroquine, quinine.
   - Other substance: Methanol.

Some Chemicals that may Cause the Change in Skin Colour

- Pink, hot skin: Atropine like medicines, amphetamines, and borax.
- Yellow skin caused by jaundice: Carbon tetrachloride, iron-containing medicines, paracetamol, pentachlorophenol, trichloroethylene, and some poisonous mushrooms.
- Yellow or orange stain: Dinitrophenol, dinoseb, DNOC, rifampicin (the stain washes off).
- Blue skin: Dapsone, naphthalene, paradichlorobenzene, phenol, sodium chlorate, sodium nitrite.

Some Chemicals that may Cause Unconsciousness

- **Medicines:** Amitriptyline and other tricyclic antidepressants, antihistamines, atropine-like medicines, barbiturates, carbamazepine, chloroquine, chlor-

promazine and other phenothiazines, chlorpropamide-like medicines, diazepam and other benzodiazepines, insulin, iron containing medicines, meprobamate, quinidine, quinine sodium valproate.

- **Other chemicals:** Benzene, carbon monoxide, carbon tetrachloride, cyanide, ethanol ethyleneglycol, methanol, toluene, trichloroethane, trichloroethylene, xylene.
- Many other medicines and chemicals taken in large amounts.
- Other common causes of unconsciousness are head injury fainting, heavy bleeding, heart attack, stroke, lack of air, epilepsy, fits, and diabetes.
- Unconsciousness is probably caused by a head injury if the patient also has any of these signs:
  - Bleeding from the ears or nose
  - Bruises or cuts on the body or head
  - Pupils that are of different sizes.

Some Chemicals that may Cause Lung Oedema

Medicines: Aspirin and other salicylates, chlorpromazine and other phenothiazines, opiates.

Pesticides: Carbamate and organophosphorus insecticides, dinoseb, DNOC, paraquat, pentachlorophenol.

Other chemicals: Ethylene glycol, petroleum distillates, turpentine and other volatile oils, irritant gases.

Some Chemicals that may Cause Slow Pulse

Medicines: Barbiturates, digitalis, digitoxin, digoxin, meprobamate, opiates, propranolol and other β-blockers.

Pesticides: Carbamate and organophosphorus insecticides.

Some Chemicals that may Cause Fast Pulse

Medicines: Aminophylline, amitriptyline and other tricyclic antidepressants, antihistamines, aspirin and other salicylates, atropine-like medicines, ephedrine, isocarboxazide and other monoamine oxidase inhibitors, pseudoephedrine.

Some Chemicals that may Cause Fits

Medicines: Aminophylline, amitriptyline and other tricyclic antidepressants, antihistamines, aspirin and other salicylates, atropine-like medicines, chloroquine, colchicine, dapsone, ephedrine, insulin and other antidiabetic drugs, iron salts, isocarboxamide and other monoamine oxidase inhibitors, opiates, phenothiazines, propranolol and other β-blockers, pseudoephedrine, quinidine, quinine.

Drugs of abuse: Amphetamine, cocaine.

Pesticides: Arsenic, carbamate and organophosphorus insecticides, metaldehyde, sodium chlorate, strychnine, thallium.

Other chemicals: Borax, boric acid, camphor, camphorated oil, carbon monoxide, cationic detergents, ethylene glycol, methanol, sodium perborate.

Some Chemicals that may Cause Smell in Breath

Camphor, camphorated oil, carbon tetra-chloride, cyanide, ethanol, methyl salicylate, paraffin, petrol, toluene, trichloroethylene, turpentine and other volatile oils, and many pesticides.

Drugs of abuse: Amphetamines, cannabis, cocaine.

Pesticides: Arsenic, chlorophenoxyacetate weed killers, dinoseb, DNOC, penta-chlorophenol.

Other chemicals: Carbon monoxide (at first).

Some Chemicals that may Cause Confusion or Hallucinations

Medicines: Aminophylline, amitriptyline and other tricyclic antidepressants, anti-histamines, atropine-like medicines, dapsone, ephedrine, insulin, propranolol and other β-blockers, pseudoephedrine.

Drugs of abuse: Amphetamines, cannabis, cocaine.

Pesticides: Chlorophenoxyacetate weed killers, organophosphorus and carbamate pesticides.

Other chemicals: Camphor, camphorated oil, ethanol, turpentine and other volatile oils.

Some Chemicals that may Cause a Low Body Temperature (less than 35°C)

Medicines: Amitriptyline and other tricyclic antidepressants, barbiturates, chlorpromazine and other phenothiazines, meprobamate, opiates.

Other chemicals: Carbon monoxide, ethanol.

Some Chemicals that may Cause Kidney Failure

Medicines: Aspirin and other salicylates, colchicine, iron-containing medicines, isocarboxazid and other monoamine oxidase inhibitors, quinine, rifampicin.

Pesticides: Arsenic, dinoseb, dinitrophenol, DNOC, paraquat, pentachlorophenol, sodium chlorate, thallium.

Other chemicals: Boric acid, camphor, camphorated oil, carbon tetrachloride, ethylene glycol, methanol, naphthalene, phenol, sodium perborate, turpentine and other volatile oils.

Some Chemicals that may Cause Liver Damage

Medicines: Iron-containing medicines, paracetamol, rifampicin.

Pesticides: Aluminium phosphide and zinc phosphide, pentachlorophenol.

Other substances: Benzene, camphor, camphorated oil, carbon tetrachloride, phenol, tetrachloroethane, toluene, trichloroethane, trichloroethylene, xylene, and poisonous mushrooms.

Some Chemicals that may Effect Breathing

a. Shallow Breathing

Medicines: Amitriptyline and other tricyclic antidepressants, antihistamines, atropine-like medicines, barbiturates, diazepam and other benzodiazepines, meprobamate, chlorpromazine and other phenothiazines.

Pesticides: Carbamate and organophosphorus insecticides.

Other chemicals: Carbon monoxide, ethanol.

b. Slow or Irregular Breathing

Medicine: Opiates.

Pesticides: Carbamate and organophosphorus insecticides.

c. Fast Breathing

Medicines: Aminophylline, aspirin and other salicylates, cocaine, chloroquine.

Pesticides: Dinoseb, DNOC, organochlorine pesticides, pentachlorophenol.

Other chemicals: Carbon monoxide (at first), ethanol, ethylene glycol, methanol, phenol.

Antidotes

Sodium nitrite, 3% solution for intravenous injection in cyanide poisoning.

Sodium thiosulphate, 25% solution: For intravenous injection in cyanide poisoning also given by mouth, with sodium hydrogen carbonate (sodium bicarbonate), to treat methaemoglobinaemia from sodium chlorate poisoning.

Succimer (DMSA—dimercaptosuccinic acid): for arsenic poisoning and lead poisoning.

Other Medicines

Antibiotic eye ointment when there is a risk of infection after burns or injury to the eye.

Antivenoms as appropriate for snakes, spiders, scorpions and stinging fish that are found in the area.

Antihistamine such as chlorpheniramine or promethazine: For intravenous injection, in case of allergic reactions.

Diazepam: For injection, to treat fits.

Diphenhydramine: For injection or for giving by mouth, for itching rash caused by irritant plants.

Epinephrine (adrenaline) injection, 1 in 1000 (1 mg/ml) for intramuscular injection: For severe allergic reactions (for example, to insect stings).

Fluorescein to detect damage to the eye from irritant or corrosive poisons.

Metoclopramide: For intravenous injection, to stop persistent vomiting.

Morphine: For severe pain.

Salbutamol for inhalation (or theophylline for intravenous injection) for asthma or wheezing caused by severe allergic reactions (for example, to insect stings).

Information for Doctors

If vomiting does not stop, the patient may need to be given a medicine like promethazine, diphenhydramine, or metoclopramide by injection.

Medicines and antidotes that can be given by doctors outside hospital

- This is not a complete list of antidotes. It includes only those that can be given outside hospital.
- **Acetylcysteine:** Given by mouth in paracetamol poisoning and carbon tetrachloride poisoning. Acetylcysteine should be given by injection only in a hospital or medical centre, where resuscitation can be given if the patient has an allergic reaction.
- **Ascorbic acid:** Given by mouth to treat methaemoglobinaemia from sodium chlorate poisoning.
- **Atropine:** For injection in poisoning from carbamate or organophosphorus pesticides.
- **Calcium gluconate solution:** For injection under the skin when hydrofluoric acid has been in contact with skin.
- **Deferoxamine (desferrioxamine):** For injection in iron poisoning.

  Dicobalt edetate, 1.5% solution: For injection in cyanide poisoning.
- **Dimercaprol (also called British anti-Lewisite (BAL) compound):** For arsenic poisoning and lead poisoning.
- **4-Dimethylaminophenol (4-DMAP), 5% solution:** For injection in cyanide poisoning.
- **DMPS (dimercaptopropane sulfonate):** For arsenic poisoning and lead poisoning.
- **Hydroxocobalamin, 40% solution:** For intravenous injection in cyanide poisoning.
- **Methylene blue:** For cyanosis caused by methaemoglobin in dapsone poisoning.
- **Obidoxime chloride:** For poisoning from organophosphorus pesticides.
- **Penicillamine:** For lead poisoning.

- **Phytomenadione (vitamin K):** For injection in warfarin poisoning.
- **Potassium ferricyanoferrate (Prussian blue) or ferric ferrocyanide:** For thallium poisoning.
- **Pralidoxime mesylate (P2S) or pralidoxime chloride (PAM 2):** For poisoning from organophosphorus pesticides (Table 15.3).
- **Pyridoxine:** For intravenous injection in isoniazid poisoning.
- **Sodium calcium edetate:** For lead poisoning.
- **Sodium hydrogen carbonate (sodium bicarbonate):** Given by mouth with sodium thiosulphate to treat methaemoglobinaemia from sodium chlorate poisoning.

Signs showing Severity of Disease

- The patient is not breathing
- Breathing is wheezy or noisy after you have cleaned the mouth and put the patient in the recovery position.
- The patient is unconscious and does not wake up when you pinch the hand.
- The pupils do not change size when you shine a light into them.
- The pulse is very slow (less than 50 beats per minute), or very fast (more than 110 beats per minute), or irregular, or very weak.

Look at the Patient

Does the patient look ill or weak? Look at the patient's eyes to see if they are damp or stained with chemicals, urine or vomit. Look at the vomit to see whether there is blood, or pieces of tablets, plants, or food in it.

Look at the Skin

- Cuts, scratches, bruises, or bleeding may mean the patient is ill because of an injury.
- Bruises may be caused by a fall. The patient may have been dizzy, unsteady, or very drowsy because of alcohol or drugs.
- Cuts on the insides of the wrists or on the neck may have been made by the patient trying to kill himself or herself, and scar lines could mean that the patient, tried to do this in the past.
- Marks on the arms near the inside of the elbow, or on the ankles or knees, with swollen veins ulcers and abscesses may have been caused by injecting drugs. The patient may be dependent on drugs.
- Blinks and stains may have been caused by corrosive or irritant liquids. Someone who has been working with a chemical may have burns on the legs, arms, chest, back, or feet. Someone who has swallowed a corrosive substance may have burns and stains on the chin and lips, and on the chest if liquid spilt out of a bottle.

Table 15.3: Poisoning syndromes

Poisons	Symptoms and signs
• Atropine, amitriptyline, antihistamines, *Datura stramonium*, *Atropa belladonna*, some kinds of mushrooms	Dry, hot skin, fever, thirst, dry mouth large pupils, fast pulse, difficulty in passing urine, hallucinations, fits, shallow breathing, unconsciousness
• Organophosphorus and carbamate insecticides, some kinds of mushrooms	Small pupils, wet mouth, sweating, wet eyes, vomiting, slow pulse, diarrhoea, fits, unconsciousness
• Opiates	Small pupils, slow breathing, unconsciousness, low temperature, slow, weak pulse, vomiting
• Amphetamines, cocaine, theophylline	Large pupils, fever, fast pulse, hallucinations, fits, anxiety, sweating, flushed skin, overactivity, confusion
• Barbiturates, diazepam and similar drugs, meprobamate	Unconsciousness, low blood pressure, shallow breathing, low temperature
• Drug withdrawal (a sudden stop in taking ethnanol (alcohol), barbiturates, diazepam and similar medicines, opiates)	Diarrhoea, goose-flesh, fast pulse, watery eyes, yawning, cramps, hallucinations, restlessness, shaking

SEXSOMNIA
(SOMNAMBULISTIC SEXUAL BEHAVIOUR)

INTRODUCTION

i. Sexual behaviour during sleep is rarely reported in the literature and generally it is not mentioned when violence during sleep is reported.

"An automatism is an involuntary piece of behaviour over which an individual has no control. The behaviour is usually inappropriate to the circumstances, and may be out of character for the individual. It can be complex, co-ordinated and apparently purposeful and directed, though lacking in judgement. Afterwards the individual may have no recollection or only a partial and confused memory for his actions. In organic automatisms there must be some disturbance of brain functions sufficient to give to the above features".

ii. A sleepwalking episode is known as a sleep transition disorder because the episode occurs when the brain is switching over from deep slow wave sleep to **REM** sleep. Thus, many sleepwalking episodes occur between 1 and 2 hours after sleep onset.

iii. Sleepwalking runs in families and has a genetic basis. It usually appears in childhood, continues through adolescence and often stops in adulthood.

iv. Between 1% and 2% of the adult population sleepwalk. The behaviour in a sleepwalking episode can be extremely variable.

A Clinical Classification of the Major Parasomnias

Simple Motor

Sleep starts (hypnic jerks) isolated sleep paralysis.

Simple Behavioural

- Confusional awakening (sleep drunkenness)
- Sleepwalking (somnambulism)
- Sleep terrors (pavor nocturnus, incubus attacks)

Complex Behavioural

- Violence to self and/or others
- Sexsomnia (somnambulism)
- Nocturnal eating syndrome

Psychosensory

- Terrifying dreams (rapidly eye movement (REM) nightmares)
- REM—sleep behaviour disorder.

Automatic

Painful erections bed-wetting (enuresis nocturna).

Medical Guidelines for Sleep-related Violence

- There should be reason (by history or formal sleep laboratory evaluation) to suspect a bona fide sleep disorder. Similar episodes, with benign or morbid outcome, should have previously occurred.
- There is evidence of lack of awareness on the part of the individual during the event.
- The victim is someone who merely happened to be present, and who may have been the stimulus for the arousal.
- Immediately following the return of consciousness, there is perplexity without attempt to escape, conceal or cover-up the action.
- With high alcohol blood levels, some confusional behaviour on awakening might be expected.
- Other risk factors for sleep-related auto-matism are being male; having a previous history of prasomnias and sleepwalking; showing a sleep schedule disorder, e.g. shift workers; mood and anxiety disorders; occasional limb jerking while asleep; having a high daily caffeine intake; and, especially, consuming bedtime alcohol or, often, to have abused drugs.

The Diagnosis of Sleepwalking in the Forensic Context

General Fators

a. **Family history:** A family history of sleepwalking is usually found in people who sleepwalk.

b. **Childhood sleepwalking:** It is common for the onset of sleepwalking to be in childhood.

c. **Adolescent sleepwalking:** Although most sleepwalkers start sleepwalking in childhood, a few begin in adolescence.

d. **Late-onset sleepwalking:** It is rare, and usually only occurs after precipitating cause, for example head injury. Sleep experts generally regard with suspicion any episode of sleepwalking which is said to be the first episode in an adult.

Specific Factors

a. **Sleep stage:** Episodes will occur during stage 2 and 3/4 non-REM sleep and thus are most likely to occur within 2 hours of sleep onset, but may occur towards the end of the night during transitions from NREM to REM sleep.

b. There should be disorientation on awakening. A straight arousal into clear consciousness is unlikely to occur on awakening from a sleep automatism.

c. **Confusional automatic behaviour** should occur. Any witness to the entire event should report inappropriate automatic behaviour, preferably with an element of confusion.

d. **There must be amnesia for the event:** Memories are poorly recorded during stage 4 sleep and equally poorly recalled. It is, however, possible for fragments of distorted memory to be retained.

e. **Trigger factors** are important. Drugs, alcohol, excessive fatigue, sleep deprivation, tiredness and stress can all precipitate a sleep automatism.

f. **Concealment:** Attempts to conceal the incident should not have occurred.

g. **Out of character behaviour:** The behaviour is almost always out of character for the individual.

Previous Sexual Symptoms in Sleep

JB reported that about a month prior to the incident he and his former girl-friend had returned to his flat after a night out drinking, going to sleep in separate bedrooms. A few days later she informed him that he had entered her room that night, and had inserted his fingers into her vagina. She also told him that when asked to stop his actions he did so and left the room without incident. She was shocked and surprised by his actions but thought that he was not fully conscious due to a glazed look in his eyes and previous witnessed sleepwalking episodes.

The statements by the complainant revealed that JB had helped her to his bed as she was inebriated. He had then gone to sleep on the sofa in a separate room. Approximately an hour later she was woken suddenly feeling a hand fondling her breasts and then, in rapid succession, she felt his erect penis penetrating her anally, vaginally and then being forced orally. Subsequent to this, JB left the room and she dressed herself, walked to leave the flat and she was leaving, saw JB in the corridor with a glazed look in his eye. JB's only recollection after going to sleep on the sofa, is that of waving goodbye to the complainant as she left the flat. The forensic evidence fonfirmed that the complainant's tissue was found on JB's penis. It also confirmed that there was no attempt by JB to conceal any evidence. The jury acquitted him on the basis of sexsomnie.

Nocturnal polysomnography (PSG): Involves the detailed study of the overnight sleep patterns of an individual. The PSG measures a variety of physiological parameters (hence poly) including brain waves (electroencephalogram or EEG); muscle tone and movement (electromyelogram or EMG) inebriated eye movements (electrooculogram or EOG); cardiovascular rhythms (electrocardiogram or ECG); respiratory parameters such as airflow, chest and abdominal movements; arterial oxygen levels (oximetry); and body position. The reasons for undertaking PSG in cases of suspected sleep-related automatism are several folds. In the first instance, to diagnose an underlying sleep disorder such as sleep disordered breathing or obstructive sleep apnoea; periodic leg movement disorder; an arousal disorder; and nocturnal epilepsy that may be responsible for precipitating a sleepwalking episode or account for the nocturnal behaviours. In the second instance, provocative manoeuvres include alcohol ingestion prior to the sleep study or sleep deprivation prior to the study. In the final instance, the sleep studies are undertaken to see whether a sleepwalking episode occurs spontaneously. Internationally accepted criteria for these studies are utilized and a three-night protocol is use with the first night being an acclimatization night, the second night is used as a baseline of the person's usual sleep pattern and the third night as a provocative night.

- Increased rate of macroarousals
- The hypersynchronous high-voltage delta waves arousal (HSDWA)

- Lower levels of slow-wave activity (delta, stage 3 and 4) in the first sleep cycle and a failure to show the decrease in delta activity across the night that is typical of normal subjects.

Suggested Reading

1. Rechtshaffen A, Kales A, editors. A manual of standardized terminology: techniques and scoring system for sleep stages of human subjects. Los Angeles, (CA): UCLA Brain Information Service/Brain Research Institute; 1968.
2. Schenck CH, Pareja J, et al. Analysis of polysomnographic events surrounding 252 slow-wave sleep arousals in thirty-eight adults with injurious sleepwalking and sleep terrors. J Clin Neurophysiol 2003;15:159–66.
3. Shapiro CM, Fedoroff JP, Trajanovic NN. Sexual behavior in sleep, a newly described parasomnia. *Sleep Res* 1996;25:367.
4. Shapiro CM, Trajanovic NN, Feddoroff JP. Sexsomnia—a new parasombia. Can J Psychiat 2003;48(5):311–7.

CHAPTER 16

Forensic Psychiatry

- Psychiatry is a special branch of medical practice which deals with the mental state (illness).
- Social behaviour and human diseases are connected with the body or diseases of soma.
- Some diseases are related to mind or the diseases of psyche, but there are some diseases which go by the name of psychosomatic diseases.
- The body can affect the mind and the mind can affect the body.

Common diseases causing mental illness are:
- Schizophrenia
- Manic depressive psychosis (MDP) or bipolar disorder.
- Anxiety neurosis

Every mentally ill person need not have unsoundness of mind.

Schizophrenia (Schizen—Split; Phren—Mind)

- Schizophrenia is a mental illness, where the person suffering, withdraws himself from the reality.
- He lives without bothering for the environment.
- There is a loss of orientation in time, place and person.
- The person suffers from delusions and hallucinations.
- He hears and experiences voices commanding him to do certain actions. Under such command, he is liable to commit crime like murder.
- He may become dangerous to himself or others.

Symptoms of Schizophrenia

- Anhedonia—inability to experience pleasure.
- Alogia—absence of speech.
- Affect—feeling of person in wakeful state.
- Asociality—person is not social.
- Aolition—absence of desire to work.
- Autism—withdrawal from playmates and treating them like machines or nonliving objects.

Positive and Negative Features

- Lack of motivation.
- Handles money poorly.
- Shows poor grooming and personal care.
- Has unnatural eating and sleeping habits.

Types of Schizophrenia

- Paranoid
- Hebephrenic
- Catatonic
- Simple (differentiated) (Tables 16.1 and 16.2)
- Talks without making sense
- Forgets to do things
- Argues too much
- Refuses to take medication
- Thinks that people talk about him

Table 16.1: Schizophrenia

	Paranoid	Hebephrenic	Catatonic	Simple (undifferentiated)
Age of onset	20–30 years	15–25 years	15–25 years	Not specific
Thought disturbance	Mild	Prominent	Prominent	+
Delusions	Prominent	Less	Less	+
Affect	According to delusions	Purposeless giggling unconnected with delusions	Unconnected with delusions	+
Hallucinations	Present	Present	Present	+
General behaviour	Nearly normal, hostile argumentative	Shabby, unkempt, poor social contact	Stupor excitement	+ /–
Negative symptoms	Very few	Prominent	–	+

Table 16.2: Differences between schizophrenia and maniac depressive psychosis (MDP) or bipolar disorder

	Schizophrenia	MDP (bipolar disorder)
Nature	Introvert (aloof)	Extrovert (outgoing)
Onset	Insidious	Acute
Disorder	Thought, feelings, behaviour	Mood
Actions	May not be related to thoughts	Actions related to mood
Relation to Interviews	Does not relate	Relates well
Inter-episodic interval	Not totally free	Free or lucid

- Hear voices, breaks and damages things:
  - There are periods of complete normal state of mind in-between.
  - During the excitement phase the person has flight of ideas, he may think that he is the richest person on the earth.
  - He suffers from lack of sleep.
  - Becomes hyperactive and energetic.
  - He may beat people and turn violent on his near and dear persons.

Depression Stage

- During this stage, the depression can go to any extreme. He avoids friends, he withdraws from social activities, he feels very weak and tired. He becomes gluminous and personified. Suicide attempt may be done or a well planned suicide may be committed.
- The person may suffer from guilt complex. Loss of appetite and loss of libido occurs. After sleep he or she may not feel fresh.
- The normal phase of maniac depressive psychosis is known as lucid interval.
- During this phase a person is normal for all purposes.
- He is responsible for his civil and criminal actions during this period.

BIPOLAR DISORDER

- In bipolar or maniac depressive psychosis, the individual suffers from mood disorder.
- The mood variation goes to the extremes of sadness and cheerfulness.

ANXIETY NEUROSIS (ANXIETY DISORDER)

Symptoms of Anxiety Neurosis

- Apprehension
- Irritability
- Fears of impending disaster
- Tremors
- Frequent urination
- Diarrhoea
- Sweating
- Palpitation
- Breathlessness
- Chest pain
- Headache, dizziness
- Lack of concentration
- Delay in getting sleep.

Differential Diagnosis of Anxiety Neurosis

- Hyperthyroidism
- Hypoglycaemia
- Phaeochromocytoma
- Alcohol withdrawal syndrome
- Temporal lobe epilepsy
- Atrial arrhythmias (paroxysmal type).

Illusion

It is a false interpretation by the sense of an external object, or a stimulus which really exists. For example, mistaking a rope for a snake in dim light.

Delusion

It is a false belief contrary to fact.

Types of delusion

Types of delusion are grandiose, delusion of persecution, delusion of reference, delusion of infidelity, nihilistic delusions, delusion of self reprochment, delusion of influence, hypochondriacal delusions.

- **Delusion of grandiose:** A poor man starts believing and behaving like rich man.

- **Delusion of persecution:** The sufferer believes that his friends and relatives are behind him to trouble him. They may give him poison.

- **Delusion of reference:** The person starts believing that everybody is talking about him.

- **Delusion of infidelity:** Here a man ultimately believes that wife is not faithful to him.

- **Nihilistic delusions:** The sufferer is basically a very strong pessimist so he is convinced that nothing exists around him in the real sense of the term.

- **Delusion of self reprochment:** The sufferer feels lot of repentance thinkings that he has committed many sins and misdeeds leading to failures.

- **Delusion of influence:** He has a strong feeling that he is guided by some supernatural power by telepathy or some external agency.

- **Hypocondriacal delusions:** He suffers from body disease though he does not have that ailment.

- Delusion has been the basis of legal test of insanity.

- The famous McNaughten rule is based on the delusion of McNaughten that the British Prime Minister Sir Robert Pill was against his religious section that he was persecuted in the religious order and under the delusion of persecution Mr Daniel McNaughten shot at Mr Edward Drummond private secretary of the Prime Minister at Charrie Cross, London, presuming that he was the Prime Minister. He was acquitted on the reason of unsoundness of mind.

- McNaughten rule states that in order to establish defence on the ground of insanity, it must be clearly proved that at the time of committing the Act, the accused was suffering under such a defect of reasoning due to disease of mind that he did not know the nature and quality of Act he was doing or if he did know it, he was not aware that what he was doing was wrong and contrary to law.

Diagnosis of Mental Illness

- **History of the patient:** Name, age, sex, marital status, education, occupation, address, religion, socioeconomic status, identification marks (at least two).

- **Accompanying person's particulars:** Nature of relationship, statement of the person accompanying the patient, identification marks.

- **Chief complaints:** With particular reference to:
  - Onset of present illness
  - Duration
  - Course
  - Precipitating factors
  - Aggravating maintaining or relieving factors.

- **History of present illness:** With reference to:
  - Time of onset.
  - Evolution of symptoms in chronological manners.
  - Any disturbance of sleep, appetite, sexual functions, etc.
  - Suicidal tendencies.

- **Past history**
  - History of similar illness, serious medical, neurological, surgical illness, drug abuse.

- **Treatment history:** Treatment taken for present and previous episodes.

- **Family history:** Family structure, family history of psychiatric and medical illness, drug abuse, suicide.

- **Personal history**
  - *Perinatal*: Date of birth, nature of delivery, any complications.
  - *Clildhood* : Who brought up, breast fed, bottle fed, relationship with mother, father and family members.
  - *Educational history*: Beginning and completion of formal education, academic achievements.
  - *Puberty*: Age of secondary sexual character development, masturbatory activities, menstrual emissions.
  - *Menstrual and obstetric history*: Regularity, duration, LMP, number of children delivered, abortions, etc.
  - *Occupational history*: When started working, jobs held, jobs changed, ambitions, present income.
  - *Sexual and marital status*: Nature of sexual activity preferred, details of

marriage, duration, relationship with spouse, divorce, separation.
  - *Premorbid personality*: Details of predominant mood, attitude to self and others, attitude to work, fantasy life habits.

- **General examination:** Detail general physical examination.

- **Mental status examination**
  - General appearance and behaviour.
  - Speech
  - Mood and affect
  - Thought
  - Cognition assessment
  - Insight
  - Judgement

- **Investigations:** Medical, toxicological, drug level, electrophysiological tests, brain-imaging tests, psychological investigations.

- **Diagnostic formulation:** After complete psychiatric assessment, a diagnostic formulation must be made along with DID and treatment plan.

IMPULSE

It is an irresistible desire to do an action without any motive or thought. Some of the impulses are:

- **Kleptomania**—steals object which has no use to him.
- **Pyromania**—sets fire to things.
- **Mutilomania**—starts disfiguring or destroying animals like insects, pets, etc.
- **Dipsomania**—drinks excess of alcohol.
- **Nymphomania**—women involve resorts to sexual intercourse.
- **Satyriasis**—man resorts to sex.
- **Corpophagia**—person resorts to eating parts of dead body.
- **Necrophagia**—cutting and tearing out genitals and other body parts and devours the flesh to obtain sexual gratification.
- **Coprolalia**—Compulsion to use obscene words, e.g. *surti lala*.

In all these activities, the person is unable to control the impulse and the irresistible desire, forces him to do the things.

HALLUCINATIONS

It is false sense of perception caused without any external object or any stimulus. The types of hallucinations are:

- **Visual:** In visual hallucination, a person see an object like a tiger about to attack.
- **Auditory:** In auditory hallucination, the person hears voices out of nothing. He may receive orders asking him to some actions ending up in doing some criminal actions.
- **Olfactory:** In olfactory hallucination, the person starts getting smell of sweet in bad odour while other around do not smell anything.
- **Gustatory:** In gustatory hallucination, the person feels the taste of food or drink without anything.
- **Tactile:** Tactile hallucinations show the presence of insects crawling. In the case of chronic cocaine poisoning tactile hallucinations are common.
- **Psychomotor:** In psychomotor type, the person starts feeling movement of parts of his body while in reality there is no movement.
- **Sexual:** In sexual hallucination, the person feels sexual pleasure without any sexual object.
- **Microptic:** In microptic hallucinations, the person starts seeing a man in a very insignificant lilliput type.
- **Macroptic:** In macroptic hallucination, a small insect like mosquito starts appear like a huge animal like dinosaurs.
- **Synesthesia:** Here the person sees the music hear the dances.
- These hallucinations lead an individual to do actions which look abnormal to the observer.
- He may even commit crimes like homicide or assault. However, the person is still punishable except when unsoundness of mind is proved.

OBSESSIONS

- It is an idea continuously striking the mind of the person compelling him to do an act, though he tries his best to overcome and stop the idea and the action, i.e. like closing the door in the night throughout the night.
- **Morbid washing of hands:** Any number of times he washes the hands he feels something is left in his hands which he should wash.

Some Obsessions end up in Phobias

These are like

- Hydrophobia—fear of water
- Agoraphobia—fear of open space
- Claustrophobia—fear of closed space
- Nicktophobia—fear of darkness
- Acrophobia—fear of heights
- Mysophobia—fear of dirt or uncleanliness
- Simple phobia—fear of some objects like insects, lizards, cockroach.
- Social phobia—fear of opposite sex (fear of rejection or humiliation)
- Zoophobia—fear of animals.

Responsibility of Mentally Ill Person

- When a person is unable to take care of himself and his surroundings, it becomes too much for him to shoulder other responsibilities of greater importance.
- A normal person is responsible for all his actions like taking care of himself, family, property, entering into business contracts, giving evidences, etc.
- A person who is suffering from mental illness and not able to understand the nature and consequences of his performing. The legal responsibilities become difficult for him. Therefore, the law withdraws the responsibility from such person in the interest of himself, his family and the society.

Civil Responsibilities

- Testamentary capacity
- Management of property
- Marriage contract
- Business contract
- Competency as a witness
- Custody of minor children
- Consent

Criminal Responsibility

- Basic principle of criminal law in India is *Actus non facit reum nisi mens sit rea* (*actus*— deeds, *reum*—forbidden, *mens*—mind, *rea*—criminal). For a person to commit crime, he needs a normal state of mind, i.e. compos mentis.
- Any crime committed when the state of mind is not normal, e.g. when a person is of unsound mind becomes subject to legal scrutiny as to whether such a person is required to be punished or not for the criminal act carried out by him.
- A person in state of unsound mind and not capable of judging the nature and consequence of the Act which he/she is committing cannot be treated in the same manner in which a person of sound mind is treated by law.
- Sometimes by reason of unsound mind a person is not aware of what he is doing is either wrong or contrary to the law.
- So, in the eyes of Indian law makers, essentially a person should be of sound mind before he is held criminally responsible for his actions.
- A normal presumption is that every person is of sound mind unless it is proved otherwise.
- So, there is need to prove the unsoundness of mind to the satisfaction of the court of law.
- Before the court can take a decision that the person is not criminally responsible.
- An individual who fails in this legal test cannot derive the benefits of legal lineage.
- If the person passes the legal test then he is ordered to be put in a psychiatry hospital or a suitable place of safe custody.
- The personal history
- The absence of motive
- The absence of secrecy
- Loss of control.

1. McNaughten's Rule

2. Durham Rule (1954)

An accused person is not criminally responsible if his unlawful act is the product of mental diseases or mental defect.

3. Curren's Rule (1961)

An accused person is not criminally responsible if at the time of committing the act, he did not have the capacity to regulate his conduct to the requirements of the law, as a result of mental diseases or defect.

4. Irresistible impulse test (New Hampshire doctrine)

An accused person is not criminally responsible, even if he knows the nature and quality of his act and knows that it is wrong, if he is capable of restraining himself from committing the Act because the free agency of his will has been destroyed by mental disease.

5. American law institute (ALI) test:
A person is not responsible for criminal conduct if at the time of such conduct, as a result of mental diseases or defect, he lacks adequate capacity of his conduct, or to adjust his conduct to the requirements of the law.

Civil Responsibility

- Management of property and affairs of insane.
- Insanity and contracts.
- Insanity and marriage contract.
- The competence of insane to be a witness
- Consent and insanity.
- Insanity and testamentary capacity.

Testamentary Capacity

- It is the capacity of an individual to make a valid will, disposing his movable and immovable assets.
- The person who is making will is called *testator*. The testator must be major. He must have sound and disposing mind. He should be fully conscious. He should know about his property and how he can dispose off.

Can a Person of Mental Illness Make a Valid Will?

- During a period of lucid interval he is eligible to make a valid will.

- If the person is unable to manage his property, the court can appoint a manager to take care of property and the dealings.
- Any person of mental ill health cannot contract for his marriage. If the marriage is contracted it can be declared null and void.
- Divorce can be obtained by the partner if the person becomes unsound by mind provided a period of two years of treatment is tried.
- He cannot give a valid consent.
- He cannot take care of his children, so custody of the child is given to other partner.
- He is not considered as a competent witness in court of law for the simple reason that he may not be able to understand the meaning of taking oath (Table 16.3).

The Legal Test (Section 84 of IPC)

- Here the person must have committed or alleged to have committed a crime.
- At the time of committing the crime the person is of unsound mind.
- He has not been aware of the nature and consequence of the Act.
- Even, if he has been aware of nature and consequences of the Act he is not aware that his act is wrong.
- He is not aware whether it is wrong or contrary to the law because of unsound mind. On a close observation by the doctor, if the doctor comes to the conclusion that the person is of unsound mind.
- On a very close scrutiny and observation by the doctor of the above criteria for the legal test, if the doctor comes to the conclusion that the person is of unsound mind:
  - That he is dangerous to himself.
  - That he is dangerous to others.
  - That he is dangerous to himself and others.

Then the MO recommends for the suitable restraint of the person of the unsound mind.

If the doctor is unable to come to a conclusion on examination of the patient, the patient is placed under observation of the doctor for a period of 10 days. If this period is not sufficient he may be examined for a second period of 10 days or even 3rd period of 10 days up to a maximum of 30 days. At the end of this period of examination, the doctor has to issue the certificate regarding the state of the mind.

Types of Admission

Once the doctor is sure that the patient is of unsound mind then he can recommend for his admission:

- Voluntary admission
- Admission under special circumstances.
- Reception order on application (petition).

Table 16.3: Differences between a person of unsound mind and a pretender

True unsoundness of mind	Feigned unsoundness of mind
Onset—true unsoundness of mind present before the onset of crime	Occurs after the crime
Motive—motiveless	Motivated by the crime
Symptoms and signs—present whether seen by an observer or not	Present or exaggerated when he knows that he is being observed
Food, hygiene, clothings, sanitation, lack of sleep, behaviour—follow the pattern of illness, whether observed or not observed	Follow the pattern for sometime very strictly when he knows that he is being observed
Exposure—since there is no presentation, excessive energy, lack of sleep, disinterest in eating, bad sanitation continue	The pretention is exposed. He may sit in a corner which is clean. He may change his clothes. He may eat his food. He may go to sleep

- Reception order without application (wandering dangerous patient).
- Admission as inpatient after judicial inquisition.
- Admission of a person of unsoundness of mind who is a criminal or a prisoner.
- **Voluntary admission** of a major patient can be carried out by the doctor incharge of a psychiatric hospital.
- If the patient is minor, the guardian's consent should be taken.
- A patient can be kept is psychiatric hospital for a period of 90 days maximum on the request of relatives of the patient.
- Admission is given by magistrate by an application of the husband/wife/relative/friend. The patient is then referred to a doctor.
- In case of dangerous and wandering patients, the person is presented by a police before magistrate, the magistrate passes the admission order into psychiatric hospital.
- In the case of criminals in prison or those who are acquitted because they are insane, the hospital stay is reviewed 6 monthly. In the case of escaped patient, he is readmitted.

Assessment of Dangerousness

Dangerousness is the threat that a person poses to society in general or to other persons in particular. Many forms of danger, both to people and to object, social danger, political danger, moral danger, physical danger, etc.
- Factors relating to offence and behaviour at the time.
- Environmental factors
- Internal factors of specific characteristic of the offender.

Discharge of the patients of unsound mind
- The patient admitted voluntarily may also be discharged at request within 24 hours.
- A patient admitted on request of relatives also can be discharged if found to be fit.
- Even if a person is not fully cured, if he is not dangerous to others he can be discharged if the relatives are ready to take care of the patient.

- In the remaining cases discharge is granted on approval by the magistrate.

Other Defences Against Criminal Responsibility
Irresistible desire or impulse
It is a desire to do an action without any motive or thought.

Somnambulism
Walking during sleep, e.g. a sleep walking man was caught by his wife mowing the lawn naked at 2 AM in London. She was woken by a noise coming from the garden.

Somnolence
It is a state of sleepiness. During this state whatever action of the person performs is liable for somnolentia.

Certain Features of Criminal Act Performed by a Person of Unsound Mind
- There is no motive
- There is no accomplices
- There is no secrecy
- He may not conceal the weapon
- He may not conceal the dead body
- He may not try to escape from the place
- He may not deny the action
- Victim of his action may be very close to him or may be a total stranger.

Five Levels of Mental Subnormality

1. Borderline	Intelligence	Quotient	84–70
2. Mild	Intelligence	Quotient	69–55
3. Moderate	Intelligence	Quotient	54–40
4. Severe	Intelligence	Quotient	39–25
5. Profound	Intelligence	Quotient	24–0

Intelligence Quotient
- The mental age is calculated by using test of mental performance.
- The commonly used tests are called Binet-Simon tests.
- Below 25—idiot
- 25–50—imbecile
- 50–75—feeble-minded.

Important features of the ACT rights of persons with mental illness: Every person has the right to access mental health care by both public and private services. Right to access of mental health care includes availability, affordability and accessibility.

Advance directive: A mentally ill person shall have the right to choose the way of treatment and can nominate a person who can take decision on their behalf.

Central and state mental health authority: Authority has the responsibility:

- To maintain register of all mental health establishments
- To develop quality service
- To train law enforcement officials
- To receive complains
- To advise the govt, on the matters relating to mental health.

Mental Health Review Commission and Board: It will be quasi-judicial body that will review the use and the procedure for making advance directives and the advice the government on protection of the rights of mentally ill persons.

Decriminalizing suicide and prohibiting electroconvulsive therapy: A person attempting suicide is given mental treatment at that particular time and it is not considered as a crime under Indian Penal Code. Electroconvulsive therapy is allowed with the use of muscle relaxants and anaesthesia which is prohibited for minors.

Insurance: Bill will facilitate insurance facility for both medical insurance as well as physical illness.

Drawbacks of the ACT (below matter as pointwise): **This Act only recognizes mental illness as a clinical issue which can only be treated by medicines and clinical procedures. The important issue of prevention and promotion of mental well-being has been neglected.**

Narrow interpretation of definition of a 'mental health professional' is a matter of conflict which create discussion to include psychotherapists, counselors and psychoanalysts.

No clear procedure is set in amended bill for 'Advance Directive'.

Once a person is admitted to mental hospital he is termed insane or mad by the society. There were no provisions in the Act to educate the society against these misconceptions. The Act fails to provide for the full list of treatment options available, so that a decision can be taken by the individual without information asymmetry.

Neither the Act nor the Rules define the constitution, procedure and terms of reference of the expert committee made for periodic review and effective implementation of the Act.

No provision for hearing of cases submitted before drafting of the Act. Although the Act provides for a simpler discharge procedure but no provisions were made for after discharge care and rehabilitation, of patients.

Much stress had been laid on hospital admission and treatment. This again increases the cost of health care. No provisions are made for home treatment.

Forensic Toxicology

CHAPTER 17

General Toxicology

TOXICOLOGY

- **Toxicology** is the study of substances which are toxic to human body causing illness, disease, deformity or death.
- **Forensic toxicology** is application of knowledge of toxicology in a court of law for the purpose of administration of justice.
- **Poisons** are those substances which are harmful to human body after entering through any route of administration.
- Poison is any substance which when administered by any route causes disease, deformity or death (injury, infirmity or death).
- Any substance is a poison when administered with the intention to cause bodily pain or disease or death.
- It is the intent which is more important than the dose or route of administration.
- Antidotes: Substances which neutralize the poison or toxin effect and make it harmless are called **antidotes.**

Common Routes of Administration

- Inunction: By rubbing over skin
- Ingestion: Taken through mouth
- Inhalation: Taken through respiratory tract
- Injection: Introduction through syringes and needle
- Intracutaneous (into the skin)
- Subcutaneous (under the skin)

- Intramuscular (into the muscles)
- Intravenous (into the vein)
- Intracardiac (into the heart)
- Intra-articular (into the joint)
- Intrathecal (into the menniges)
- Intraventricular (directly into the ventricles)
- Intraocular (into ocular chamber)
- Intraperitoneal (into the peritoneum)
- Subconjunctival (below the conjunctiva)

Others

- Per vaginal (into the vagina)
- Per rectal (into the rectum)
- Per urethral (into the urethra)
- By instilling into nasal cavity
- By sublingual administration
- By drops into ear, nose, throat, eyes, mouth
- By application on nipple, through sucking.

CLASSIFICATION OF POISONS (BASED ON ACTIONS) (Figs 17.1 to 17.12)

1. Corrosives
2. Irritants
3. Vegetable alkaloidal poisons
4. Vegetable cardiac poisons
5. Irrespirable gases
6. Inebriant poisons
7. Anaesthetic substances
8. Miscellaneous groups
9. Food poisoning
10. Insecticides
11. Environmental toxicity
12. Chemicals

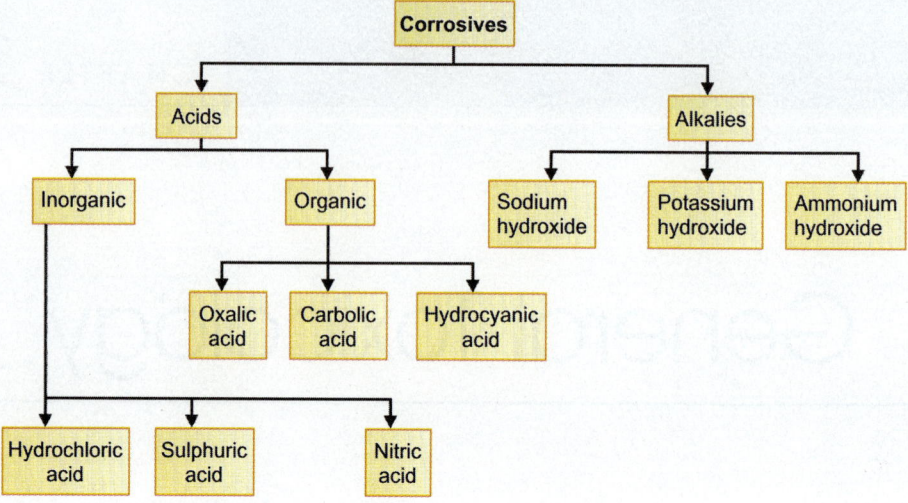

Fig. 17.1: Corrosives

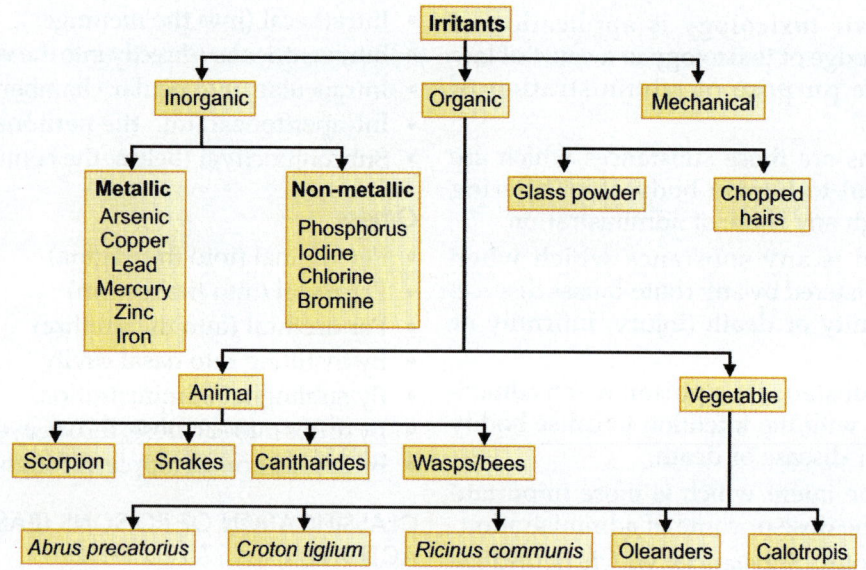

Fig. 17.2: Irritants

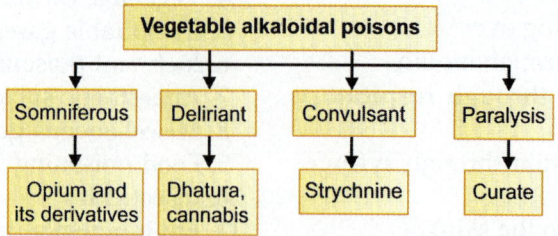

Fig. 17.3: Vegetable alkaloidal poisons

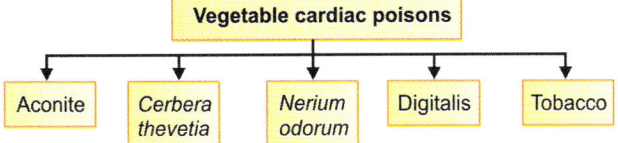

Fig. 17.4: Vegetable cardiac poisons

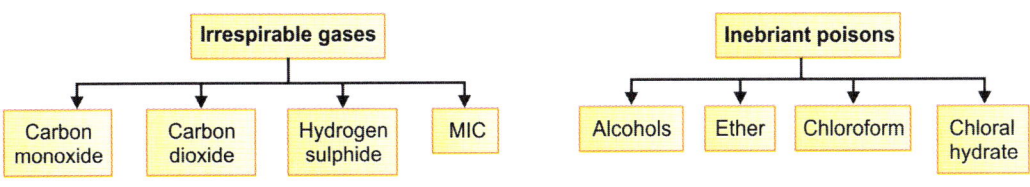

Fig. 17.5: Irrespirable gases

Fig. 17.6: Inebriant poisons

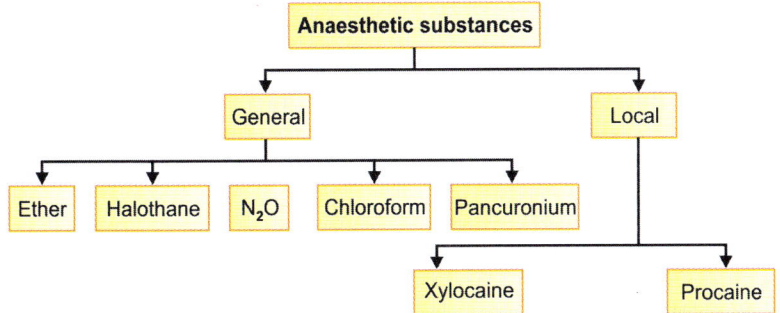

Fig. 17.7: Anaesthetic substances

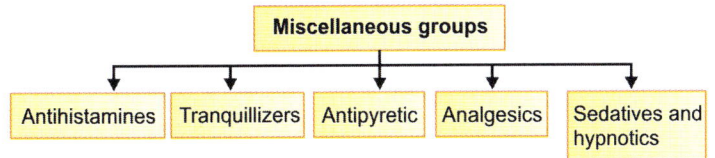

Fig. 17.8: Miscellaneous groups

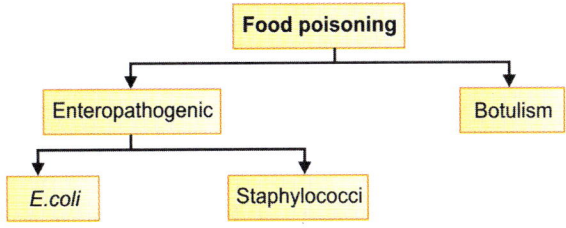

Fig. 17.9: Food poisoning

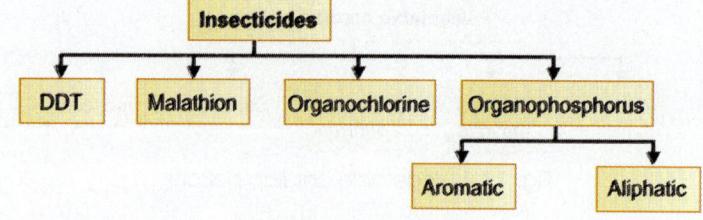

Fig. 17.10: Insecticides

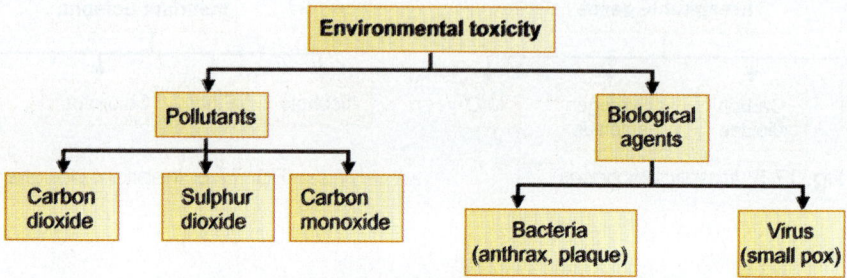

Fig. 17.11: Environmental toxicity

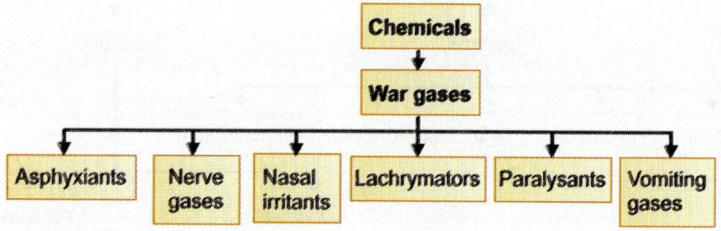

Fig. 17.12: Chemicals

DUTIES OF DOCTOR IN CASES OF POISONING

Doctors who are registered medical practitioners (registered with state medical council) and engaged in general practice or hospital service as physicians, come across poisoning cases during their practice.

First duty of a doctor is to make diagnosis of the poison.

- Once the diagnosis is made, the immediate duty is to save the life of the patient.
- The patient should be removed from the source of poisoning.
- If necessary a professional colleague's opinion is taken.
- If poisoning is due to contaminated food or drinking water the concerned health authorities must be notified.
- Once the patient is stabilised, the medicolegal issues can be considered, i.e

a dying declaration, if the patient is conscious.

- Materials like vomit, urine, faeces, stomach wash contents are collected in clean containers, labelled, sealed, preserved and transmitted to forensic science laboratory for chemical analysis. If there is any material like syringe, empty vessel, glass, half consumed food, etc. they are also to be collected and transmitted to FSL for chemical analysis.
- In private practice, a case of suicidal poisoning may not be informed to the police, however, when police or magistrate enquire for investigation, the doctor must furnish all information.
- In homicidal poisoning, information should be given to the nearest police station.
- In government and quasi government hospitals all poisoning or suspected

poisoning cases are to be informed to police.

- Inspite of the treatment if the patient dies, death certificate should not be issued and police should be informed for further action.

TREATMENT OF POISONING

- Removal of poison from the stomach by stomach wash or using emetics.
- Inactivation or neutralisation of the poison by using antidotes.
- Hastening the elimination of poison from the system by using diuretics, purgatives, dialysis or other means.
- Giving relief to the symptoms by symptomatic treatment like pain relieved by giving pain killers, convulsions relieved by anticonvulsants.
- Taking care of life supporting measures.

Life supporting measures include

- **Blood pressure:** Maintenance: Recording BP frequently.
- **Blood care:** By giving blood transfusion if required.
- **Balance** of fluids to be maintained by taking care of output and input.
- **Bladder** care by putting an indwelling catheter which also helps in noting the real and exact output of urine.
- **Bowel care** is taken by administering enema if required in patients flatus tube and doing other required measures.
- **Back care or bedsores prevention:** This is required in patients who are bed ridden by using waterbeds or beds which have inflation-deflation facility.
- **Bed position:** The bed is raised at the head end or foot end depending upon the case.
- **Body position:** The body is kept in a lateral position or inclined position with back rest or by adjusting the angle of the bed.
- **Breathing management:** By keeping a patent airway using an intubation tube or doing a tracheostomy, if necessary. Intermittent positive pressure may be maintained in **Bird's** respirator.

- **Bread care:** Should not be forgotten, i.e. required nutrients should be given by nasogastric tube or IV alimentation depending upon the situation.
- **Balance of mind:** In cases of attempted suicide, psychiatric attention is required to drain the pressure to cope up with the situation that has led to the consumption of poison.
- In majority cases, the poison is consumed by ingestion. Even now in India, people consume poisons of vegetable origin like *dhatura, Nerium odorum, Cannabis, Clistanthus colonis*, agriculture connected substances like baygon, aluminium phosphide, opium and its derivatives.
- Elimination or removal of poison from the stomach is necessary in cases where the patient has consumed poison less than 3 hours before the person is brought to hospital.
- **By washing the stomach,** the unabsorbed poison comes out as it is and prevents further increase in the levels of the poison in system.
- **Stomach wash** is carried out by using the stomach tube, it is also known as **Boas** tube.
- It is a flexible rubber tube, 1½ metre long, 1 cm in diameter.
- It has a blunt-rounded end which is pushed into the stomach (stomach end).
- The other end contains a funnel and it is held nearer to the mouth (mouth end).
- Near the tip of the stomach end there are large holes through which the fluid enters the stomach.
- The stomach tube has a mark 50 cm above the stomach end (lower end) so when tube reaches this mark we know that the tube has entered the stomach.
- Vaseline or glycerine is applied to the stomach tube as lubricant.
- The stomach tube is passed through a mouth gag.
- The tongue is pressed with a depressor and the tube is pushed gently.
- The patient is kept in the prone position.
- The head is near the end of the cot so that the throat is at lower level.

- This prevents the regurgitated matter or the fluid from entering the respiratory passages.
- The funnel is held above the head. The first liquid to be passed through tube is plain warm water 500 ml. The fluid enters the stomach by gravity.
- The funnel is then lowered below the level of stomach. The stomach contents come out from funnel.
- They are collected in a clean container and kept preserved for chemical analysis purpose.
- These returns are observed for the presence of capsules, tablets, vegetables, shreds of blood or mucous membrane, colour, smell of the fluid, etc.
- Efforts are to be made to identify the poison by colour, smell, etc.
- Based on the symptoms and signs of the patient what is to be added in the stomach wash is decided. Each time 500 ml fluid is used containing a suitable antidote.
- Stomach was is continued until the clear fluid coming from stomach and the fluid which we are pushing inside the stomach are same in colour.
- This suggests that there is no further action between antidote and poison in stomach.
- In other words, the poison inside the stomach is neutralised.
- Then instead of leaving the stomach empty some more quantity of antidote should be left in the stomach.
- If there is any chance of poison remaining inside the stomach, that is also neutralised.

Stomach wash is contraindicated in cases of

- Children
- Convulsions
- Corrosive poisoning
- Comatose patients
- In convulsion cases like strychnine poisoning the convulsion is controlled, patient is anaesthetised and then gastric lavage is done.
- In case of corrosive acids like sulphuric acid and corrosive alkalies, there is danger of perforation of stomach and oesophagus, so stomach wash is not recommended.

- In children, the stomach tube being wider in diameter it is not used. However, a Ryle's tube which has shorter length and narrow calibre is utilized.
- In case of coma, after intubation of the patient, a nasogastric tube is passed and the stomach contents are removed by the tube with due care.

Emetics

Emetics are those substances which induce vomiting.

The various domestic emetics are

- Large quantities of warm water.
- 15 gm of mustard powder mixed in 200 ml of warm water.
- Two spoons of common salt in 200 ml of warm water. All these are available in house so we can call them as household emetics.

Other emetics are

- 0.5 gm of copper sulphate in 10–15 ml of warm water.
- Tartar emetic 25 gm in 200 ml of warm water.
- Apomorphine hydrochloride given as a SC injection in dose 1–2 gm. *It is a central emetic and causes projectile vomiting.*
- Zinc sulphate 1–2 gm in 200 ml of water.
- Ammonium carbonate 1–2 gm in 200 ml of water.
- Tincture ipecac in 30 ml dose for adults and 15 ml for children.

Contraindications

- Poisoning in corrosive acids and alkalies.
- In volatile poisoning like kerosene and gasoline.
- Strychnine poison
- Comatose patient
- Advanced pregnancy.

Complications of Stomach Wash

- Aspiration pneumonia
- Laryngospasm
- Stomach/oesophagus perforation.

ANTIDOTES

Antidotes are those substances which are used to nullify or neutralize the action of poisons.

Types of Antidotes

- Universal antidotes
- Physiological antidotes
- Chemical antidotes
- Mechanical antidotes

Universal Antidotes

Universal antidote is a general antidote used in cases of unknown poisons. Commonly known antidote contains:

- One part of milk of magnesia
- Two parts of powered charcoal
- One part of strong tea
- Milk of magnesia neutralizes acid, strong tea precipitates alkaloids and charcoal (activated) adsorbs poisonous substances.
- In many places, in place of universal antidotes people are using only activated charcoal in doses of 4–8 gm.

Physiological Antidotes

Physiological antidotes are those substances which produce manifestations diametrically opposite to the poison consumed.

Examples

Atropine and physostigmine—in cases of atropine poisoning physostigmine is given as antidote. Physostigmine causes pupillary contraction, lowers the heart rate, increases the secretions of glands.

Other Examples

- Atropine and morphine, strychnine and barbiturates.
- PAM in organophosphorus compounds.
- Cyanides and nitrates.

Chemical Antidotes

The chemical antidote acts with poison to form harmless, nontoxic compounds.

Examples

- In corrosive acid poisoning aluminum hydroxide gel is given.
- In alkali poisoning vinegar (acetic acid dilute) is used.
- In oxalic acid poisoning lime is used.
- In lead poisoning sodium sulphate is used.
- In carbolic acid poisoning magnesium phosphate is used.
- In phosphorus poisoning copper sulphate is used.

Potassium permanganate is an oxidizing agent. It is used as a good chemical antidote in cases of opium and its alkaloids, phosphorus, cyanides, barbiturates, etc. Hydrated ferric oxide is used in arsenic poisoning.

Mechanical Antidotes

Mechanical antidotes are those substances which act as simple physical agents without any chemical reaction.

Examples

- 4.8 gm finely powdered activated charcoal causes absorption through the active pores.
- It is useful in alkaloid poisons.
- Demulscent substance like albumin makes a coating on stomach mucosa. It is useful in cases of phosphorus, phenol, kerosene poisoning, etc.
- Bulky food, e.g. bananas or gruel also act as mechanical antidote in case of glass pieces or diamond dust consumption.

Chelating Agents

These are substances which inactivate a metallic poison. They form nontoxic, stable and soluble compounds with heavy metals like lead, mercury, zinc, cobalt, arsenic, etc.

- BAL—2,3-dimercaptopropanol or dimercaprol or British antilewisite.
- EDTA—ethylenediaminetetra-acetic acid.
- Penicillamine (cuprimine)
- Desferrioxamine

BAL

- BAL is used against heavy metal poisoning like arsenic, mercury, gold, antimony,

thallium, lead, etc. Heavy metals have a great affinity for – SH radicals in the cells and tissue enzymes.
- They displace hydrogen and deprive the body of tissue enzymes.
- Dimercaprol forms stable compound with heavy metals.
- It is excreted outside the body in urine. It does not cause damage to excretory organs like liver and kidney.
- It is contraindicated in cadmium poisoning and in cases of pre-existing liver damage.
- BAL is administered in doses of 3–4 mg/kg body weight. It is in oily base of peanut oil or arachis oil with 20% benzyl benzoate solution.
- This injection should not be given intra-venously, it is given deep intramuscular, in gluteal region.
- Higher doses of BAL can cause BAL poisoning effects.
- The effects are restlessness, salivation, lacrymation, a sense of constriction of chest, rise of temperature, fall of blood pressure, vomiting, etc.

Ethylenediaminetetra-acetic Acid (EDTA)

- EDTA is useful as an antidote in heavy metals like lead, zinc, magnesium, iron, cadmium, copper, etc.
- Calcium disodium versenate is a very good chelating agent against lead poisoning.
- It is given by slow IV drip. It should not be given orally.

Penicillamine (Cuprimine)

- Hydrolysis of penicillin produces penicillamine. It has stable – SH group. It is useful in copper, mercury, zinc poisoning and also in lead poisoning. *It is taken orally.*
- It may cause pyridoxine deficiency, therefore B$_6$ should be given usually 4 times in a day for a period of 8–10 days.
- Adverse reactions like skin rash, leuko-penia, thrombocytopenia, agranulocytosis may occur. So, relevant blood test should be done during penicillamine usage.

Desferrioxamine

- It is a water-soluble compound. It is a specific chelating agent in iron intoxication. It is used by oral, intramuscular or intravenous route.
- **Oral dose:** 8–10 gm dissolved in 80–100 ml of distil water.
- **IM dose:** 1 gm
- **IV dose:** 1–2 gm dissolved 5% glucose saline 500 ml.

Hastening the elimination of poison from system by

- Diuresis
- Dialysis
- Diaphoresis
- Catharsis

Diuresis: 20% mannitol in 500 ml for 12 hours. Mannitol diuresis helps in phenobarbitone poisoning. It also relieves cerebral oedema. Frusemide or lasix is used to give forced alkaline diuresis.

Dialysis: Peritoneal dialysis is useful in salicylate and aspirin poisoning among children.
- *Haemodialysis* is useful in cases of bar-biturate, methyl alcohol, bromide poisoning, etc.
- Exchange transfusion is useful in children in case of poisonings like barbiturate, carbon monoxide, etc.

Diaphoresis: Induction of sweating, sometimes useful in hyperpyrexia.

Catharsis: Helps in the elimination of poisonous material while passing the stool. Sodium sulphate is preferred over others.

Factors Influencing the Action of a Poison in the Body

- Age of the person
- State of the body
- Health of the person
- Presence of any illness
- Intoxicated or otherwise
- State of sleep
- State of exertion or exercise
- Mental alertness

- Route of administration
- Quantity of the poisonous substance
- State of the substance—physical, chemical and concentration
- Tolerance
- Adverse reactions
- Cumulative effect
- Idiosyncrasy
- Stomach condition—empty or full, sick or well, absence or presence of hydrochloric acid.

Age

Elderly persons can tolerate opium and its derivatives more than the children and infants. Children tolerate better than grown ups in the case of atropine and related substances.

State of the Body

A person who is in good physical health and well-built tolerate poisons better than a sick person.

Presence of any Illness

- A person suffering from disease of liver or kidney shows increased effect of the poison.
- Patients who are recently ill like delirium can tolerate sedatives and tranquillizers more than others.

Intoxicated or Otherwise

- When a person is in a state of intoxication the action of the poisonous substance is delayed in sleep.
- Slow absorption occurs due to low metabolic status.
- When the person is highly active as in exercise, action of some poisons is delayed, like alcohol.

Mental Alertness

- When a person consumes any poison unknowingly, the poison may not show action for sometimes.
- In some cases if the person knows about the substance, this manifest is less as in the case of LSD.

Route of Administration

A substance inhaled causes fast effects. In the order of decreasing activity we can mention IV, IM, intracutaneous or subcutaneous, oral, introduction through open wound or inunction or rubbing over skin.

Quantity of Poisonous Substance

In larger doses ordinarily the effect is more, but sometimes as in case of $CuSO_4$, a larger dose produces vomiting and takes out the poison.

State of the Substance

- In the gaseous form poisons are absorbed faster than liquid or solid forms. Some seeds when swallowed intact come out intact without any manifestation, but on crushing they show poisonous symptoms, e.g. nux vomica seeds.
- When a strong acid is consumed it acts as corrosive and on dilution it may function as an irritant, e.g. hydrochloric acid.
- Sometime, a dilute solution may be absorbed faster and symptoms may occur fast, e.g. oxalic acid solution.

Tolerance

- Alcohol is the best example of substance which creates **tissue tolerance.**
- **Adverse reaction:** Some substances may cause adverse reactions instead of the expected reaction, e.g. penicillin injection.

  Cumulative effect: Substance like digitalis gets accumulated in the body and causes unexpected toxic effect.

Idiosyncracy

- Human beings react to drugs in different ways.
- Unsuspected and unexpected adverse action can occur in individuals, potassium iodide, aspirin, sulpha drugs, food materials like eggs, prawns, mushrooms and even chocolates can create problems like urticaria, server aromatic action and even haemorrhages in skull bone.

- What we call ordinary quantity and which does not cause bad effects in the person may be fatal at times. *Just 1 gm of aspirin* may kill a person.

Stomach Condition

- By far the commonest culprit or victim for all the unwanted stuff is the stomach. It is the most insulted organ next to skin.
- If the mucous membrane of stomach is ulcerated or eroded the poison my be absorbed faster, if there is mucus coating on the stomach wall the absorption may be delayed.
- If the production of hydrochloric acid is less, substances like cyanides are not absorbed.
- If stomach is full, the poison absorption may be delayed.
- Kidney disease may also sometimes delay excretion of poison and prolongs the poisonous manifestations.

POISONING RELATED VARIOUS SYMPTOMS

Substances Causing—Pinpoint Pupils

- Carbolic acid
- Opium
- Morphine
- Organophosphorus compounds

Substances Causing—Dilated Pupils

- *Dhatura*
- Ethyl alcohol
- Cocaine
- Cyanide
- Carbon monoxide

Substances Causing—Jaundice

- Phosphorous
- Arsenic
- CCl_4 (Carbon tetrachloride)
- Chloroform

Substances having Odour or Smell

- Carbolic odour: Phenol
- Bitter almond odour: Cyanide
- Garlic odour: Phosphorous, thalium, arsenic.
- Fishy odour: Aluminium phosphide, zinc phospide
- Rotten egg odour: Hydrogen sulphide
- Apple-like odour: Chloroform, acetone
- Spirituous odour: Ethyl alcohol
- Vicks odour: Methyl salicylate (nilgiri oil)

Substances Causing—High Blood Pressure

- Cocaine
- Amphetamines

Substances Causing—Low Blood Pressure

- Opium
- Organophosphorus compounds
- Carbon monoxide
- Cyanide

Substances that Increase Pulse Rate (Tachycardia)

- Caffeine
- Cannabis
- Carbon monoxide
- Cocaine
- Amphetamines

Substances that Decrease Pulse Rate (Bradycardia)

- Opium
- Organophosphorus compounds

Substances that Decrease Respiratory Rate

- Opium
- Nicotine
- Strychnine
- Ethyl alcohol
- Barbiturates

Substances that Increase Respiratory Rate

- Salicylates
- Amphetamine
- Cocaine

Substances Causing—Hypoglycaemia

- Insulin
- Ethyl alcohol
- Salicylates
- Isoniazid

Substances Causing—Acidosis

- Methanol
- Paraldehyde
- Salicylates
- Ethylene glycol

Substances Causing—Alkalosis

- Ingestion of large quantities of sodium carbonate
- Loss of hydrochloric acid
- Uraemia with vomiting

Substances that Increase Temperature

- *Dhatura*
- Belladonna
- Atropine
- Arsenic

Substances that Decrease Temperature

Opium

Substances Causing—Abortion (Abortifacients)

- Calotropis
- Ergot
- Quinine

Stupefying Agents

- *Dhatura*
- Cannabis
- Chloral hydrate

Cattle Poisons

- *Abrus precatorius*
- Calotropis

Cardiac Poisons

- Aconite
- Nicotine
- Quinine
- Digitalis
- Cyanides
- Oleander

Nephrotoxic Poisons

- Mercury
- Oxalic acid
- Cantharides

Aphrodisiac Substances

- Vyagra
- Cocaine
- Penegra
- *Cannabis indica*
- Arsenic
- Cantharides

Depilatories (Hair Removers)

- Salts of arsenic
- Thallium, barium sulphide

Arrow Poisons

- Aconite
- *Abrus precatorius*
- Curare
- Strychnine
- Snake venom
- Croton oil

Skin Colours/Pigmentation

Yellowish	Picric acid
	Sodium nitrate
	Carotene
	Chloroquine
Red	Borate
	Rifampicin
Blue	Tetracycline, naphthalene
	Bismuth
	Silver
	Mercury
Brown	Nitrates and nitrites
	Arsenic
Orange	Dinitrophenol

Discolouration of Teeth

Brownish	Tetracycline
Yellowish	Nitric acid
Chalky white	Sulphuric acid
Blue-line of gums	Lead poisoning

Colour of Vomiting

Brown colour	Arsenic
White colour	Antimony
Green colour	Digitalis
Black colour	Sulphuric acid
Slate grey colour	Corrosive sublimate

Bleached Mouth Appearance

- Corrosive acid
- Corrosive sublimte

Poisons Causing Pulmonary Oedema

- Opiates
- Aspirin
- Carbamates
- Organophosphorus compounds
- Ethylene glycol
- Irritant gases

Poisons which Cause Fits

- Aspirin
- *Dhatura*
- Chloroquine
- Insulin
- Quinine
- Organophosphorus insecticides
- Strychnine
- Carbon monoxide
- Methanol
- Ethylene glycol

Adverse Effects of Some Drugs

1. **Gingival hyperplasia**

   Phenytoin   Lamotrigine
   Calcium antagonists Cyclosporine
   Sirolimus

2. **Pancreatitis**

   Asparaginase   Didanosine
   Stavudine   Zalcitabine
   Azathioprine   Ethacrynic acid
   Sulfonamides   Furosemide
   Corticosteroids   Opioids
   Thiazides   Estrogens
   Mercaptopurine   Pentamidine
   Valproic acid   Oral
                                      contraceptives

3. **Erythromycin estolate**

   Anabolic steroids   Acetohexamide
   Chlorpropamide   Androgens
   Nitrofurantoin   Phenothiazines
   Oral contraceptives Gold salts
   Cyclosporine   Flucloxacillin
   Co-amoxyclav   Methimazole

4. **Altered taste**

   ACE inhibitors   Acetazolamide
   Biguanides   Lithium
   Griseofulvin   Rifampicin
   Metronidazole

5. **Metallic taste**

   Metronidazole   Acetazolamide
   Disulfiram   Auranofin
   Vincristine

6. **Pulmonary fibrosis**

   Bleomycin   Mitomycin
   Amiodarone   Busulfan
   Chlorambucil   Cyclophos-
                                       phamide
   Methysergide   Vinblastine
   Methotrexate

7. **Pulmonary eosinophilia**

   Amiodarone   Bleomycin
   Captopril   Gold salts
   GM-CSF   Nitrofurantoin
   Contrast media   L-tryptophan
   Phenytoin   Iodine
   Carbamazepine   Aspirin
   Sulfasalazine   Nilutamide
   Propylthiouracil   Penicillamine
   Methotrexate   Minocycline

8. **Edation**

   Clonidine   Methyldopa
   Antihistaminics   Barbiturates
   Benzodiazepines   Reserpine
   TCAs

9. **Extrapyramidal reactions**

   Metoclopramide   Methyldopa
   Phenothiazines   Reserpine
   Amitriptyline   L-dopa
   Butyrophenones, e.g. haloperidol

10. **Seizures**

    INH   Nalidixic acid
    Amphetamines   Imipenem
    Local anaesthetics   Pethidine
    Penicillins   Phenothiazines
    TCA   Vincristine
    Bupropion   Clozapine
    Physostigmine   Quinolones
    (IV)
    Theophylline

11. Tremors
TCAs
Theophylline
Lithium
Sympathomimetics (β_2-agonists)

12. Peripheral neuropathy

INH	Didanosine
Stavudine	Zalcitabine
Paclitaxel	Nitrofurantoin
Cisplatin	TCAs
Ethambutol	Nalidixic acid
Chlorpropamide	Demeclocycline
Ethionamide	Hydralazine
Metronidazole	Polymyxin B
Procarbazine	Phenytoin
Tolbutamide	Vincristine
Chloroquine	Chloramphenicol
Amiodarone	Clofibrate
Methysergide	

Aminoglycosides, e.g. streptomycin

13. Pseudotumor cerebri (raised ICT)

Sympathomimetics	Nalidixic acid
Oral contraceptives	Tetracyclines
Hypervitaminosis A	Glucocorticoids
Amiodarone	

14. Hypertension

Cocaine	MAO inhibitors
Cyclosporine	Glucocorticoids
Oral contraceptives	TCAs
Rofecoxib	Valdecoxib
Clonidine withdrawal	Sympatho-mimetics

15. Hypotension

Theophylline	Adenosine
Morphine	Quinidine
Fosphenytoin (IV)	Amiodarone
IL-2	Levo-dopa
Alpha blockers	Guanethidine
Bretylium	β-blockers (IV)
Glyceryl trinitrate	Chlorpromazine
Diuretics	Clonidine
Calcium channel blockers	

16. Congestive heart failure

Minoxidil	CCBs
β-blockers	Carbenoxolone sodium

Diazoxide	Estrogens
Indomethacin	Mannitol
Phenylbutazone	Corticosteroids
Verapamil	

17. First dose phenomenon

Prazosin	Muromonab-CD3

Sargramostim
ACE inhibitors especially captopril

18. Exacerbation of angina

α-blockers	Withdrawal of β-blockers
Ergotamine	Thyroxine excess
Methysergide	Sumatriptan
Minoxidil	Hydralazine
Vasopressin	Oxytocin
Nifedipine	

19. Cardiomyopathy

Daunorubicin	Emetine
Lithium	Phenothiazines
Sympathomimetics	Trastuzumab
Doxorubicin (adriamycin)	

20. Hyperglycaemia

Thiazides	Furosemide
Glucocorticoids	Oral contraceptives
Diazoxide	L-asparaginase
Glucagon	Cyclosporine
Phenytoin	Propranolol
Tacrolimus	Protease inhibitors
Niacin	Encainide

Pentamidine (late in therapy)

21. Hypoglycaemia

Oral hypoglycaemics	Quinine
Insulin	β-blockers
Ethanol	Octreotide

Salicylates (late in overdose)
Pentamidine (early in therapy)

22. Hypertriglyceridaemia

Corticosteroids	Protease inhibitors
β-blockers (non-ISA)	Ethanol
Estrogens	Oral contraceptives
Thiazides	

23. **Hyperkalaemia**

NSAIDs	SCh
ACE inhibitors	

Potassium sparing diuretics (spiro-nolactone, amiloride and triamterene)

Salt substitutes	ARBs (losartan)
Lithium	Pentamidine
Digoxin overdose	Cyclosporine
Heparin	β-blockers (initially)
Cytotoxics	Trimethoprim

24. **Hypokalaemia**

Thiazides	Furosemide
Carbenoxolone	Lithium
Corticosteroids	Amphotericin B
Gentamicin	Insulin
Mannitol	Theophylline

Carbonic anhydrase inhibitors

25. **Hyperuricaemia**

Cyclosporine	Diuretics
Pyrazinamide	Low dose salicylates
Nicotinic acid	Cytotoxics

26. **Hypercalcaemia**

Cholecalciferol	Thiazides
Calcium (IV)	

27. **Hypocalcaemia**

Calcitonin	Bisphosphonates
Plicamycin	Phenytoin
Gallium nitrate	

28. **Lactic acidosis**

Phenformin	Metformin
Zidovudine	Zalcitabine
Spironolactone	Acetazolamide
Salicylates	

29. **Gynaecomastia**

Digitalis	Spironolactone
Testosterone	Ketoconazole
Ethionamide	Calcium antagonists
Estrogens	Griseofulvin
INH	Methyldopa
Reserpine	Phenytoin
Cimetidine	Flutamide
Cyproterone acetate	Goserelin
Clomiphene	

30. **Hyperprolactinaemia**

Phenothiazines	Butyrophenones
TCAs	Reserpine
Methyldopa	Metoclopramide
Domperidone	

31. **Hyperthyroidism**

Amiodarone	Iodides

32. **Hypothyroidism**

Lithium	Iodides
Sulfonamides	Amiodarone
Phenylbutazone	Carbimazole
Acetazolamide	Phenytoin

33. **Nephrogenic diabetes insipidus**

Lithium	Demeclocycline
Methoxyflurane	

34. **Colour vision alteration**

Sulfonamides	Thiazides
Barbiturates	Digitalis
Ethambutol	Quinine
Streptomycin	

35. **Glaucoma**

Mydriatics	TCAs
Sympathomimetics	Corticosteroids

36. **Ototoxicity (vestibular)**

Aminoglycosides	Mustine
Quinidine	Quinine
Chloroquine	Vancomycin
Furosemide	Ethacrynic acid

Salicylates (high dose)

37. **Ototoxicity (auditory)**

NSAIDs	Vancomycin
Ethacrynic acid	Aminoglycosides

38. **Aplastic anaemia**

Chloramphenicol	Phenytoin
Gold salts	Carbamazepine
Phenylbutazone	Sulfonamides
Zidovudine	Colchicine
Carbimazole	Quinacrine

Felbamate
Cytotoxics
Thioamides
Trimethadione

39. Haemolytic anaemia in G6PD deficiency

Primaquine	Furazolidone
Chloramphenicol	Dapsone
Aspirin	Quinidine
Procainamide	Nalidixic acid
Quinine	Cotrimoxazole
Nitrofurantoin	Sulfonamides
Phenazophridine	

40. Megaloblastic anaemia

Pentamidine	Methotrexate
Trimethoprim	Cotrimoxazole
N_2O	Oral contraceptives
Metformin	Primidone
Phenobarbitone	Phenytoin
Triamterene	

41. SLE-like syndrome

Hydralazine	Acebutolol
Asparaginase	Barbiturates
Bleomycin	Cephalosporins
Iodides	Sulfonamides
Thiouracil	Methyldopa
Phenytoin	INH
Quinidine	Procainamide

42. Myopathy

Statins	Clofibrate
Daptomycin	Amphotericin B
Carbenoxolone	Chloroquine
Cimetidine	Oral contraceptives
Corticosteroids	

43. Skeletal muscle tremors

B$_2$-agonists	Zaleplon

44. Erythema multiforme/Stevens-Johnson syndrome/toxic epidermal necrolysis

Sulphones	Allopurinol
Cephalosporins	Chlorpropamide
Codeine	Ethosuximide
Lamotrigine	Nalidixic acid
Phenylbutazone	Piroxicam
Quinolones	Tocainide
Valproic acid	Penicillins
Tetracyclines	Salicylates
Barbiturates	Carbamazepine
Phenytoin	Thiazides

45. Hirsutism

Anabolic steroids	Minoxidil
Cyclosporine	Phenytoin

46. Decreased libido/impotence

β-blockers	Antipsychotics
Lithium	Clonidine
Diuretics	Methyldopa
Oral contraceptives	Sedatives
TCAs	

47. Interstitial nephritis

Cephalosporins	Ciprofloxacin
Allopurinol	Furosemide
NSAIDs	Methicillin
Phenindione	Rifampicin
Sulfonamides	Thiazides

48. Syndrome of inappropriate ADH secretion

Vinca alkaloids	Cyclophosphamide
Desmopressin	Oxytocin

49. Disulfiram-like reaction

Metronidazole	Cefamandole
Cefotetan	Cefoperazone
Moxalactam	Chlorpropamide
Procarbazine	

50. Osteoporosis

Glucocorticoids	Heparin
Thyroxine	

51. Prolonged QT interval

Terfenadine	Astemizole
Cisapride	Sparfloxacin
Gatifloxacin	Grepafloxacin
Amiodarone	Bretylium
Disopyramide	Procainamide
Quinidine	Sotalol
Mefloquine	Pentamidine
Thioridazine	Ziprasidone

Table 17.1: Street names of some drugs of abuse

Drug of abuse	Street name
Gamma hydroxybutyrate (GHB)	Liquid ecstasy grievous bodily harm
Phencyclidine and ketamine	Angel dust
Special K	Hog
Cocaine	Crack (vapour to be smoked)
Rush	
Coke	
Snow	
Blow	
Peruvian marching powder	
Methylene dioxymethamphetamine (MDMA)	Ecstasy Rave drug
Lysergic acid diethylamide (LSD)	Windowpane
	Twenty-five

CHAPTER 18

Corrosives

SULPHURIC ACID (H₂SO₄)

- Pure sulphuric acid is deceptive in appearance.
- It is colourless and oily liquid.
- It looks innocent.
- It does not emit fumes on exposure to air.
- It may be mistaken for liquid paraffin or water and glycerine.
- When it comes into contact with skin it becomes black.
- Cloth and paper turn to reddish brown in colour, burn and then leave holes.
- It is a highly corrosive substance.
- When mixed with water it generates lot of heat.

Manifestations of Sulphuric Acid Poisoning

Symptoms and Signs

- Burning pain in mouth, throat, gullet up to stomach.
- Spitting of content causes staining, brownish discolouration of angle of mouth, chin and chest.
- If the person touches it with fingertip, it gets discoloured and burnt (Fig. 18.1).
- Lips, mouth become softened, excoriated and covered with dirty white necrotic material.
- It turns into blackish brown colour.
- The mouth may be filled with thick brown, viscous material consisting of saliva and excoriated mucus patches.

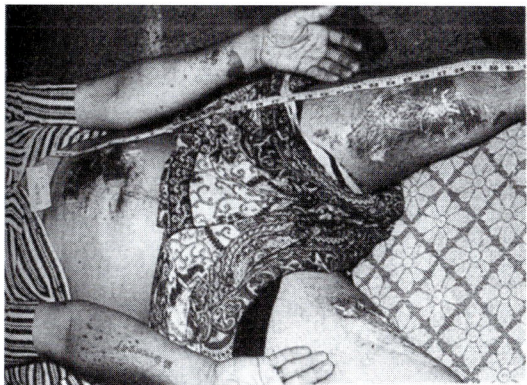

Fig. 18.1: Acid burns

- This substance causes difficulty, in speaking and swallowing.
- It may prevent respiration and cause of death due to asphyxia.
- The patient suffers from retching and vomiting.
- The vomited substance causes effervescence of earth (earth alkaline).
- Patient has lot of thirst.
- If the drinks water it further stimulates retching and vomiting.
- Lot of saliva is secreted which passes along angle of mouth and causes staining.
- The throat is swollen, swallowing becomes painful and difficult.
- Abdomen becomes distended and board like rigidity occurs when there is perforation of stomach.
- There may be loss of voice, frequent coughing occurs.

- Oedema of glottis causes respiratory obstruction and anoxia.

Causes of Death

- Shock
- Anoxia due to oedema glottis
- Exhaustion
- Perforation of stomach
- Toxaemia
- Peritonitis
- Stricture oesophagus.

Postmortem Appearances

- Angle of the mouth gets brownish black salivary stain.
- Lips—excoriated, mucosa of mouth—corroded.
- Tongue—distorted.
- Teeth—chalky white, oesophagus mucosa corroded.
- Stomach—internally almost black in colour with perforation.
- Dark brown or black liquid in the stomach.
- Mucous membrane detached.
- Stomach wall soft and pulpy.
- The perforated material enters into viscera of abdomen or thorax causing blackening of heart, lungs, spleen, liver, kidney, etc.
- Death is generally immediate.
- Delayed deaths are due to starvation because of oesophageal stricture.

Treatment

- **Mild alkalies:** Aluminium hydroxide gel.
- **Demulscents:** Milk or egg albumin.
- Tracheostomy to overcome oedema glottis.

   Fatal dose: 5–10 ml

   Fatal period: 18–24 hours

Medicolegal Issues

May be pushed into vagina to punish a woman for infidelity to cause severe vaginal stenosis.

Vitriolage

- Persons seeking malice, jealousy and hatred, maim or disfigure their enemy by throwing the oil of vitriol or sulphuric acid.
- This is called vitriolage.
- It causes burns on the face and corrosion of eyes.
- It is treated by immediate irrigation of eyes with plain water then with aqueous solution of sodium bicarbonate.
- A few drops of olive oil are instilled into the eyes.
- **The acid burns** can be differentiated from other burns by:
   - Absence of vesication.
   - Discolouration caused on the skin.
   - The presence of chemical on skin and clothing (confirmed by chemical analysis).

NITRIC ACID (HNO$_3$)

- It is a colourless, fuming liquid.
- It has a peculiar chocking odour.
- When it comes into contact with the organic matter it produces **xanthoproteic reaction** deep yellow colour is due to xanthoproteic acid yellow in colour.
- Burning pain, salivation, difficulty in swallowing and violent vomiting are seen.
- The vomit is yellowish brown in colour.
- The teeth look yellow.
- It causes irritation of eyes, nose and air passages, with lacrimation, difficulty in breathing, sneezing, coughing, dyspnoea and photophobia.
- Oedema glottis may lead to anoxia and death.
- Death may occur due to pulmonary oedema.

   Fatal dose: 10–15 ml

   Fatal period: About one day

Postmortem Appearances

- Yellow frothy mucus from mouth and nose, yellow staining on mouth, chin and cheeks.
- Stomach mucosa yellowish brown, soft, friable, ulcerated.
- Perforation rarely seen.

Treatment

It is same as in sulphuric acid.

Medicolegal Issues

- It is used by Goldsmiths.
- Used as suicidal poison among Goldsmiths more than others.
- It may be used for vitriolage purpose.

HYDROCHLORIC ACID (HCl)

- It is a colourless fuming liquid.
- It attacks respiratory passage more than the nitric acid and sulphuric acid.

Fatal dose: 15–30 ml

Fatal period: 18–30 hours

Symptoms and Signs

- The fumes cause cough, dyspnoea, cyanosis and anoxia due to oedema glottis.
- Bronchopneumonia occurs.
- Mucosa of mouth and tongue turn greyish white.
- Those exposed constantly to HCl fumes suffer from conjunctivitis, corneal ulcer, coryza, pharyngitis, laryngitis glossitis, stomatitis and gastritis, convulsions, delirium, etc.

Postmortem Appearances

- Buccal and oesophageal mucosa are ash grey in colour.
- Stomoch mucosa shows greyish-white patches.
- Stomach contains brownish acidic fluid.
- Lungs inflamed and show congestion and patchy consolidation.

Medicolegal Importance

- May be used for vitriolage.
- For cleaning the drains.

ORGANIC ACIDS

OXALIC ACID (ACID OF SUGAR)

- It is colourless, crystalline substance mistaken for magnesium sulphate.
- It is used as ink remover, bleaching agent in book binding, metal cleaning and dyeing industry.

Symptoms and Signs

- Due to precipitation of ionised calcium, manifestations of hypocalcaemia are seen.

- Tetanic convulsion, bradycardia, cardiac irregularities seen.
- Due to nephrotoxicity scanty urine containing albumin, oxalate crystals, blood is seen.
- Ventricular fibrillation, renal failure and death occur.

Fatal dose: 15–30 gm of oxalic acid, even 4 gm may cause death.

Fatal period: 1–2 hours

Treatment

- Stomach wash with calcium gluconate.
- 10 ml of 10% calcium gluconate IV.
- Dialysis or exchange transfusion to combat renal failure.
- Irrigation of eyes and washing of skin.

Postmortem Appearances

- Corroded angles of mouth and chin.
- Stomach walls friable and soft.
- Kidneys congested with tubules showing oxalate crystals.

Medicolegal Issues

- It is suicidal agent and an abortifacient.
- People are using oxalic acid for long time in calcoprinting, cleaning brass and copper articles, etc.
- Develop white, opaque, brittle nails.

CARBOLIC ACID

- Phenol is monohydroxybenzene.
- It is an alcohol.
- It occurs as colourless needle shape crystals.
- Absorbs moisture from atmosphere and turns pink.
- It has typical pungent smell and phenol-like odour.
- It reacts with alkalies to form carbolates.
- It is used as antiseptic, disinfectants and preservative.

Fatal dose: 15 gm

Fatal period: 1–4 hours

Symptoms and Signs

- It is locally a corrosive.
- In reaction to skin, it causes coagulation of cell proteins.

- It is local anaesthetic.
- It has central narcotic effect.
- It acts on the cells of brain, heart and kidneys.
- On the mucous membrane it causes irritation, inflammation, necrosis and sloughing.
- It affects medullary centres and higher centres causing rapid loss of senses.
- The urine in carbolic acid poisoning when first passed looks normal in colour.
- After some time the colour changes to olive green due to formation of hydroquinone and pyrochetacol.
- The urinary manifestation of carbolic acid is known as carboluria. The pupils are pin-pointed and catracted.

Treatment

- Stomach wash with sodium or magnesium sulphate.
- Olive oil or 10% glycerine are also used.
- The sodium or magnesium sulphate react with phenol and produce insoluble sulphocarbolates.
- Phenol burns on skin are treated with 10% alcohol. Demulcents like milk or egg white.
- Shock and collapse treated with IV normal saline and sodium bicarbonate.

Causes of Death

- Metabolic acidosis
- Renal damage
- Failure of respiratory centre

Oochronosis

- This is a chronic poisoning of phenol when it is used as a daily skin disinfectant by medical personnel.
- The features are anorexia, headache, vertigo, dark colour urine, pigmentation of skin and sclera, loss of weight.

Postmortem Appearances

- Phenol like odour around mouth and other contents.
- Corrosion of angles of mouth and chin.
- Brown leathery discolouration of stomach.

- Greyish white patches.
- Kidney shows haemorrhagic nephritis.
- Liver and spleen congested.
- Brain oedematous and congested.
- Viscera in this case is preserved in saturated solution of common salt for purpose of chemical analysis.

ACETYLSALICYLIC ACID (ASPIRIN)

- It is odourless, white, crystalline powder.
- It is medically used as analgesic, anti-pyretic and anti-inflammatory agent.
- In small doses or low dose it is used for prophylaxis of cerebrovascular ischaemic attacks in migraine.

Fatal dose: 5–10 gm

Fatal period: 2 minutes to many hours.

- Idiosyncrasy to aspirin or hypersensitivity occurs in persons who are prone to allergy.
- It causes skin rashes, swelling of face and eyelids, conjunctivitis, rhinitis, bronchospasm, tinnitus, deafness, per-spiration, diarrhoea, abdominal pain, anoxia, haemorrhage, neoplasm, dyspnoea, coma, terminal hyperpyrexia and haemo-rrhage due to capillary damage.

General Symptoms and Signs

Bloodstained vomiting, haematemesis, dyspnoea and acidosis. Death may be due to acidosis and uraemia. Early death due to shock and delayed death due to respiratory failure.

Treatment

- Stomach wash with plain warm water followed by 5% sodium bicarbonate solution.
- Lactate solution IV to combat with acidosis.
- Activated charcoal
- O_2 inhalation
- 20% mannitol 500 ml
- Dialysis or exchange transfusion.
- Noradrenaline drip to combat circulatory collapse.
- Vitamin K to combat hypoprothrom-binemia 5 mg/day.

Postmortem Appearances

- Skin rashes
- Erosion of gastric mucosa
- Petechial haemorrhages in pleura and pericardium.
- Pulmonary and cerebral oedema.

Reye's Syndrome

- In children below 15 years of age Reye's syndrome is sometimes observed on consumption of aspirin.
- Acute onset hepatic failure and ence-phalopathy with residual neurological manifestations.
- When Reye's syndrome is suspected mannitol drip is given IV to relieve cerebral oedema followed by symptomatic management.

Medicolegal Issues

Accidental aspirin poisoning especially in children is more common.

ALKALIES

- Strong alkalies extract water from tissues and precipitate proteins.
- Common alkalies are potassium hydroxide, sodium hydroxide.

Ammonium Hydroxide

- Ammonia has its own characteristic odour.
- Hydroxides of potassium and sodium are used as ripe cleaners.
- Alkalies are soapy and bitter.

Fatal dose

- Sodium hydroxide   5 gm
- Potassium hydroxide   15 gm
- Sodium carbonate   30 gm
- Ammonium hydroxide   30 ml of 25% concentration solution

Treatment

Alkalies are neutralised by weak acids like vinegar.

Symptoms and Signs

- Soapy taste in mouth.
- Excoriation and corrosion of mouth, gullet.
- Strongly alkaline vomiting.
- Purging is seen accompanied by tenesmus.
- Stool contains lot of mucus with blood.

   In the case of ammonia: Sneezing, coughing lacrimation, visual disturbances, acute dyspnoea, tightness in chest, frothy sputum due to pulmonary oedema. Death may occur due to shock, pulmonary oedema, pneumonia or bronchopneumonia.

Postmortem Examination

- Softening of mucosa of mouth, lips oesophagus.
- Deep chocolate or dark black colour.
- Stomach congested, blackish brown in colour.
- Congestion and oedema in glottis.
- Lungs show bronchopneumonia.

Medicolegal Issues

Accidental poisoning is more common.

CHAPTER 19

Non-Metallic Irritant Poisons

IRRITANTS

Irritants are poisons cause inflammation of gastrointestinal tract, the respiratory tract or the skin. There is a delay of ½ hour to 1 hour between consumption and manifestations. Difficulty in swallowing, burning pain, constriction in throat, pain in gullet, stomach, thirst, nausea and repeated vomiting. The diarrhoea is accompanied with pain and tenderness in abdomen, painful urination and cramps in the legs. The person may die to dehydration and shock.

The differential diagnosis of irritants or poisoning:
- Gastroenteritis
- Cholera
- Peritonitis
- Perforation of stomach

Postmortem Appearances

The mucous membrane of stomach is intensely congested.

PHOSPHORUS

- Phosphorus is a non-metallic irritant or poison. It is hepatotoxic and is also called protoplasmic poison. White or yellow phosphorus catches fire on exposure to air, so it is always preserved under H_2O in amber colour bottles.
- On exposure to light, white PO_4 changes to yellow.
- It has garlic like odour. It glows in darkness (phosphorescence).

- Pure red phosphorus is not poisonous, but commonly available red phosphorus is contaminated with yellow phosphorus and hence becomes poisonous.
- Yellow phosphorus was used before lucifer matches but nowadays red phosphorus is used because yellow phosphorus is not very safe for domestic matches.
- The sides of a matchbox contain thin layers of red phosphorus mixed with glass particles.
- The match stick does not contain red phosphorus.
- It only contains potassium chloride and antimony sulphide.

Manifestations of Phosphorus Poisoning

- When a person consumes white or yellow phosphorus, there is garlic-like odour from mouth.
- The gastritis causing nausea and vomiting is followed by diarrhoea with painful passing of stool.
- If the vomit contains yellow phosphorus, it shines in darkness. After the initial phase of symptoms the patient reaches the stage of liver toxicity and renal failure.
- The liver and spleen are enlarged and tender.
- The diarrhoea is severe, with bleeding from nose, urethra, vagina and uterus.
- There may be abortion in pregnant women and dysuria followed by anuria (painful urination and scanty urine formation).
- Liver toxicity causes hypoglycaemia.

- The liver cell metabolism is disturbed leading to fatty degeneration.
- When a person consumes large dose of phosphorus he/she develops delirium followed by coma and even death. Peripheral circulatory collapse may also occur.

Symptoms and Signs

- Garlic-like odour from mouth.
- Gastritis causing nausea and vomiting is followed by diarrhoea with painful passing of stool.
- Liver toxicity and renal failure.
- Liver and spleen are enlarged and tender.
- Diarrhoea is severe with bleeding.
- Large doses will cause coma and death.

  Fatal dose: 30–120 mg

  Fatal period: 4–10 hours

Treatment

- Stomach wash with $KMnO_4$ in water or 0.1% Cu_2SO_4 solution.
- Shock and dehydration are treated with 5% glucose saline.
- Vitamins C and K, B complex, Ca salts.

Postmortem Appearances

- Garlic smell, yellow discolouration of skin, phosphorescence of stomach content.
- Stomach and intestine yellowish colour.
- Liver shows necrobiosis
- Petechial haemorrhage
- Acute yellow atrophy of liver
- Liver is smaller, greasy, like wrinkled capsule.

Phossy Jaw

Chronic necrotizing chemical osteomyelitis due to chronic exposure to yellow phosphorus. Teeth are painful with swelling and necrosis of lower Jaw. The mucous membrane of mouth is congested. The patient feels tired, suffer from joint pains and emaciation.

Treatment

- Shifting the person from source of phosphorus.

- The teeth are examined and carious teeth are filled up.
- Sodium carbonate mouth wash is prescribed.

Medicolegal Issues

- Used to commit suicide
- Criminal abortion
- Detected in dead body, advance state of decomposition
- Incendiary bomb
- PO_4 is mixed with wet cowdung and thrown on huts, when it dries it catches fire.

PHOSPHINE (PH$_3$)

- It is a rat poison and has like fish. This gas causes sudden death in human being.
- Pain in chest, nausea, vomiting, diarrhoea, pulmonary, oedema, tremors, delirium, coma and death.
- Death is due to peripheral circulatory collapse.

Postmortem Examination

- Congestion of brain, liver, lungs, etc.
- Aluminium phosphide and zinc phosphide poisonings cause death due to release of phosphine.

Poison	Pattern of mucosa
Arsenic	Red velvety mucosa of stomach
H_2SO_4	Brown or black with erosion, perforation and carbolization
Carbolic acid	Green white or brown—white or grey leathery and thickened
HNO_3	Mucosa
HCl	Yellow
Ammonia	Pink
HCN	Perforated
KCN	Pink
KOH, NaOH	Brick red to brown
Phosphorus	Deeply congested, black-yellow or grey-white

CHAPTER 20

Metallic Irritant Poisons

Arsenic compounds, antimony, mercuric compounds, bismuth, copper, thalium, zinc, chromium and aluminium are considered as inorganic metallic irritants.

ARSENIC

Actually Arsenic is a metalloid, though it is generally taught here.

Compounds of Arsenic

- White arsenic or arsenious oxide (*sankhya*) is a white crystalline powder.
- It is also available in the form of solid mass. The opaque mass looks like porceline so it is also called vitreous arsenic.
- White arsenic dissolves slowly in water and soon gets precipitated at the bottom.
- It freely mixes in boiling milk.
- It is used in the manufacture of fly paper, rat poisons, sometimes in complexion powder and also in the preservation of timber and leather.
- It is also used in Ayurveda and Unani medicines for skin diseases, joint pains, syphilis and impotence.

Acute Arsenic Poisoning

- Symptoms start after half an hour or late if other than oral route is used.
- Arsenic inhibits – SH enzyme system, thus the cellular metabolism is hampered.
- It is also a capillary poison and dilates the capillaries.

- Vomiting, diarrhoea, pain, anoxic convulsions, coma and death.
- A large dose causes rapid death due to shock without producing any symptoms or it may cause severe vomiting so that all the poisons go out of stomach so that the patient may survive.
- In arsenic poisoning, the patient passes rice water stools resembling cholera.
- Patient is restless and dehydration is fast, collapse and death occurs due to peripheral circulatory failure.

Fatal dose: 180 mg

Fatal period: 12 hours to 48 hours.

Arsenic poisoning has to be differentiated from cholera.

Treatment

Stomach wash with warm milk and water, then with freshly prepared hydrated ferric hydrochloride. It will convert arsenious acid into a harmless and insoluble salt ferric arsenite. Half a glass of water, 45 ml of ferric chloride and 15 g of sodium carbonate or magnesium oxide are mixed well. It is filtered and administered to the patient.

BAL: BAL (2, 3-dimercaptopropanol) in a dose of 2.5 mg/kg body weight is given as deep IM. Injection every 4 hours for 2 days, then 2 times a day on third day and daily 1 dose till the symptoms completely disappears.

Postmortem Appearances

- Stomach contains white gritti sand-like particles of arsenic. Stomach wall is soft, swollen and congested. White particles of arsenic are embedded in the mucus. On scrapping, mucous membrane is found highly congested and inflamed.
- Heart—subendocardial haemorrhage in the left ventricle. Petechial haemorrhages are also seen in the pericardium, auricles and left ventricle. Myocardium shows fatty degeneration and swelling.
- Liver, spleen, kidneys show enlargement, congestion, fatty infiltration and degeneration. Lungs congested and oedematous.

Chronic Arsenic Poisoning

Gastrointestinal and nutritional manifestations: Loss of appetite, swollen gums, abdominal swelling, diarrhoea, foul smelling stools.

Changes in Eyes, Skin, Hair and Nails

- There are patchy areas of brownish discolouration in abdomen, face, limbs and joints.
- Eczematous lesions are also seen.
- Hyperkeratosis of palm and feet which may later on undergo malignant change into basal cell carcinoma or carcinoma *in situ*. Hairs become lustureless and falls off.
- Nails show Aldrich-Mee's lines. Transverse lines across the nails 1–2 mm broad. If a person consumes poison intermittently these lines are also seen intermittently.

Nervous system manifestation: Tingling, numbness, cutaneous hyperaesthesia, arthralgia, peripheral neuropathy, impotence, bone marrow depression—thrombocytopenia, anaemia. **Liver damage** may cause jaundice.

Folic Acid Deficiency

Megaloblastic anaemia.

State of Paralysis

- High stepping gait, paralysis, atrophy of extensor muscle, wrist and foot drop, become bedridden with impaired vision.

- Death occurs because of heart failure or infections. Chemical analysis of hair, skin, nails, long bone detects poison.

Treatment

- Withdraw arsenic from the patient.
- BAL: 100–300 mg, IM 6 hourly first three days, once a day for next 10 days, until the toxic manifestations are freed.
- Vitamins B_1, B_6, B_{12}—injections.

Postmortem Appearances

- Liver—fatty degeneration.
- Kidneys—parenchymatous glomerulonephritis.
- Muscles—greasy, wasted.
- Heart—myocardial fatty changes.
- GIT—inflammation reactions.

D/D of Chronic Arsenic Poisoning

- Peripheral neuritis
- B_1 deficiency (beriberi)
- Addison's disease
- Chronic alcoholic disease.

Arsenophagia/Arsenophagist

- Persons who take arsenic are known as arsenophagists.
- People take arsenic for improving the complexion, for increasing the libido (aphrodisiac).
- Slowly these people are capable of taking large dose without acute poisoning manifestations due to tolerance.

Medicolegal Issues

- Popular homicidal poison.
- It is administered into the food without the knowledge of victim.
- The accused can vanish before the symptoms appear.
- The manifestations resemble with natural disease.
- Disadvantage of arsenic as homicidal poison. It can be detected from hair, nails, bones even long time after death or even years after the person dies.

Some Facts About Arsenic

- Abortifacient
- Aphrodisiac
- Not a normal constituent of the body.
- Mixed with H_2O of wells and ponds to cause mass homicide.
- White arsenic is mistaken for baking powder, salt or sugar.
- Used as love philter by women who want to keep their lovers on their spell.
- Quack medicines containing arsenic can lead to arsenic poisoning.

DIFFERENCE BETWEEN ARSENIC POISONING AND CHOLERA

Mercury

- It is a liquid metal. It has bright silvery lusture.
- It evaporates to some extent even at room temperature.
- Its fumes are invisible and odourless. Pure metallic mercury is non-poisonous.
- The vermillion used by Hindu married woman on hair parting consists of mercuric sulphide in the form of red crystalline powder.
- Mercuric chloride or corrosive sublimate available as greyish white crystalline powder is a commonly used poison. It is a homicidal poison. It is used as germicide and is available in the form of tablets also.

Mercuric chloride: Also known as corrosive sublimate inactivates sulphydryl enzymes, interferes with cellular metabolism and functions.

Manifestations of Acute Poisoning

- Metallic taste, choking sensation in throat, difficulty in breathing, hoarseness of voice, nausea, wretching, vomiting.
- The vomiting is greyish, salivary, mucoid material and also bloodstained stool passed.
- Urine scanty, there is greyish white coating of mouth, tongue and fauces.
- There is renal tubular necrosis.
- Circulatory collapse occurs.

Fatal dose: 1 gm in adult.

Fatal period: 3–5 days commonly. Death may also occur due to uraemia in 2–3 days.

Treatment

- Stomach wash with warm water followed by milk, egg albumin.
- 5–10% freshly prepared sodium formaldehyde sulfoxylate with 5% sodium bicarbonate.
- BAL (British antilewisite) 300 mg IM (3–4 mg/kg body weight).

Postmortem Appearances

- Greyish white stomach surface, swollen, diffusely corroded with patches of submucous haemorrhage, perforation also occurs.
- Gangrenous colitis
- Liver shows hydropic degeneration.
- Heart shows fatty degeneration.
- Glomeruli show acute degeneration.
- Cortex pale and pyramids are deeply congested.

Medicolegal Issues

- Homicidal poison.
- When applied to vagina to induce abortion it may cause stomatitis, haemorrhagic, colitis, nephritis and death due to uraemia.

Chronic Mercuric Chloride Poisoning

It is characterized by

- Hatter's shakes
- Mercurial erethism
- Mercuria lentis
- Loss of weight
- Chronic nephritis
- Gingivitis, loss of teeth
- Foul breath
- Inflamed salivary glands
- Childish behaviour
- Stammering
- Hyperkeratosis of hand and feet
- Hatter's shakes are seen in chronic mercury poisoning. There is shaking of fingers leading to shapy and shaky handwritings. Tremors are also seen on the tongue and

face muscles. Staggering gait and stammering speech are noticed. Peripheral neuritis occurs. At a later stage paralysis of limbs may occur.

Mercuria lentis

- Deposition of mercury in anterior part of lens through the cornea.
- Deposit is brownish in colour.

Mercurial erethism: Here the patient exhibits timidity, shyness, loss of confidence, insomnia, loss of memory (amnesia), sometimes illusion, delusions and hallucinations. Skin eruptions of erythema are eczema type. Blue-black lines on the gums are seen.

Treatment

- Removal from place of contamination.
- Feeding liberal quantity of good milk.
- Gargling of mouth with borax or potassium chlorate.
- Intravenous injection of sodium thiosulphate
- 0.4–0.6 gm in 5 ml of normal saline on alternate days.

Medicolegal Issues

- Murderers use corrosive sublimate in milk, lassi, etc.
- In children, *pink diseases* may be caused by grey mercury powders (calomel).
- It is manifested by swelling and dermatitis of hands and feet with necrotic ulcers in mouth.

Minamate bay diseases

- This is the epidemic poisoning which occurs in fisher's families near Minamate-Bay in Japan by eating fish containing mercuric chloride coming out of a chemical factory as effluent.
- Similar problem occurred in Goa also.

Mercurous chloride or calomel

- Converted into mercuric chloride on exposure to chlorine in water.
- Eliminated through saliva, urine, faeces, milk and sweat. It crosses the placental barriers and passes in fetus and uterus also.

- Deposited in hair, fingernails and kidneys.
- **Therapeutic dose:** 30–180 mg.
- Calomel is used as skin antiseptic, diuretic and purgative.

Copper Sulphate (Blue Vitriol)

- Copper sulphate poisoning is more common than other salts.
- They are large blue crystals, freely soluble in water.
- In small doses it acts as astringent and in big doses it acts as emetics.
- In large doses it acts as irritant poisoning.
- **Emetic dose:** 0.3–0.6 gm
- **Fatal dose:** 15 gm
- **Fatal period:** 1–3 days

Manifestations of Acute Poisoning

- Symptoms start within ½ hour.
- Metallic taste, burning mouth, pain in abdomen, repeated vomiting, bluish tinge on gums and tongue, blue or green vomiting.
- Repeated diarrhoea brown liquid, oliguria, anuria, albuminuria, haematuria, anaemia, muscular cramps, convulsions, limb paralysis.
- Jaundice due to hepatotoxicity causing centrilobular necrosis and stasis of bile.
- Death occurs due to coma, liver failure and kidney failure.

Treatment

- Stomach wash with 1% potassium ferro-cyanide, with copper it forms cupric cyanide.
- Egg albumin precipitates copper so it is given in food.
- Milk is also given.

Postmortem Appearances

- Skin is yellowish due to jaundice.
- Bluish green froth from mouth and nostrils.
- Stomach content blue/green, mucosa green.
- Liver soft, fatty and enlarged.
- Haemolysis of blood, degeneration of proximal convulsated tubules are seen.

Chronic Poisoning

It causes haemochromatosis or bronze diabetes or pigment cirrhosis. Green or chronic poisoning is characterised by green or purple line of gums. Coppery taste in mouth, dyspepsia, abdominal colic, renal damage, Greenish colour of hair, urine and sweat.

Treatment

- Removal from the source
- Nutritious diet, milk and eggs
- EDTA and penicillamine as per the need.

MLI

- Suicidal poison
- Rarely used as cattle poison
- Introduced in vagina for criminal abortion
- Copper salts are used as antidote in phosphorus poisoning
- As an emetic. It is eliminated through bile, saliva, milk and faeces.

Lead

Chronic lead poisoning is more common than acute poisoning. It is known as plumbism.

Plumbism is characterised by

- Anemia
- Asthenia—weakness
- Arthralgia
- Amenorrhoea
- Anosmia
- Ataxia
- Atrophy of optic nerve
- Anorexia
- Aggressive behaviour
- Abdominal colic
- Abortion
- Blue line on gums
- Belly ache—abdominal colic/lead colic
- Blood pressure—systolic raised
- Constipation
- Colic
- Convulsions
- Clonic

- Tonic
- Cerebral oedema
- Cerebral palsy
- Drop—wrist drop/foot drop
- Dysmenorrhoea
- Demyelination
- Delerium
- Encephalopathy—lead
- Foul smelling breath
- Foetal changes
- Gliosis
- Hypertrophy of heart
- Halitosis
- Impotence
- Infertility
- Interstitial nephritis
- Mental retardation
- Vertigo

The manifestations can be grouped as gastrointestinal, neurological, renal, haematological and other.

Blood Findings in Lead Poisoning

- Punctate basophilia
- Hypochromic microcytic anaemia
- Anisocytosis
- Poikilocytosis
- Thrombocytopenia
- Polychromasia

Detection of early cases of poisoning can be done by the estimation of coproporphyrin in the urine.

Treatment

It is a cumulative poison (digitalis is another cumulative poison):

- Removal of the person from source.
- Parathyroid hormone—this hormone causes deleading and decreases stored lead and facilitates its excretion.
- Diet low in calcium favours mobilisation of lead.
- Liberal quantities of milk, vitamins C and D.
- Calcium versanate, calcium EDTA for deleading given by slow IV drip.
- 5 ml of 20% solution of EDTA added to 500 ml of normal saline or 5% glucose

saline. It is given twice daily for 5 days. It is repeated after 2 days rest.

- Diethylenetriamine penta-acetic acid (DTPA) 2–4 ml in 25% solution. It is given once in 2 weeks.

Postmortem Appearances

- Blue lines in the gums, foot, wrist drop, paralysed muscles, liver, kidneys are hard and degenerated.
- Heart hypertrophy, atheromatous changes in aorta and aortic valves, hyperplasia of bone marrow. Cerebral oedema, petechial haemorrhages in brain, sometimes meningitis.

Acute Lead Poisoning

Lead inhibits tissue enzymes by combining with sulphydryl groups by accumulation of coproporphyrin, ALA, protoporphyrin.

Fatal dose: 30 gm

Fatal period: 2–3 days

Manifestations

Burning mouth, constricted throat, salivation, coated tongue, offensive breath. Blue line in gum margins, vomiting, constipation, scanty urine. Punctate basophilia, big joint pains, flexor muscle cramps, stupor, coma and death.

Treatment

- Stomach wash with 1% $MgSO_4$, then with plain water.
- Inject morphine with atropine for pain relief.
- EDTA 2% solution in normal saline
- Mannitol IV drip to relieve cerebral oedema.

Postmortem Appearances

These are not characteristic features. The mucous membrane of small intestine and stomach inflamed.

Zinc Phosphide

- Bluish white metal has garlic odour.
- It is used as rat poison.

- Characterised by vomiting, respiratory distress, tremors, drowsiness, collapse, coma, death.
- The poison acts slowly. It reacts with HCl in stomach and produces phosphine.
- Phosphine acts as a respiratory depressant.

Treatment

- Stomach wash with warm water
- Activated carcoal
- Penicillamine 250 mg—2 gm daily
- 5% glucose saline.

Postmortem Appearances

Blood is cherry red, steel grey powder in stomach, liver, lungs and kidneys congested.

Metal Fume Fever

Occurs due to chronic inhalation of zinc, fever with rigor, severe respiratory distress, cyanosis.

Aluminium Phosphide (Celphos)

Used as fumigant to control rodents in food-grains and fields. Vomiting mixed with blood, dyspnoea, rapid pulse, clonic convulsion, corrosion of mouth and throat due to precipitation of proteins, clonic convulsion and death.

Hepatic Manifestations

Jaundice, hepatitis, hepatomegaly.

Cardiac Manifestations

Myocarditis, pericarditis, arrhythmia and cardiac shock.

Respiratory Manifestations

Pulmonary oedema, cyanosis, dyspnoea.

CNS Manifestations

Convulsions, encephalopathy. Involvement of various systems depend upon dose and severity of poisoning.

Fatal dose: 100–500 mg

Fatal period: Within 24 hours

Treatment

- Stomach wash with warm water
- Activated charcoal 100 gm by mouth

- Liquid paraffin.
- $MgSO_4$ 1 gm repeated after 2 hours, then 1 gm every 6 hourly for 6–7 days by IV drip.

Medicolegal Issues

Common suicidal poison.

THALLIUM (THALLOTOXICOSIS)

- Used in ringworm paste, hair removers and depilatory creams.
- It is also used in preparation of rat pastes, depilators, paints and dyes.
- Patient suffers from thalotoxicosis.

Manifestations

- Loss of appetite, abdominal colic, loss of large bunches of hair, outer 2/3rds of eyebrow, axilla, amenorrhea in women and aspermia in men.
- Retrobulbar neuritis, polyneuritis.

Treatment

- Stomach wash with potassium iodide.
- Prussian blue 25 mg/1 kg body with 15% mannitol introduced in duodenum as a drip through stomach tube.

Postmortem Appearances

Submucosal gastric haemorrhage, fatty degeneration of heart and liver, kidneys, necrosis of cells of convoluted tubule.

Medicolegal Issues

- Industrial poison used as homicidal poison, is easily soluble and is odourless, tasteless, can be given in food and drink.
- Thallium can be recovered from roots of hair, nails and bone.

Radioactive Substances

- Radium, thorium, uranium and their salts constantly emits radiation.
- Nuclear fission is used in India for production of electricity by atomic power stations.
- Radiation causes cellular damage, carcinogenesis and even death. Fetuses are highly susceptible to radiation. Exposure to 1000 radiation is fatal.
- By inhalation, injection or handling, radioactive substances produce poisoning symptoms.

Manifestations

Fatigue, nausea, emaciation, aplastic anaemia, ulceration, haemorrhage, perforation in gastrointestinal tract. Testes and ovaries show degenerative changes, eyes with cataract, mandibular necrosis, carcinoma in lungs, malignancy of bones, loss of hair, opportunistic infections.

Treatment

Depends on symptoms

- Antibiotics
- Haematinics
- Fresh blood, marrow cell transfusion.

Postmortem Appearances

Presence of radioactive substance in soft tissue, bones.

Precautions to be Taken during Autopsy

- Lead rubber gloves should be used.
- Radioactive fluid like urine, ascites fluid should be sent for analysis.
- The doctor should check his own radio-activity from time to time.
- Cremation may be permitted, however, the best way is by burrying deep in the seabed.

Lead

- First metal known to man (Dom, Ind, Thera)
- Abundant in soil
- It is a heavy, steel grey metal
- All salts of lead are poisonous.

Lead Salts

- Lead acetate—therapeutics (hair dyes)
- Lead carbonate—white lead paints
- Tetraethyl lead—in petrol as an antiknock to prevent internal combustion.
- Lead tetraoxide—cosmetics (vermilion).
- Lead sulphide—collyrium for the eyes by muslims
- Lead oleate—to procure abortion (tonic contractions of uterus).
- Lead metal when melted toxic fumes
- Lead salts crayons

Toxicokinetics

- Inhalation
- Ingestion
- Intradermal
- Stored in bones—phosphate and carbonate.
- In gums lead sulphide + H_2S **blue line/lead line.**

Signs and Symptoms of Acute Poisoning

- Metallic taste in the mouth.
- Burning sensation in the throat and gullet.
- Abdominal pain, nausea, vomiting.
- The vomit may contain streaks of blood.

Signs and Symptoms of Acute Lead Poisoning

- Diarrhoea or sometimes constipation
- Stools are black in colour
- Finally, collapse precedes death.

Treatment

- Stomach wash with 10% magnesium sulphate in water.
- EDTA 2% in normal saline (chelating agent)
- Slow intravenous drip.

Chelating Agents

- With takes away the poison from the blood and tissues by combining with metallic ions, to form an inactive, water soluble complex which is readily excreted in the urine.
- Pencillamine (2 gm) daily orally
- PM stomach, intestines inflammed large intestines, black coloured stools.
- Symptoms start after half an hour or late if other than oral route is used.
- Arsenic inhibits – SH enzyme system thus the cellular metabolism is hampered.
- It is also a capillary poison and dilates the capillaries.
- Vomiting, diarrhoea, pain, anoxic convulsions, coma and death.
- Large dose causes rapid death due to shock without any symptoms, it may cause severe vomiting so that all the poisons go out of stomach so that the patient may survive.
- Patient passes rice water stools resembling cholera.
- Restless and dehydration is fast, collapse and death occurs due to peripheral circulatory failure.

CHAPTER 21

Vegetable Irritant Poisons

EXAMPLES OF VEGETABLE IRRITANTS

- *Abrus precatorius*
- *Calotropis giganta*
- *Semicarpus anacardium*
- *Croton tiglium*
- *Ricinus communis*
- *Capsicum annum*
- *Claviceps purpurea* (ergot).

The plants produce alkaloids, glycosides, resins, glycoproteins, etc. These may be found in leaves, fruits, flowers, seeds, roots, stem, etc. Toxalbumins or phytotoxins are toxic proteins. They cause agglutination and lysis of red cells. Toxalbumin is antigenic in nature. It is capable of producing antibody when injected into body. It is seen in:

- *Abrus precatorius*—abrin
- *Croton tiglium*—crotin
- *Ricinus communis*—ricin
- Semicarpus—semicarpol, bhilawinal
- Calotropis—calotropin, calotoxin, calactin, gigantin, procerin, uscharin, calotroxin.
- *Capsicum annum*—capsicin
- *Lal chitra*—plumbagin (glycoside)
- Ergot—ergotamine

Abrus precatorius

- The seeds are egg-shaped, scarlet in colour with black bottom. Indian goldsmiths used it for weighing silver and gold.

- The active principle in seed is abrin (toxalbumin).
- It also contains abrusic acid and haemagglutinin.
- Symptoms and signs resemble those of viperine snakebite.

Fatal dose: 90–120 mg

Fatal period: 3–5 days

Crushed and powdered seeds are poisonous, cooked seeds are not poisonous. It is a popular cattle poison.

The pieces of sui/sutari are needles, which are sharp and pointed. They are made by mixing the powder of *Abrus precatorius* with dough (*atta*) and water. Small sharp needles are made out of this paste and are dried under sun. The pieces of sui are inserted into holes made into stick. The victim animal is given a blow with the stick. The sui enters the flesh, causes pain and swelling. Oozing of blood occurs at site. Animals become drowsy, stop eating becomes weak, drops down becomes unconscious and finally dies. The death may be mistaken for snakebite.

Abrus precatorius is also used as an arrow or spear poison for hunting or in tribal wars. Other arrow poisons are strychnine, curare, snake venom.

Lethal dose: Two crushed seeds.

Treatment

Sui, symptomatic.

Autopsy shows

Swelling, necrosis, at the site, oozing of blood, pieces of sui under the skin, congestion of gastric intestinal mucosa and other organs.

Calotropis giganta (Akdo, Madar)

- It has two varieties having purple and white flowers. Leaves are thick.
- When leaves and stem are cut, milky white juice exudes.

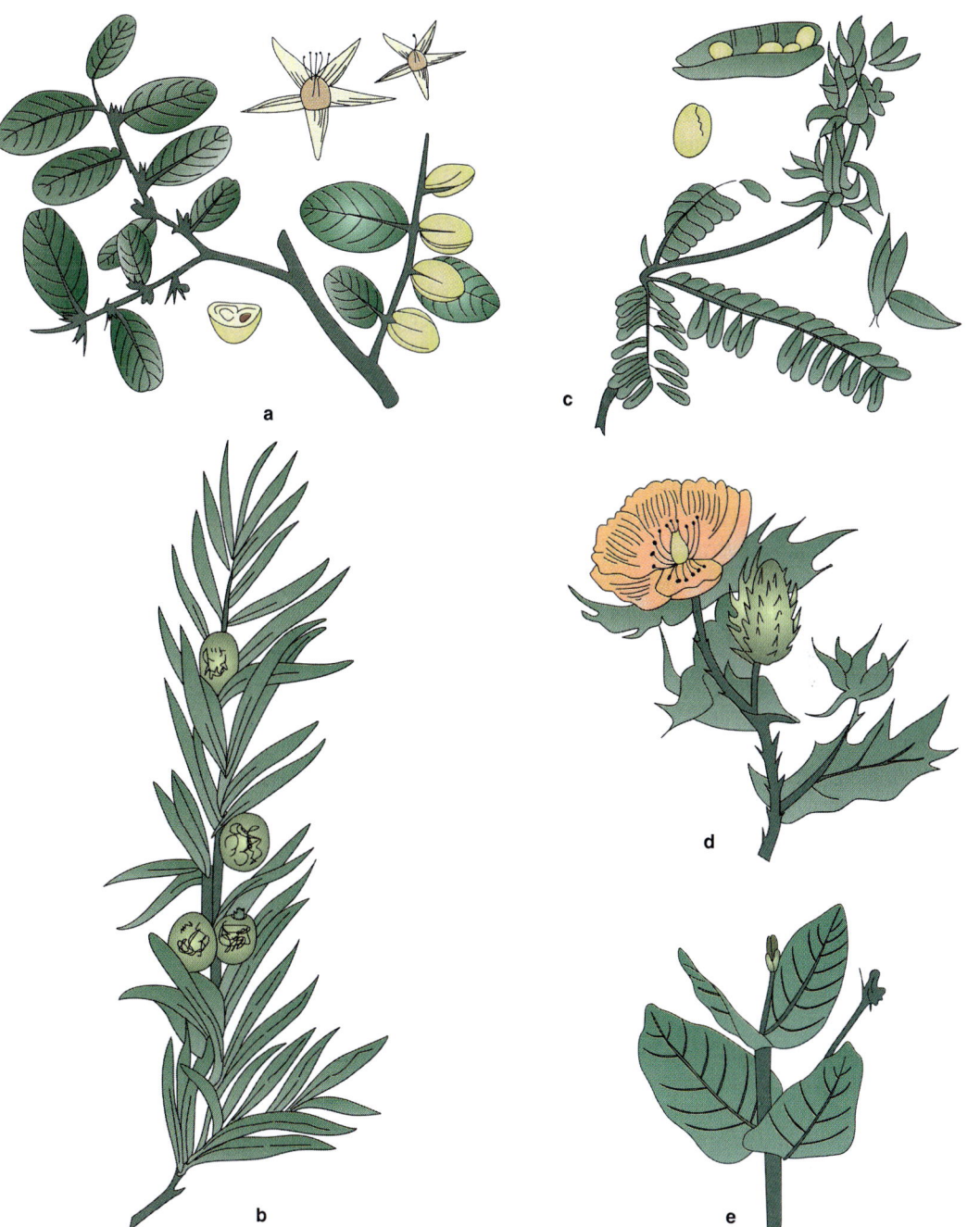

Figs 21.1a to e: Vegetable irritants: (a) *Clestanthus collinus;* (b) *Taxus baccata;* (c) *Abrus precatorius* with fruit and seeds; (d) *Argemone mexicana;* (e) *Calotropis giganta*

- The juice is called madar juice. Juice causes redness and blister formation on skin.
- On ingestion, nausea, vomiting, diarrhoea, collapse and death may follow. In eye, it causes purulent ophthalmitis.
- The leaves are heated and applied as poultice to relieve pain.
- The powdered bark is used as emetic.
- Madar juice is used for criminal abortion in the form of abortion stick.

Treatment

- Stomach wash with warm water.
- Demulscents
- Stimulants

Postmortem Findings

Acute inflammation of gastrointestinal tract and congestion of abdominal organs.

Semicarpus anacardium (Marking Nut)

- Fruit is called Bhilawa or marking nut. It has shape-like cashewnut.
- The juice of marking nut is used as marking ink by dhobis.
- When the juice is applied on skin it creates irritation and painful blisters.
- The main blister is surrounded by small vesicles. The skin turns black.
- There is itching, along the line of scratching. Due to itching, fresh eruptions erupt.
- The skin lesion looks like bruise, but on careful examination the blister is surrounded by vesicles and satellite blisters which helps in differentiation.
- The blister fluid is sent to Forensic Science Laboratory for chemical analysis which can show the presence of active principle, semicarpol and bhilawinal. When thrown into eyes causes irritant congestion, when thrown on face out of jealousy, hatred, it causes disfiguration. It is used as abortifacient by applying the juice to abortion stick. It is thrown on genitals as a punishment for infidelity. On ingestion it causes severe gastrointestinal tract irritation.

Treatment

- Stomach wash with warm water.
- Demulscents

  Fatal dose: >5 gm

Postmortem Appearances

Severe inflammation of gastrointestinal tract, congestion of organs of abdomen.

Ricinus Communis

- Castor oil (arandi) is used as a preservative of pulses like gram, tuver dal, wheat.
- Ricin is the phytotoxin and active principle.
- Raw seeds are poisonous when eaten (chewing). Swallowing or choking does not cause poisoning. Castor oil is a purgative.
- Accidental poisoning in children is common due to chewing of seeds.

Clinical Manifestations

Abdominal colic, nausea, vomiting, laryngeal collapse, death.

Treatment

- Stomach wash
- Demulscents
- Stimulants

  Fatal dose: 10 seeds.

Autopsy shows

- Gastrointestinal tract is inflamed. Seeds of castor may be seen in stomach and mistaken for croton seeds.
- Castor seeds are big, large, red, brown with blotches or small grey seeds with brown polish, bright and mottled.
- Croton seeds are dull oval, dark brown or brownish grey.

Croton tiglium (Jamalgota)

- Seeds are very poisonous, contain toxalbumin, crotin and a glycoside called crotonaside.
- Croton oil consists of crotonolic acid, methyl crotonic acid and crotonol.

Clinical Manifestations

Nausea, vomiting, diarrhoea (bloodstained), tachycardia, vertigo, salivation, circulatory and respiratory collapse and death.

Medicolegal Issues

- Croton oil used as on abortifacient.
- As arrow poison by some tribes. It is used as purgative.

  Fatal dose: 4 seeds.

Treatment

- Stomach wash with warm water
- Demulscents
- Stimulants
- IV glucose saline to combat dehydration.

Autopsy shows

- Severely inflamed gastrointestinal tract.
- Croton seeds may be detected from stomach.

Capsicum annum (Chillies)

- Chilly seeds resemble *dhatura* seeds. They can be differentiated without difficulty.
- *Dhatura* seeds are thick, kidney shaped, have a double-edged convex border.
- Chilly seeds are thin yellow, with single edged convex border.
- Chillies are used to torture a person or to obtain confession by force, by applying seeds to eyes, nose, throat, vagina and anus. Powder is used to throw on face and eyes to facilitate robbery.

Treatment

- When thrown into eyes, must be washed with plenty of cold water and sterile saline water.
- Bland eye drops, e.g. olive oil.

Medicolegal Issues

- To facilitate robbery
- To cause torture
- Women can use chilly spray toward off sexual attacks
- Chilly bombs are used by police to dispel mobs.

Plumbago rosea, Plumbago zeylanica (Lal Chitra or Chitra)

- The active principle is plumbing.
- It is a glycoside occurs in crystal form as golden yellow, shining needles.

- It causes death due to respiratory failure if taken in large doses.
- On external application the root causes irritation and blisters.
- The paste of crushed root is applied on uterus or painted on abortion stick to procure criminal abortion.

Argemone mexicana

- It is also known as *pila dhatura*.
- It has yellow flowers and spiny leaves.
- The seeds resemble black mustard seeds.
- It is, therefore, adulterated with mustard seeds and mustard oil.
- It has two alkaloids—berberine and protopine.
- The oil contains sanguinarine.

Clinical Manifestations

- The seeds on consumption produce oedema of legs, breathlessness, liver enlargement and sometimes diarrhoea.
- Argemone oil contains alkaloids sanguinarine and dihydrosanguinarine.

  Epidemic dropsy is seen in many states from time to time in India—Gujarat, Bihar, Orissa, UP, MP. Vomiting, diarrhoea and oedema of lower limbs occur on consumption of adulterated oils. In some cases heart failure may occur.

Treatment

- Symptomatic
- Withdrawl of adulterated oil.

Lathyrus sativus (Kesari Dal)

- It is used as food in Reva and Satna districts.
- The local name of this pulse is kesari dal.
- It is adulterated with red gram (besan).
- Lathyrism is the manifestation of use of kesari dal.
- It causes spastic paraplegia.
- The toxic principle is BOAA, it is B-(N) oxalylamino-L-alanine.

Clinical Manifestations

- Suddenly there may be severe agonizing calf muscle pain.

- Slowly the patient notices weakness in limbs, even while sitting.
- Insisted to walk without stick, till he finally develops spastic gait, walking on toes with crossing of legs like scissors. He may end up in total paraplegia of lower limbs.

Treatment

- Stop using this pulse
- Symptomatic

Ergot

- It is the compact mycelium of parasitic fungus *Claviceps purpurea*. It attacks oats, wheat, barley, bajra and rye.

- The diseased grain is deep purple in colour tapered at both ends. The alkaloids of ergot are:
  - Ergotoxin
  - Ergotamine
  - Ergometrine

Ergotism is the manifestation of chronic poisoning. It consists of two forms:

1. Gangrene type
2. Convulsion type

1. Gangrene type: Severe pain in the limbs, tingling and numbness, swelling,

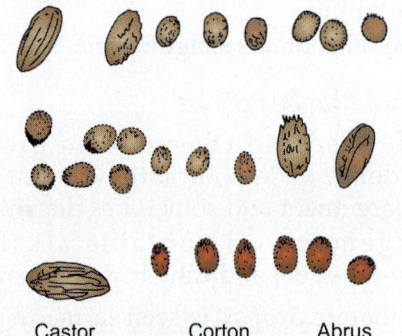

Castor   Corton   Abrus

Fig. 21.2: Seeds containing phytotoxins

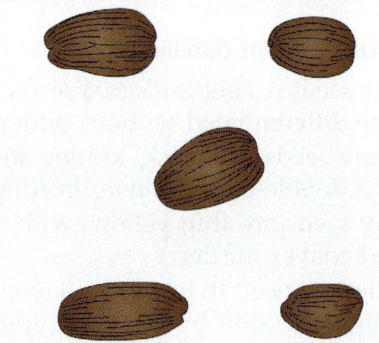

Fig. 21.4: *Semicarpus anacardium*

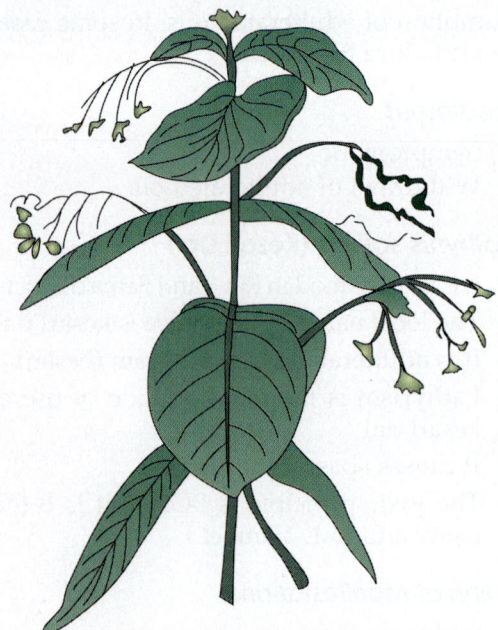

Fig. 21.3: *Calotropis giganta*

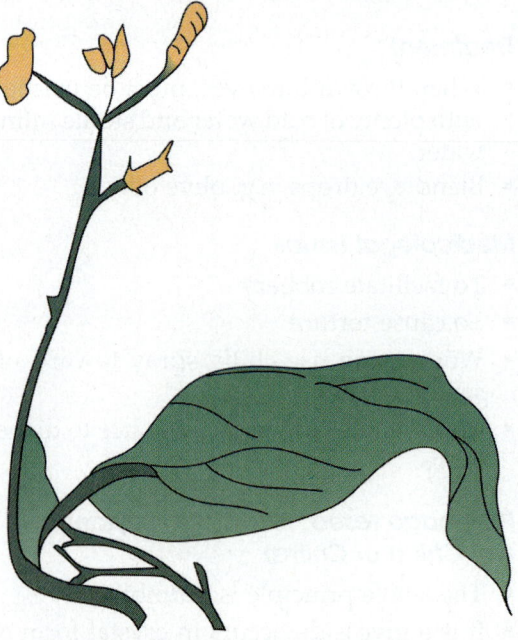

Fig. 21.5: *Plumbago zeylanica*

dry gangrene of fingers and toes extending up to elbow or knees.

2. **Convulsion type:** Itching, tactile hallucinations, periodic painful violent convulsions, dim vision, dilated fixed pupils. Death due to spasm and weakness of respiratory muscles.

Ergot has got specific action on uterine muscle and causes contraction so it is used during initial stage of labour. It is also used as abortifacient.

Treatment

- Stomach wash with warm water.
- Amyl nitrite inhalation, if the patient complains of angina or chest pain.
- Peritoneal dialysis.
- In chronic poisoning, sodium nitroprusside is used to counteract vasoconstriction.
- Priscolin (tolazoline) is also used for vasodilation.

Medicolegal Issues

Abortifacient to procure criminal abortion.

CHAPTER 22

Mechanical Irritants

IRRITANTS

- Mechanical injury is also seen among psychosomatic patients who try to hurt themselves due to fear or agony with some sharp instrument or by ingesting harmful non-edible things which causes internal bleeding, haemorrhage, abdominal pain and irritation in colon.
- Inflammation of the mucous membrane of stomach and intestine is caused by irritating factors.
- The anxiety state, depression of mood, sleep disorder and unaware state of mind the individual can behave abnormal and ingest the following.

Substances Involved

- Pins and needles swallowed.
- Hair's plucked and nails chewed.
- Accidental intake of glass pieces.
- Ceramics

- Dust and debris from older building under renovation.
- Leaded foil wine bottle caps.

Manifestations

- The **manifestations** are abdominal cramps, fever, pain, nausea, vomiting, diarrhoea, headache and sometimes perforation of stomach.
- Out of the mechanical poisoning mentioned above the poisoning caused by powdered glass is dangerous and if broken in the mouth accidentally can cause stomach ulcer (e.g. magician showing magic show and chewing glass tubes).

Treatment

- Easily digested food like gruel and banana should be prescribed.
- In some novels or stories the characters try to hurt themselves by ingesting diamond which can be fatal due to mechanical injury in the alimentary canal.

CHAPTER 23

Poisonous Creatures

SKINK OR STRIPED SKINK

These are rarely seen lizards mistaken as snakes, easily recognized by the pale stripes running down the length of its body. Though there is common belief that the skinks are non-poisonous, but it is not true, as the poisoning cases are also reported. It belongs to family **Scincidae**.

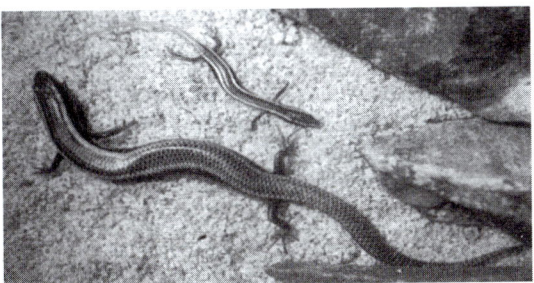

Fig. 23.1: Skink

OPHITOXAEMIA: SNAKEBITE POISONING

There are two main types of snakes—Viperidae and Colubridae. Colubridae family includes king cobra, cobra and krait. Viperidae family includes Russell's viper or saw-scaled viper.

Besides there are land snakes or terrestrial snakes, and the sea snakes. These are poisonous snakes and this chapter deals with the manifestation of poisonous snakebite.

Non-poisonous snakes are more in number than the poisonous snakes. 3500 species of snakes are found in the world, out of which only 300 species are poisonous to human beings. A poisonous snake can be easily distinguished from non-poisonous snake.

COBRA

Characters of King Cobra (*Ophiophagus hannah*)

It has a hood but not the spectacle mark. On the head, there are two big occipital shields behind the parietals. It is yellow, green, brown or black in colour.

The throat is of cream colour. Towards the end, the tail shield are divided.

Characters of Cobra (*Naja naja*)

Cobras are found throughout India. They are 5–6 feet long and usually are of black colour. They have well-marked hood and spectacle mark, monocular or binocular on the back. Sometimes it has an oval spot. Only when it is angry, it expands its neck in the form of a hood.

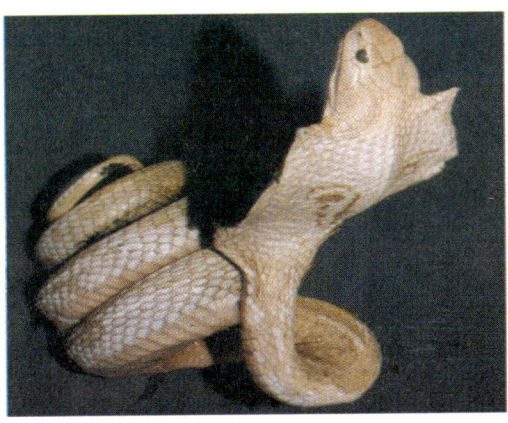

Fig. 23.2: Cobra (naja)

The third supralabial shield is big, it extends from the eye to nasal shield. The caudal scales are double.

KRAIT

Characters of Common Krait (*Bungarus caeruleus*)

The head shields are large, four shields are seen on either side of lower lip. On the back, there is a central row of hexagonal scales. The tail is round and belly is creamy white. The belly and tail scales and not divided.

The banded krait is of jet black colour with alternate yellow bands on its back. Common krait is of shining steel black colour.

SEA SNAKES

All sea snakes are poisonous. Their bite causes severe weaknes due to muscular damage. Their eyes are very small, and the tail is flattened. Belly scales are narrow, back scales are trabeculated. Commonest sea snakes are *Hydrophis caerulescens*.

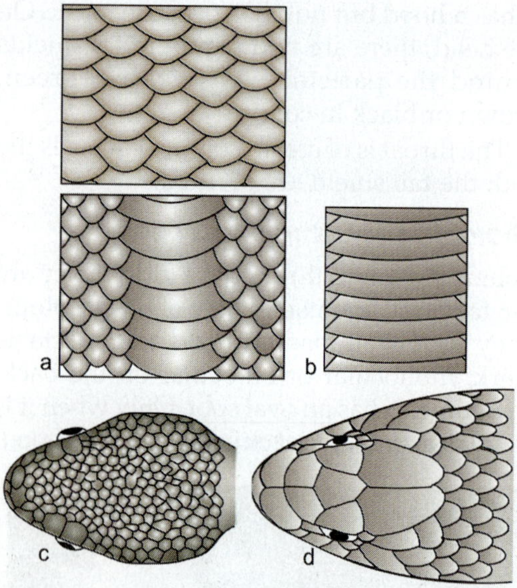

VIPER

The viper belongs to Viperidae family. They have broad lozenge-shaped head, narrow neck and short tail. Pupils are vertical. They give birth to young ones, i.e. they are viviparous. Vipers are of two types:
1. Pit viper.
2. Pitless viper.

In pit vipers, there is deep depression or pit between head and eyes.

The pitless vipers in India are dangerous. They are ***Daboia elegans*** (Daboi is on the outskirts of Vadodara, Gujarat. These vipers are common so the name Daboi as come) or Russell's viper and *Echis carinatus* or saw-scaled viper (Figs 23.4 and 23.5).

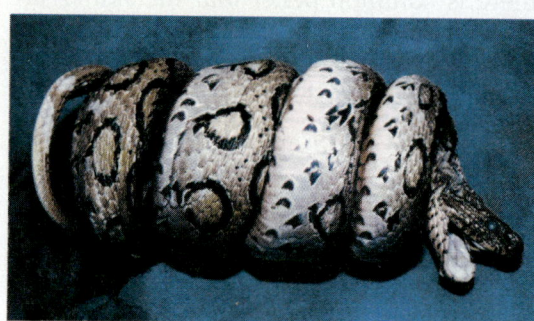

Fig. 23.4: Russell's viper

Fig. 23.3: Differences between poisonous and non-poisonons snakes:
(a) If the belly scales are small like those on the back of are moderately large, but do not cover the entire breadth of the belly (non-poisonous).
(b) If the belly scales are large and cover the entire breadth (poisonous or non-poisonous).
(c) If the scales on the head are small (poisonous, viper).
(d) If the scales on the head are large (poisonous or non-poisonous).

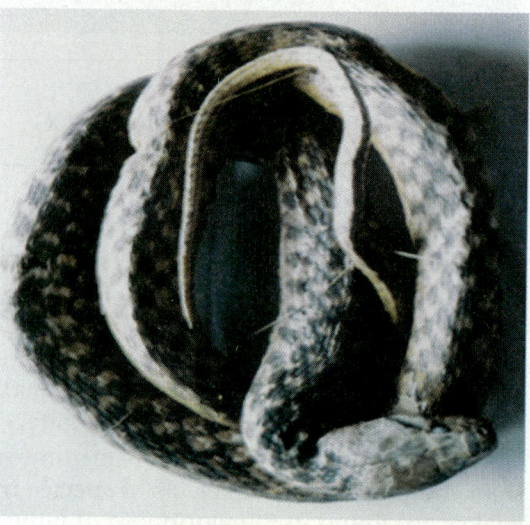

Fig. 23.5: Saw-scaled viper

Russell's viper is buff coloured, 4–5 ½ feet long, stout, tail short, head flat, heavy and triangular. It has three rows of brown spots on the back. Before it attacks, it causes a lot of hissing noise. The belly plats are broad and the caudal shields are bifid.

Echis viper or saw-scaled is small brown or brownish grey in colour, grows about 1– 1 ½ feet.

On the back, it has a continuous wavy line. Between the upper curves of wavy lines, there are diamond-shaped areas of dark shades. The back is covered with scales which are keel (ridge down the centre, making them rough to touch) and rough. When it moves, the scales cause rustling sound. Each scale is dented like a saw, therefore, it is called saw-scaled viper.

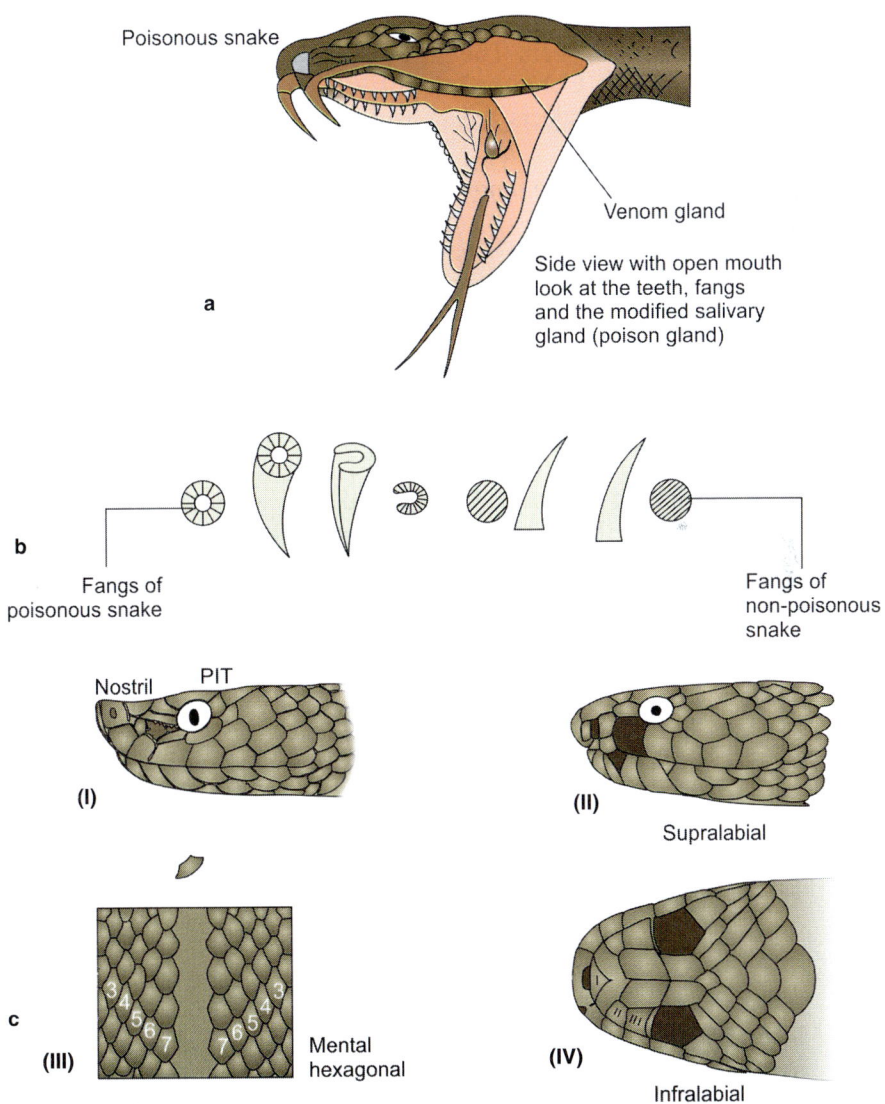

Fig. 23.6: Poisonous snakes: (a) Side view with open mouth—the teeth, fangs and the modified salivary gland (poison gland); (b) Fangs/teeth of poisonous and non-poisonous snkes; (c) Head and body scales of poisonous snakes (I, II, III and IV)

Fangs

Fangs are seen in poisonous snakes. There are two-groved, tubular teeth connected to glands secreting venom by a communicating duct. These glands are situated below and behind eyes. When the snake attacks a victim, the fans penetrate the skin and the venom is discharged into the victim. Fangs of cobra are short and fine. Fangs of viper are strong and long. The fangs leave on the victim two clear punctured wounds and the skin lacerate due to movement of clothing. The site of bite shows oedema. In viper bite, oozing of blood is seen. The viper can bite with open mouth. Cobra has to close the lower jaw before it injects the venom.

Non-poisonous snakes do not have fangs (Table 23.1).

SNAKE VENOM

- The venom of viper is haemolytic, but the venom of cobra and krait is neurotoxic.
- The neurotoxic effect is like curare. It can lead to paralysis also.
- The snake venom consists of neurotoxin, haemolysin, proteolysin, fibrinolysin, cholinesterase, coagulase, cardiotoxin, hyaluronidase, ophioxidase.

Action of Venom

- Local action—local inflammatory oedema and ecchymosis.
- Systemic action—starts in about 10 minutes time.

The manifestations depend upon the amount of venom entering the body. The venom is harmless when taken orally but when there is an ulcer in mouth, it can be absorbed and cause poisonous symptoms. In Colubridae bite (cobra, krait), there is irritation, redness and swelling at the site of bite followed by giddiness, muscular weakness, drwosiness, paralysis of lower limbs spreading up to trunk and head. Breathing decrases and it may finally stop.

In the case of viper bite, the swelling is more with ecchymosis and oozing of blood. The patient collapses with cold, clamy skin, rapid thrady pulse, dilated pupils and loss of consciousness. Haemorrhages are seen through various orifices of the body.

Fatal dose: About—12 mg of cobra venom; 40 mg of viper venom.

Table 23.1: Snakes—features

Feature	Elapids – Cobra – Coral – Krait	Vipers	Sea snakes
Type of venom	Neurotoxic	Vasculotoxic	Myotoxic
Site of action	Motor nerve cells and resembles curare	Endothelial cells and RBC 1/t haemolysis	Muscles
Local symptoms at site of bite	Minimal	Severe, i.e. severe swelling oozing of blood and cellulitis	Minimal
Clinical presentation	Muscle weakness of legs and face. Cobra venom produces convulsions while krait venom produces only paralysis	Venom causes enzymatic destruction of cell walls and coagulation disorder	Venom produce generalized muscle pain, weakness polymyositis (limb girdle type) myoglobinuria increased K$^+$ and muscle enzymes f/b renal and respiratory failure

Treatment

- Local application of ointment above the wound.
- Incision of local punctures caused by the bite and sucking the poison with a breast pump or suction machine.
- The wound is washed with 1% solution of potassium permanganate.
- Administration of antivenom—polyvalent antisnake venom is available. It is useful against cobra, krait, Russell's viper and saw-scaled viper.

It is available as lyophilized (freeze/dried) powder in an vial. The distilled water is also supplied. It is prepared at the Hafkin's Institute, Mumbai. Its potency is maintained for 10 years.

Snake venom antiserum is a sterile preparation containing equine immunoglobulin fragments F (ab') 2. Freeze-dried powder is reconstituted in 10 ml of sterile water for injection IP supplied along with the vial. Each ml has power to specifically neutralize the venoms of following species of snakes:

- 0.60 mg of dried Indian cobra (*Naja naja*) venom
- 0.45 mg of dried common krait (*Bangarus caeruleus*) venom
- 0.60 mg of dried Russell's viper (*Vipera russelli*) venom
- 0.45 mg of dried saw-scaled viper (*Echis carinatus*) venom

Reconstitution of lyophilized antivenom: The antivenom is supplied in liquid and freeze-dried form as well. The freeze-dried powder is reconstituted with 10 ml of sterile water for injection IP supplied with the pack. The whole content of freeze-dried powder dissolves into a clear colorless or pale yellow liquid.

Sensitivity test: A preliminary sensitivity test is done by giving 0.1 ml of 1 in 10 dilutin of the serum intracutaneously. The reactin is observed. If there is no allergic response, intravenous injection of the polyvalent antisnake serum is given.

If the patient is sensitive, slow desensitization is done before administering the larger dose.

- Adrenaline, calcium chloride, corticosteroids and antihistamines are given depending on the requirement.

Medicolegal Issues

Orally it is non-poisonous. It is poisonous through SC, IM or IV routes.

Postmortem Appearances

The bite marks are deeper in vipers. Swelling and cellutitis, ulceration and gangrene are seen at the viper bite site. Different organs show congestion and petechial haemorrhages. Necrosis of liver, haemorrhages into orifices, haemorrhagic interstitial nephritis and intracerebral haemorrhage can be seen.

In cobra bite, respiratory paralysis causes death, so manifestations, like cyanosis, Tardieu's spots, and cerebral oedema are seen.

SCORPION STING

The scorpions are arthropods with eight legs. At the end of the tail, there is hollow sting, communicating with poisonous glands. Scorpion poison contains neurotoxin acting on respiratory and vasomotor centre, nerve terminals, and end plates of striated and unstriated muscles.

It also contains agglutinins, lecithin, haemolysins, etc.

Clinical Manifestations

A person stung by scorpion suffers from severe pain. He may develop pulmonary oedema, cardiac arrhythmias, muscular fasciculation, convulsions and death.

Treatment

- Application of tourniquet above the sting site.
- Multiple incisions and sucking of venom.

- Local instillation of insulin is found to be very useful. This treatment is supported by WHO monograph on scorpion bite by Prof. KRK Murthy of Sion Medical College, Mumbai.
- Local infiltration of emitine hydrochloride is also helpful.
- Calcium gluconated IV relives oedema and pain.
- Atropine prevents pulmonary oedema. Barbiturates help in convulsions (however, barbiturates should be discouraged).

Scorpion anitvenom when required: Venom from a single scorpion may contain several neurotoxins such as histamine, serotonin and enzymes. The most important clinical effects of envenomation are neuromuscular, neuroautonomic and local tissue effects.

Grades of Clinical Picture Serverity

- Grade 0: No local or systemic signs.
- Grade I: Local signs, pain, and/or paraesthesia at the site of sting.
- Grade II: Local signs and pain + remote pain and/or paraesthesia.
- Grade III: Local pain + cranial, autonomic or somatic neuromuscular dysfunction.

In grades I, II and III, the dose may be repeated after 1–2 hours, if improvement has not occurred. The dose should be increased, if the interval between the sting and the treatment is prolonged or the site of the sting is on the head, neck or shoulders. Place ice on the sting site and immobilize the stung limb to reduce pain and venom extension.

Reconstitution of the Lyophilized Antiserum

Remove the flip off on the seal over the diaphragms of the vials of antivenin and diluents. Sterilize the rubber diaphragm with alcohol. Withdraw the diluent in a sterile syringe. Insert the needle through the stopper of the vial containing antiserum and point the diluent jet to the center of lyophilized pellet to be dissolved and in order to prevent floating. Swirl the vial gently for one to five minutes and do not shake to avoid foaming.

CANTHARIDES

Spanish fly: *Cantharis vesicatoria*

Blister beetle: It is a fly with a shining metallic green colour head, legs and wings. The powder of the dried body contains cantharidin.

The Indian variant giving cantharidin is *Mylabris cichorii*. It is seen during rainy season in Kashmir and northern parts of India. The other Indian species are *Mylabris pustulata* and *Mylabris macilanta*.

Cantharidin hair oil is used for hair protection. It is a skin irritant and causes redness followed by small vesicles which unite to form a large blister.

Poisonous manifestations occur through skin absorption also. The person suffers from blisters swollen tongue, has difficulty in swallowing and salivations. Mucous blood vomiting with shining green particles observed. Bloody stools, painful loin, difficulty in urination, oliguria, haematuria, painful priapism, seminal emissions, abortion in pregnant women. Death occurs due to respiratory failure.

Fatal dose: 1.5–2 g of cantharide powder.

Fatal period: 1 day—11/2 days.

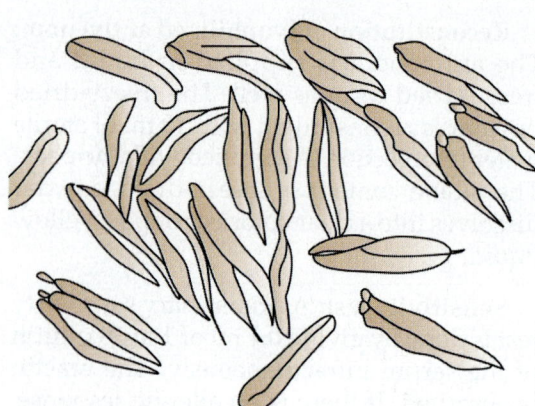

Fig. 23.7: Animal irritant: *Cantharis (lytta) vesicatoria* or Spanish fly

Treatment

- Early stomach wash to eliminate poison.
- IV glucose and blood transfusion.

Postmortem Features

Stomach mucosa may show green particles of canthrides. Stomach mucosa is blood-stained, soft, ulcerated, sometimes with area of necrosis. Kidneys—blood in pelvis, ureter, bladder. Acute tubular necrosis seen. Pulmonary oedema present.

Medicolegal Issues

- Cantharide is an aphrodisiac.
- Used as an abortifacient.

CHAPTER 24

Food Poisoning

POISONOUS MUSHROOMS (FUNGI)

- With popularity of Chinese and fast food, more and more Indians are eating mushrooms.
- There are some poisonous varieties of mushrooms which may accidentally mixup with food and cause poisoning.

Poison Mushrooms

Amanita muscaria   It is white in colour. It grows in sandy places.

Amanita phalloides   It is called *death cap*, it is also white in colour. It grows in woody places.

Muscarine and muscaridine occur in *Amanita muscaria*, whereas phylloidin, phallon and Amanita occur in *Amanita phalloides*.

The manifestations are of two types

- Irritant group.
- Neurotoxin group.

Manifestations occur 6–10 hours after consumption. Nausea, retching, vomit, diarrhoea, bloody stool, cyanosis, jaundice, dehydration, peripheral circulatory failure and death.

The neurological manifestations are headache, delirium, contracted pupils, twitching of limbs, bradycardia, wheezing and coma.

Treatment

- Stomach wash with potassium permanganate.
- Fine powdered activated charcoal.
- Atropine as physiological antidote for muscarine.
- Vitamin E, B-complex, vitamin K and other symptomatic treatment.

Postmortem Features

- In irritant type, signs of gastrointestinal tract irritation is seen.
- Fatty degeneration of liver and heart necrosis of renal tubules.
- **In neurotic** type poisoning, the necrosis and haemorrhage in brain is significant feature.

Medicolegal Issues

- People working in the mushroom farms suffer from respiratory troubles.
- Mushroom intoxication may be mistaken for alcoholic intoxication.
- In mushroom intoxication, pupils are contracted.

BOTULISM OR ALLANTIASIS

- It refers to the manifestation caused by exotoxin of *Clostridium botulinum*. This type of food poisoning occurs due to canned vegetables, fruits, meat, tinned fish, etc.
- The manifestations occur within 24 hours of consumption of food. The neurological manifestation predominates dilated pupils, ptosis, diplopia, aphonia (loss of voice) dysphagia, suffocation, cyanosis, delirium, coma, and death.

Treatment

- 5–10 thousand units IV antibotulinum serum.
- Symptomatic test.

TYPES OF FOOD POISONING

- Food poisoning includes any type of illnes suffered by a person after consuming food.
- Bacterial food type:
  - Infection type.
  - Toxin type.

Infection Type

- Salmonella group
- *Bacillus proteus*
- *E. coli*
- Haemolytic streptococci.
- Staphylococci
- Shigella group
- This occurs due to consumption of unhygienic, imperfectly cooked and uncooked food.

Clinical Manifestations

Depends on the type of organism. Fever, diarrhoea and vomiting are common symptoms.

Treatment

Depends on isolation and drug sensitivity of the organism. Appropriate antibiotic given.

- Symptomatic management.

Toxin Type

- Toxin of *Staphylococcus*
- Phytotoxin
- *C. welchii*
- Vibrio group
- *E. coli*
- Mycotoxins in Reye's syndrome

Clinical Manifestations

Violent vomiting but rapid recovery with prompt treatment.

Treatment

- 5% glucose saline
- Stomach wash warm water
- Symptomatic management.

CHAPTER 25

Cerebral Poisons

Cerebral poisons are of the following four main types

1. Somniferous
2. Deliriant
3. Inebriant
4. Convulsant

SOMNIFEROUS (OPIUM AND ITS ALKALOIDS)

- Opium is a derivative of unripe poppy capsule—*Papaver somniferum.*
- Opium is obtained by making multiple incisions on unripe poppy capsules.
- The acrid juice coming out on drying becomes dark brown to black mass of opium.
- Opium contains two main groups of alkaloids: Phenanthrene and isoquinoline group.

Phenanthrene group consists of
- Morphine 10%
- Codeine 0.5%
- Thebaine 0.3%

Benzyl isoquinoline group consists of
- Papaverine 1%
- Narcotine 6%
- The synthetic derivatives are meperidine or pethidine, heroin or diacetyl-morphine.
- Standard opium produced in Ghazipur factory contains 10% morphine.

Manifestations of Acute Opium Poisoning

They occur in three stages:

1. Stage of excitement
2. Depression
3. Narcosis

- These three stages may be intermixed.
- A sense of physical and mental well-being, talkativeness, headache, numbness of limbs, drowsiness, giddiness, sleep, contracted pupil, cyanosis of lips and finger-tips, opium smelling breath, slow pulse, and slow breathing.
- The patient enters the stage of coma, from stage of sleep through stage in narcosis, no response to stimuli.
- Cold, clamy skin, dried up secretions, body temperature below normal, pale face, deep cyanosis of lips and finger-tips, fall of blood pressure, 3–4 minutes respiration rate, pin-point contracted pupils, and full bladder.
- Up to this stage, with proper and prompt treatment, recovery can occur.
- If the treatment is not given, cyanosis increases, pulse slows down, respiration goes down till it is not counted, pupils become contracted.
- Fine-lather like froth seen at mouth and nostrils due to pulmonary oedema, temperature goes down, breath smells opium, a few convulsions may occur before death.
- Death may be due to respiratory centre failure.

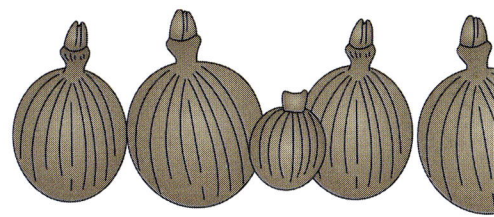

Fig. 25.1: Poppy capsules

Differential Diagnosis

Cerebral haemorrhage	Meningitis
Epileptic coma	Encephalitis
Head injury	Carbolic acid poisoning
Uremic coma	Barbiturate poisoning
Diabetic coma	CO poisoning
Alcoholic coma	Heat hyperpyrexia
Cerebral malaria	Hysteric coma

Treatment

- Stomach wash (through) and repeat 1:5000 solution of potassium permanganate until the returning fluid becomes pink in colour.
- Afterwards also about 500 ml of this solution is left behind in the stomach because opium is resecreted or secreted in stomach.
- $KMnO_4$ acts as physiological antidote.
- *Specific antidote N-acyl morphine hydrobromide.*
- It is given in IV dose of 5 mg repeated every 15–30 minutes until the pupils begin to dilate or rate of respiration increases.
- Nowadays, a true morphine antagonist is available.
- It is the drug of choice.
- It is naloxone hydrochloride (narcan) and is given IV 0.4–0.8 mg repeated as per the requirement.
- The patient is constantly watched. General care of patient in coma is to be observed.
- Even if the opium and derivatives are taken in injectable form, gastric lavage with $KMnO_4$ solution should be done because these substances are secreted or excreted in stomach.

Postmortem Features

- Cyanosis of fingers and lips.
- Fine froth-like lather near the mouth and nostrils, contracted pupils, opium smell.

- Congested stomach mucosa.
- Trachea, bronchial congestion with fine froth.
- Lungs oedematous, brain congested, bladder full. There are no pathognomonic signs.

Medicolegal Issues

- Popular suicidal agent.
- Pethidine abuse common among doctors and nurses.
- It is used for infanticide, sometimes by applying to breast and feeding.
- It is used for doping of the race horses.
- As an aphrodisiac, though in the long run it causes impotence.
- Opium dependence is very common.
- Even Taliban of Afghanistan was selling opium to run its government.

Chemical Test for Opium

- The suspected material is treated with 3 ml of H_2SO_4 and 3 drops of formalin.
- A change of colour from red to violet to blue indicates presence of opium.

PETHIDINE (MEPERIDINE)

- It has been very popular drug of abuse among doctors and nurses.
- Meperidine hydrochloride or pethidine given parentally is equivalent to 10 g of morphine, regarding the analgesic effect produced.
- Meperidine is a phenylpiperidine. The effects are similar to morphine.
- It does not cause constipation like opium.
- It has a mild stimulation effect on uterus.
- It is metabolized in liver.
- Pethidine may not cause nausea or vomit like morphine.
- Large doses of repeated injections cause tremors, muscle twitches, dilated pupils, exaggerated reflexes and convulsions.
- When death occurs it is due to respiratory depression.

  Therapeutic dose: 50–150 mg IM or IV administration.

  Fatal dose: 1–2 g.

  Fatal period: 24 hours.

Treatment

- Stomach wash with $KMnO_4$.
- IV administration of stimulants like coramine.

Case Example

- The author has seen a case brought for autopsy in Tirupathi Medical College in 1970.
- The person was found hanging from a tree near the railway crossing on the outrisks of Tirupathi.
- Autopsy findings were those of anoxia with a ligature mark round the neck suggestive of hanging.
- Viscera was sent for chemical analysis and pethidine was detected by chemical analysis.
- In 1974, there was a sensational case of a gang consisting of pharmacists, polytechnic fellow, a driver, etc. who committed a series of murders.
- The Tamil Nadu government established special court to try all such cases together.
- This particular person was a Malaysian civilian about to embark a bus, when he was trapped by the gang.
- Later injection of pethidine was given to him. The gang brought him to Andhra border, hanged the body by a tree and disappeared.
- Conviction of death sentence was awarded to the members of the gang.

HEROIN

- It is diacetylmorphine, very popular drug of abuse, it is known as brown sugar, 2–3 times more effective than morphine.
- It is most dangerous among all the drugs of abuse. Within days tolerance occur.
- Skin popping, i.e. markings of SC injections, main lining, i.e. markings of the IV injections are commonly seen among these users.
- It gives a 'Kick' or 'Rush' with flushing of face and pleasurable sensation sometimes related to sexual organs.

CODEINE

It is methyl morphine and is commonly used as cough remedy. It is also an analgesic. Children suffer from harmful effects in toxic dose, like convulsions and delirium.

Fatal dose: 500–600 mg.

Management: Similar to morphine poisoning.

ETHYL ALCOHOL

- *"What wonders alcohol does not do! It provokes and unprovokes. It provokes the desire, but take away the performance"*

  — William Shakespere.
- When we say alcohol, it is commonly ethyl alcohol. Western civilization is alcohol-based civilizaiton. In contrast, Eastern civilization of China is opium user.
- Many books are written and much research has been done on good effects and bad effects about alcohol.
- It is a common proverb that in the beginning man consumes alcohol, but later on alcohol consumes man.
- A chronic alcohol user develops changes even in the personality.
- The simplest problem is suspicion about the fidelity of his wife.
- Serious things include sex assaults, cruelty to spouse and children, violent crimes, drunken driving, etc.

Common preparations of alcohol with the contents of alcohol:

Ginger beer	1–3%
Beer	5–6 %
Champhagne	10–15%
Wine	10–20%
Brandy	40–45%
Gin	40%
Whisky	40–50%
Rum	50–60%
Vodka	60–65%

- Absolute alcohol contains 99.95% of alcohol.
- Rectified spirit contains 90% alcohol.
- Methylated spirit (denatured alcohol) 95% alcohol and 5% methyl alcohol.

- Proof spirit, at 10.5°C temperature, the concentrations of alcohol in water is such that 12 parts of distilled water and 13 parts of alcohol by spirit and contains 57.10% by volume of ethyl alcohol. Anything over is called over proof and anything below it is called under proof.
- **Fatal dose:** 150 ml of absolute alcohol.
- **Fatal period:** 12–24 hours.
- **Food value of alcohol:** 7 calories/gram.

Symptoms and Signs

Zero order kinetics of alcohol

- Irrespective of blood alcohol concentration (8–12 ml of absolute alcohol/hour is degraded) in unit time. So, if a person consumes alcohol at a very low-pace, he may not be drunk at all.

Synergistic effects of alcohol

- Synergism occurs with opioids, hypnotics, tranquilizers, antidepressants and antihistamines.
- **Acute alcoholic intoxication** is characterized by gastric irritation, low blood pressure, hypoglycaemia, dilated pupils, respiratory depression, collapse, coma and death.
- **Chronic alcoholic disease** is characterized by nutritional deficiencies, malabsorption, polyneuritis, pellagra, tremors, convulsions. Wernicke's encephalopathy, cirrhosis of liver, cardiomyopathy, high blood pressure, congestive heart failure, cardiac arrhythmias, skeletal myopathy, Korsakoff's syndrome.
- **Korsakoff's syndrome is** characterized by disorientation, amnesia for recent events, talks half truths and distorted facts, polyneuritis with paraesthesias, weak limbs, unsteady gait, loss of deep reflexes.
- **Wernicke's encephalopathy is** characterized by acute confusion, delirium and stupor due to heavy drinking. It involves brain or spinal cord.

Acute alcoholic hallucinosis: The person hears derogatory and condemning types of remarks.

Mallory-Weiss syndrome: In this, the patient suffers from mediastinitis with oesophageal rupture.

Marchiafava's syndrome: In chronic alcoholics, degeneration of the corpus callosum occurs.

Saturday night paralysis: It so-called because the week end relaxation over drinks may end up with pressure on the radial nerves due to arm hanging over a chair.

Alcoholic blackout: Here the patient loses memory. Normally he is unable to recall anything that happened during that period.

Delirium tremens: In this state, the alcoholic person suffers from insomnia, restlessness, loss of memory, coarse muscular tremors of face, hand and tongue, a tendency to commit assault or homicide or even suicide.

- He suffers from disorientation of time and place. Delirium of horrors.
- It is treated as a state of unsoundness of mind.
- Delirium tremens occurs in chronic alcoholics after acute infection, trauma, temporary excess use of alcohol or a sudden withdrawal of alcohol.

Treatment

- Hypertonic glucose infusion.
- Antibiotics (if required).
- Multivitamins: Examples vitamins K, B_1, B_6, B_{12}.
- Chlorpromazine has a beneficial tranquilising effect.

In vivo veritas: There is an old Roman saying, "It speaks that a person under alcoholic influence speaks truth and reveals his real personality."

McEwan's sign: In deep alcohol coma, the pupils tend to contract. On pinching or slapping on the neck, the pupils slowly dilate and return to earlier state. This finding appears to have been not seen by doctors examine alcohol cases.

AGN or alcohol gaze nystagmus: Due to reduced visual effect and dilated pupils, the person who consumed alcohol stares and tries to steady his gaze leading to alcoholic gaze nystagmus.

Drunk: A person who has consumed alcohol is said to be drunk when he is so much under the influence of alcohol that he is unable to execute action in which he is engaged at the material time.

Proof spirit: This was the proof for the strength of spirit, e.g. whisky. When whisky is poured on gunpowder and ignited, it explodes. When water is mixed to it, the gunpowder does not get ignited (Table 25.1).

When alcohol is 49.29% W/W or 57.1% V/V, it is called 100% proof spirit.

Disulfiram or antabuse: This is administered to chronic alcoholics to get rid of the alcohol abuse, by an aversion technique.
- First the choice drink is given and then disulfiram.
- Over night drink is not given.
- Disulfiram causes aldehyde syndrome manifested by many distressing symptoms like dizziness, vomiting, mental confusion, throbbing headache, visual disturbances, flushing, tightness of chest and circulatory collapse. These manifestions last for 2–4 hours.

First day: 1 g

Second day: 0.75 g.

Third day: 0.50 g.

Followed by –0.25 g per day and continued till the physician is satisfied with the result. The treatment should be under a caring physician.

Citrated calcium carbide (CCC) has rapid and short duration of action.

Scheme for Examination of Alcohol Intoxication

(Based on British Medical Association, Special Committee, 1954 report).
- Name:
- Age:
- Sex:
- Address:
- Date and time of examination:
- State of clothing: Solid by vomiting/urine/any other/none.
- Character of speech: Thick/slurred/over precise.
- Evidence of self-control:
- Memory:
- Mental alertness:
- Sample of handwriting:
- Its character: (ask the person to write N, M, W).
- Pulse: Tachycardia/normal/any other
- Temperature:
- Skin: Dry/moist/flushed.
- State of tongue: Dry/moist/bitten/furred/any other.
- State of teeth: Dentures/broken/bleeding/anyother.
- Smell of breath: Smell of alcohol (yes/no)
- Hiccups: Present/absent.

Table 25.1: Symptoms and signs of alcohol poisoning

Blood concentration	Symptoms	Condition of person
0.05% (50 mg/100 ml)	Loss of inhibition, impaired judgement	Delighted and devilish
0.1% (100 mg/100 ml)	Staggering gait, loss of coordination, slurred speech	Delinquent and disgusting
0.2% (200 mg/100 ml)	Person needs help; extremely emotional	Delirious and dizzy
0.3% (300 mg/100 ml)	Stuporous, totally helpless	Dazed and dejected
0.4% (400 mg/100 ml)	Comatose	Dead drunk
0.6–0.7% (600–700 mg/100 ml)	Death due to respiratory centre paralysis	Dead

- **Conjunctiva:**
- **Pupils:** Dilated/constricted
- **Reaction to light:**
- **AGN (fine lateral nystagmus):** Present/absent
- **Hearing:** Normal/impaired
- **Gait:**
  - Walking in a straight line
  - Walking along a circle
  - With eyes open/with eyes closed
- **Muscular coordination:**
  - Finger-to-finger/finger-to-nose test
  - Buttonning or unbuttonning clothes
  - Picking up a coin from the floor
- **Reflexes:** Knee, ankle jerks: Loss/normal/exaggerated.
- **Blood pressure:**
- **State of heart:**
- **State of lungs:**
- **State of abdomen:**

Opinion: Based on the above examination the person examined:

- Has not consumed alcohol.
- Has consumed alcohol, but not under the influence.
- Has consumed alcohol and under the influence.

Samples for Analysis

Blood

- Cleaned with water (not spirit) and washed with soap.
- 10 ml blood collected in a bottle containing 10 mg sodium fluoride and 30 mg potassium oxalate.

Or

- Readily made available EDTA bulbs are used.
- The bottle sealed, labelled and transmitted immediately.

Breath analysis: 60 to 100 ml of air is collected in the balloon breath analysis kit and the colour change noted for the rapid test for drunken driving (2100 ml air contains same amount as 1 ml of blood).

Saliva: 10 ml of saliva is collected and sent for analysis.

Urine: Two samples are required. One as soon as the person is seen by doctor, second 30 minutes later. If alcohol level is more in second sample, he is in *absorption phase.*

If the first sample shows more alcohol, he is in *elimination phase.* If the value is almost the same, it is in the peak state.

Urine and blood ratio: 1.3:1.0 (at equilibrium).

Widmark's formula: a = c p r.

- a = amount of alcohol expressed in grams.
- c = amount of alcohol in g/kg estimated in blood.
- p = the weight of the person in kg.
- r = it is a factor. ± 0.85 for men.
          ± 0.055 for women.

Contents of denatured spirit: 0.5% caoutchoucine, 0.5% pyrione and 0.5% naphthalene, methyl alcohol and ethyl alcohol.

Differential diagnosis of acute alcoholic coma

- Barbiturate poisoning
- Paraldehyde poisoning
- Cardiovascular accidents
- Hypoglycaemia
- Head injury
- Schizophrenia

METHYL ALCOHOL

- Methyl alcohol is added to rectified spirit to make it unfit for drinking.
- However, from time to time, tragedies occur due to consumption of methylated spirit.
- Methyl alcohol is converted to formaldehyde and formic acid by alcohol dehydrogenase.

Clinical Manifestations

- Methyl alcohol poisoning results in retinal damage (due to formic acid), blurred vision, optic disc congestion, blindness, acidosis (due to formic acid). Bradycardia, hypotension, headache, vomiting, delirium, dyspnoea, coma, death.

Treatment

- Stomach wash with sodium bicarbonate solution.
- Ethanol 10% in water through nasogastric tube for several days till total relief is obtained.
- IV sodium orally bicarbonate drip to combat acidosis.
- Potassium chloride infusion.
- 50 ml 5% ethyl alcohol orally 4–5 days.

Specific Antidotes

- Calcium leucovorin (hastens formic acid metabolism).
- 4-methyl pyrazole (alcohol dehydrogenase inhibitor).

Medicolegal Issues

- The Supreme Court of India (EK Chandrasenan, State of Kerala) ordered an enhanced sentence of life imprisonment to the perpetrators of illicit liquor tragedy in 1982 in which 70 people lost life and 24 others lost eyes (became blind).
- 60–70% methyl alcohol was mixed with ethyl alcohol and sold to consumer.

Postmortem Features

- Stomach mucosa congested, lungs congested and oedematous.
- Degenerative changes in optic disc and retina.
- Brain and meninges congested.
- Kidney tubular degeneration seen.
- Liver shows fatty change.

Fatal dose: 60–140 ml

Fatal period: 1–4 days.

Association of Alcoholic Anonymous (AAA)

All over the world, alcoholics willing to overcome the habit or those who gave up alcohol communicate with each other and meet to explain the desire and dissociation from alcohol.

BARBITURATES

- Barbiturates are hypnotics which cause sleep.
- All barbiturates are derivatives of barbituric acid or malonyl urea.
- They are used as hypnotics, sedatives depending upon potency, duration of action and route of administration.
- They have synergistic effect with alcohol.
- The dose dependent effects are → sedation → sleep → anaesthesia → coma → death.

Classification

- Ultrashort acting
- Short acting
- Intermediate acting
- Long acting

Ultrashort Acting

Action starts within 5 minutes. Examples, pentothal sodium, thiopentone sodium.

- **Therapeutic dose:** 250–500 mg IV
- **Fatal dose:** 5–20 gm.

Short Acting

Action starts within 3–6 hours.

- **Example:** Seconal (quinol barbitone).
- **Evipan:** Cyclonol.
- **Therapeutic dose:** 75–150 mg.
- **Fatal dose:** 15–20 g.

Intermediate Acting

- **Example:** Soneryl (butabarbitone), nembutal (pentobarbitone).
- **Therapeutic dose:** 100–200 mg
- **Fatal dose:** 15–30 gm
- **Duration of action:** 4–8 hours

Long Acting

Duration of action: 8–16 hours

- **Example:** Phenobarbitone sodium (gardinal)
- **Therapeutic dose:** 60–120 mg
- **Fatal dose:** 30–50 gm

Characteristic Features

- Stage of excitement
- Stage of confusion
- Stage of coma

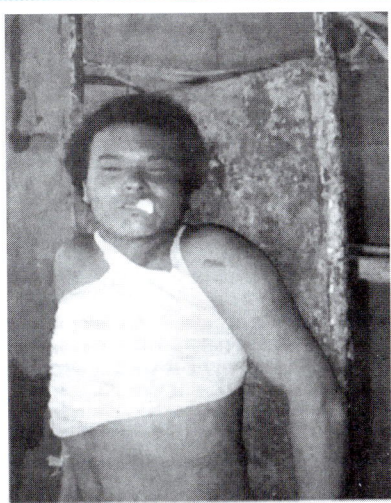

Fig. 25.2: Fine, white, lathery froth coming out from mouth (barbiturate poisoning)

The main effects are on

- The central nervous system
- Respiratory system
- Thermoregulatory system
- Gastrointestinal system
- Genitourinary system
- Cutaneous lesion
- The manifestations start with excitement, pass through confusion and end in varying levels of coma before death.
- The patient slowly goes into sleep, pupils dilated, blood vessels dilated, respiration becomes slow and deep, body temperature falls.
- Emptying time of stomach delayed.
- Oliguria, glycosuria.
- Blood shows, leukopenia, thrombocytopenia.
- There is a direct myocardial toxicity with barbiturates.
- Skin shows bullous lesions.
- Death occurs due to respiratory failure or ventricular fibrillation in early stages, bronchopneumonia or irreversible anoxia and pulmonary oedema in later stages.

Management

Intensive supportive therapy is the corner stage of therapy.

- Stomach wash with $KMnO_4$
- 5% glucose IV drip

- Oxygen
- Noradrenaline drip
- Dialysis and exchange transfusion
- Forced diuresis using 25% solution of mannitol 200 ml, followed by 5% solution of 500 ml.
- It is continued alternating with 5% dextrose solution for 24 hours.
- The aim is to maintain a urine volume of 4–6 litres in 24 hours.
- Sodium bicarbonate is added depending upon requirement.

Postmortem Features

- Barbiturate blisters when they are present.
- Cyanosis, presence of barbiturate lumps or mass; crystals in stomach.
- Congested, oedematous lungs.
- Petechial haemorrhage on lungs, pleura, heart.
- Kidney shows convoluted tubule necrosis.
- Brain oedema.

Medicolegal Issues

- These are most commonly used substances of abuse.
- Suicides with barbiturates are more common among doctors and paramedical personnel.
- Nowadays, this is very rare.

Barbiturate Automatism

- It is a common phenomenon among people who take barbiturates as a routing matter in the treatment of epilepsy.
- In barbiturate automatism, the person swallows one tablet, after sometimes he forgets that he has taken the tablet so takes next tablet.
- Every time he takes the tablet, he forgets that he has already taken one tablet, so automatically he enters the phase of swallowing.
- The barbiturate is taken in excess by the individual and the person dies due to respiratory depression.
- Sometimes the question arises as the person dies due to automatism or he commits suicide.
- In suicide, there is intentional gulping of a number of tablets at the same time.

- On the outskirts of Dhoraji, Rajkot in Gujarat, one mother and two daughters found dead in a farmhouse.
- They were bought for autopsy to Irwin Hospital, Jamnagar.
- On opening the stomach, lumps of white material (Gardinal) were found in all the three bodies.
- Even their pet dogs on autopsy showed similar material.
- A case of Pact/Mass suicide.

NON-BARBITURATES

- **This group includes:** Chloral hydrate, carbromol, glutethimide, methaqualone, methylpentynol.

Chloral Hydrate

- It is the oldest synthetic hypnotic.
- It has its own aromatic smell.
- It is a safe hypnotic.

Toxic Manifestations

- Central nervous system depression.
- Irritation to skin and gastric mucosa.
- Deep cyanosis, urticarial rash, convulsions, coma and death due to respiratory centre paralysis and heart failure.

Treatment

- Stomach wash with warm water
- Cardiorespiratory stimulants
- Analeptics
- Vitamin C
- Oxygen

Postmortem Appearances

- Chloral hydrate smell
- Fatty change in liver, heart, kidneys.
- Delayed chemical analysis shows negative results due to rapid deterioration after death.

Medicolegal Issues

It is known as *Sukha Sharab* (dry liquor).

Fatal dose: 10 g.

Fatal period: 8–12 hours. It is banned in India.

Mandrax (Methaqualone)

- It causes paraesthesia and euphoria.
- It is said to be aphrodisiac.
- Patient looses consciousness, myoclonic jerks, extensor plantar response, papilloedema, myocardial damage, thrombocytopenia.

Treatment

- Haemoperfusion with charcoal.
- Bilateral up going plantar response is a characteristic feature.
- It is banned in India.

Fatal dose: 5 g.

Fatal period: 12–24 hours.

Postmortem Features

All organs are congested

Medicolegal Issues

- It is a substance of abuse.
- It is banned in India.

BROMIDES

Manifestation of bromide poisoning are: Vertigo, mental confusion, staggering gait, fall of BP, feeble pulse, low temperature, shallow breathing, myasthenia, muscular paralysis, collapse, coma, death (clinical picture resembles alcohol intoxication).

Other examples: Dhatura, chloral hydrates.

Fatal dose: 30–45 g.

Fatal period: 6–18 hours.

Treatment

- Gastric lavage
- Normal saline drip (chloride displaces bromide and removes the symptoms of bromide).

Bromism

- It is chronic exposure to bromine or bromides.
- It causes muscular weakness, incoordination, blunting of memory, hallucinations, delusions.

Case Example

Exposure to bromine fumes caused irritation and skin blisters on exposed parts of body and face of 14 pharmacy students in the laboratory of Institute of Technology, BHU.

PARALDEHYDE

- It is a potent hypnotic.
- It causes severe CNS depression.
- It is converted into acetaldehyde and finally into CO_2 and H_2O in the liver.
- It has a typical odour.
- It causes acidosis, liver and kidney damage.
- Pupils are dilated, death is due to respiratory failure.

  Fatal dose: 100–150 ml.

  Fatal period: 12–24 hours.

Treatment

- Stomach wash with Na_2CO_3.
- IV calcium and dextrose.

Postmortem Features

- Characteristic odour.
- It has been very popular drug for convulsions to children.
- Stomach mucosa congested.
- Liver, kidneys congested.
- Bronchopneumonia.

TRANQUILIZERS

Benzodiazepines overtook, overshadowed and displaced barbiturates as hypnotics and sedatives, though they are introduced as antianxiety drugs (Table 25.2).

Table 25.2: Major and minor tranquilizers

Benzodiazepines	Example	Therapeutic dose
Slowly eliminated	Flurazepam	15–30 mg
	Diazepam	5–10 mg
Relatively slowly eliminated	Nitrazepam	5–10 mg
	Flunitrazepam	1–2 mg
Relatively rapidly eliminated	Timazepam	10–20 mg
	Trizolam	0.25 mg
Ultrarapidly eliminated	Midazolam	7.5 mg

Toxic Manifestations

Myocardial depression, orthostatic hypotension, contracted pupils, decreased sweating, corneal opacities, priapism, urticaria, dermatitis, grey blue pigmentation.

Treatment

- Gastric lavage
- Activated charcoal
- Fulmazenil 0.3 mg IV injections control the overdose of BZD derivatives.

Medicolegal Issues

- Death is rare with treatment.
- These can become substances of abuse, so need constant supervision of physician.

CHAPTER 26

Deliriant Poisons

DHATURA (DATURA)

- *Dhatura* poisoning is very common in India.
- It is used as **stupefying agent** to facilitate robbery by preparing snacks containing *dhatura* powder and administering to fellow passenger in trains.
- They offer biscuits, pakoda, bhajiya, etc. In Mehsana region of Gujarat and in other parts of North India like Bihar, UP, this type of poisoning is common.
- *Datura alba* has white flowers.
- *Datura niger* has black flowers.
- *Datura tatula* has purple flowers.
- The fruit of *dhatura* bears thorns, so it is called thorn apple.
- The flowers are bell shaped.
- It is also called Devil's weed.

Other Varieties

- *Datura atrox* has white flowers.
- *Datura metel* has white flowers.
- *Datura ferox* has white flowers.
- *Dhatura* is used as an abortifacient and a homicidal agent.
- It is also used as aphrodisiac.
- It is sometimes used as a roadway poisons to facilitate robbery or rape.

Fatal dose: About 100–125 seeds

Fatal period: About 24 hours.

Clinical Manifestations

- Dry skin
- Dryness of mouth
- Difficulty in swallowing (dsyphagia)
- Dizziness
- Delirium
- Dilated pupils
- Diplopia
- Drunken (staggering) gait
- Difficulty in speech
- Drowsiness
- Dreadful hallucinations
- Dry hot skin
- Depression of vomiting centre
- Depression
- Dark or yellowish brown seeds in stomach
- Double-edged convex border of seeds
- Dilatation of capillaries.

Character of hallucinations of *dhatura*: He pulls imaginary threads from tip of his fingers and he threads imaginary needles.

Eye manifestation in *dhatura*: Widely dilated pupils, loss of accommodation, photophobia, diplopia (double vision), temporary blindness, light reflex sluggish in the beginning and absent later.

Differences between chilly seeds and dhatura seeds: See Table 36.29.

Dhatura intoxication

- Flushy face, dilated pupils, confused mind, bizzare behaviour, staggering gait, dry and difficult talk, double vision, dazed appearance and when these people enter in police stations,

- **They are mistaken for cases of alcoholic intoxication,** even their story that they have been robbed of valuables is viewed with doubt or suspicion.

The clinical stages of poisoning are

- The stage of delirium.
- The stage of coma.
- **The manifestations are summarized by Mortan "Hot as a hare (dry skin), blind as a bat (eye changes), dry as a bone (dryness of skin), red as a beet and mad as a wet hen" (low muttering delirium).**

ALKALOIDS

- Atropine (traces)
- Hyoscine
- Hyoscyamine

Treatment

- Stomach wash with $KMnO_4$.
- Physostigmine 0.5 mg IV repeated hourly as per need.
- Pilocarpine 5 mg SC.
- Rest—symptomatic management.

Postmortem Appearances

Congestion of gastrointestinal tract, recovery of *dhatura* seeds from stomach is possible even in decomposed bodies because they resist decomposition.

Other poisons which resist decomposition are: Strychnine, nicotine, endrin, phosphorus, arsenic, antimony, yellow oleander, etc.

CANNABIS SATIVA

- It is said to be the favourite of the Lord Shiva.
- It is used as a traditional drink during the Holi festival.
- About 10% of the world population is said to be using in one or other form.
- *The various preparations of cannabis are*: A hand-fold cigarette reefers.
- A reefer contains 0.5–2 gm of Marijuana (Marihuana).
- This is popular in North America, Europe.
- It is also known as the herb of pleasure **(Hashish-El-Khif Arabic).**

- They carried out the religious assassinations.
- The word Hashish is derived from assasin.

Charas

- Smoked in water-cooled pipes, i.e. Hooka also known as hubble-bubbles.
- A sweet preparation made from charas is called *majun*.
- Charas is the dried resin.
  - *Ganja*—is the dry flowering tops. It is smoked as a cigarette.
  - *Bhang*—is the crushed leaves.
- It is taken in a form of round crushed paste like ball (gola) with almond and milk known as thandai in Varanasi.
- Cannabis has about 61 active principles called canabinoids.
- Tetrahydrocanabinol and its variant Delta-9 THC cause most of the typical effects.

Manifestations of Acute Cannabis Poisoning

- The manifestations are related to mind and body.
- The mental manifestations are a sense of detachment, dreaminess, disinhibition, depersonalization, euphoria, fleeting emotions.
- Laughing without any reason, feeling sleepy, irrelevant thoughts, disorientation, decreased concentration.
- Seeing non-existing objects, hallucinations and illusions.
- Tightness of chest, fear of death, altered sense of time and space, impaired judgment, irresponsible conduct, rapid speech, talkative.

Physical Manifestations

- Hunger, thirst, nausea, dizziness, restlessness, dry mouth, tremors, frequency of urine and red eyes.

Fatal dose: Charas 2 g, ganja 8 g, bhang 10 g/kg body weight

Fatal period: Death is rare.

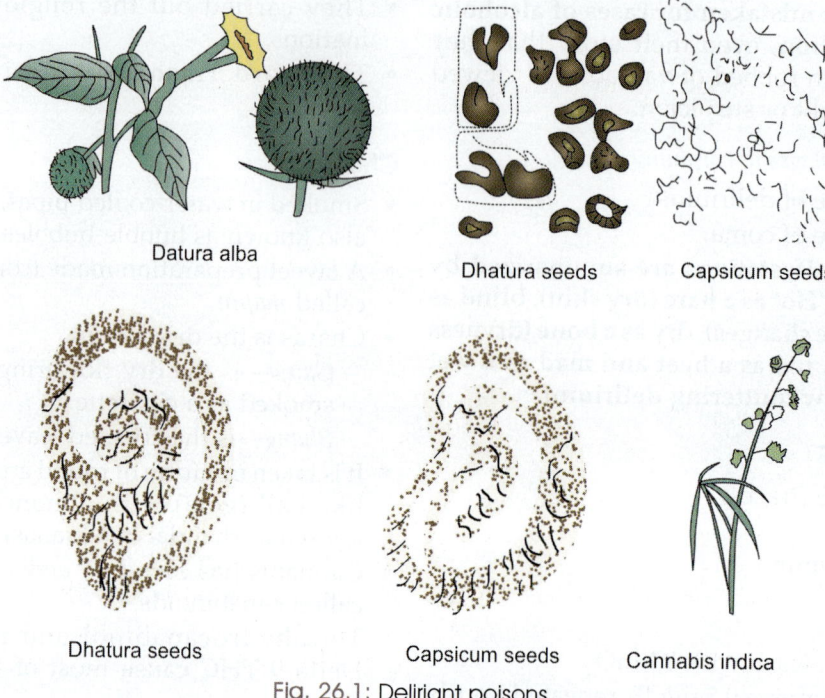

Datura alba   Dhatura seeds   Capsicum seeds

Dhatura seeds   Capsicum seeds   Cannabis indica

Fig. 26.1: Deliriant poisons

Treatment

- Stomach wash.
- 5–10 mg of diazepam.

Chronic Poisoning

- It is a popular substance of abuse.
- In chronic users, there is loss of appetite, weakness, **vacant look, tremors, impotence,** moral deterioration, **hallucinations** and **delusions** of **persecution**.

Runamok

- A chronic user of cannabis develops an impulse to kill.
- The persons first kills a person on whom he has real or imaginary enemity, then he goes on a killing spree, **killing anyone who comes across and finally surrenders himself or commits suicide.**

Postmortem Appearances

- Not characteristic.
- Individual may show evidence of bronchitis and wasting of muscles, organs congested.

Medicolegal Issues

- As an aphrodisiac, supposed to increase the duration of sexual act.
- Long-term users are likely to become impotent.

PSYCHEDELIC SUBSTANCES

- Lysergic acid diethylamide (LSD)
- Dimethyl amine (DMT)
- Psylocybin
- Mescaline
- Methylene dioxymethomphetamine: Ecstasy (MDMA).
- LSD is the most potent. Even 25–50 µg can cause psychedelic effects.

Clinical Manifestations of LSD Consumption

- **Mood changes:** Like elation and depression, arousal and panic, hallucinations, distortions of perception, dilated pupils, high blood pressure, salivation, lacrimation, increased reflexes, darker colour, altered shapes.
- **Bad trip:** It is characterized by severe depression and suicidal thoughts.

Ecstasy (MDMA)

It enhances insight, helps knowledge. It causes dry mouth, jaw clenching, jaw pain, visual hallucinations, hyperthermia, panic attacks.

Medicolegal Issues

- It is a popular substance of abuse.
- Run amok—homicide and/or suicide.
- Popular for pleasant feeling and sense of detachment which helps a person to live in his own world of ecstasy.
- It is a banned substance.

COCAINE

- It is a naturally occurring alkaloid, extracted from the levels of *Erythroxylum coca*.
- It is regarded as a gift from the God.
- It is used as an aphrodisiac, as a real anaesthetic.
- It is used in pain.
- Chronic poisoning is known as cocainism.

Manifestations

- Magnan's symptom (cocaine bugs).
- These are tactile hallucinations.
- The person feels a sense of bugs crawling under the skin.
- Pupils are dilated.
- **Acute cocaine poisoning** causes within a few minutes a feeling of faintness, collapse and death. Acute cocaine poisoning can cause also myocardial infarction.

Fatal dose: 1–15 g.

Fatal period: Few minutes to few hours.

Treatment

- Stomach wash with $KMnO_4$
- Control of convulsions.
- Amylnitrate inhalations.

Postmortem Appearances

- Are those of anoxic death.
- Cocaine has a fast rate of decomposition.

Medicolegal Issues

- It is banned under the Narcotic and Psychotropic Substances Act.
- It is an aphrodisiac.
- **Crack:** It is a preparation containing baking soda and water. It is suitable for smoking.
- Cocaine produces a **dose-dependent increase in heart rate and blood pressure followed by a sense of a self-confidence and well-being and improved performance of talks of vigilance and alertness.**
- Higher dose causes stereotyped behavior and tendency for violence.
- Cocaine is used as a snuff in the eastern part of India, Orissa and Bihar.
- It produces ulceration and perforation of the nasal septum.
- It also causes blackening of gums and teeth.

CHAPTER 27

Substance Abuse

- **People become dependent on certain substances for various reasons.**
- **Habit formation occurs when a person becomes dependent.**
- Common habits like taking coffee or tea are not associated with any serious withdrawal symptoms.
- However, once the habit occurs as in the case of opium, barbiturates, alcohol or nicotine, individual suffers from manifestations of withdrawal, either psychological or physical or both.

Substances forming dependence are not always used as drugs, e.g. solvents, like:
- Gasoline (petrol)
- Toluence (glue sniffing)
- Xylol
- Benzene
- Carbon tetrachloride

These cause dependence or solvent abuse, therefore the term substance abuse appears to be more appropriate than drug abuse.

Factors Affecting Abuse of Substances

Agent factors (drug or substance)
- Easy availability
- Low cost
- Good potency
- Easy way like chewing, snuff of consuming inhalation, oral and parenteral.
- Quickness of effect and duration of effect.

Host factors (user factors)
- Tolerence (hereditary or acquired)
- Enjoyment like intoxication
- Mental manifestations
- Earlier pleasant experience

Environmental factors
- Attitude of community or culture, e.g. western countries have a culture of alcohol, eastern countries have a culture of taking opium and cannabis.
- **Social group:** In a group of smokers or alcoholics, the non-user is tempted, induced, prompted or forced.

Pharmacological Actions
- Development of tolerence.
- As tolerence develops, the addict takes more and more quantity and becomes more and more dependent.

Groups of Drugs of Abuse

Stimulants: Amphetamine group of drugs.

Depressants: Hypnotics and narcotics (barbiturates, mandrax, opium, pethidine, heroin).

Psychotropic and psychedelic substances: Alcohol, cocaine, cannabis, LSD and psylocybin.

Types of Tolerance
- Innate tolerance, i.e. pre-existing.
- Acquired tolerance
  - Pharmacokinetic
  - Pharmacodynamic

- Learned tolerance { Behavioural / Conditioned }
- Acute tolerance
- Reverse tolerance (sensitization)
- Cross-tolerance

WITHDRAWAL SYNDROMES

Withdrawal syndrome occurs because of the non-availability of the drug or substance. Hyperarousal of the CNS for the purpose of readaptation because of the absence of the drug.

Alcohol Withdrawal Syndrome

Manifestations

- Craving for alcohol
- Irritability
- Tremors
- Nausea
- Lack of sleep
- Altered sleep behaviour
- Tachycardia
- Hypertension
- Convulsions
- Delirium tremors
- Severe agitation
- Confusion
- Visual hallucinations
- Dilated pupils.

Opium/Morphine Withdrawal Syndrome

Manifestations

- Craving for the substance
- Restlessness
- Irritability
- Muscular cramps, aches
- Anxiety, insomnia
- Yawning
- Sweating
- Vomiting
- Gooseflesh (piloerection: Erection of hair)
- High BP
- Dilated pupils
- Fever

Cannabis Withdrawal Syndrome

Manifestations

- Restlessness
- Irritability
- Insomnia
- Muscular cramps
- Nausea

Cocaine Withdrawal Syndrome

Manifestations

- Depression
- Fatigue
- Sleepiness
- Bradycardia

Nicotine Withdrawal Syndrome

Manifestations

- Anger
- Impatience
- Irritability
- Depression
- Lack of concentration
- Low heart rate
- Increased appetite and weight gain

Benzodiazepines Withdrawal Syndrome

Manifestations

- Anxiety
- Tingling and numbness
- Muscular cramps
- Sleep disturbance

DRUG ABUSE DEATHS

- In a suspected case of death due to or related to drug or substance abuse, the doctor performing autopsy has to carefully look for multiple needle marks or scars in front of the elbow, back of the wrist, forearms, lower limbs, and hands.
- The scars are circular, depressed, hyper-pigmented or hypertrophied.
- Evidence of acute, chronic or healed ulcer or abscesses seen.
- Phlebothrombosis, thrombophlebitis or subcutaneous scaring can be seen.
- Recent injection marks, used or unused needles, vials, capsules, half-smoked or non-smoked reefers may be found in the person's clothes or the place where the body was found. Plastic bag or plastic sheet acrosal can be seen.

- In the case of drug stuffing or drug bagging, the drug may be found in small packets or condoms and swallowed by the person. It can be seen on X-ray examination (he may be a drug pusher or a drug carrier.)

Postmortem Appearances

- Autopsy features include self neglect in the form of malnutrition
- Bad hygiene
- Dental lesions
- Fungal infections
- Respiratory infections, STD
- Tuberculosis including AIDS

The doctor should look for manifestations of routine drug abuse, complications like bronchopneumonia, encephalitis, pyaemic abscess. Acute muscular necrosis should also be looked for. Injection sites, empty vials, stomach contents, blood, urine, organ tissues required should be subjected and collected for chemical analysis in FSL.

Management of Drug Abuse

- Motivation
- Immediate treatment of withdrawal
- Treatment of drug abuse with drugs, psychotherapy in patient rehabilitation programme and out-patient treatment.

Medicolegal Issues

- Drug dependence is a global problem.
- Banned drugs are traded across the nations by smuggling.
- Prevention and control of drug trafficking by rule of law includes even death sentence for drug traffickers.
- The drug trade causes homicides, accidents and even suicides by innocent victims and carriers.
- Nowadays terrorist organisations amass wealth through drug trade and use that money for buying weapons for terrorism. Recent example of Taliban regime in Afghanistan should be an eye opener to the civilized world.
- Drug use and drug abuse have been coexisting.

- Total eradication of drug abuse by punitive and retributive measures appears to be a distant dream.

I. Cocaine

- Cocaine has replaced heroin as the illicit drug of choice in many areas of the United States.
- It is being seen in greater frequency in individuals dying suddenly of heart disease, apparently acting as a precipitating agent.
- Cocaine is snorted, injected and, as 'crack', smoked.

II. Methamphetamine

- After cocaine, methamphetamine is the most commonly used illegal stimulant. It is sometimes sold as cocaine. It is extremely cheap and easy to manufacture.
- When methamphetamine is illegally manufactured, a small amount of its parent compound amphetamine is also produced.

III. MMDA, MDMA (Ecstasy), Phentermine, Propylhexedrine

Phenmetrazine just like methamphetamine are all derivatives of amphetamine with more or less of the same actions.

IV. Opiates

Opium is derived from the poppy plant, *Papaver somniferum*. It contains three alkaloids of interest to the field of toxicology: Morphine, codeine and heroin.

V. Fentanyl

Fentanyl is one of a number of synthetic versions of the opiates.

- Fentanyl was developed as an anaesthetic agent. It has both anaesthetic and analgesic properties.
- It is approximately 200 times as potent as morphine with rapid onset of action and short duration.
- Popsinger Michael Jackson is said to have died of Fentanyl overdose and his doctor is charged for the offence of homicide.

CHAPTER 28

Pesticides

Pesticides include insecticides, rodenticides, fungicides, herbicides, fumigants and insect repellants.

INSECTICIDES
Metallic Inorganic Insecticides

	Fatal dose	Antidotes
Arsenic trioxide	10 mg	Dimercaprol
Copper acetoarsinate	10 mg	Dimercaprol
Tartar emetic	10 mg	Dimercaprol
Corrosive sublimate	07 mg	Dimercaprol
Hydrogen cyanide	30 mg	Amylnitrite

Synthetic Organic Insecticides

Fatal dose and antidote

1. Chlorinated hydrocarbons:

DDT	30 g	Pheno-
Gammexane	28 g	barbitone and
Endrin	5–6 g	calcium carbonate

2. Organophosphorus compounds:

Aliphatic (alkyl) compounds
Malathion	60 g	Atropine
Aromatic (aryl) compounds		PAM
Parathion	1 g	DAM
Diazinon	25 g	

Carbamates: Baygon

Rodenticides	Fumigants
Zinc phosphide	Napthalene
Thallium sulphate	Paradichlorobenzene
Strychnine	
Herbicides	*Insect repellants*
Sodium arsenite	Sulphuric acid
Dinitro phenol	Diesel oil

FUNGICIDES
- Dithiocarbamates.
- Pentachlorophenol.
- Hexachlorobenzene (gammexene).

Classification Based on Severity of Toxicity
Virtually harmless: Fungicides like petroleum wash, copperoxide.

Relatively harmless: 20% sulphuric acid used as weed killer. Sodium chlorate used as road side herbicide.

Mildly toxic: Chlorinated hydrocarbons (gammexane organochloro compounds—dieldrin, endrin).

Highly toxic
- Alkyl phosphates
- Aryl phosphate
- Hydrocyanic acid
- Nicotine
- Paris green

ORGANOPHOSPHORUS COMPOUND POISONING

- These are popular suicidal poisons in India, however, replaced by aluminium phosphide and baygon.
- **Clinical manifestations of organophosphorus poisoning:**
  - **Muscarine like symptoms:** Pinpoint contracted pupils, salivation and sweating.
  - **Nicotine like symptoms:** Twiching of eyelids, neuromuscular block and paralysis.

  Central nervous system: CNS stimulation followed by:

- Depression
- Headache
- Giddiness
- Tremors
- Slurred speech
- Disorientation

  Difficulty in breathing, cyanosis, pulmonary oedema, hypertension, convulsions, coma, death (Salivation, lacrimation, urination, diarrhea, giddiness, emesis—SLUDGE).

  Blood porphyrins: Porphyrins in blood cause **chromolachryorrhoea** where the person sometimes sheds **red tears.**

  Fatal dose: 50 mg to 1 gm.

  Fatal period: 1 to 24 hours.

Treatment

- Removal from the source of exposure.
- Removal of clothes.
- Washing the body with soap and water.
- Atropinisation: Atropine sulphate 2 mg, IV repeated every 10 minutes until the pupils are dilated.
- Specific cholinesterase reactivators, e.g. PAM, DAM (diacetyl monoxime).

Dose

1 g IV 5% solution in water slow injection for 5 minutes repeated depending on requirement. Remaining treatment is symptomatic.

Medicolegal Issues

- Spraying of organophosphorus compound in agricultural purpose causes accidental death in farmers.
- Suicidal poisoning is common.

DDT (DICHLORODIPHENYLTRICHLOROETHANE)

It has been used to kill mosquitoes, flies, bugs, etc. 2% solution is also poisonous for human beings.

Clinical Manifestations

- Salivation
- Nausea
- Vomiting
- Nervousness
- Vertigo
- Tinnitus
- Blurred vision
- Muscular tremors
- Incoordination, paralysis of extremities pulmonary oedema and death due to respiratory failure.

  Fatal dose: 30 gm.

  Fatal period: 1 to 2 hours.

Treatment

- Stomach wash with 0.2% $KMnO_4$.
- Thiopentone sodium IV 100–250 mg.
- 10%–10 cc IV calcium gluconate.

Postmortem Appearances

- Congestion of organs
- Liver
- Lung
- Spleen and fatty change in heart

ENDRIN

- It is insoluble in water so it is dissolved in aromax (solvent with kerosene-like smell).
- It has kerosene-like smell.
- It is available in 20% aromax solution.
- It is known as plant penicillin as it is used extensively against pests of plants.

Clinical Manifestations

- Nausea
- Vomiting

- Salivation
- Froth at mouth and nostrils
- Dyspnoea
- Restlessness
- Spasm of muscles and convulsions
- Coma and death due to respiratory failure.

Treatment

- Stomach wash with 0.2% $KMnO_4$
- 10% calcium gluconate 10 ml with glucose in IV drip.
- Thiopentone sodium IV 100–250 mg.
- Remaining symptomatic treatment.

  Fatal dose: 5–6 gm

  Fatal period: 1 to 2 hours.

Postmortem Appearances

- Cynosis of lips
- Finger tips
- Dilated pupils, kerosene-like smell.
- Stomach contents may be blood stained.
- Congestion of stomach mucosa.
- Respiratory tract, subpericardial and subendocardial haemorrhage.
- Congestion of brain, liver, kidney, etc.
- Pulmonary oedema with voluminous lungs.

Medicolegal Issues

In agricultural areas, toddy mixed with endrin is used for homicidal purposes.

CARBAMATES

- Baygon is the commonest carbamate used.
- Baygon spray is common household.
- So it is a tempting domestic poison.
- It is a cholinesterase inhibitor.

Clinical Manifestations

- These are similar to organophosphorus compound poisoning, however, the action here is rapid.
- Atropine is the antidote of choice.
- The difference in the treatment between baygon and organophosphorus poisoning

is that in organophosphours poisoning, pralidoxime is given, in baygon it should not be given.

Benzyl Hexachloride (BHC)

- It is benzyl hexachloride ($C_6H_6Cl_6$) or **gammexane or lindane.**
- It is an aromatic chlorinated benzene compound.
- It is a popular agricultural spray used against the pests.

  Manifestations: Similar to DDT

  Treatment: Same as in DDT poisoning

NAPHTHALENE

- Naphthalene balls are commonly used as a household preservative for clothes.
- They are known as **moth balls.**
- They are attractive to children so they may swallow them, if they are in reach.
- It is toxic substance and death occurs with 2 gm.

  Fatal dose: 2 gm.

  Fatal period: 2 to 3 hours.

Clinical Manifestations

- Those of acute nephritis.
- Haemolytic anaemia and jaundice.
- The liver is enlarged, patient shows cyanosis, delirium, drowsiness, collapse, coma and death.
- Opacities of lens are seen.
- Death occurs fast in this poisoning.

Treatment

- Stomach wash with plain water and $MgSO_4$.
- Sodium bicarbonate 15 g orally every 4 hrs.
- Haemodialysis and exchange transfusion, if required.

Postmortem Appearances

- Jaundice
- Congested kidneys
- Enlarged liver with necrosis
- Haematuria
- Hb and albumin casts in tubules

Case report

- A teen-aged Muslim girl swallowed naphthalene balls as her parents did not accept her love affair.
- In the N.C. Hospital Surat, she was treated and discharged after recovery.
- The naphthalene ball smell was coming out of her breath during examination.

KEROSENE (GASOLINE)

- Kerosene or gasoline poisoning must be discussed because of the organophosphorus
- Compounds which have kerosene-like smell.

  The kerosene-like smell is due to solvent aromax.
- **In DDT, the solvent is kerosene, so kerosene smell in DDT is due to kerosene only.**
- Kerosene is accidentally consumed thinking that is water especially by children.

Clinical Manifestations

- The breath smells of kerosene
- Pupils initially contracted, but later dilated, lungs congested.
- Patient suffers from difficulty in breathing.

Postmortem Appearances

- Lungs become heavy.
- Firm on cutting, blood-stained froth
- Kerosene smell is present.

  Fatal dose: 15–30 ml.

  Fatal period: Less than 24 hours.

Treatment

- In children with kerosene poisoning, stomach wash should not be given to avoid aspiration pneumonic.
- Treatment of choice is antibiotic crystalline penicillin.

HAIR-DYE POISONING

Introduction

- In India, the most of the suicides are committed by ingestion of poisons, mainly pesticides.
- Nowadays, hair dye has been established as a preferred means of suicide, particularly in females.
- In the Indian subcontinent, hair dye poisoning either suicidal or by toxic overuse has been emerging as a very common poisoning due to its:
  - Extensive use
  - Low cost
  - Easy availability without any difficulty.
- All hair dyes irrespective of their brands and company contain PPD, as its key toxic component but can also be used for color enhancement

Types of Hair Dyes

- Vegetable hair dyes (Henna)
- Temporary hair dyes (water-soluble)
- Semipermanent hair dyes

- Permanent hair dyes (PPD, resorcinol)
  - Oxidation hair dyes
  - Progressive hair dyes (lead acetate/ Bismuth citrate)

Poisonous Ingredients

Permanent Dyes

- Paraphenylene diamine
- Resorcinol
- Propylene glycol
- Ethylenediaminetetraacetic acid (EDTA), sodium.

PARAPHENYLENE DIAMINE (PPD) $(C_6H_4(NH_2)_2$

- It is an aromatic amine not found in nature.
- It is available in the form of white crystals when pure and rapidly turns brown when exposed to air. It is used in most of the hair dyeing preparations, in almost all commercially available dyes as it:
  - Accelerates the dyeing process
  - Enhances color
  - Provides permanent results

- It is also used in industrial products such as:
  - Textile or fur dyes
  - Dark-colored cosmetics
  - Temporary tattoos
  - Photographic development

Clinical Features of Poisoning

Angioedema or Cervicofacial Oedema

- Early manifestations of oral PPD intake (usually within 4–6 hrs of ingestion) include respiratory distress due to swelling of upper airway and angioedema.
- **Angioedema:** It is defined as abrupt swelling of dermis and subcutis associated with occasional pain rather than pruritus and skin returning to normal usually within 72 hrs.

Angioedema is

- Immunologically mediated
- Anatomically limited
- Non-pitting oedema

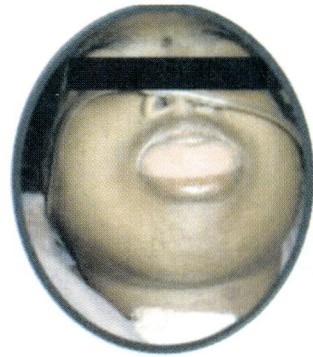

Fig. 28.1: Angioedema

Stages of angioedema (Pishoo et al)

Stage	Feature
Stage 1	Facial and lip oedema
Stage 2	Soft palate oedema
Stage 3	Lingual oedema
Stage 4	Laryngeal oedema

Rhabdomyolysis

- Appearance of cola-colored urine is the initial sign of rhamdomyolysis which is due to myoglobinuria.

- Majority of the patients present with back pain, limb pain and generalized myalgia.
- Acute muscle necrosis is the cause of tenderness and local oedema of muscle apart from myalgia.
- A positive urine dipstick test for haeme, with absence of red cells on microscopic examination confirms myoglobinuria.
- Dissolution of striated muscle fibres occurs with leakage of muscle enzymes myoglobin, potassium, calcium sometimes leads to adverse outcomes.
- CK levels are the most sensitive indicators of myocyte injury.

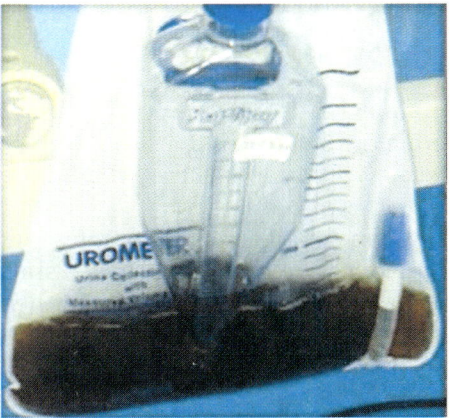

Fig. 28.2: Cola-colored urine

Myocarditis

- It is rhabdomyolysis of myocardium
- It was reported in 15% of total cases with mortality rate of 29%.

Renal failure

- It signifies severity of intoxication.
- It occurs due to a combination of hypovolemia, toxic injury and myoglobinuria.

Management

- There is no specific antidote available for PPD.
- Treatment is aimed at rapid identification of potentially life-threatening complications and prevention of renal failure.
- Gastric lavage may be useful, if the patient presents within 1 hour of ingestion but

contraindicated, if airway protective reflex is lost.
- Activated charcoal: Because of low molecular weight and hydrophilic nature of PPD, it has low adsorbability.
- Airway protection is the most important consideration with laryngeal angioedema % mainly done by endotracheal intubation or tracheostomy.

Medical Treatment

- Mainly by steroids and antihistamines.
- In the event of life-threatening reaction involving utricaria with laryngeal oedema or angioedema, epinephrine may be tried to stabilize patient.

For rhabdomyolysis

- Aggressive fluid resuscitation with isotonic fluids to restore renal perfusion and increased urine flow is necessary to prevent acute kidney injury.
- In case of oliguria, haemodialysis is the treatment.

For myocarditis: Continuous cardiac monitoring is essential to prevent any arrhythmia.

PARAQUAT POISONING

Introduction

- Paraquat is a rapidly acting, non-selective herbicide; inexpensive.
- Dermal/spray exposure (inhalation)—limited localized injury.
- Ingestion—high case fatality rate
- Diquat is a related herbicide—similar mechanism, clinical features, treatment
- Coformulated with an antiemetic/alginate to reduce absorption.

Pharmacology and Cellular Toxicology

- Chemically—bipyridyl compounds
- Absorption—concentrated inside cells. Redox cycling (repetitive enzyme mediated cycling between paraquat and its radicals)
- Byproduct—superoxide radical
- Redox cycling—consumes NADPH (antioxidant)
- Oxidative stress—cellular damage
- Secondary inflammatory response
- Multiorgan failure—organs with high blood flow, oxygen tension and energy requirements—lungs/heart/kidneys/liver

Kinetics

- Highly polar and corrosive
- Ingestion—rapid absorption—rapid distribution
- Max tissue levels 6 hrs
- Active uptake by cell membrane transporters (e.g. spermidine/putrescine)

- High conc—in liver, lungs, kidney, muscle
- No significant phase 1/phase 2 biotransformation
- Elimination—kidneys
- Minor—most ingested will appear in urine by 24 hrs.
- Severe-kidney function impaired—elimination delayed; elimination half life can exceed 100 hrs.

Clinical Features

History

- Formulation, strength and dose are important—>30 ml of 20% paraquat can be lethal.
- Kidney disease and age >50 yrs—bad prognosis
- Time of ingestion
- Painful mouth, difficulty in swallowing, nausea, vomiting, abdominal pain
- Burning skin sensation
- Respiratory complaints—systemic poisoning

Physical Examination and Basic Monitoring

- Mouth, pharynx—necrosis, inflammation, ulceration—may be delayed to up to 12 hours, peak severity in some days later
- Dehydration (vomiting)
- Monitor respiratory rate, pulse oximetry—O_2 only if SpO_2 <90%

- Heart rate, BP—progressive refractory hypotension
- Chest—dyspnoeic, tachypnoeic, crackles (alveolitis) subcutaneous emphysema—mediastinitis
- Abdominal pain, diffuse tenderness
- Topical contact—corneal ulceration, non specific dermatitis

Lab Evaluation

- *General testing*
  - Blood tests—on admission, every 6 to 12th hourly for first 48 hours, then based on clinical severity—vomiting, diarrhoea, kidney injury.
  - If prognosis is poor—palliative measures
  - Serum electrolytes—may be altered due to vomiting, diarrhoea, acute kidney injury and multiorgan dysfunction.
- *Renal function*
  - AKI suggests significant poisoning—acute tubular necrosis/volume depletion—increased mortality
  - Serum creatinine-rate of increase correlates with survival—<0.034 mg%/hr over 5 hrs (survival); >0.049 mg% hr/over 6 hrs (death)
  - Serum cystatin C—>0.009 mg/L/hr over 6 hours (death)
- *Blood gas*
  - Alkalaemia—vomiting, early in the course
  - Acidaemia—respiratory acidosis (alveolitis, pneumonitis) and metabolic acidosis (diarrhoea, AKI, mitochondrial toxicity, hypotension)
- Respiratory index >1.5 (death)
- Arterial lactate—MODS, hypotension, ARDS. Lactate concentration >40 mg%—fatal outcome—helps determine prognosis
- Chest radiograph—for assessing acute lung injury (hypoxia/hyperventilation/crackles)—direct effect of paraquat (bilateral)/aspiration (focal—mostly right lung).
- Early phase (1–2 weeks)—diffuse alveolar infiltrates—ARDS
- Late phase—reticulointerstitial infiltrates—progressive fibrosis

- Toxicology screen—for patients in altered mental status—usually not caused by paraquat-but by acetaminophen exposure, etc.
- *Specific testing*
  - Urine paraquat—inexpensive; based on color change after addition of dithionite solution to urine—positive within 6 hrs after large ingestion, remains positive for several days.
  - Positive test—40% mortality. Negative-100% survival.
  - Methods—100 mg sod. dithionite to 10 ml of 2 M sodium hydroxide—200 µl of this to 2 ml urine—blue (paraquat), green (diquat)—darker the color, more the concentration.
  - Serum paraquat—nomograms—correlate serum paraquat concentration with mortality risk.
  - The proudfoot nomogram, best cut off for the severity in paraquat poisoning (SIPP).
  - SIPP score—paraquat concentration (mg/dl) × time since poisoning (hrs). Score <10 survival is likely.
  - Challenges—imprecise time of exposure, paraquat assay within a relevant time frame.
  - Qualitative serum paraquat—in patients with positive urinary dithionite test.
  - Solution prepared as before—but added to 2 ml of plasma instead of urine-equivocal color change—50% mortality, definitive color change—100 % mortality.
  - Topical exposure—no need of investigations.
  - If in doubt—urinary dithionite at 6 and 12 hrs for reassurance.

Diagnosis

- History of ingestion/exposure
- Physical examination—oropharyngeal burns, etc.
- Subsequent development of—AKI, metabolic acidosis, or ARDS.
- Lab confirmation—urine dithionite test

Differential Diagnosis

- No other pesticide makes such severe oral burns.

- Most corrosives do not cause acute systemic toxicity.
- Previously was mistaken for HIV-related infections—oral candidiasis/*Pneumocystis jirovecii* pneumonia.

Management

- Determined on an individual basis based on amount ingested, time elapsed since exposure.
- None of the current treatments is effective in severe poisoning.
- Symptoms/signs manifest in 6 to 12 hrs—need monitoring at least for this duration.
- Negative urinary dithionite test at 6 hrs—minimal exposure.
- GI decontamination to limit systemic exposure.
- Hemoperfusion followed by hemodiafiltration/repeated hemoperfusion may be beneficial, if commenced within 4 hrs of exposure.
- Antedotes—antiiflammatory and antioxidant therapies—limited data to support efficacy.
- For severe poisoning—better approach may be palliative care.
- Titrated fentanyl/morphine.

Initial Resuscitation

- Follows standard guidelines.
- O_2 should not be administered unless SpO_2 <90%.
- Hydration—2 to 3 L of isotonic crystalloids or more.
- Continuous pulse oximetry
- For severe systemic illness—active management may be futile, but decision can be taken based on history/prognostic tests/clinical signs.
- Gastrointestinal decontamination:
  - If presented within 2 hrs of exposure: Activated.
  - Charcoal 1 g/kg in water, max dose 50 g; per oral or via NG tube.
  - Gastric lavage and forced emesis are contraindicated—caustic injury.
  - NG tube aspiration prior to charcoal administration.

- Topical/inhalational exposure:
  - Wash with soap and water for 15 min.
  - Staff should use universal precautions.
  - Ocular exposure—standard treatment for corrosive exposure—rinsing for 30 min.
- Monitoring: Pulse oximetry.

Specific Treatment

- *Indications for extracorporeal therapies*
  - Hemoperfusion for 4 hrs, if initiated within 4 hrs of ingestion.
  - Haemodialysis/hemofiltration may be used—paraquat has less protein binding.
  - Rebound in plasma paraquat following hemoperfusion can be minimized with continuous extracorporeal technique.
- *Antiinflammatory and immunosuppressive therapy*
  - Cyclophosphamide + glucocorticoid—not validated by studies
  - Antioxidant therapy—acetylcysteine, sodium salicylate, deferoxamine, vitamin C, vitamin E.

Ongoing Management

- Avoid O_2 unless hypoxic.
- Correct electrolyte abnormalities.
- Monitor blood lactate concentrations, renal function.
- Acute hepatic injury/pancreatitis—do not influence prognosis.
- The likely outcome is generally apparent within a day or two:
  - Either critically ill with severe poisoning
  - Mild to moderate poisoning but adequately compensated without intervention
  - Asymptomatic.
- Renal failure resolves in weeks.
- Lung injury becomes progressively more severe for several weeks.
  - Lung transplant ineffective—paraquat injures the allograft
- Diquat—may be associated with MODS and rapid death similar to paraquat.
  - But survivors are most likely to recover and not experience delayed or progressive respiratory failure.

CHAPTER 29

Poisons Affecting Cardiovascular System

- **Cardiac poisons** include alkaloids or inorganic chemicals.
- Nicotine, nicotinine (*Nicotiana tobaccum*)
- Digitoxin (*Digitalis purpurea*)
- Nerin (*Nerium odorum*)
- Cerebrin thevetin (*Cerbera thevetia*)
- Aconitin, aconine (*Aconitum napellus*)
- Quinine (*Cinchona* sp.) and hydrocyanic acid.

NICOTIANA TOBACCUM (TOBACCO)

- Worldwide there are 30 million adult deaths per year, out of it three million deaths are tobacco related.
- Among people in their seventies, heart attacks are double in smokers than non-smokers.
- Among people in 50s, heart attacks are four times more common.
- Among people in 30s and 40s, heart attacks are five times more common, if compared to non-smokers (British Heart Foundation, 1995).
- Lung cancer is more common among smokers.
- Palate cancer is more common in people who smoke till burning end of cigarette inside the mouth.
- The alkaloids of tobacco are nicotine and nicotinine.

Acute Poisoning

- Contracted pupils, high temperature, headache in early stage followed by nausea, vomiting, excessive salivation, abdominal pain, tachycardia and hypertension.
- Bradycardia, respiratory depression, dilated pupils, convulsions, coma in later stage and death.

Fatal dose: 1–2 drops of pure nicotine orally can cause death.

Fatal period: Nicotine when swallowed causes death within no time, even within 5–10 minutes.

Treatment

- Stomach wash with warm water and 1:10,000 $KMnO_4$ solution.
- Maintenance of airway.
- Oxygen inhalations.

Postmortem Appearances

- Tobacco odour in breath and from body.
- Leaf fragments inside stomach, mucosa congested.
- Lungs, liver and brain congested.

Tobacco and malingering: People who want to escape duty especially in police and army keep tobacco in armpit to get fever and obtain sick certificate.

DIGITALIS PURPUREA

- It is a cardiac poison.
- The alkaloids are—digitoxin, digitalin, digitonin.
- Digoxin is obtained from leaves of *Digitalis leniata*.

Toxic Manifestations

- Anorexia
- Vomiting
- Diarrhea
- Vertigo
- Headache
- Precordial pressure
- Heart block
- Ventricular tachycardia
- Dilated pupils
- Yellow or green vision
- Delirium
- Hallucinations, convulsions
- Death occurs due to cardiac arrest or ventricular fibrillation.

    Fatal dose: 2–3 g, powdered leaves.

    Fatal period: Up to 24 hours.

Treatment

- 0.6 mg atropine intravenously.
- 50 mg IV lignocaine.
- Disodium acetate to lower blood calcium.
- High potassium diet.
- Diuretics like lasix.

Postmortem Features

Features of hyperacute congestive heart failure.

NERIUM ODORUM (KANER)

It has white or pink flowers. Active principle is neriine having digitalis-like action.

Manifestations

Similar to digitalis.

    Fatal dose: 16.6 g of root.

    Fatal period: 1–1½ days.

Treatment

Antiarrhythmic drugs like lignocaine 50 mg IV.

    Postmortem appearances: Not characteristic.

Medicolegal Aspects

- The root is used as abortifacient.
- The root juice is used as cattle poison.

CERBERA THEVETIA (PEELA KANER)

- It has large yellow bell-shaped flowers and green globular fruit.
- It contains a single light brown triangular shaped nut with two pale yellow seeds inside. Active principles are **cerebrin and thevetin.**

Clinical Manifestations

- Burning mouth
- Dry throat, tongue tingling, numbness and headache
- Dilated pupils
- Muscular weakness
- Fainting
- Rapid weak pulse
- Heart block
- Collapse
- Peripheral circulatory failure and death

    Fatal dose: Upto 10 seeds.

    Fatal period: 2–3 hours.

Treatment

- Stomach wash
- Symptomatic test

Medicolegal Importance

- The seeds and roots are used as abortifacients.
- Seeds are used as cattle poison.

Cerbera Odollam

- Its action is similar to *Cerbera thevetia.*
- It has white flowers and lanceolate leaves.
- The fruit resembles unripe mango.
- Active principle is cerebrin.
- It has digitalis-like action hence treatment is similar to digitalis.

ACONITUM NAPELLUS (ACONITE)

Also known as *mitha jahar*. The dry root is conical and tapering with longitudinal wrinkles, dark brown externally, on cutting whitish starchy material which turns dark brown on exposure.

The active principles are:

- Aconitin
- Picra-aconitine

- Aconine
- Pseudoaconitine
- Pseudoaconine

Clinical Manifestations

- Sweet bitter taste
- Burning and tingling of tongue, lips, mouth and throat.
- Salivation, dysphagia, vomiting, alternate contraction and dilatation of pupils.
- Vertigo, muscular weakness, twitching and spasms.
- Slow feeble irregular pulse.
- Low blood pressure.
- Rapid shallow respirations.
- Subnormal temperature.
- Death due to ventricular fibrillation.

  Fatal dose: 1 g of powder of root.

  Fatal period: 1–6 hours.

Treatment

Stomach wash with tannic acid; atropine to maintain temperature and bradycardia 0.1/ novocaine 50 ml.

Postmortem Appearances

Congestion of stomach and small intestine, frothy mucous in bronchi, features of anoxic death.

Medicolegal Issues

- Considered as an ideal homicidal poison because it can be given in **sweet pan** (betel leaf) or fruit juice.
- Death is certain. It disappears fast from the system, so chemical analysis may be negative.
- It is used as arrow poison.
- It is used as abortifacient.
- In homeopathy, extractum aconitum liquidum is used in treatment of heart problems.
- Professor Sharma of Banaras Hindu University (BHU) was a popular homeopath in the campus.
- He had chest pain and administered himself homeopathic medicine aconite.
- He developed cardiac poisoning.

- Symptoms disappeared after prompt treatment at SS hospital, BHU.

CHLOROQUINE

- It is a popular antimalarial drug. Parenteral administration causes hypotension, arrhythmias, convulsion and death in some cases.
- Excess of dose can cause loss of vision due to retinal damage.
- Skin rashes, loss of hair and retinal damage can occur, if given for longer duration.

  Chemical dose chloroquine phosphate: 2.5 g.

  In children, parenteral chloroquine can cause convulsions and death.

Postmortem Appearances

- History of injection of chloroquine.
- Myocardial congestion, petechial haemorrhages, skin rashes, sometimes porphyrias.

QUININE/QUINIDINE

Quinine is derived from the cinchona bark. The other alkaloid is cinchonidine. It is a strong protoplasmic poison.

Toxic Manifestations

- Headache
- Giddiness
- Bitter taste
- Tinnitus
- Deafness
- Fixed dilated pupils
- Urticarial rash
- Methaemoglobinaemia
- Tachycardia
- Low blood pressure
- Cyanosis
- Delirium
- Coma and death
- It has direct effect on endometrium and can cause abortion
- It releases insulin causing hypoglycaemia.

Treatment

Stomach wash with magnesium sulphate procainamide.

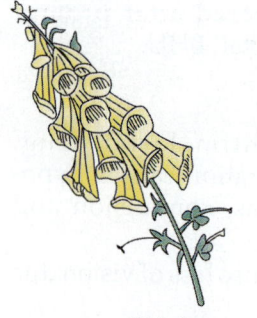

Digitalis purpurea

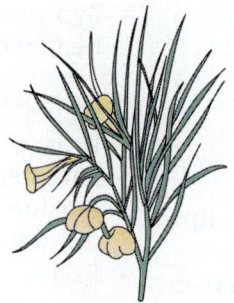

Cerbera thevetia

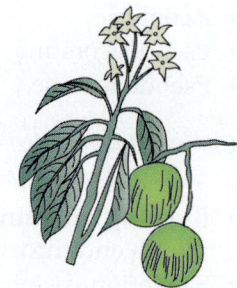

cerebra odollam

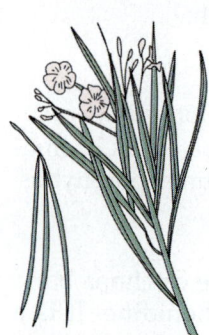

Nerium odorum

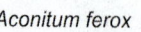

Aconitum ferox

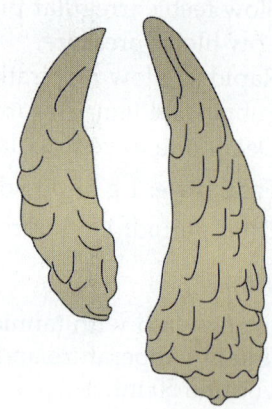

Dried roots of Aconitum napellus

Fig. 29.1: Poisons affecting cardiovascular system

Cinconism

- It is chronic poisoning with quinine. Ringing in ears, nausea, vomiting, headache, vertigo, difficulty in hearing and seeing.
- Sometimes even with a single therapeutic dose, the patient may suffer from itching, rashes, oedema of face, bronchocon-striction.

HYDROCYANIC ACID

- It is also called 'cyanogen' in gaseous state. It has smell like bitter almonds.
- Some persons cannot smell hydrogen cyanide due to sex-linked defect (recessive trait).
- Cyanide acts on cytochrome oxidase.
- It prevents the formation of ATP.
- It forms a compound with haemoglobin and prevents intracellular oxidation.

Clinical Manifestations

- Cyanogen gas inhalation causes the most rapid death
- Headache
- Vertigo
- Confusion
- Drowsiness
- Trismus (inability to open mouth due to clenching of teeth)
- Hyperthermia
- Convulsions
- Odour of bitter almonds in the breath, bright red blood
- Sinus arrhythmia
- Hypotension
- Cardiovascular collapse and death
- Pupils dilated
- **Eyes are glassy and prominent**
- Pupils dilated and unreactive

Principles of Management

- Cytochrome oxidase + cyanide = cytochrome oxidase cyanide.
- Cyanide + haemoglobin = cyanhaemoglobin.
- Cynide + methaemoglobin = cyanmethaemoglobin (non-toxic).

Treatment

Eli Lilly Approach:

- 0.2 ml of amyl nitrate ampule is broken in a handkerchief and held near the patient's nose and the patient is allowed to breathe in.
- Sodium nitrite 300 mg in 10 ml of distilled water given intravenous. There is a competition between methaemoglobin and cytochrome oxidase for cyanide ion. Since cyanide ion is taken up by methaemoglobin, cytochrome oxidase is left out freeing the celluler respiration.
- Infusion of 50% solution of sodium thiosulphate (25 g) also helps in the treatment.

- Dicobalt acetate reacts with cyanide and forms a harmless product which is excreted in urine. Slow IV 600 mg of Dicobalt acetate is given. This is better than nitrites. (Cobalt—EDTA)

- 100% oxygen is given (Hyperbaric O_2).

Postmortem Appearances

- Dilated pupils with **clear glassy eyes.**
- Fine froth at mouth.
- Cherry red colour hypostasis.
- **Bitter almonds** smell in the breath.
- Oedematous lungs.
- Red congested stomach and intestinal mucosa.

Medicolegal Issues

- Execution in cyanogen gas chambers was done by Nazis in Germany.
- It is a popular suicidal poison.

CHAPTER 30

Irrespirable Gases

Carbon dioxide, carbon monoxide, hydrogen sulphide (sewer gas), nitrous oxide, and war gases act as irrespirable gases and cause problem for continuation of breathing.

CARBON MONOXIDE

- Carbon monoxide is formed whenever there is incomplete combustion of any carbonaceous material.
- It is produced by diesel engines, in exhaust fumes of motors, motor cars and trucks.
- Carbon monoxide is odourless, colourless, tasteless, non-irritative gas.
- It is highly poisonous gas.
- It has 240 times more affinity to haemoglobin than oxygen.
- It combines with Hb to produce carboxyhaemoglobin.
- It knocks away the oxygen carrying capacity at cellular level.
- The effect of carbon monoxide concentration in blood is given as follows.

Level of Carbon Monoxide in Blood

Clinical Manifestations

- Below 10% No signs
- Below 20% Headache, dizziness
- Below 25% Throbbing headache
- Below 30% Nausea, giddiness ringing in ears, dimness of vision, slurred speech, drowsiness.
- Below 40% Incoordination, muscular weakness.
- Below 50% Collapse.
- Below 55% Paralysis and coma.
- Above 60% Coma and death.

Treatment

- Keep the patient away from source.
- 95% oxygen and 5% carbon dioxide mixture administered.
- Symptomatic management.

Postmortem Features

- Bright red lips and nails.
- Bright cherry red blood.
- Pulmonary oedema.
- Hemorrhagic necrotic heart lesions.

Medicolegal Issues

- Accidental poisoning is more common than suicide or homicide.
- 15–30% blood level causes symptoms similar to 'drunk', alcoholism.

HYDROGEN SULPHIDE (SEWER GAS POISONING)

- Sewers, cess pools, unused wells cause decomposition of organic material and generate hydrogen sulphide.
- It has smell of rotten eggs.

Clinical Manifestations

- Photophobia
- Lacrymation

- Pulmonary oedema
- Vertigo
- Weakness
- Muscle cramps
- Respiratory depression
- Cardiovascular collapse and death.

Postmortem Features

- Early appearance of greenish disco-louration of body.
- Other findings are those of anoxic deaths.

  Fatal dose: Exposure to 2,000 ppm causes death immediately.

Medicolegal Issues

When a person falls into a manhole, abandoned well or cess pool, death results due to hydrogen sulphide poisoning.

Treatment

- Remove the person from source
- Fresh air
- Inhalation of oxygen
- IV respiratory stimulants, like coramine 1–2 ml of 25% solution.

Sewer Gas

Sewer gas consists of hydrogen sulphide, carbon dioxide and methane. It interferes with cytochrome oxidase system and causes anoxic death.

CARBON DIOXIDE

It is natural component of atmospheric air. Atmospheric air contains 0.4% of carbon dioxide (Table 30.1).

Table 30.1: Percentage of CO_2 in atmosphere

% in atmosphere	Manifestations
5%	Respiratory rate increased, nausea, headache, giddiness, loss of muscle power
10%	Hyperapnea, sweating, visual disturbances, tremors, loss of consciousness
25–30%	Convulsions and death

With 95% oxygen and 5% carbon dioxide, stimulation of respiratory center occurs. Solid carbon dioxide is sold as **dry ice.**

Treatment of Carbon Dioxide Inhalation

- Patient is removed to open air.
- Administration of oxygen.
- Cardiac stimulants, if required.

Postmortem Features

- Congestion, dilated pupils.
- Marked cyanosis.
- Petechial haemorrhages.

Medicolegal Importance

Accidental deaths occur when people enter into unused wells.

WAR GASES

- These are chemical compounds employed on enemy forces to produce poisonous effects. **They are:**
  - **Vesicants:** Blistering gases (mustard gas, lewisite).
  - **Asphyxiants:** Lung irritants and chocking gases (phosgene, diphosgene, chloropicrin).
  - **Lachrymators:** Tear gases (CAP, BBC, KSK).
  - **Paralysants:** HCN, H_2S.
  - **Sternutators:** Nasal irritants (diphenyl chloramine).
  - **Nerve gases:** Phosphate esters.

Treatment

- **Blister gases:** Washing in the part thoroughly, eye wash with sodium bicarbonate solution. BAL 2 ml of 5% solution.
- **Asphyxiants:** Oxygen inhalation. Atropine for pulmonary oedema. Antibiotics to prevent pneumonia.
- **Lachrymators:** Eyewash with boric acid solution. Sodium bicarbonate for local skin ulcers.
- **Paralysants:** Look into treatment of HCN and H_2S.
- **Sternutators:** Sodium bicarbonate, nasal drops.

- **Nerve gases:** Atropinization: PAM, if required.
- The Skripals were poisoned with a substance that was part of the Novichok group of nerve agents developed by the Soviet Union's military in the 1970s and 80s.
- Novichok agents are believed to be 5 to 10 times more lethal than more commonly known nerve agents VX and sarin poison gases. (*Recent Russian spy death in Salisbury England 2018.*)

Atropine

Genus name of belladonna, a poisonous, crystalline alkaloid, C_{17}, H_{23}, NO_3, obtained from belladonna.

CHAPTER 31

Spinal and Peripheral Nerves

STRYCHNINE POISONING (SPINAL)

- Strychnine is highly poisonous crystalline alkaloid obtained from *Strychnos nux-vomica* seeds. Fruits are globular and seeds are disc shaped. Other alkaloid is brucine. It acts on ventral (anterior) horn cells of spinal cord.
- The seeds are flat, circular or concavo-convex with ash grey colour.
- Strychnine present in the body does not change due to decomposition and hence detected even years after death from the dead body tissues.
- It is used as *nervine* tonic and is a rodenticide too.
- Acute strychnine poisoning is chara-cterized by bitter taste in the mouth when taken orally.
- Symptoms are choked throat, stiff neck and face, twitching of muscles.
- Strychnine causes excitation to all areas of nervous system.
- All the muscles affected at the same time show convulsions clonic and tonic.
- A grin on the face called *risus sardonicus* is seen.
- The body is arched in hyperextension known as *opisthotonus*.
- Sometimes forward bending called *emprosthotonus* occurs.
- Side bending is occasionally seen and is known as *pleurosthotonus*.
- **The mind is clear till impending death.** Pupils are dilated.

- Cyanosis occurs.
- A ray of light can throw the body into convulsions so the patient should be kept in a closed dark place.
- Death results from mechanical interference with breathing and anoxia.
- Strychnine poisoning differs from tetanus.
- In tetanus, there is history of injury.
- Lock-jaw occurs first.
- Muscles are rigid in between convulsions whereas in strychnine poisoning, muscles relax in between convulsions.

Treatment

- Patient is kept in closed dark space to minimize convulsions.
- Convulsions are controlled with short-acting barbiturate like phenobarbitol sodium.
- After convulsions are controlled, stomach is washed with warm water containing 1:1000 $KMnO_4$ solution.
- Diazepam, pentobarbitone, and pancuro-nisum, if required.
- O_2 administered as per requirement.
- Other symptoms are managed as per the requirement.

Postmortem Features

- Rigor mortis onset early and lasts longer.
- Postmortem heating of the body (post-mortem caloricity).
- Cadaveric rigidity may occur without preliminary relaxation.
- Stomach mucosa, liver, kidney and lungs congested, brain, membranes

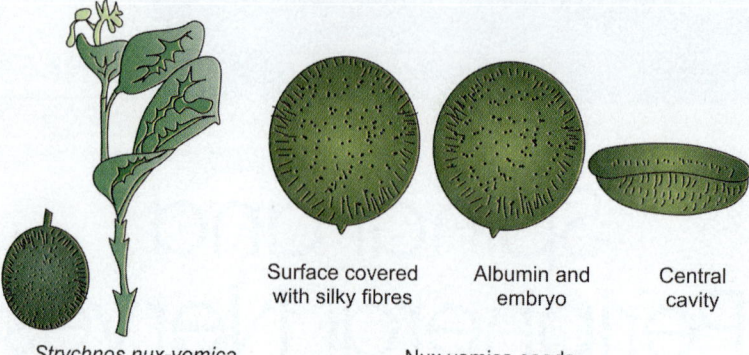

Surface covered with silky fibres   Albumin and embryo   Central cavity

Strychnos nux-vomica   Nux vomica seeds

Fig. 31.1: Poisons affecting nervous system

and upper part of spinal cord also get congested.

Fatal dose: Powder from one seed.

Fatal period: One to two hours.

Medicolegal Issues

- It is a deadly poison.
- Accidental poisoning occurs from dispensing mixtures.
- Nux vomica seeds are used as cattle poison. It has a false reputation as an aphrodisiac.

POISONS AFFECTING PERIPHERAL NERVOUS SYSTEM

Curare

- It is the active principle found in *Strychnos toxifera*.
- **It is very poisonous but when swallowed it is not poisonous (like snake venom).**
- Curare acts on the motor end plates and causes voluntary muscles paralysis from legs in upward direction to diaphragm.
- Drooping eyelids, diplopia, dilated pupils, limb paralysis, paralysis of neck and chest are the symptomatic features.
- Consciousness is not lost till the end.

Treatment

Neostigmine 1 mg and edorphonium chloride 10 mg act as antidote.

Autopsy

Features are those of anoxic death due to diaphragmatic paralysis.

Medicolegal Issues

Used as an arrow poison.

Hemlock

- *Conium maculatum* or spotted hemlock was presumedly used to kill Socrates. Acts on neuromuscular junction and nicotinic effect on autonomic ganglion, crushed leaves give mousy odour.
- The alkaloids are coniine, methyl coniine, conhydrine.
- It was used in ancient Greece as a **state poison,** to kill condemned persons.

Manifestations

- Bitter taste
- **Mousy odour**
- Constriction of throat
- Salivation
- Headache
- Staggering gait
- Ascending paralysis of limbs
- Dilated pupils
- Ptosis
- Clear state of mind till death
- Convulsions
- Cyanosis
- Death due to paralysis of respiratory muscles

  Fatal dose: 30–60 mg coniine.

  Fatal period: In a few minutes (sometimes a few hours).

Treatment

- Stomach wash with tannic acid.
- Control of convulsions by anticonvulsants.
- Oxygen supplementation.

Medicolegal Issues

Accidental poisoning may occur.

Medical Jurisprudence

CHAPTER 32

Medical Jurisprudence

INTRODUCTION

- Medical jurisprudence is the knowledge of law required for proper medical practice (*juris*—law—*prudence*: knowledge).
- The legal knowledge required for a medical practitioner in his day-to-day affairs must be updated so that he may not be unaware about the clutches of law.
- Only a qualified and registered medical practitioner is eligible to practice.
- He is permitted to practice in the system of medicine in which he has obtained his degree and registration.
- A homeopathic doctor is not eligible to practice allopathy.
- An allopathic doctor in the same way is not permitted to practice homeopathy or ayurveda. This is clearly made out in the judgement of Dr AK Patel by the Supreme Court of India.
- In this case, the homeopathic doctor who was indulged in allopathy was declared to have committed negligence *per se*.

REGISTERED MEDICAL PRACTITIONER

- A registered medical practitioner is one who has passed his MBBS, completed internship and registered himself with the State Medical Council or with the Medical Council of India. He enjoys certain rights and responsibilities.
- He has a right to choose his patients.
- He is permitted to practice the allopathic medicine.
- He can seek government/public/state/ trust or any other undertaking services.
- He can prescribe the medicine listed under Dangerous Drugs Act.
- He can give evidence as an expert in court of law.
- He can issue certificate like birth, death, sickness, etc.
- He has a right to claim his fees from the patients, if required through the court of law.
- He is permitted to carry out medicolegal autopsy, if required. In Gujarat, the doctors who are MBBS or those with higher qualifications are permitted to do the medicolegal autopsy.
- He can perform a surgical operation.
- He can practice midwifery.
- He must show due care and skill in treating the patients.
- He should not guarantee cure.
- He cannot desert the patient in middle. If he is going out of station, he should keep a colleague to take care till he returns.
- In case of emergency, a doctor cannot reject the patient, he must take the immediate care before he handover the case to some other doctor.
- He should not do experiments on the patient, he should only do the treatment carried out by his colleagues of similar qualification practicing in the same area.
- Doctor should take consent of the patient before examining him/her.

- No female patient should be examined in the absence of a female attendant.
- The doctor's behavior towards the patient should be polite and sympathetic.
- He should take the opinion of a senior colleague or a specialist in all cases of doubt or difficulty.
- The secrets of personal nature that he comes to know should not be carelessly talked about.
- Professional secrecy should be maintained unless forced under law to give the information. Even that it should be revealed under protest.
- He should give death certificate free of cost.
- A doctor should not take fee (money) from his professional colleagues.
- A doctor should not share his fees with any other unqualified person.
- A doctor should not talk loosely about his professional colleague, however, any criticism can be carried out about the academic matter, in a professional meeting or conference.
- In cases of homicidal poisoning, he must inform the police.
- He has no right to hold information from the police regarding the matters pertaining to police investigation in suspected crimes.

Patient's Duty Towards the Doctor

- The patient has no right to withdraw from the doctor without informing the doctor.
- He should follow all the instructions given by doctor regarding investigation and treatment.
- He must pay the fees to the doctor.
- He must give all the details about the disease that he already knows and should not hide anything from the doctor.

Duties of Doctors Towards State Government

- A registered medical practitioner must inform the health officer of the concerned area about the infectious disease/notifiable disease.

- He should inform the police regarding the patient in whom he suspects criminal involvement, rape, murder, criminal abortion, etc.
- He should inform about birth/death to the concerned office.

MEDICAL COUNCIL OF INDIA (MCI)

- Medical Council of India (MCI) is a national body governing the medical profession in the country. The Medical Council of India Act 1956 amended in 1964 provides for formation of MCI.
- The composition of MCI is made of one member from every state, nominated by Central Government in consultation with State Government, one member from each university elected by the members of senate of each university from the medical faculty, one member from each state maintaining the state medical register, seven members elected by the registered medical practitioners (RMP), eight members nominated by the Central Government.
- The headquarters of MCI is in New Delhi.
- The council members elect the president and vice president for five years.
- The members of the council are also elected or nominated for a term of five years.

Functions of Medical Council of India

- Maintaining the standard of undergraduate and postgraduate medical qualification in the country.
- It recognises foreign medical qualifications.
- It can make Central Government to withdraw recognition of a medical qualification.
- It recognises the medical qualification, medical degrees, diplomas, etc.
- It maintains a medical register.
- It can issue warning notices from time to time to the practitioners.
- It deals with the appeals made by persons punished by the state medical councils and advises the Central Government regarding the action to be taken.

STATE MEDICAL COUNCIL

- The state medical council is formed by the members elected from registered medical practioners of the state and members nominated by the state government.
- The members elect president and vice-president.

Functions of State Medical Council

- It maintains state medical register.
- Registration is granted to medical practitioners possessing degrees or diplomas as mentioned in the first and second schedule of Medical Council of India Act.
- The disciplinary action committee of State medical council shoulders the responsibility of exercising the disciplinary control over the registered medical practitioners on the state.
- The council has a power to remove the name of the person form the register, when he is convicted for a crime in a court of law.
- After doing a proper enquiry, if a registered medical practitioner is found guilty of infamous conduct.
- The removal of name may be temporary or permanent. Permanent removal of he name from state medical register amounts to professional death sentence.
- State medical council can also give warning notices from time-to-time to the registered medical practitioners regarding unethical practices.

Disciplinary Actions on the Registered Medical Practitioners

- By itself, the state medical disciplinary committee does not take into cognizance regarding the conduct of the registered medical practitioners.
- However, when a complaint is lodged by somebody, the disciplinary action committee informs the accused person in writing and gives him time to reply regarding the allegations made against him.
- After the reply received, if the committee wants to proceed further, it issues a notice to the practitioner and directs him to appear on a particular day and time for hearing purpose.
- After the due process, if it is felt that the registered medical practitioner is at fault, then the committee may recommend any of the following punishment:
  - Giving a warning to the doctor not to repeat in future.
  - A temporary removal of the name from the register (penal erasure).
  - Permanent penal erasure (professional death sentence).

Warning Notice

- Every registered medical practitioner is expected to follow a certain code of medical ethics. From time-to-time, violation of the code leading to professional misconduct causes infamous acts.
- The state medical council or the Medical Council of India from time-to-time issues a warning notice incorporating the infamous acts and warns the registered errant medical practitioners about the penal action likely to be carried out.

Infamous Conduct

- **Any conduct** on the part of a registered medical practitioner which is considered as disgraceful and dishonorable by professional brotheren of good repute is called as infamous conduct or professional misconduct. The following are commonly considered as infamous acts:
  - **Adultery**—having sex relations with a married woman or with married female.
  - **Association** with quacks, unqualified persons.
  - **Alcoholism**—attending patients under the influence of alcohol.
  - **Abortion**—which is considered criminal in nature.
  - **Abuse of drugs (addiction)**
  - **Advertisement**
  - **Abuse of dangerous drugs**
  - **Avoiding a patient to see when** called.

- **Avoiding to consult** another colleague when in doubt of poisoning or danger of it.
- **Infamous conduct** is also known as ethical malpraxis. Lord Justice Lopes laid down the definition of infamous conduct in the year 1894, "If a registered medical practitioner during his medical practice has done something which is reasonably regarded as disgraceful by his fellow registered medical practioners, who are reputed and competent, then he is guilty of infamous conduct".

Different Codes of Ethics

- The history of the first use of code of ethics in the practice of medicine can be traced as back as in the 5th and 4th century BC.
- Hippocrates recommended certain principles for those who choose to practice medicine.
- These principles with some modifications are accepted by the new practitioners in the form of oath.

The Oath of Hippocrates

- I swear by Apollo Physician, by Asklepios, by Heatlh, by Panacea, and by all the Gods and Goddesses, making them witnesses, that I will carry out, according to my ability and judgement, this oath and this indenture.
- To regard my teacher in this art as equal to my own parents; when he is need of money to share mine with him; to consider his offspring as my own brother; to teach them this art, if they require to learn it, without fee or indenture.
- To impart precept, oral instruction, and all other learning to my sons, to the sons of my teacher, and to pupils who have signed the indenture and sworn obedience to the physicians' law, but to none other.
- I will use treatment to help the sick according to my ability and judgement, but I will never use it to injure or wrong them.
- I will not give poison to anyone though asked to do, nor will I suggest such a plan.

- Similarly, I will not give a pessary to a woman to cause abortion. But in purity and holiness I will guard my life and my art.
- I will not use the knife either on sufferers from stone, but I will give place to such as art craftsman therein.
- Into whatsoever houses I enter, I will do so to help the sick, keeping myself free from all intentional wrong-doing and harm especially from fornication with woman or man, bond or free.
- Whatsoever in the course of practice I see or hear (or even outside my practice in social intercourse) that ought never to be published abroad, I will not divulge, but consider such things to be holy secrets.
- Now, if I keep this oath and break it not, may I enjoy honour in my life and art, among all men for all time; but if I transgress and forswear myself, may the opposite befall me.

The Declaration of Geneva, 1948

The World Medical Association at its third general Assembly at Geneva in September, 1948, adapted certain codes of ethics, in the form of oath to be taken by all members of the profession, at the time entering into medical profession.

The declaration of Geneva is as follows

1. I solemnly pledge myself to consecrate my life to the service of humanity.
2. I will give to my teachers, the respect, and gratitude which is their due.
3. I will practice my profession with conscience and dignity.
4. The health of my patient will be my first consideration.
5. I will respect the secrets which are confided in me.
6. I will maintain by all the means in my power, the honour and the noble traditions of the medical profession.
7. My colleagues will be my brothers.
8. I will not permit considerations of religion, nationality, race, party, politics or social standing to intervene between my duty and my patient.

9. I will maintain the utmost respect for human life from the time of conception. Even under threat, I will not use my medical knowledge contrary to the laws of humanity.

10. I make these promises solemnly, freely and upon my honour.

MALPRAXIS (MALPRACTICE/NEGLIGENCE)

- Malpraxis (wrong practice) is defined as want of reasonable care, judgement and skill or willful negligence on the part of doctor during the treatment of the patient that results in injury or loss of life to the patient. *The following are the ingredients of malpractice:*
  - Doctor–patient relationship
  - Duty on the part of doctor
  - Dereliction of duty
  - Damage to the patient
- This damage is due to the dereliction of duty or dereliction of the duty is the direct cause of damage. When a patient comes to a doctor for his professional guidance, the doctor and patient develop the professional relationship.
- In this relationship, the patient comes with faith in the doctor, he develops devotion towards the treatment of the patient. Once the doctor–patient relationship is established, the doctor is expected to discharge his professional duties towards his patient without any reservations.
- The doctor should not default in the discharge of his duties towards his patient. He is expected to bestow, upon his patient, reasonable care and skill that is expected from him, appropriate to the qualification, experience and knowledge.

- The standard of practice expected from his is the same as that of standard or expertise exhibited by his professional colleagues of similar qualification, experience and knowledge of practicing in the same area in which he is practicing.
- The skill expected from the MBBS doctor is of MBBS level. The skill expected from MD or MS is not of MBBS, but of MD or MS standard.
- In other words, the patient and public are entitled to demand reasonable care and skill from their doctor in the treatment.
- When the doctor fails to show reasonable care and skill or when he acts carelessly or rashly in his work, then due to his acts of omission or commission, the patient may suffer injury directly because of the action or inaction of the doctor.
- Once the damage has occurred in the form of defect or deformity or death or some complication due to the doctor's fault, the patient can demand compensation from the doctor for the damage caused to him.
- When no criminal law is violated then, to demand in forms of financial compensation, the patient can file a civil case against the doctor.
- When the negligence is very gross, suggesting the recklessness on the part of doctor, it becomes criminal malpraxis.
- Here, the state gets involved, the state prosecutes the doctor for offence like when

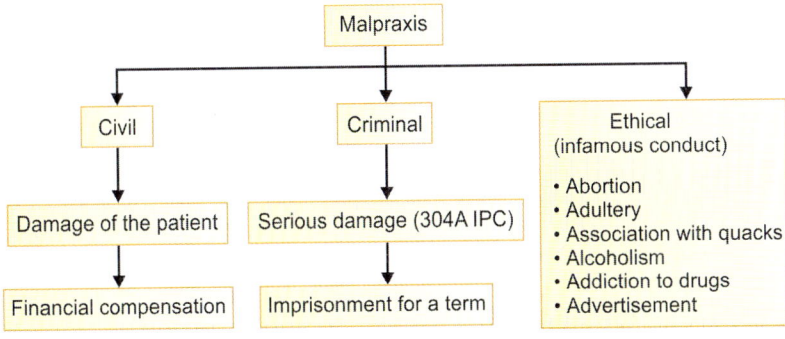

Fig. 32.1: Types of malpraxis

the patient dies by the negligent act of the doctor, the doctor may face a criminal case attracting imprisonment for a term in such cases.

- **When the code of medical ethics is violated, the doctor is involved in ethical malpraxis.**
- The patient who files the case has to shoulder the burden of proof in civil cases.
- However, sometimes when a swab or surgical instrument is forgotten in the abdomen and is recovered after other surgery, the very act of negligence stares at us.
- This is known as *Res Ipsa Loquitor,* which means that the thing speaks for itself.
- In such an event, the result is because of action of the doctor, this is called post-HoC of ergo Propter HoC which means that the thing that is happened and a consequence of the thing which has been done.

Negligence

- Doctor–patient relationship → doctor's duty to patient → damage to patient → damage due to patient's suffering → dereliction of duty → demand for compensation → proof of negligence → compensation or punishment or both.

Setup of Consumer Forum

↓

District level forum—District consumer redressal forum (up to 20 lakhs)

↓

State level forum—State consumer redressal forum (up to one crore)

↓

National level forum—National consumer grievance (more than one crore) redressel forum

↓

Supreme Court

- Sometimes when a senior doctor gives instruction to a junior, the junior person during his dealing with the patient causes damage to the patient.
- In such case, the damage suffered by the patient is not directly due to the dereliction

of duty on the part of doctor, but it is because of the negligent act of his junior or subordinate or assistant.

- Here the *maxim qui facit per oleun facit per second,* meaning one who acts through another acts himself, i.e. when somebody is acting through another person it amounts to actions by himself, this is also known as vicarious responsibility, the responsibility of the superior for the negligent act of juniors, this is also called respondent superior, i.e. let the superior be responsible.
- This becomes applicable only when, there is master–servant relationship between the senior and the junior.
- In a ship, whenever something happen wrong for all the activities, the captain of the ship is wholly responsible.
- In the same way, the head of the team the doctor becomes responsible for the negligence of the nurses and other assistant. This is known as the *doctrine of the captain of the ship.*
- In these cases of negligence, the doctor also gets some defences on his part, in other words like the doctor has duties to the patient and the patient also has duties to the doctor.
- The patient must give full history.
- He should not hide anything from the doctor.
- He should follow the advice of the doctor regarding investigation and treatment.
- He must obey instructions about, medicine, exercise, diet, etc.
- He should not desert the doctor and go away without informing the doctor.
- The act of negligence on the part of patient, in the doctor–patient relationship becomes critical for the doctor to plead defence in case of negligence suit.
- *Contributory negligence* is the negligence on the part of patient that has contributed to the damage and he suffers from his own fault.
- If he suffers bodily damage or death on account of such contribution, the doctor cannot be held responsible.

- In the same way, when the patient has not taken the medicine as directed by the doctor or when patient has not revealed history to the doctor or if he fails continuation of treatment as prescribed, if the patient does not get investigated as directed and consequently, he suffers damage, the doctor can plead defence on these grounds in case of a negligence suit.

CONSUMER PROTECTION ACT AND DOCTOR

- Before the Consumer Protection Act came into existence, negligent acts of the doctors were liable for civil and criminal cases and their proceedings were carried out in the relevant court of law.
- The Consumer Protection Act 1986 brought a change in this scenario.
- The Supreme Court of India vide its clear verdict, explicitly brought a change service rendered by the doctor for a consideration under preview of the CPA in the year 1995.
- As per the judgement of Supreme Court of India on 13th November 1995, the medical services delivered on payment basis can be questioned under the CPA before the Consumer Grievance Redressal Forum by the patients who feel aggrieved by the treatment meted to them from the doctor.

Who is a Doctor?

- The word doctor is derived from the Latin word *Docere* which means to teach. So, every doctor has a duty to teach the patient about his illness and its consequences besides giving treatment.
- A doctor is a registered medical practitioner (RMP) who is registered under the Medical Council of India Act and authorized to practice in this system in the authorized area by the said registration.

Who is a Patient?

A patient is any person who goes to the doctor for the relief of suffering or pain as a result of disease or illness or any other cause.

Who is a Consumer?

A consumer is a person who takes services from a doctor by paying a consideration in the from of money or otherwise or by promising to pay the consideration or by paying part of money with a promise to pay remaining consideration.

What is Deficiency?

Deficiency means fault, imperfection, short-comings or inadequacy of the quality, nature and manner of performance, needed by the doctor and/or a hospital.

What is Damage?

- Damage is the suffering on the part of the patient as a result of the deficiency in services rendered by the doctor.
- When a patient as a consumer by paying charge for the services rendered by the doctor suffers damage as a result of the deficiency in service due to the negligence of the doctor during his duty towards his patient, the patient can approach for compensation, the Consumer Protection Act.

How Patient will Approach the Forum?

- Before lapse of two years after suffering the damage, the patient as a consumer under the CPA becomes a complainant, the complainant can submit his complaint, in writing even by a simple postal letter giving details of his grievance.
- The procedure is simple. There is no court fees. On receiving the complaint, the Consumer Forum issues notice to the doctor who is accused of deficiency of services.
- The doctor gets 30 days time to reply to the notice from the forum.
- After receiving the reply or if he fails to reply, the forum proceeds further, it goes to the whole matter like whether there is doctor–patient relationship, whether the doctor has rendered services for considerations, whether there is deficiency in service or whether the patient has suffered from any damage?

- Whether the damage is due to deficiency in service, if the forum is satisfied that the patient as a consumer has suffered a deficiency in service, satisfying the provision of CPA, the doctor is asked to pay the penalty.
- The penalty to be paid by the doctor is decided by the forum.
- If he wants to contest the penalty and appeals against the judgement of the forum, he can apply for the permission of appeal and on getting permission, he can approach the higher forum.
- The district forum can try a case where the claim is up to rupees 5 lakhs.
- The state forum when the claims between rupees 5 and 20 lakhs and the national forum when the claim is more than rupees 20 lakhs.
- The consumer forum is expected to complete the hearing in 90 days and pass an order.
- If it wants to get some laboratory reports or laboratory test, the period may be 150 days.
- The appeal should be filed within 30 days after an order is passed by a district commission, a state commission or national commission, before the higher forum.
- Under the Consumer Protection Act, after going through the complaint, if it is found by the forum that the service provider (doctor) is not deficient and on the contrary, if the complaint filed by the complainant is a frivolous or ficticious, then not only the complaint may be dismissed but also a penalty may be imposed on the complainant up to an amount of Rs. 10,000.
- If the provider (doctor) or the complainant (patient) fails to obey the order of the forum, then such person is punishable with imprisonment for a period of not less than one month or up to 3 years or with fine not less than Rs. 2000, up to Rs. 10,000 or with both imprisonment and fine.

Composition of Forum

- The district forum consists of three members.
- The Chairman is of the rank of district judge and one lady must be present.
- The state commission also consists of three members.
- The national commission consists of five members.
- The Chairman of the state commission is the rank of high court judge and the Chairman of the national forum of the rank of Supreme Court judge.

Who cannot File under this Act?

- When the patient receives free treatment from a doctor or a hospital, the services rendered are free of cost, in such cases the patient cannot complain under this Act.
- However, a case may be filed in a civil court for compensation under civil malpraxis.

CONSENT

- When two persons come to an agreement about an act and both of them understand about it with the same meaning and the action is carried on one or the other or both carry out the act together, the said act is said to be carried out with consent.
- In fact, this is *mutual consent* brought about after understanding everything about the act being carried out and after knowing about the nature and consequences of the act once it is carried out.
- Here in relation to medical practice, the doctor carries out some action, the patient agrees to that action.
- Physical examination, anaesthesia, investigations, and surgical procedures are commonly performed activities performed by the doctors upon the patients.
- The doctor has to explain about the procedure and consequences of the procedure namely the benefits and side effects and complications which are likely to occur, if any.
- Thus, the doctor informs the patient about the pros and cons of the Act for which the patient is giving his agreement.
- In other words, the patient is being fully informed, such a consent where the

patient is made aware by the doctor about the benefits, and side effects of any procedure, the patient agreeing the consent is called *informed consent.*

Valid Consent

- A valid consent is one which is agreed upon by a patient after he/she is informed about the various aspects of the act and the patient agrees after understanding them.
- A legally valid consent is one wherein a valid consent is given by the person who is above the age of legally permitted age.
- Any person in sound state of mind *who is above 12 years* can give a valid consent.
- A person below the age of 12 years cannot give a valid consent, so the consent of *parent or guardian* is required to be taken.
- A consent can be *implied or express consent.*
- An implied consent is a consent which is implied in the very act of the patient.
- When a patient enters the doctor's clinic, there is an implied consent for a routine medical examination and treatment.
- An express consent is an consent which is specifically expressed in writing or orally.
- An express consent is written in most of the cases. A written consent is risk free and legally easily acceptable.
- A consent is invalid, when it is given by a person below the age of 12 years, a person who is of unsound mind, a person who is legally banned from giving a consent, consent which is not an informed consent, any consent obtained by putting a person under fear of death, hurt, impersonation or intoxication.
- Any consent, which is obtained without following rules and regulation, laid down by statute or law for examinations or actions that are bound by such statue or laws, e.g. consent by a girl below 18 years or sexual intercourse.
- A consent is not considered as a valid consent when it is given unknowingly.

Consent is obtained in relation to

- Medical examinations
- Injury certificates
- Organ experimentation
- Human experimentation
- Examination of victim in rape case or examination of victim in any case.

In all medicolegal examinations, a written consent is required

- Medical examination without consent is allowed to be carried out by a doctor when an accused person is brought for examination under arrest (Section 53, CrPC).
- In the case of persons of unsound mind who are suffering from mental illness, a consent is not only allowed, but it is valid during the remission phase or lucid interval.
- At this time, the patient has clear and sound mind and is capable of making reasonable judgements and, therefore, becomes responsible for actions carried out.
- The consent given during this lucid interval, therefore, becomes valid.
- After death, a consent for autopsy or for transplantation of organs is necessarily obtained from the legal custodian of the body.

TRANSPLANTATION OF HUMAN ORGANS

- Human Organs Act, 1994 brought into force from 4th Feb 1995, provides for the regulation of removal, storage and transplantation of human organs for therapeutic purposes.
- This Act also aims at the prevention of commercial dealings in human organs and for matters connected with it.
- According to this Act, a deceased person is one in whom there is permanent disappearance of life due to brainstem death.
- A donor is any person who is above 18 years of age.
- He willingly gives consent and authorizes for removal of organ for therapeutic purpose.
- A recipient is a person who receives the organ to be transplanted.
- Transplantation means grafting of human organ from any living or deceased person

to some other living person for therapeutic purpose.

- Only a board of medical experts is permitted to certify brainstem death for the purpose of removal of any organ.

The board consists of

- Hospital incharge
- One independent registered medical practitioner whom the hospital incharge calls.
- A neurologist or neurosurgeon nominated by the incharge.
- The registered medical practioner treating the patient in whom brainstem death has occurred.
- Removal of human organs are not authorized in which inquest is likely to be carried out on the body for purpose of law.
- No hospital other than the registered for the purpose can carry out removal, storage or transplantation of organs.
- No removal of organs is allowed for any other purpose except the therapeutic purpose.
- When the applicant for registration of the hospital is not happy with the decision of appeal to the central government or state government, depending upon whether the rejecting committee is of central or state government, within 30 days of receiving the order.
- Any unauthorized person removing the organs is punishable for a term of 5 years and a fine of Rs. 10,000.
- If a registered medical practitioner receives punishment for unauthorized removal of organs, then the authority also can inform the state medical council to remove the name from the register for 2 years for the first offence, for a subsequent offence permanent removal of the name from register is done.
- Any action of commercial nature connected with human organ transplantation is liable to be punished for an imprisonment up to 7 years and fine up to Rs. 20,000.
- The minimum punishment in such cases is 2 years imprisonment and Rs. 10,000 fine.

- The court has a power to give less punishment but it has to give the reason in the judgement, if it gives less than the minimum punishment.
- The cases under this Act are tried by a first class judicial magistrate or a metropolitan magistrate.
- The magistrate takes cognizance of the offence after receiving complaint from appropriate authority.

Duties of Registered Medical Practitioner

The registered medical practitioner should see:

- The donor has given authorization or not.
- The donor is in proper health and fit to donate the organ.
- The donor should be a near relative of the recepient.
- On the donor and the recipient, test has to be carried out for HLA and genetic compatibility.
- First DNA test with two multilocus gene probe is carried out, if the routine tests do not establish the relationship between donor and recipient; in such cases, tests are done using at least two multilocus gene probe; if this also fails, then DNA polymorphism with five multilocus gene probe should be done.
- If the husband or the wife is the donor, then a certificate to that effect is taken from both of them.
- In the case of removing organs form dead body, the registered medical practitioner should satisfy that the donor has clearly authorized the removal and did not withdraw authorization before death otherwise the legal custodian can give the permission.
- The registered medical practitioner also should be satisfied that if the donor is in brainstem death, all the members of the board should sign the certificate; if the donor is below 18 years of age, the consent of the parents must be obtained.

MEDICAL INDEMNITY INSURANCE

- After the advent of Consumer Protection Act, the Supreme Court verdict declared that the doctors meddling with is patients on payment as services under this Act.

- The medical profession is threatened with uncertain situations of who among his patients and when converts himself into a consumer and charge him with a case demanding huge sum of money for damages suffered by him as compensation.
- So the registered medical practitioner is placed in a situation where without hesitation and confidence he can proceed with his patients.
- Something is required to reveal and regenerate confidence in the registered medical practitioner to face the consumerist patient bravely.
- To that end, the medical indemnity insurance serves the purpose.
- When claims arise out of bodily injury or death of any patient caused by or alleged to have been caused by omissions or negligence in services rendered, the registered medical practitioner who is covered under the medical indemnity insurance, enjoys the umbrella of the company which the indemnity the injured person against legal liability to pay the compensation including the defence cost, fees as expenses.
- Presently, the Oriental Insurance Company, and the General Insurance Corporation provide medical indemnity insurance cover.
- The amount of premium varies depending upon the speciality of the doctor.

PRENATAL DIAGNOSTIC TECHNIQUES ACT, 1996

- From 1st January 1996, the Government has prohibited the use of prenatal diagnostic techniques like ultrasonography, amniocentesis and others, for the purpose of determination of sex of unborn child.
- Under this Act, only authorized and registered genetic clinics, genetic counselling centres and genetic laboratories are authorized to conduct prenatal diagnostic techniques and to offer genetic

counselling. Prenatal tests are carried out for the purpose of detecting:
  - Genetic disorders
  - Metabolic disorders
  - Chromosomal disorders (abnormalities)—congenital malformations
  - Sex-linked disorders
  - Haemoglobinopathies, etc

The prenatal diagnostic tests are carried out only in cases of:

- Pregnant women above 35 years.
- Pregnant women who have undergone two or more natural abortions.
- Pregnant women who are exposed to teratogenic drugs, radiation, infection or hazardous chemicals.
- Pregnant women having family history of mental retardation or physical deformity like spasticity.
- Written consent must be obtained from the patient as per the above rules. Even after the examination, the sex of the foetus should not be told to the pregnant woman or relatives by gestures, signs or any other manner.
- There is prohibition of advertisements by any person or genetic counseling center or laboratory for prenatal determination of sex.
- Anybody who carries out advertisement of any type is liable for punishment of imprisonment up to 3 years and fine up to Rs. 10,000.
- Any doctor who informs the sex of unborn child is liable for imprisonment up to 3 years and Rs. 10,000 fine for first time. On repetition, the imprisonment is 5 years and fine Rs. 50,000.
- If a doctor is convicted for this offence, his name is recommended to be erased from the medical register for a period of 2 years of first offence and permanently for subsequent offence.
- Anybody who brings any pregnant women for prenatal diagnostic technique for any purpose other than described under this Act shall be punished for imprisonment up to 3 years and fine of Rs. 10,000; for subsequent offence imprisonment of 5 years and fine of Rs. 50,000. All records

connected with matters under this Act should be preserved for a period of 2 years.

HUMAN RIGHTS AND ABUSES

- The World Medical Association wants the members of medical profession to see that human rights violations are not conceded.
- Adequate human care should be given to all human beings irrespective of caste, creed, colour, race, sex and whether he is a free person or prisoner (legal status).
- The prisoner should get a human treatment. Doctors who are incharge of prisoners or custody persons have a duty to provide protection of their mental and physical health.
- The quality and standard of medical treatment should be the same as is given to the free persons.

Rights of Victims

- We come across various types of victims in medicolegal practice, i.e. victims of rape, dowry and torture (cruelty), abortion, patient as a victim (as a consumer).
- All these victims have right to approach the police and file a case against the persons victimising them and seeking redressal of the grievance.

Torture Victims

Torture is of two types—physical and psychological.

1. **Physical torture** includes beating, heating, electrocution, suspending in normal or abnormal positions, using irritants, roller torture, sexual torture, mutilation, asphyxial torture.
2. **Psychological torture** consists of deprivation, coercion, communication.
   - **Deprivation:** Includes social, sleep, sensory and perception deprivation, deprivation of nutrition, hygienic deprivation and deprivation of health services.
   - **Coercion:** Humiliation, threat, sexual torture, etc.
   - **Communication:** By giving wrong information, distortion of perception.

Treatment of Torture

- Remove the torture source or agent.
- Treat the patient for physical and psychological relief.

Medicolegal and Ethical Aspects of Torture

- The doctor should not associate himself with any type of torture on human beings.
- The doctor will not provide any place or instruments to help the torture practice.
- The doctor should not be present when any torture proceedings are going on.
- Doctor should have clinical independence in deciding what went wrong.
- If a prisoner refuses food, he cannot be forced to take nourishment, but when a patient is unable to make voluntary decision about refusal, he should be fed with force.

Table Deaths (Deaths on Operation Table)

Deaths during and after surgery wake-up the patient's relatives to file a case against the surgeons and anaesthesiologist.

The surgical reasons for table deaths are:

- Death due to injury or disease.
- Death due to diseases other than for which operation is carried.
- Death due to disease not diagnosed before operation.
- Major blunder like cutting of large vessel or rupturing the respiratory passage.
- Surgical complications like, shock, haemorrhage, embolism, etc.
- Other cases like electrocution due to leaking cautery during surgery.
- Injuries due to fall from operation table.
- Injuries due to shifting from one place to other.
- During surgery, on wrong patient, wrong organ.

Causes Connected with Anaesthesia

- Giving anaesthesia to a wrong patient.
- Wrong posture of the patient causes paralysis of a part of limb.

- Faulty anaesthetic equipments
- Failure to recognize impending danger while monitoring the vital signs.

Anaesthetic Complications

Coughing, cardiovascular complications, airway obstruction, bronchospasm, hypoventilation, arrhythmias, hypertension, hypotension, regurgitation of gastrointestinal tract contents, anaphylactic reactions, due to anaesthetic agents, barbiturate, succinylcholine (muscle relaxant), malignant hyperthermia.

Medicolegal Issues

- Table death enquiry is to be carried out by a magistrate.
- The anaesthesist, surgeon and hospital are likely to face litigation for negligence under Section 304A (Rash and Negligent Act).
- The anaesthetist, surgeon, and hospital also face civil compensation case under the civil law of negligence.
- The anaesthetist, surgeon, and hospital are liable to face a suit for damage under the Consumer Protection Act.

HOSPITAL WASTE MANAGEMENT

- On March 1, 1997, the Supreme Court directed the government to see that every hospital and nursing home, if more than 50 beds, dispose hospital waste by incinerator or alternate methods.
- Biomedical wastes should not be mixed with other wastes. Maintenance of the records of disposal is compulsory.
- It is subjected to inspection and verification by the environment pollution control board.

Categories of Hospital Waste

- General waste
- Clinical waste
- Chemical waste
- Radioactive waste
- Pressurized containers
- Usually the hospital wastes are 80–85% non-infectious wastes, 10% infectious wastes, and 5% hazardous wastes.

- The amount of waste generated is 1–10 kg/bed/day. The biomedical waste is disposed as follows:
  - Black bags—food waste, paper, dry waste.
  - Blue bags—crushed syringes, needles.
  - Red bags—IV sets, urobags, catheters.
  - Yellow bags—dressing material, body parts, placenta, plaster cast, etc.

Method of Disposal

- **Black bags:** The material is disposed off in a secured land, filling place.
- **Blue bags:** Disposed by autoclaving, microwave, chemical treatment.
- **Red bags:** Autoclaving, microwave, chemical treatment.
- **Yellow bags:** Incinerator or deep burial.
- Microbiology and biotechnology wastes (wastes from laboratory cultures, specimens of microorganism, vaccines, human and animal cell culture, infectious agents from research, etc.) are treated and disposed by heat autoclaving, microwave and incineration.
- If the hospital waste is not disposed in safe manner, government from time-to-time checks the institutions under Section 15 of the Environmental Protection Act.
- Government has the power to punish the defaulter. The punishment is imprisonment up to 5 years or penalty up to Rs. 5 lakhs or both.
- If the default continues then for everyday a fine of Rs. 5000/day up to one year afterwards imprisonment up to 7 years.
- By the end of 2002, every clinic and hospital in India is completely covered under this Act, so every doctor should know the severe punishment, liable to pay for disobeying the rules of biomedical waste disposal.

Health Hazards of Hospital Waste

- Injuries from sharp objects can occur to all categories of hospital staff and those who are handling the waste. These injuries can cause tetanus, AIDS, hepatitis 'B' and 'C', septicemia and infections.

- Risk of infections outside hospital for people handling waste and the general public like hepatitis, AIDS, typhoid and gastroenteritis, etc.
- Recycling of disposable material, like syringes, needles, etc.
- Parasitic infections can occur from hospital waste.

DEATH AND EUTHANASIA

- Death can occur in a painless and sudden fashion.
- However, it is not in every case, there are many patients who suffer from pain and severe structural and functional disabilities for long time.
- Such types of frustrations create loss of confidence on one's own self and also on the medical system.
- Doctors in practice face these situations frequently, but they should not be tempted to short circuit the lifespan.
- If any person including a doctor tries to carry out any procedure or advise the patient to use certain types of drugs or chemicals not with intention of relieving of suffering but with an intention of relieving of suffering but with an intention to hasten the death or precipitate the death, then death is precipitated by the action of the doctor even with the consent of the patient thinking that this is the only way of relieving the suffering, it amounts to euthanasia.
- Euthanatos (Eu: well; Thanatos: Death). When a doctor tries to give a good death to the patient by his actions, it becomes euthanasia or mercy killing.
- This is positive or active euthanasia.
- When the doctor remains silent and withdraws life-saving methods to hasten the death, it becomes passive euthanasia. The Nagoya High Court in 1986 stated:
  - That the victim must be suffering an incurable illness and that death is imminent.
  - That he must suffer from unbearable pain obvious to anyone.
  - That the purpose of the mercy killing is the relief of pain.
  - That the ailing person's conscience is clear and that he, in all seriousness arises for or approves the mercy killing.
  - That it is performed by a physician, unless that is not possible.
  - That the method of killing is morally accepted.
  - In USA, Dr Jack Kevorkian started assisted suicide openly to help voluntary euthanasia.
  - In 1999, he was sentenced to 10–25 years imprisonment for causing death of Thomas Yonk suffering from motor neuron disease. *In India, euthanasia is not legal.*

However, passive euthanasia, i.e. on advance directive by patient and with a DNR (do not resuscitate order), the patient can be allowed to breath his last. This is now permitted. Attempt to suicide is considered as psychiatric need for counselling and prevention and so this is considered not a crime. However, abetment continuous to be a crime.

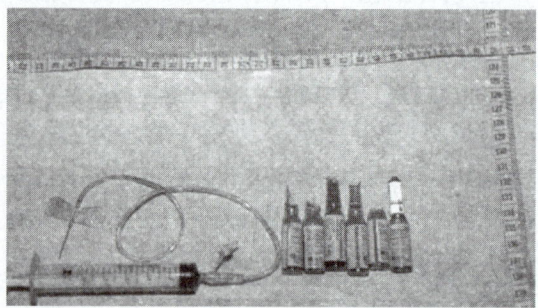

Fig. 32.2: Preparation of suicide

Medicolegal Issues of Medical Records

- Medical records are the properties of hospital, nursing homes or clinics.
- The confidentiality of the medical record must be maintained by the hospitals.
- Hospitals must keep the records as per the international rules laid down for the maintenance of the records.

- A discharged patient should be given discharge summary even when he is discharged against medical advice (DAMA) and death summary should be issued to the next of kin.
- Courts have the power to summon any medical record.

Medicolegal Importance of Medical Records

- Insurance cases
- Consumer protection cases
- Personal injury claim cases
- Workmen compensation claim cases
- Dying declaration
- Injury certificates
- Autopsy records
- There are a number of insurance claims in relation to death, injuries and disability. When the insurance company asks for certificate from the doctor, this certificate should be given.
- When a patient turns into a litigant and files a case against the doctor in consumer grievance redressal forum, the hospital has to provide the record to the forum.
- Personal injury claims are made in vehicular accidents of third party nature and comprehensive nature cases.
- The insurance company seeks the medical record. The company has to be provided with the certificate concerning the injuries.
- Workman Compensation Act 1923 involving the issue for the workman suffering loss during the work in which the person is engaged.
- The employer or the labour court secures the records or certificates.
- Dying declaration, injury certificates, autopsy records, and the recorded documents in relation to these issues are required in the court of law.
- They are received by the investigating officer and the court for the said purpose.
- The party involved in this case can obtain the copy from police or court.

Hospital Emergency Service

The Supreme Court of India gave the directions to be followed in these cases. These are:

- The doctor on emergency duty should admit the patient who is in serious condition.
- He should consult the concerned specialist.
- Patient should not be left unattended.
- The medical record should be preserved in the medical record department.
- The hospital register should contain the name, age/sex, address and the illness of the patient.
- Date and time of medical attention should be maintained.
- A copy of the roster duty of the doctor should be available in the medical superintendant's office.
- The medical officers should write their names clearly and also put signatures.
- From time-to-time, and the emergency drugs, instruments must be checked and kept in working order.

ARTIFICIAL INSEMINATION

- Artificial insemination is not natural insemination.
- It is insemination or introduction of semen in female genital tract artificially, by means of instruments.
- When the husband's semen is used it is called homologus AIH.
- If other than husband semen is used, it is called AID (donor insemination).

Indications of Artificial Insemination

- When the husband is impotent, but fertile, AIH is done.
- When the husband is infertile, when there is Rh incompatibility between husband and wife, AID is done.

Selection of Donor for AID

- The donor or recipient or family should not know the identity of the donor or recipient.

- The donor must be below 40 years.
- He must be having already living and healthy children.
- Consent of husband and the recipient must be taken for pregnancy.

Selection of Recipient

- She must be around the ovulation period.
- She must be in good health and must not have gynaecological problems that disturb the pregnancy.

Procedure

- One ml of semen is deposited just above the internal is by sterile instrument as soon as the sample is collected.
- The semen sample should have normal sperm count and morphology.
- The semen sample is collected after 3 days of abstinence.
- After injection, the woman is asked to lie down in same position for about 6 hours.
- Throughout the procedure, a lady attendant must be present.

Legal Issues of Donor Insemination

- As long as the husband does not raise issue, there is no problem including legitimacy.
- **Assisted reproduction:** *In vitro* fertilisation and embryo transfer back into the woman's uterus can help in conception, this helps in cases where there is some problem for women.
- In cases when there is some problem for man like quantity and quality of spermatozoa, a micromanipulation.
- This facilitates fertilisation and conception in women who have no problem.

Surrogate Mother or Borrowed Womb

- It is used in cases of women who cannot carry on the pregnancy.
- The fertilised ovum is installed into mother who carries on further pregnancy till delivery and hands back the child to the biological mother.
- Medicolegal problem that can arise is that, the surrogate mother refuses to handover the child to the biological mother.

STERILISATION

- In government hospitals, sterilisation is provided free of cost for both men and women.
- The husband should be above 25 years and below 50 years of age.
- The wife should be above 20 years and below 40 years of age.
- They should have two children at the time of operation.
- In males, vasectomy is done and in women tubectomy is carried out.
- Written consent of the partners is required.
- Permanent sterilisation is vasectomy in male and tubectomy in female and temporary sterilisation is by using hormones, lippes loop, etc.

Quality Family Planning

New Facilities for Doctors and Patients

- Millions of couple in our country plans their families by opting for tubectomy, vasectomy or other methods of contraception.
- The Government of India has taken special steps to improve the quality of family planning services and provide insurance cover to them.

All health facilities providing family planning services will ensure:

- Empanelled doctors, qualified and trained, to provide sterilisation services.
- Doctors to screen the acceptor's fitness through a checklist before the operation.

Benefits under the scheme arising out of sterilisation:

- Failure of sterilisation: RS. 30000/–
- Complications up to 6 days from the date of discharge: Rs. 25000/–
- In the unlikely even of loss life.
- During operation in the hospital or within 7 days of discharge from the hospital: Rs. 2 lakh.
- Within 8 to 30 days from the date of discharge from the hospital: Rs. 50000/–
- Indemnity cover to all government and accredited private doctors/health facilities rendering family planning services up to a maximum amount of

Rs. 2 lakh doctor/health facility/case, maximum up to 4 cases per year.

Medicolegal Importance

- Cases of failure of vasectomy and tubectomy are known.
- They cause marital disharmony and allegations of infidelity.
- The doctor who has operated may face a case demanding compensation.

MEDICAL TERMINATION OF PREGNANCY

- Medical termination of pregnancy (MTP) is permitted in India after the MTP Act was introduced in 1971.
- Under this Act, MTP is permitted on the following grounds:
  - Therapeutic
  - Eugenic
  - Humanitarian
  - Social
- **Therapeutic:** When the woman is likely to suffer serious injury or death, if the pregnancy is allowed to continue.
- **Eugenic:** If the mother has suffered during the first trimester of pregnancy from infections like rubella virus, herpes, CMV or toxoplasmosis. If the child is allowed to be born, it may suffer from physical or mental abnormalities.
- **Humanitarian:** When rape is followed by pregnancy, such pregnancy can be terminated.
- **Social:** In married woman, the pregnancy has resulted due to failure of contraceptives.

Who can do medical termination of pregnancies (MTPs)?

A gynaecologist or any other doctor who has assisted in at least 25 such cases and authorised by the government to do MTPs.

Where medical termination of pregnancies (MTPs) can be done?

- They can be carried out in government hospitals or non-government institutions who are authorized for the purpose by the government.

- Written consent can be obtained from the women above 18 years, in women below 18 years or of unsound mind case, consent of guardian is required.

At what time of pregnancy, it is done?

- A single doctor can decide and perform less than 12 weeks, and between 12 and 20 weeks, a second medical officer's opinion is required.
- After 20 weeks, termination is not allowed except in emergency to save the life of mother.

Methods of Medical Termination of Pregnancies (MTP)

- Dilation and curettage
- Vacuum aspiration method
- Hysterotomy

Complications of Medical Termination of Pregnancies (MTPs)

- Immediate—shock and haemorrhage perforation, peritonitis, embolism.
- Delayed complication—infertility, PID.

NULLITY OF MARRIAGE

Marriage is declared null and void under the following circumstances:

- When the marriage is performed below the age of legally valid marriage age. 18 years in case of female, 21 years in case of male. When one of the married partners is of unsound mind at the time of marriage.
- Consumation of marriage has not taken place due to refusal to Sexual Act or impotence.
- When a women is proved to have been pregnant by another man at the time of marriage.
- When it is found out that either the man or woman was already legally married before this marriage.
- In nulity of marriage, the law declares that no marriage has been registered in law between the two persons in question.

DIVORCE

Divorce differs from nullity of marriage. In the case of divorce, the existing legally valid marriage is legally dissolved and divorce is granted.

- By mutual consent.
- When the husband is doing actions like sodomy, bestiality.
- When the husband is found guilty of rape.
- In case of unsoundness of mind which appears to have no cure.
- In leprosy or sexually transmitted diseases. In the partner, if a communicable form existing for three years.
- In case of adultery.

BLOOD BANKS

- The blood banks in India are permitted to operate with a licence from the authority at the national level after due recommendation from the state level authority.
- Blood banks are required to possess sufficient space as per the rules and regulation, for reception, taping, refreshment, storage and distribution.
- Platelet separation is to be done by the blood banks as per the recommendations of NACO and drugs controller.
- Commercial donors are prohibited. Only voluntary donors are permitted.
- Any donor cannot repeat the donation before the lapse of 2 months after first donation.
- Each taping is not permitted to exceed 300 ml normally (8 ml/kg body weight).
- Emergency drugs and oxygen should be available in the blood bank to help the donor and recipient, if and when required.
- The donor is allowed to leave the place after satisfying that he is normal.
- The recipient is permitted to receive blood carefully and without permitting overloading.
- Immediate blood transfusion reactions sometimes occur, so without crossmatching blood should not be transferred.
- Those whose weight is less than 35 kg are not entitled to donate. Blood transfusion reactions can occur in the recipient immediately when there is mismatched blood transfusion.
- The patient develops rigor, compression of chest, presence of free haemoglobin in the blood, high levels of bilirubin, haemoglobinuria, with positive urobilinogen and urobilirubin.
- Mismatched blood transfusion causes immediate death, sometimes the patient may survive.
- Blood transfusion can lead to infections, to serious disease like AIDS, hepatitis 'B', malaria, syphilis, etc.
- Blood bags of 150, 300 and 450 ml are used. Maximum amount collected is 450 ml.
- Air embolism may occur, if about 100 ml of air enters the vessel during the transfusion.
- Excess volume transfusion can cause pulmonary oedema and overloading over heart.

PRESUMPTION OF SURVIVORSHIP

- Law presumes that a person is alive unless he is not heard off for a period of seven years by the nearest and dearest with whom he is in communication, after he lived for a period of 30 years, otherwise the law presumes that the person is alive.
- The problem of presumption of survivorship can also occur in disasters like plane crash, mines caving, shipwreck, earthquake, war, etc.
- There is no specific law in country for this.
- The factors to be into consideration are—age, sex, health, injuries, mode of death like drowning, asphyxia, starvation, cold, heat, burns, suffocation, and delivery.
- Adults survive better than young and old persons. Males survive longer than females.
- Healthier persons, swimmers survive over non-swimmers.
- In stampede, people nearer to surface and with less injuries, survive more to deeper and with more injuries.
- Adults tolerate cold more than children and older people. Heat is tolerated more by old people.
- When the oxygen is less, women survive more than men.

- *All the presumptions are useful when the time of death is in doubt.*

Presumption of Death

- The question of presumption of death occurs in cases of:
  - Property
  - Insurance
  - Inheritance, etc.

- This question arises when a person is believed to be dead and the body is not seen after death.

- A person who is living for the last 30 years and he is not heard for a period of 7 years by his near and dear ones, the presumption is in favour of death unless proved otherwise.

WORKMEN'S COMPENSATION ACT, 1923

SCHEDULE 1

(See sections 2(1) and 4)

Part I

List of injuries deemed to result in permanent total disablement

Serial no.	Description of injury	Percentage of loss of earning capacity
1.	Loss of both hands, or amputation at higher sites	100
2.	Loss of hand and a foot	100
3.	Double amputation through leg or thigh, or amputation through leg or thigh on one side and loss of other foot	100
4.	Loss of sight to such an extent as to render the claimant unable to perform any work for which eyesight is essential	100
5.	Very severe facial disfigurement	100
6.	Absolute deafness	100

Part II

List of injuries deemed to result in permanent partial disablement

Serial no.	Description of injury	Percentage of loss of earning capacity
	Amputation case—upper limbs (either arm)	
1.	Amputation through shoulder joint	90
2.	Amputation below shoulder with stump less than 8 inches from tip of acromion	80
3.	Amputation from 8 inches from tip of acromion to less than 4½ inches below tip of olecranon	70
4.	Loss of a hand or of the thumb and four fingers of one hand or amputation from 4½ inches below tip of olecranon	60
5.	Loss of thumb	30
6.	Loss of thumb and its metacarpal bone	40
7.	Loss of four fingers of one hand	50
8.	Loss of three fingers of one hand	30
9.	Loss of two fingers of one hand	20
10.	Loss of terminal phalanx of thumb	20

(Contd.)

List of injuries deemed to result in permanent partial disablement *(Contd.)*

Serial no.	Description of injury	Percentage of loss of earning capacity
	Amputation cases—lower limbs	
11.	Amputation of both feet resulting in end-bearing stumps	90
12.	Amputation through both feet proximal to metatarsophalangeal joint	80
13.	Loss of all toes of both feet through the metatarsophalangeal joint	40
14.	Loss of all toes of both feet proximal to the proximal interphalangeal joint	30
15.	Loss of all toes of both feet distal to the proximal interphalangeal joint	20
16.	Amputation at hip	90
17.	Amputation below hip with stump not exceeding 5 inches in length measured from tip of great tronchanter	80
18.	Amputation below hip with stump exceeding 5 inches in length measured from tip of great tronchanter but not beyond middle thigh	70
19.	Amputation below middle thigh to 3½ inches below knee	60
20.	Amputation below knee with stump exceeding 3½ inches but not exceeding 5 inches	50
21.	Amputation below knee with stump exceeding 5 inches	40
22.	Amputation of one foot resulting in end-bearing	30
23.	Amputation through one foot proximal to the metatarsophalangeal joint	30
24.	Loss of all toes of one foot through the metatarsophalangeal joint	20
	Other injuries	
25.	Loss of one eye, without complications, the other being normal	40
26.	Loss of vision of one eye, without complications or disfigurement of eye-ball, the other being normal	30
	Loss of fingers of right or left hand—index finger	
27.	Whole	14
28.	Two phalanges	11
29.	One phalanx	9
30.	Guillotine amputation of tip without loss of bone	5
	Middle finger	
31.	Whole	12
32.	Two phalanges	9
33.	One phalanx	7
34.	Guillotine amputation of tip without loss of bone	5
	Ring or little finger	
35.	Whole	7
36.	Two phalanges	6
37.	One phalanx	5
38.	Guillotine amputation of tip without loss of bone	2
	Loss of toes of right or left foot—great toe	
39.	Through metatarsophalangeal joint	14
40.	Part, with some loss of bone	3
	Any other toe	
41.	Through metatarsophalangeal joint	3
42.	Part, with some loss of bone	1

(Contd.)

Serial no.	Description of injury	Percentage of loss of earning capacity
	Two toes of one foot, excluding great toe	
43.	Through metatarsophalangeal joint	5
44.	Part, with some loss of bone	2
	Three toes of one foot, excluding great toe	
45.	Through metatarsophalangeal joint	6
46.	Part, with some loss of bone	3
	Four toes of one foot, excluding great toe	
47.	Through metatarsophalangeal joint	9
48.	Part, with some loss of bone	3

List of injuries deemed to result in permanent partial disablement (Contd.)

HUMAN DISABILITY EVALUATION

Necessity for evaluation of human disability arises for the purposes of:
- Workmen compensation
- Admission to schools and colleges
- Recruitment in service
- A ward of petrol pumps, ration shops, etc.
- Concession in railway travel
- Concession in bus travel
- Exemption from professional tax
- Concession in income tax
- Claims from accident—claims tribunals in cases of accidents
- Admission to special schools—deaf and dumb, blind, mentally retarded.

Types of Disabilities/Types of Challenges

- Physically handicapped or challenged
- Mentally handicapped or challenged
- Visually handicapped or challenged
- Hearing handicapped or challenged
- Mutism or vocally handicapped or challenged
- Evaluation under each category is carried out by the concerned specialist and certified by the authorized official in a government hospital.
- The benefits provided for handicapped persons are being availed more and more these days, awareness and education of the challenged persons by NGOs, etc.

MAINTAINING GOOD MEDICAL PRACTICE

- The principal objective of the medical profession is to render service to humanity with full respect for the dignity of profession and man.
- Physicians should merit the confidence of patients entrusted to their care, rendering to each a full measure of service and no devotion.
- Physicians should try continuously to improve medical knowledge and skills and should make available to their patients and colleagues the benefits of their professional attainments.
- The physician should practice methods of healing founded on scientific basis and should not associate professionally with anyone who violates this principle.
- The honoured ideals of the medical profession imply that the responsibilities of the physician extend not only to individuals but also to society.

Membership in Medical Society

- For the advancement of his profession, a physician should affiliate with associations and societies of allopathic medical professions and involve actively in the functioning of such bodies.
- A physician should participate in professional meetings as part of continuing medical education programmes, for at least 30 hours every 5 years, organized by reputed professional academic bodies or

any other authorized organisations. The compliance of this requirement shall be informed regularly to Medical Council of India or the state medical councils as the case may be.

Maintenance of Medical Records

- Every physician shall maintain the medical records pertaining to his/her indoor patients for a period of 3 years from the date of commencement of the treatment.
- If any request is made for medical records either by the patients/authorized attendant or legal authorities involved, the same may be duly acknowledged and documents shall be issued within the period of 72 hours.
- A registered medical practitioner shall maintain a register of medical certificates giving full details of certificates issued. When issuing a medical certificate, he/she shall always enter the identification marks of the patient and keep a copy of the certificate. He/she shall not omit to record the signature and/or thumbmark address and at least one identification mark of the patient on the medical certificates or report. Efforts shall be made to computerize medical records for quick retrieval.

Display of Registration Numbers

- Every physician shall display the registration number accorded to him by the state medical council/medical council of India in his clinic and in all his prescriptions, certificates, money receipts given to his patients.
- Physicians shall display as suffix to their names only recognized medical degrees or such certificates/diplomas and memberships/honours which confer professional knowledge or recognizes any exemplary qualification/achievements.
- These regulations may be called the Indian Medical Council (Professional Conduct Etiquette and Ethics) Regulations, 2002.
- They shall come into force on the date of their publication in the official Gazette 1st April 2002.

Code of Medical Ethics

Duties and Responsibilities of the Physician in General

- Character of physician (doctors with qualification of MBBS or MBBS with postgraduate degree/diploma or with equivalent qualification in any medical discipline)—a physician shall uphold the dignity and honour of his profession.
- The prime object of the medical profession is to render service to humanity.
- Reward or financial gain is a subordinate consideration.
- Whosoever chooses his profession, assumes the obligation to conduct himself in accordance with its ideals.
- A physician should be an upright man, instructed in the art of healing. He shall keep himself pure in character; discharging his duty without anxiety; conducting himself with propriety in his profession and in all the actions of his life.
- No person other than a doctor having qualification recognized by Medical Council of India and registered with Medical Council of India/state medical council(s) is allowed to practice modern system of medicine or surgery. A person obtaining qualification in any other system of medicine is not allowed to practice modern system of medicine in any form. If any one does as per the Supreme Court judgment, it becomes negligence *per se*.
- **Use of generic names of drugs:** Every physician should, as far as possible, prescribe drugs with generic names and he/she shall ensure that there is a rational prescription and use of drugs.
- **Highest quality assurance in patient care:** Every physician should aid in safeguarding the profession against admission to it of those who are deficient in moral practice. Any attendant who is unregistered or unqualified and shall not be permitted such persons to attend, treat or perform operations upon patients wherever professional discretion or skill is required.
- **Exposure of unethical conduct:** A physician should expose without fear or favour,

incompetent or corrupt, dishonest or unethical conduct on the part of members of the profession.

- **Payment of professional services:** The physician, engaged in the practice of medicine shall give priority to the interests of patients. The personal financial interests of a physician should not conflict with the medical interests of patients. A physician should announce his fees before rendering service and not after the operation or treatment is underway. Remuneration received for such services should be in the form and amount specifically announced to the patient at the time the service is rendered. It is unethical to enter into a contract of 'no cure no payment'. Physician rendering service on behalf of the state shall refrain from anticipating or accepting any consideration.

- **Evasion of legal restrictions:** The physician shall observe the laws of the country in regulating the practice of medicine and shall also not assist others to evade such laws. He should be cooperative in observance and enforcement of sanitary laws and regulations in the interest of public health. A physician should observe the provisions of the state acts like Drugs and Cosmetics Act, 1940; Pharmacy Act, 1948; Narcotic Drugs and Psychotropic Substances Act, 1985; Medical Termination of Pregnancy Act, 1971; Transplantation of Human Organ Act, 1994; Mental Health Act, 1987; Environmental Protection Act, 1986; Prenatal Sex Determination Test Act, 1994; Drugs and Magic Remedies (objectionable advertisement) Act, 1954; Persons with Disabilities (equal opportunities and full participation) Act, 1995 and Biomedical Waste (Management and handling) Rules, 1998 and other such Acts, Rules, Regulations made by the Central/ State Governments or local administrative bodies for the protection and promotion of public health.

Duties of Physicians to their Patients

Obligations to the Sick

- Though a physician is not bound to treat each and every person asking his service,

he should not only be ever ready to respond to the calls of the sick and the injured, but should be mindful of the high character of his mission and the responsibility he discharges in the course of his professional duties. In his treatment, he should never forget that the health and the lives of those entrusted to his care depend on his shill and attention. A physician should endeavour to add to the comfort of the sick by making his visits at the hour indicated to the patients. A physician advising a patient to seek service of another physician is acceptable, however, in case of emergency, a physician must treat the patient. No physician shall arbitrarily refuse treatment to a patient. However, for good reason, when a patient is suffering from an ailment which is not within the range of experience of the treating physician, the physician may refuse treatment and refer the patient to another physician.

- Medical practitioner having any incapacity detrimental to the patient or which can affect his performance vis-à-vis the patient is not permitted to practice his profession.

- **Patience, delicacy and secrecy:** Patience and delicacy should characterise the physician. Confidences concerning individual or domestic life entrusted by patients to physician and defects in the disposition or character of patients observed during medical attendance should never be revealed unless their revelation is required by the laws of the state. Sometimes, however, a physician must determine whether his duty to society requires him to employ knowledge, obtained through confidence as a physician, to protect a healthy person against a communicable disease to which he is about to be exposed. In such instance, the physician should act as he would wish another to act towards one of his own family in like circumstance.

- **Prognosis:** The physician should neither exaggerate nor minimize the gravity of a patient's condition. He should ensure himself that the patient, his relatives or his responsible friends have such knowledge of the patient's condition as this will serve the best interests of the patient and the family.

- **The patient must not be neglected:** A physician is free to choose whom he will serve. He should, however, respond to any request for his assistance in any emergency. Once having undertaken a case, the physician should not neglect the patient, nor should he withdraw from the case without giving adequate notice to the patient and his family. Provisionally or fully registered medical practitioner shall not willfully commit an act of negligence that may deprive his patient or patients from necessary medical care.

- **Engagement for an obstetric case:** When a physician who has been engaged to attend an obstetric case is absent and another is sent for delivery accomplished, the acting physician is entitled to his professional fees, but should secure the patient's consent to resign on the arrival of the physician engaged.

Duties of Physician in Consultation

- **Unnecessary consultations should be avoided:** However, in case of serious illness and in doubtful or difficult conditions, the physician should request consultation, but under any circumstances such consultation should be justifiable and in the interest of the patient only and not for any other consideration.

- Consulting pathologists/radiologists or asking for another diagnostic laboratory investigation should be done judiciously and not in a routine manner.

- **Consultation for patient's benefit:** In every consultation, the benefit to the patient is of foremost importance. All physicians engaged in the case should be frank with the patient and his attendants.

- **Punctuality in consultation:** Utmost punctuality should be observed by a physicians in making themselves available for consultations.

- **Statement to patient after consultation:** All statements to the patient or his/her representatives should take place in the presence of the consulting physicians, except as otherwise agreed. The disclosure of the opinion to the patient or his/her relative or friends shall rest with the medical attendant.

- Differences of opinion should not be divulged unnecessarily, but when there is irreconcilable difference of opinion, the circumstances should be frankly and impartially explained to the patient or his relatives or friends. It would be open to them to seek further advice as they so desire.

- **Treatment after consultation:** No decision should restrain the attending physician from making such subsequent variations in the treatment, if any unexpected change occurs, but at the next consultation, reasons for the variations should be discussed/explained. The same privilege, with its obligations, belongs to the consultant when sent for in an emergency during the absence of attending physician. The attending physician may prescribe medicine at any time for the patient, whereas the consultant may prescribe only in case of emergency or as an expert when called for.

- **Patients referred to specialists:** When a pataient is referred to a specialist by the attending physician, a case summary of the patient should be given to the specialist, who should communicate his opinion in writing to the attending physician.

- **Fees and other charges:** A physician shall clearly display his fees and other charges on the board of his chamber and/or the hospitals he is visiting. Prescription should also make clear, if the physician himself dispensed any medicine.

- A physician shall write his name and designation in full along with registration particulars in his prescription letter head.

Note: In gvernment hospital where the patient load is heavy, the name of the prescribing doctor must be written below his/her signature.

Responsibilities of Physicians to Each Other

- **Dependence of physicians on each other:** A physician should consider it as a pleasure and privilege to render gratuitous service to all physicians and their immediate family dependants.

- **Conduct in consultation:** In consultations, no insincerity, rivalry or envy should be indulged in. All due respect should be observed towards the physician incharge of the case and no statement or remark be made, which would impair the confidence reposed in him. For this purpose, no discussion should be carried on in the presence of the patient or his representatives.
- **Consultant not to take charge of the case:** When a physician has been called for consultation, the consultant should normally not take charge of the case, especially on the solicitation of the patient or friends. The consultant shall not criticize the referring physician. He/she shall discuss the diagnosis and treatment plan with the referring physician.
- **Appointment of substitute:** Whenever a physician requests another physician to attend his patients during temporary absence from his practice, professional courtesy requires the acceptance of such appointment only when he has the capacity to discharge the additional responsibility along with his/her other duties. The physician acting under such an appointment should give the utmost consideration to the interests and reputation of the absent physician and all such patients should be restored to the care of the latter upon his/her return.
- **Visiting another physician's case:** When it becomes the duty of a physician occupying an official position to see and report upon an illness or injury, he should communicate to the physician in attendance so as to give him an option of being present. The medical officer/physician occupying an official position should avoid remarks upon the diagnosis or the treatment that has been adopted.

Duties of Physician to the Public and to the Paramedical Profession

- **Physicians as citizens:** Physicians, as good citizens, possessed of special training should disseminate advice on public health issues. They should play their part in enforcing the laws of the community and in sustaining the institutions. That advance the interests of humanity. They should particularly cooperate with the authorities in the administration of sanitary/public health laws and regulations.
- **Public and community health:** Physicians especially those engaged in public health work, should enlighten the public concerning quarantine regulations and measures for the prevention of epidemic and communicable deseases. At all times, the physician should notify the constituted public health authorities of every case of communicable disease under his care, in accordance with the laws, rules and regulations of the health authorities. When an epidemic occurs, a physician should not abandon his duty for fear of contracting the disease himself.
- **Pharmacists/nurses:** Physicians should recognize and promote the practice of different paramedical services such as, pharmacy and nursing as professions and should seek their cooperation wherever required.
- **Unethical acts:** A physician shall not aid or abet or commit any of the following acts which shall be construed as unethical.
- **Advertising:** Soliciting of patients directly or indirectly, by a physician, by a group of physicians or by institutions or organisations is unethical. A physician shall not make use of him/her (orhis/her name) as subject of any form or manner of advertising or publicity through any mode either alone or in conjunction with others which is of such a character as to invite attention to him or to his professional position, skill, qualification, achievements, attainments, specialities, appointments, associations, affiliations or honours and/or of such character as would ordinarily result in his self aggrandisement. A physician shall not give to any person, whether for compensation or otherwise, any approval, recommendation, endorsement, certificate, report or statement with respect of any drug, medicine, nostrum

remedy, surgical, or therapeutic article, apparatus or appliance or any commercial product or article with respect of any property, quality or use thereof or any test, demonstration or trial thereof, for use in connection with his name, signature or photograph in any form or manner of advertising through any mode nor shall he boast of cases, operations, cures or remedies or permit the publication of report thereof through any mode. A medical practitioner is, however, permitted to make a formal announcement in press regarding the following:

– On starting practice
– On change of type of practice
– On changing address
– On temporaty absence from duty
– On resumption of another practice
– On succeeding to another practice
– Public declaration of charges.

- Printing of self photograph, or any such material of publicity in the letter head or on sign board of the consulting room or any such clinical establishment shall be regarded as acts of self-advertisement and unethical conduct on the part of the physician. However, printing of sketches, diagrams, picture of human system shall not be treated as unethical.

- **Patent and copyright:** A physician may patent surgical instruments, appliances and medicine or copyright applications, methods and procedures. However, it shall be unethical, if the benefits of such patents or copyrights are not made available in situations where the interest of large population is involved.

- **Running an open shop (dispensing of drugs and appliances by physicians):** A physician should not run an open shop for sale of medicine for dispensing prescriptions prescribed by doctors other than himself or for sale of medical or surgical appliances. It is not unethical for a physician to prescribe or supply drugs, remedies or appliances as long as there is no exploitation of the patient. Drugs prescribed by a physician or brought from

the market for a patient should explicitly state the proprietary formulae as well as generic name of the drug.

- **Rebates and commission:** A physician shall not give, solicit, or receive nor shall he offer to give, solicit or receive any gift, gratuity, commission or bonus in consideration of or return for the referring, recommending or procuring of any patient for medical, surgical or other treatment. A physician shall not directly or indirectly participate in or be a party to act of division transference, assignment, subordination, rebating, splitting or refunding of any fee for medical, surgical or other treatment.

- The above shall apply with equal force to the referring, recommending or procuring by a physician or any person, specimen or material for diagnostic purposes or other study/work. Nothing in this section, however, shall prohibit payment of salaries by a qualified physician to other duly qualified person rendering medical care under his supervision.

- **Secret remedies:** The prescribing or dispensing by a physician of secret remedial agents of which he does not know the composition, or the manufacture or promotion of their use is unethical and as such prohibited. All the drugs prescribed by a physician should always carry a proprietary formula and clear name.

- **Human rights:** The physician shall not aid or abet torture nor shall he be a party to either infliction of mental or physical trauma or concealment of torture inflicted by some other person or agency. If he does, it is clear violation of human rights.

- **Euthanasia:** Practicing euthanasia shall constitute unethical conduct. However, on specific occasion, the question of withdrawing supporting devices to sustain cardiopulmonary function even after brain death, shall be decided only by a team of doctors and not merely by the treating physician alone. A team of doctors shall declare withdrawal of support system. Such team shall consist of the doctor incharge of the patient, chief medical officer/medical officer in-charge of the hospital and a doctor nominated by the incharge of the hospital from the hospital staff or in accordance with the provisions of the Transplantation of Human Organ Act, 1994.

- **Misconduct:** The following acts of commission or omission on the part of a physician shall constitute **professional misconduct** rendering him/her liable for disciplinary action.

- If he/she **does not maintain the medical records** of his/her indoor patients for a period of three years and refuses to provide the same within 72 hours when the patient or his/her authorised representative makes a request for it.

- If he/she **does not display the registration number** accorded to him/her by the state medical council or the Medical Council of India in his clinic, prescriptions and certificates, etc. issued to him.

- **Adultery or improper conduct:** Abuse of professional position by committing **adultery or improper conduct** with a patient or by maintaining an improper association with a patient will render a physician liable for disciplinary action as provided under the Indian Medical Council Act, 1956 or the concerned state medical council act.

- **Conviction by court of law:** Conviction by a court of law for offences involving moral turpitude/criminal acts.

- **Sex determination tests:** On no account, sex determination test shall be undertaken with the intent to terminate the life of a female foetus developing in her mother's womb, unless there are other absolute indications for termination of pregnancy as specified in the Medical Termination of Pregnancy Act, 1971. Any **Act of termination of pregnancy of normal female foetus amounting to female foeticide shall be regarded as professional misconduct** on the part of the physician leading to penal erasure besides rendering him liable to criminal proceedings as per the provisions of this Act.

- **Signing professional certificates, reports and other documents:** Registered medical practitioners are in certain cases bound by law to give or may from time-to-time be called upon or requested to give certificates, notification, reports and other documents of similar character signed by them in their professional capacity for subsequent use in the courts or for administrative purposes, etc. **Any registered practitioner who is shown to have signed or given under his name and authority any such certificate, notification, report or document of a similar character which is untrue, misleading or improper, is liable to have his name deleted from the register.**

- A registered medical practitioner shall not contravene the provisions of the Drugs and Cosmetics Act and regulations made thereunder. Accordingly:

- **Prescribing steroids/psychotropic drugs when there is no absolute medical indication.**

- **Selling Schedule 'H' and 'L' drugs and poisons to the public except to his patient** in contravention of the above provision shall constitute **gross professional misconduct on the part of the physician.**

- **Performing or enabling unqualified person to perform an abortion or any illegal operation for which there is no medical, surgical or psychological indication.**

- A registered medical practitioner shall not issue certificates of efficiency in modern medicine to unqualified or non-medical person.

Note: The foregoing does not restrict the proper training, the instruction of bonafide students, midwives, dispensers, surgical attendants or skilled mechanical and technical assistants and therapy assistants under the personal supervision of physicians.

- A physician should not contribute to the lay press article and give interviews regarding diseases and treatments which may have the effect of advertising himself or soliciting practices; but is open to write to lay press under his own name on matters of public health, hygenic living or to deliver public lectures, give talks on the radio/TV/internet chat for the same purpose and send announcement of the same to lay press. An institution run by a physician for a particular purpose such as a maternity home, nursing home, private hospital, rehabilitation centre or any type of training institution, etc. may be advertised in the lay press, but such advertisements should not contain anything more than the name of the institution, type of patients admitted, type of training and other facilities offered and the fees.

- It is improper for a physician to use **an unusually large sign board** and write on it anything other than his name, qualifications obtained from a university or a statutory body, titles and name of his speciality, registration number including the name of the state medical council under which registered. The same should be the contents of his prescription papers. It is improper to affix a sign-board on a chemist's shop or in places where he does not reside or work.

- The registered medical practitioner **shall not disclose the secrets of a patient** that have been learnt in the exercise of his/her profession **except:**
  - **In a court of law under** orders of the presiding judges.
  - **In circumstances where there is a serious** and identified risk to a specific person and/or community.

- **Notifiable diseases**
  - In case of **communicable/notifiable diseases,** concerned public health authorities should be informed immediately.

- The registered medical practitioner **shall not refuse on religious grounds** alone to give assistance in or conduct of sterility, birth control, circumcision and medical termination of pregnancy when there is medical indication, unless the medical practitioner feels himself/herself incompetent to do so.

- Before performing an operation, the physician should obtain in writing the consent from the husband or wife, parent or guardian in the case of **minor,** or the patient himself as the case may be. In an operation which may result in sterility, the consent of both husband and wife is needed.

- A registered medical practitioner shall not publish photographs or case reports of his/her patients without their permission, in any medical or other journal in a manner by which their identity could be made out. If the identity is not to be disclosed, the consent is not needed.

- In the case of running a nursing home by a physician and employing assitants to help him/her, the ultimate responsibility rests on the physician.

- A physician shall not use touts or agents for procuring patients.

- A physician shall not claim to be specialist unless he has a special qualification in that branch.

- No act of *in vitro* fertilisation or artificial insemination shall be undertaken without the formal consent of the female patient and her spouse as well as the donor. Such consent shall be obtained in writing only after the patient is provided, at her own level of comprehension, with sufficient information about the purpose, methods, risks, inconveniences, disappointments of the procedure and possible risks and hazards.

- **Research:** Clinical drug trials or other research involving patients or volunteers as per the guidelines of ICMR can be undertaken, provided **ethical considerations are borne in mind. Violation of existing ICMR* guidelines** in this regard shall **constitute misconduct. Consent taken** from the patient for trial of drug or therapy which is **not as per the guidelines** shall also be **construed as misconduct**.

- If a physician posted in a **rural area is found absent on more than two occasions** during inspection by the head of the district health authority or the Chairman, Zila Parishad, the same shall be **construed as a misconduct,** if it is recommended to

*(ICMR—Indian Council of Medical Research).

the Medical Council of India/state medical council by the state government for action under these regulations.

- A physician posted in a medical college/institution both as teaching faculty or otherwise shall remain in hospital/college during the assigned duty hours. If they are 'found absent' on more than two occasions during this period, the same shall be construed as a misconduct, if it is certified by the Principal/Medical Superintendent and forwarded through the state government to Medical Council of India/state medical council for action under these regulations.

Punishment and Disciplinary Action

- It must be clearly understood that the instances of offences and of professional misconduct which are given above do not constitute and are not intended to constitute a complete list of the infamous acts which calls for disciplinary action and that by issuing this notice the Medical Council of India and/or state medical councils are in no way precluded from considering and dealing with any other form of professional misconduct on the part of a registered practitioner. Circumstances may and do arise from time-to-time in relation to which there may occur questions of professional misconduct which do not come within any of these categories. Every care should be taken that the code is not violated in letter or spirit. In such instances as in all others, the Medical Council of India and/or state medical councils have to consider and decide upon the facts brought before the Medical Council of India and/or state medical council.
- It is made clear that any complaint with regard to professional misconduct can be brought before the appropriate medical council for disciplinary action. Upon receipt of any complaint of professional misconduct, the **appropriate medical council** would **hold an enquiry** and **give opportunity to the registered medical practitioner to be heard in person or through pleader.** If the medical practitioner is **found to be guilty** of committing professional misconduct, the appropriate medical council **may award** such **punishment as deemed necessary or may direct the removal altogether** or **for a specified period, from the register of the name** of **the delinquent registered practitioner. Deletion** from the register shall be **widely publicised in local press as well as in the publications of different** medical associations/societies/bodies.

- In case, the punishment of removal from the register is **for a limited period,** the appropriate council may **also direct that the name** so removed **shall be restored** in the register **after the expiry of the period** for which the name was ordered to be removed.
- **Decision on complaint** against delinquent physician shall be taken **within a time limit of 6 months.**
- **During the pendency of the complaint, the appropriate council may restrain the physician from performing the procedure or practice which is under scrutiny.**
- **Professional incompetence shall be judged by peer group as per guidelines prescribed by Medical Council of India.**

DOCTOR AND TORTURE

Types of Torture

The process of torture usually starts after sunset in an isolated/remote/confined place with a formidable display of power associated with unnecessary unsystematic violence. This initial 'softening phase' continues for a couple of days and is followed latter by systematic violence/torture methods, when the torturer recognises the weak spots of the victim to make him/her breakdown. Torture has become a science where not only medical doctors, but also psychologists have been involved in developing new and even, more brutal methods to breakdown the victims.

The systematic torture can be divided into three basic categories:
1. Physical torture
2. Sexual torture
3. Psychological torture

It has been observed frequently that there is combination of different types of torture in a single individual. Physical/sexual torture is invariably associated with psychological torture in the form of 'torture syndrome'.

1. Physical Torture

The Human Rights Commission of El Salvador published a list of 40 different methods and the Chilean Human Rights Commission lists 85 different types of physical torture. However, some of the common methods of physical torture are:

- Beating on different body parts from head to toe can be accomplished by hands, rod, stick, chain or any other similar object, falanga is a special type of beating carried out by suspending a victim upside down and then beating over the soles by a rod/stick.
- Heat torture can be inflicted by means of cigarette, cigar, candle, hot iron or any other similar hot object placed on or very close to body especially over sensitive and/or concealed part of body.
- Electrical torture is done by giving electric shocks by placing the electrodes over concealed parts of body such as genitals, oral cavity, nipples, anal canal, armpits, nasal cavity, etc. so that it cannot be detected easily.
- Pulling and/or twisting of nails, hairs, tongue, teeth, breast or nipples or genitals by hands or through some device.
- Irritant torture is done by application of an irritant substance like chilly powder in eyes, genitals or anal region.
- They may also be asked to eat or drink irritants.
- The victim may be asked to walk on a thorny surface or over broken glasses barefooted.
- Ear torture is inflicted by beating both ears simultaneously with the palm of hands and is called 'telephone'.
- It causes rupture of tympanic membrane causing intense pain and bleeding with loss of hearing.
- Cold torture is done by making a person to walk barefooted on ice or in very cold water or making him lie down naked on ice or icy water for long time. One can also be submerged in ice-cold water.
- Suspension either by hands or legs for a sufficiently long time.

- Abnormal position that can be in sitting or standing or even lying down.
- Roller torture is done by applying roller, over the body in lying position.
- Asphyxial torture is accomplished by suffocating the victim either in a closed chamber or submerging in water called wet submarine or water asphyxiation.
- Pharmacological torture is done by administering drugs and chemicals that produce unpleasant symptoms. It is mostly conducted under medical supervision.
- Mutilation is done by inflicting very severe type of injuries all over the body so that it becomes difficult even to identify the individual.
- Piercing torture is done by pushing needles under nails or in tongue.
- Rope bondage is done by complete bondage of rope tightly either over extremities or all over the body.

2. Sexual Torture

The prevalence of sexual torture in different studies varies 14 to 16% among all torture cases. The sexual torture can be in the following forms:

- Violence on the sexual organs like injury/mutilation, etc. It can be performed by burning sensitive parts, by penetrating vagina and/or anus by inserting batons, rods, bottles, etc.
- Physical sexual assault, i.e. sexual act being performed by torturer on victim, by forcing sexual act among victims or performing sexual act by animals on the victims using different ways.
- Mental sexual assault can be done by forcing nakedness, asking to watch sexual torture, sexual humiliations or even sexual threats.
- Combination of above.

3. Psychological Torture

- The psychological torture has a very high prevalence rate varying from 33 to 77% in different series of torture cases.
- The different techniques used for psychological torture are:

– Deprivation techniques
- Social deprivation
- Sensory deprivation
- Perceptual deprivation
- Sleep deprivation
- Nutritional deprivation
- Hygienic deprivation
- Medical care deprivation

– Coercion techniques
- Impossible choice situation
- Humiliation
- Threats
- Blind obedience of rules

– Communication techniques
- Counter effect
- Double binding
- Disinformation
- Distortion of perception
- Conditioning to new reflexes

The effects of the physical torture can be appreciated and documented by a doctor when such examination is conducted:

- Carefully
- Using proper procedure and equipment
- Within a reasonable time after the incident
- The method of examination depends whether the victim is alive or dead.
- Examination of a live victim is not very much different from other medicolegal examinations.
- However, it can be modified depending upon the requirement of the case infrastructure available with the doctor.
- Basically, such an examination includes:
  - History taking
  - Examination
  - Evaluation
  - Conclusion
- A scheme of examination in torture cases on important points based upon Istanbul Protocol is given in (Table 32.1).
- Examination of cases of death due to torture. (Table 32.2) is one of most difficult cases for doctors that usually require expertise and integrity of the highest order.

Table 32.1: Examination of body parts in torture cases

Body part	Procedure and important lesions
1. Skin	Look for generalised skin diseases, pretorture lesions, torture lesions—abrasions, contusions, puncture, stab wound, and burns of any type, hair and nail removal. Describe their localisation, symmetry, shape, size, colour and surface. Opine whether self-inflicted or otherwise
2. Face	Palpate for evidence of fracture, crepitation swelling or pain. Look for deformity, swelling examine cranial nerves. CT is better option than routine radiography for diagnosing facial fractures
3. Eyes	Look for conjunctival haemorrhage, lens dislocation, subhyaloid haemorrhage, retrobulbar haemorrhage and visual field loss. Take an opinion from ophthalmologist. CT/MRI/high resolution ultrasound be used depending upon availability and indication
4. Ear	Examine tympanic membrane for rupture using an otoscope. Otorrhoea may be present in recent cases. Investigate for hearing loss, fracture of temporal bone or disruption of ossicular chain. Ultrasound can be used depending upon availability and indication
5. Nose	Examine for alignment, crepitation and deviation of septum. Simple fracture can be diagnosed by standard nasal radiography. For complex fractures, CT is recommended and if rhinorrhoea is present, CT and/or MRI should be done
6. Jaw, oropharynx and neck	Look for mandibular fracture/ dislocation, temporomandibular joint syndrome, crepitation and hyoid bone or laryngeal cartilages, cervical spine injuries, gingival haemorrhage and gum morphology

(Contd.)

Table 32.1: Examination of body parts in torture cases *(Contd.)*

Body part	Procedure and important lesions
7. Oral cavity and teeth	Examine for tooth avulsions, fractures of teeth, dislocated fillings and broken prostheses, dental caries and gingivitis, traumatic lesions in mouth, help of radiography and MRI may be taken depending upon the lesions type, extent and location
8. Chest and abdomen	Examine for pain, tenderness or discomfort, look for possibility of intramuscular, retroperitoneal and intra-abdominal haematomas. US, MRI and/or CT scan should be used, if intra-abdominal lesion is suspected
9. Genitourinary	Look for external lesions and foreign body. The equipment that can be used for internal examinations are colposcope, urethroscope, proctoscope, ultrasound and dynamic scintigraphy depending upon the signs/symptoms or allegations
10. Central/peripheral nervous system	Evaluate cognitive ability and mental status, look for raticulopathies, neuropathies, cranial nerve deficits, hyperalgesia, paraesthesias, hyperaesthesia, change in position and temperature sensation, motor functions like gait, muscle co-ordination and power. Apart from conventional radiography of skull, CT and/or MRI should be used to exclude intracranial trauma
11. Musculoskeleta	Look for pain, tenderness, haematomas in joint spaces and muscles, evidence of compartment syndromes, fresh or old fractures, osteomyelitis, deformities and dislocations. Investigations that can be used are routine radiography, arthoscopy, arthography, CT and bone scintigraphy

Table 32.2: Postmortem detection of torture case

Torture technique	Physical findings
Beating	
1. General	1. Scars, bruises, lacerations, multiple fractures at different stages of healing, especially in the unusual locations, which have not been medically treated.
2. To the soles of the feet ('falanga', 'falaka', 'bastinado') or fractures of the bones of the feet	2. Haemorrhage in the soft tissues of the soles of the feet and ankles. Aseptic necrosis
3. With the palms on both ears simultaneously ('el telefone')	3. Ruptured or scarred tympanic membrane. Injuries to the external ear
4. On the abdomen, while lying on a table with the upper half of the body unsupported ('operating table','el quirofano')	4. Bruises on the abdomen. Back injuries. Ruptured abdominal viscera
5. To the head	5. Cerebral cortical atrophy, scars, skull fractures, bruises, haematomas
Suspension	
6. By the wrists ('la bandera')	6. Bruises or scars about the wrists. Joint injuries.
7. By the arms or neck	7. Bruises or scars at the site of binding. Prominent lividity in the lower extremities
8. By the ankles ('murcielago')	8. Bruises or scars about the ankles. Joint injuries
9. Head down, from a horizontal pole placed under the knee with the wrists bound to the ankles ('parrot's perch', 'jack', 'pau de arara')	9. Bruises or scars on the anterior forearms and back of the knees. Marks on the wrists and ankles
Suffocation	
10. Forced immersion of the head in water, often contaminated ('wet submarine', 'pileta', 'latina')	10. Faecal matter or other debris in the mouth, pharynx, trachea, oesophagus or lungs, intrathoracic petechiae

(Contd.)

Table 32.2: Postmortem detection of torture case *(Contd.)*

Torture technique	Physical findings
11. Tying of a plastic bag over the head ('dry submarine')	11. Intrathoracic petechiae
Sexual abuse	
12. Sexual abuse	12. Sexually transmitted disease. Pregnancy. Injuries to the breasts, external genitalia, vagina, anus or rectum
Forced posture	
13. Prolonged standing ('el planton')	13. Dependent oedema. Petechiae in the lower extremities
14. Forced straddling of a bar ('saw horse', 'el cabellete')	14. Perineal or scrotal haematomas
Electric shock	
15. Cattle Prod ('La picana')	15. **Burns:** Appearance depends on the age of the injury. Immediately red spots, vesicles and/or black exudate *Within a few weeks*: Circular, reddish, mascular scars *After several months*: Small, white, reddish or brown spots resembling telangiectasis
16. Wires connected to a source of electricity	16. Perianal or rectal burns
17. Heated metal skewer inserted into the anus ('black slave')	17. Vitreous humour electrolyte abnormalities
Miscellaneous	
18. Dehydration	18. Bitemarks
19. Animal bites (spiders, insects, rats, mice, dogs)	

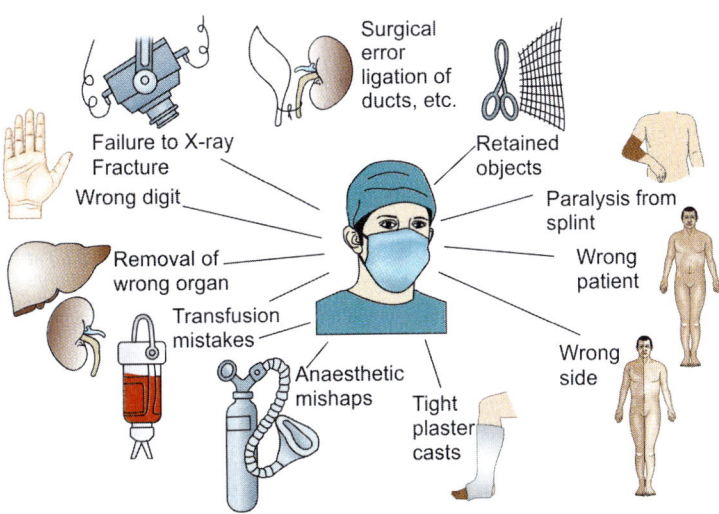

Fig. 32.3: Medical negligence: Some causes

- The goals for such an examination are:
  - What torture has taken place?
  - What types of injuries are present on the body?
  - How much is the duration of injuries?
  - What could be the possible mode of causation of injuries?
  - What is the nature of injuries?
  - What is the nature of weapon used?
  - Which injuries are fatal in ordinary course of nature?
  - What is the cause of death?
  - What are the contributing factors in causing the death?
- The examination should not be confined to that of the body alone, but should also include the history and death scene examination as they may provide vital clue to arrive it.

HOMEOPATHY—CENTRAL COUNCIL ACT, 1973
(No. 59 of 1973) (Extracts)

An Act provided for the constitution of a Central Council of Homeopathy and the maintenance of a Central Register of Homeopathy and for matters connected therewith. Be it enacted by Parliament in the twenty-fourth year of the Republic of India as follows:

Short Title, Extent and Commencement
- This Act may be called the Homeopathy Central Council Act, 1973.
- It extends to the whole of India.

Definitions
- In this Act, unless the context otherwise requires:
  - "Board" means a board, council, examining body or faculty of homeopathy (by whatever name called) constituted by the state government under any law for the time being in force regulating the award of medical qualifications, in, and registration of practitioners of homeopathy.
  - "Central Council" means the Central Council of Homeopathy constituted under Section 3.
  - Central Register of Homeopathy" means the register maintained by the Central Council of Homeopathy under this Act.
  - "Homeopathy" means the homeopathic system of medicine and includes the use of biochemic remedies.
  - "Medical Institute" means any institution within or without India which grants degrees, diplomas or licences in homeopathy.
  - "Prescribed" means prescribed by regulations.
  - "Recognised Medical Qualification" means any of the medical qualifications, in homeopathy, included in the second or the third schedule.
  - "Regulation" means a regulation made under Section 33.
  - "State Register of Homeopathy" means a register or registers maintained under any law for the time being in force in any State regulating the registration of practitioners of homeopathy.
  - "University" means any university in India established by law and having a faculty of homeopathy and includes a university in India established by law in which instruction, teaching, training or research in homeopathy is provided.
- Any reference in this Act to a law which is not in force in the State of Jammu and Kashmir shall, in relation to that state, be construed as a reference to the corresponding law, if any, in force in that State.
  a. The Central Government shall, by notification in the official Gazette, constitute for the purposes of this Act, a Central Council consisting the following members namely.
  i. Such numbers of members not exceeding five as may be determined by the Central Government in accordance with the provisions of the first schedule from each state in which, State Register of Homeopathy is maintained, to be elected from amongst themselves by persons enrolled on that register as practitioners of homeopathy.
  ii. One member from each university to be elected from amongst themselves by the members of the faculty or department (by whatever named called) of homeopathy of that university:
  - Provided that until any such faculty or department of homeopathy is started in at least seven universities, the Central Government may nominate such number of members not exceeding

seven as may be determined by the Central Government from amongst the teaching staff of medical institutions within India, so however, that the total number of members so nominated and elected under this clause shall in no case exceed seven.

iii. Such number of members, not exceeding 40% of the total number of members elected under clause (a) and (b), as may be nominated by the Central Government, from amongst persons having special knowledge or practical experience in respect of homeopathy or other related disciplines:
– Provided that until members are elected under clause (a) or clause (b) in accordance with the provisions of this Act and the rules made thereunder, the Central Government shall nominate such number of members, being persons qualified to be chosen as such under the said clause (a) or clause (b), as the case may be, as that government thinks fit; and references to elected members in that Act shall be construed as including references to members so nominated.

b. The President and the Vice-President of the Central Council shall be elected by the members of the Central Council from amongst themselves in such manner as may be prescribed.
– Provided that two years from the first constitution of the Central Council, the President and the Vice-President shall be nominated by the Central Government from amongst the members of the Central Council and the President and the Vice-President so nominated shall not withstanding anything contained in sub-section (1) of Section 7 hold office during the pleasure of the Central Government.

Incorporation of Central Council
The Central Council should have perpetual succession and a common seal, with power to acquire, hold and dispose of property, both movable and immovable and to contract and shall be a body corporate by the name of the Central Council of Homeopathy having by the said name sue and be sued.

Recognition of Medical Qualification Granted by Certain Medical Institutions in India
• The medical qualifications granted by any university, board or other medical institution in India which are included in the second schedule shall be recognised medical qualifications for the purpose of this Act.
• Any university, board or other medical institution in India which grants a medical qualification not included in the second schedule may apply to the Central Government to have any such qualification recognised and the Central Government, after consulting the Central Council, may, by notification in the official Gazette, amend the second schedule so as to include such qualification therein and any such notification may also direct that an entry shall be made in the last column of the second schedule against such medical qualification only when granted after a satisfied date.

Recognition of Medical Qualifications Granted by Medical Institutions in States or Countries Outside India
• The medical qualifications granted by medical institutions outside India which are included in the third schedule shall be recognised medical qualifications for the purposes of this Act.
a. The Central Council may enter into negotiations with the authority in any state or country outside India, which by the law of such state or country is entrusted with the maintenance of a register of practitioners of homeopathy, for setting of a scheme of reciprocity for the recognition of medical qualifications in homeopathy and in pursuance of any such scheme. The Central Government may, by notification in the official Gazette, amend the third schedule so as to include therein any medical qualification which the Central Council has decided should be recognised and any such notification may also direct that any entry shall be made in the last column of the third schedule against such medical qualification declaring that it shall be a recognised medical qualification when granted after a specified date.
b. Where the Council has refused to recommend any medical qualification which has been imposed for recognition by any authority referred to in clause (a) and that authority applies to the Central Government in this behalf, the Central Government, after considering such application and after obtaining from the Council a report, if any as to the reasons for any such refusal, may, by notification in the official Gazette, declare that such qualification shall be a recognised medical qualification and the provisions of clause (a) shall apply accordingly.

Rights of Persons Possessing Qualifications Included in Second or the Third Schedule to be Enrolled

- Subject to the other provisions contained in this Act, any medical qualification included in the second or the third schedule shall be sufficient qualification for enrollment on any State Register of Homeopathy.
- No person, other than a practitioner of homeopathy, who possesses a recognised medical qualification and is enrolled on a State Register or the Central Register of Homeopathy:
  - Shall hold office as homeopathic physical or any other office (by whatever designation called) in government or in any institution maintained by a local or other authority.
  - Shall practice homeopathy in any state.
  - Shall be entitled in sign or authenticate a medical or fitness certificate or any other certificate required by any law to be signed or authenticated by a duly qualified medical practitioner.
  - Shall be entitled to give any evidence at any inquest or any court of law as an expert under Section 45 of the Indian Evidence Act, 1872, on any matter **relating to homeopathy**.
- **Nothing contained in sub-section (2) shall affect:**
  - The right of a practitioner of Homeopathy enrolled on a State Register of Homeopathy to practice homeopathy in any state merely on the ground that, on the commencement of this Act, he does not possess a recognised medical qualification.
  - The privileges (including the right to practise homeopathy) conferred by or under any law relating to registration of practitioners of homeopathy for the time being in force in any state, on a practitioner of homeopathy enrolled on a State Register of Homeopathy.
  - The right of a person to practice homeopathy in a state in which on the commencement of this Act, a State Register of Homeopathy is not maintained if, on the commencement, he has been practising homeopathy for not less than five years.
  - The right conferred by or under the Indian Medical Council Act, 1956 (including the right to practice medicine as defined in clause (f) Section 2 of the said Act) or the Indian Medical Central Council Act, 1970 of persons possessing any qualification included in the respective schedules to the said Act.
- Any person who acts in contravention of any provision of sub-section (2) shall be punished with imprisonment for a term which may extend to one year or with fine which may extend to one thousand rupess or with both.

Power to Require Information as to Courses of Study and Examinations

Every University, Board or Medical Institutions in India which grants a recognised medical qualification shall furnish such information as the Central Council, may from time-to-time, requires as to the courses of study and examinations, to be undergone in order to obtain such qualification, as to the ages at which such courses of study and examinations are required to be undergone and such qualification is conferred and generally as to the requisites for obtaining such qualification.

Withdrawal of Recognition

- When upon report by the inspector or the visitor, it appears to the Central Council:
  - That the courses of study and examination to be undergone in, or the proficiency required from candidates at any examination held by any university, board or medical institution.

OR

  - That the staff, equipment, accommodation, training and other facilities for instruction and training provided in such university, board or medical institution or in any college or other institution affiliated to the university.

Do not conform to the standard prescribed by the Central Council, the Central Council shall make a representation to that effect to the Central Government.

- After considering such representation, the Central Government may send it to the government of the state in which the university, board or medical institution is situated and the state government shall forward it along with such remarks as it may choose to make to the university, board or medical institution, with an intimation of the period within which the university, board or medical institution may submit its explanation to the state government.
- On the receipt of the explanation or where no explanation is submitted within the period fixed, then, on the expiry of that period, the state government shall make its recommendations to the Central Government.
- The Central Government, after making such further inquiry, if any, as it may think fit, may, by notification in the official Gazette, direct that an entry shall be made in the second schedule against the medial

qualification declaring that it shall be a recognised medical qualification only when granted before a specified date or that the said medical qualification if granted to students of a specified college or institution affiliated to any university shall be recognised medical qualification only when granted before and specified date or, as the case may be, that the said medical qualification shall be recognised medical qualification in relation to specified college or institution affiliated to any university only when granted after a specified date.

Maximum Standards of Education in Homeopathy

- The Central Council may prescribe the maximum standards of education in homeopathy, required for granting recognised medical qualifications by universities, boards or medical institutions in India.
- Copies of the draft regulations and of all subsequent amendments thereof shall be furnished by the Central Council to all state governments and the Central Council shall, before submitting the regulations or any amendment thereof as the case may be, to the Central Government for sanction take into consideration the comments of any state government received within three months from the furnishing of the copies as aforesaid.

The Central Register of Homeopathy

- The Central Council shall cause to be maintained in the prescribed manner, a register of practitioners of homeopathy to be known as the Central Register of Homeopathy which shall contain:
  - In Part I, the names of all persons who are for the time being enrolled in any State Register of Homeopathy and possess any of the recognised medical qualifications.
  - In Part II, the names of all persons, other than those included in Part I, who are for the time being enrolled on any State Register of Homeopathy.
- It shall be the duty of the Register of the Central Council to keep and maintain the Central Register of Homeopathy in accordance with the provisions of this Act and of any orders made by the Central Council and from time-to-time to revise the register and publish it in the Gazette of India and in such other manner as may be prescribed.
- Such register shall be deemed to be a public document within the meaning of the Indian Evidence Act, 1872 and may be proved by a copy published in the Gazette of India.

Supply of Copies of State Register of Homeopathy

Each Board shall supply to the Central Council three printed copies of the State Register of Homeopathy as soon as may be after the commencement of this Act and subsequently after the first day of April each year and each board shall inform the Central Council without delay of all additions to, and other amendments in, the State Register of Homeopathy made from time-to-time.

Registration in the Central Register of Homeopathy

The Registrar of the Central Council may, on receipt of the report of registration of a person in a State Register of Homeopathy or on application made in the prescribed manner by any person, enter his name in the Central Register of Homeopathy; Provided that the Registrar is satisfied that the person concerned is eligible under this Act for such registration.

Professional Conduct

- The Central Council may prescribe standards of professional conduct and etiquette and a code of ethics for practitioners of Homeopathy.
- Regulations made by the Central Council under sub-section (1) may specify which violations thereof shall constitute infamous conduct in any professional respect, that is to say, professional misconduct and such provision shall have effect not withstanding anything contained in any law for the time being in force.

Removal of Names from the Central Register of Homeopathy

- If the name of any person enrolled on a State Register of Homeopathy is removed therefrom in pursuance of any power conferred by or under any law relating to registration of practitioners of homeopathy for the time being in force in any state, the Central Council shall direct the removal of the name of such person from the Central Register of Homeopathy.
- Where the name of any person has been removed from a State Register of Homeopathy on any ground other than that he is not possessed of the requisite medical qualifications or where any application by the

said person for restoration of his name to the State Register of Homeopathy has been rejected he may appeal in the prescribed manner and subject to such conditions, including conditions as to the payment of a fee, as may be prescribed, to the Central Government whose decision, which shall be given after consulting the Central Government shall be binding on the state government and on the authorities concerned with the preparation of the State Register of Homeopathy.

Privileges of Persons who are Enrolled on the Central Register of Homeopathy

• Subject to the conditions and restrictions and laid down in this Act regarding practice of homeopathy by persons possessing certain recognised medical qualifications, every person whose name is for the time being borne on Part I of the Central Register of Homeopathy shall be entitled according to his qualifications to practice of homeopathy, in any part of India and to recover in due course of law in respect of such practice any expenses, charges in respect of medicaments or other appliances or any fees to which he may be entitled.

• Subject to the provisions of sub-section (3) of Section 15, any person whose name is for the time being borne on Part II of the Central Register of Homeopathy, may practise Homeopathy in any state, other than the state where he is enrolled on the State Register of Homeopathy with the previous approval or the government of the state where he intends to practice.

Registration of Additional Qualification

• If any person whose name is entered in the Central Register of Homeopathy obtains any title, diploma or other qualification for proficiency in homeopathy, which is a recognised medical qualification, he shall, on application made in the behalf, in the prescribed manner, be entitled to have an entry standing such other title, diploma or other qualification made against his name in the Central Register of Homeopathy either in substitution for or in addition to any entry previously made.

• The entries in respect of any such person in a State Register of Homeopathy shall be altered in accordance with the alteration made in the central Register of Homeopathy.

Person Enrolled on Central Register of Homeopathy to Notify Change of Place of Residence or Practice

Every person registered in the Central Register of Homeopathy shall notify any transfer of the place of his residence or practice to the Central Council and to the board concerned, within 90 days of such transfer, failing which his right to participate in the election of members to the Central Council or a Board shall be liable to be forfeited by order of the Central Government either permanently or for such period as may be specified therein.

CHAPTER 33

Subject Review

This chapter is contributed by Dr Maniganda Raj, Chennai.

DEFINITIONS

Inquest: Inquest is an inquiry into the cause of death which is clearly not due to natural causes.

Types of inquest:

- Coroner's inquest
- Magistrate's inquest
- Police inquest
- Medical examiner's system

Coroner's inquest does not exist anywhere in India now. Police inquest is conducted by a police officer not below the rank of a sub-inspector of police.

Panchas/panch witness/panchayatdars: The police inquest is conducted in the presence of two or more responsible or respectable citizens of neighbourhood where the incident has occurred. The witness is given by the panchas/citizens/inhabitants.

Panchnama/inquest report: It is the statement of all facts and circumstances relating to cause of death as observed by the panchas, being recorded on paper and designed by police officer investigating the case.

Sub-poena/summons (sub—under— poena—penalty): It is a document compelling the attendance of a witness in court of law under penalty at a particular time, date and place to give evidence on a written order from the presiding officer of a court of law.

Conduct money: It is the money that is tendered at the time of serving summons to meet the travelling expenses to and fro by the party who has summoned a person as witness, in civil cases.

Oath: It is a declaration, required by the law to be made before the court, by the witness, to speak the truth, the whole truth and nothing but the truth. The purpose of administering oath is to compel the witness to speak the truth only and if he fails to do so, he can be penalised.

Perjury: It is wilful utterance of falsehood in a court of law under oath in the witness box.

Leading question: A leading question is one which suggests its own answer.

Documentary evidence: Documentary evidence comprises all the documents to be produced before the court (includes medical certificates, ML reports, dying declarations).

Medicolegal report: It is a report drawn by a medical officer in compliance of a requisition received from a magistrate or police officer, e.g. postmortem report, injury certificate, etc.

Dying declaration: It is a statement, written or verbal, made by a person who is since deceased, relating to the cause of his conditions or circumstances which later results in his death.

In short, it is a statement made by a person (dying person) who is facing an impending death about connected circumstances.

Compos mentis: Means sound mind. It is a state of mind which is neither hilarous nor depressed, it is a balanced mind capable of understanding and judgement in a proper manner.

Dying deposition: When a dying declaration is recorded by a magistrate in the presence of accused person who is given the opportunity to cross-examine the declarant, it is called dying deposition. It is infact a bed-side court.

Hearsay evidence: It is the evidence of one who has no personal knowledge of the facts of the case, but just repeats what he has heard others say (also called indirect/second hand evidence). Hearsay evidence is not accepted as an evidence in a court of law.

Common/ordinary witness: He is the one who testifies only to the facts observed by him. He is not qualified to make inferences and draw opinions.

Expert/skilled witness: He is the one who is skilled in scientific, technical or professional matters, in any art or occupations and who on account of his professional training, experience and ability, is capable of forming opinions or conclude inferences from the facts observed by him or noticed by others. Example:
• Medical expert
• Ballistic expert
• Handwriting expert
• Finger print expert and so on.

Hostile witness: A hostile witness is one who deliberately conceals the truth or gives false evidence. One who utters falsehood in a court of law contrary to the party calling him.

Professional secrets: Professional secrets are the secrets that a doctor comes to know of, in his professional capacity (it is an implied contract between the doctor and his patient, not to reveal the latter's secrets).

Identification: It means determination of individuality or recognition of a living person or dead body.

Hermaphroditism/intersexuality: Condition that results from anomalies or external and internal sex organs. A true hermaphrodite is one who presents both testes and ovary and has both man and woman elements at a time.

Hermaphrodite/inter sex: It is one where both male and female characters extst in verying proportions resulting from disturbances in development of genitals.

True hermaphroditism (double sex): A condition where both ovaries and testes are present in same individual.

Male pseudohermaphroditism: Person possesses external genitals of female but has testes.

Female pseudohermaphroditism: Person who has external genitals of male but internally has ovary.

Attrition: The wearing away of the substance of teeth is called attrition.

Gustafson's method: Method of estimation of age from tooth from a study of attrition of teeth, secondary dentine formation, transparency of root and resorption of root and paradentosis.

Arcus senilis: Arcus is a white green ring which appears in the periphery of cornea, resulting from degenerative changes in corneal tissue, after 40 years of age.

Responsibility: Means liability of a person for his acts and if these acts are contrary to the law, then the liability to be punished for the same.
• *Actus* (deeds)
• *Non-facit reum* (forbidden)
• *Nisi mens sit rea* (criminal mind)
• *Doli* (intent) *incapax* (incapable of)

Volention fit injuria: He who consents to an act is not injured by it.

Juvenile: One who is below age of 16 years.

Reformatory school/Borstal school: A school which is meant for reforming a juvenile offender.

Scar/cicatrix: When there is a breech in continuity of skin and mucous membrane, repair of injury begins at once, culminating in formation of fibrous tissue called scar. Scar is a fibrous tissue matrix resulting from repair of an injury and normally devoid of pigment layer, hair follicles, blood, nerve supply, sweat and sebaceous glands.

Linea albicantes (striae abdominalis): Scars that result from stretching of skin during pregnancy with resultant formation of scar tissue in deeper layers of dermis suggesting previous pregnancy.

Tattoo/tattoo mark: Tatau mark/pierce (Polynesian language). It is a design made on the skin by means of a needle dipped in dye.

Anthropometry: Deals with the measurement of various parts of human body.

Dactylography: Study of fingerprint or footprint system.

Fingerprint: It is an impression of the cutaneous ridges of the fleshy portion of the distal end of finger.

Quetelet's rule: Every nature made thing shows unlimited and infinite variations of forms.

Plain fingerprint: Print is taken by simply pressing the inked finger directly on paper.

Rolled fingerprint: Print is taken by rolling the inked finger on paper from side-to-side.

Poroscopy: The papillary ridges on skin of the fingers are studded with minute pores which are mouths of ducts of sweat glands. These pores are permanent and vary in size, shape, position and number in each individual. This method of identification of an individual by examining the pores is called poroscopy.

Lanugo: These are soft, tine, downy, non-pigmented, colourless hair of newborn infant with no medulla.

Exhumation: Exhumation means to dig out, unearth or disinter a dead body after burial for legal purposes.

Cephalic index/breadth index: This index is obtained by multiplying the maximum breadth of skull by 100 and dividing this by maximum length of skull measured anteroposteriorly.

Classification:
- Dolichocephalic (long headed), CI → 70–74.9, e.g. Aryans.
- Mesaticephalic (medium headed), CI → 75–79.9, e.g. Chinese/Europeans.
- Brachycephalic (short headed), CI → 80–85, e.g Mongolians.

Height index: It is the height of skull, multiplied by 100 and the sum divided by length of the skull (height is distance between tip of mastoid process and bregma).
- Chinese: 75
- Negro: 72
- English: 71

Nasal index: It is the width of nasal aperture multiplied by 100 and the sum divided by:

$$\text{Height of nasal aperture} = \frac{\text{Width}}{\text{Height}} \times 100$$

- Negroes: 55
- Chinese: 50
- English: 46

Forensic thanatology: It is the subject which deals with the medicolegal study of death, the chemistry of death and the conditions affecting dead bodies.

Somatic death: It is defined as permanent and irreversible cessation of vital functions of circulation and respiration. The person ceasing to exist as a functional whole.

Cellular death: Defined as irreversible loss of integrity of cells as functional units.

Diaphanous/transillumination test: Web test—during life, webs of the finger appear red and translucent against bright light, because of circulation, but after death appear opaque against light.

Icard's test: A small quantity of 20% alkaline solution of fluorescein is injected intravenously which produces a greenish colouration of skin where blood is circulating (test is done in daylight).

Magnus/ligature test: A ligature is tied lightly at the distal end of a finger, which becomes blue and swollen, if circulation is going on, due to venous obstruction.

Winslow's test/mirror test: Any bright reflecting surface is placed on the chest and reflections of a beam of light focused on it will move, only if there is respiration.

Suspended animation: A condition in which life stands suspended, i.e. there is temporary stoppage of circulation and respiration. Seen in:
- Apparently drowned persons
- After anaesthesia
- Cerebral concussion
- Electrocution
- Newborn infants
- Sun stroke

Postmortem caloricity: Usually there is fall of temperature of the body after death, but rarely one may note a rise of temparature of dead body after death. This is called postmortem caloricity.
- Pulmonary haemorrhage, meningococcal meningitis.
- Sun stroke, hyperpyrexia.

Postmortem staining/lividity/cadaveric lividity/hypostatis/rigor mortis: After death, fluid blood gets collected in toneless capillaries and veins in dependent parts of the body, in obedience to law of gravity. This stasis of blood discolours or stains the skin and organs which is termed as postmortem staining.

Fixation of postmortem staining: After death, once the blood has coagulated, hypostasis remains permanent and is not affected by any further change in position of the body. This is termed as fixation of postmortem staining. Usually gets fixed in 6–8 hours.

Purple colour	Asphyxial death
Cherry red colour	CO, HCN poisoning,cold/ burns
Chocholate brown	Sodium nitrate, quinine
Bluish green	Hydrogen sulphide poisoning

Rigor mortis/cadaveric rigidity/death stiffening: After the period of primary relaxation, some hours after death, the muscles stiffen and body becomes rigid. This rigidity is called rigor mortis (rigidity of death).

Breaking of the rigor: When a limb which is stiff due to rigor mortis is forcibly flexed at a joint, the limb becomes flaccid and remains so after that. This is called breaking of the rigor. Once broke, it does not develop again.

Goose skin/goose flesh/cutis anserine: When rigor mortis affects the erectores pilorum muscles of the skin, skin papillae stand out prominently and hair of the body stand on end presenting a puckered, pimpled or granular appearance of skin called goose skin.

Cold stiffening/freezing/cold rigor/cold rigidity: This refers to stiffening of the muscles which results from solidification of muscle fat and body fluids when body is exposed to a freezing temperature.

Heat stiffening/heat rigor/heat rigidity: This refers to the stiffening of the muscles resulting from coagulation of muscle proteins when body is exposed to temperatures of over 70°C.

Cadaveric spasm/instantaneous rigor/cataleptic rigidity: This is a condition where the muscles stiffen immediately after death, there being no primary flaccidity of muscles after death.

Postmortem discolouration: This refers to the green to black discolourations of skin, organs and tissues of the body as a result of putrefaction.

Marbling of the skin: Due to decomposition of blood within vessels, the blood pigment, therefore, stains the vessel walls. The course of veins is thus visible as bluish network and forms a characteristic mosaic pattern on the skin, termed as marbling of skin.

Postmortem blisters: As a process of putrefaction, more and more gases accumulate in body which exert pressure within, resulting in formations of blebs/bullae on surface of skin in about 36 hours after death. These blebs are called postmortem blisters (contain only gas; no fluid, no evidence of vital reactions).

Skin sock/skin glove: Peeling/denuding/shedding of cuticle occurs in putrefaction as a result of which skin may peel off from hand/foot in form of a glove. This is called skin glove/skin sock.

Foamy liver: In putrefaction, the liver becomes spongy and foamy giving a honey comb appearance. This is called foamy liver.

Forensic entomology/entomology of the cadaver/entomology of the dead: A study of insects, maggots, etc. that infest a dead body.

Adipocere/saponification: It is a modification of process of putrefaction which results from postmortem hydrogenation of body fats and their hydrolysis into fatty acids.

Mummification: Refers to the postmortem dehydration and desiccation of the body.

Sudden death: Defined as death occurring suddenly and unexpectedly and not due to apparent injury or poisoning.

Vagal inhibition/reflex cardiac arrest/reflex cardiac syncope/reflex cardiac inhibition/vagal inhibition: Vagal inhibition is a condition in which sudden stoppage of heart and respiration occurs, as a result of reflex vagal stimulations and consequent paralysis of cardiac and respiratory centres. Vagal inhibition leads to instantaneous death due to vagal stimulation causing cardiac inhibition.

Wound/injury: Defined as a disruption in the anatomical continuity of tissues of the body, caused by application of mechanical violence. Wound is a disolution in the continuity of body tissues due to trauma.

Abrasion/surface scrape: An injury to the skin, resulting from scraping away of superficial layer of epidermis due to friction with a rough object or surface. Abrasion is a mechanical injury caused due to friction between body part and a rough surface leading to loss of superficial layer of skin or mucous membrane. It heals rapidly without leaving a scar in the skin unless deeper dermis is involved.

Scab/crust: It is nothing but dried up blood, lymph and injured epithelial cells.

Scab

- Wet
- Dry
- Water as circumstances of lymph and blood as soon as the injury occurs.

Crust: Crust is the encrustation due to drying up of dust, debris, lymph and blood after any injury.

Scratch abrasion: A scratch is caused by a narrow, but sharp object running across the skin, e.g. finger nail, pin or thorn.

Graze abrasion/sliding abrasion/scraping abrasion/grinding abrasion: A graze is produced whrn a broad surface of skin scrapes against or slides against a rough object or surface.

Impact abrasion/imprint abrasion: An impact abrasion is caused by the impact or stamping of an object on the skin, e.g. impact of radiator grice of motor car in road accident.

Pressure abrasion/crushing abrasion/friction abrasion: A pressure abrasion is caused by pressure of an object on the skin; e.g. ligature mark in case of strangulation. Impact abrasions and pressure abrasions are also called pattern abrasions. Therefore, the pattern of the object responsible is imprinted on the skin.

Contusion/bruise: An injury in which there is a breech in continuity of subcutaneous tissues without loss of external continuity due to applications of blunt force. (There is leakage of blood into the tissues, due to rupture of subcutaneous blood vessels.)

Haematoma: When larger blood vessels are injured a large effusion of blood collects, called haematoma.

Lacerated wound/tear/rupture: One in which the skin and sometimes even the deeper tissues are torn or lacerated, as a result of blunt violence.

Incised-like wound/apparent incised wound/split: Type of lacerated wound produced on situations where the overlying skin is tightly stretched over bone, underneath without much intervening tissue.

Avulsion: Means tearing away of the skin caused by grinding compression of a weight.

Chop wound/cut laceration: Defined as solution in continuity of tissues without loss of substance caused by a sharp heavy weapon with cutting edge.

Defence cuts/potective cuts: These are incised wounds sustained in an attempt to protect self from an attack with a sharp edges weapon.

Stab wounds/punctured wounds: One which penetrates through the skin and deeper tissues, depth being more than length and breadth and produced by a sharp/blunt stabbing weapon like dagger, sword, etc.

When a stab wound penetrates into body cavity, it is called penetrating wound.

If it has come out from the other side, then it is called perforating wound.

Forensic ballistics: Science dealing with firearms.

Barrel: Metal tube through which the bullet passes when fired from a cartridge.

Calibre/bore/guage: It is the internal diameter of barrel infront of the chamber (in rifles, revolvers, pistols, etc., it is the distance between two opposite ends and not grooves). Smooth bore firearms are called shotguns.

Choking of a firearm: Means narrowing or constriction of the barrel near the muzzle end of shortguns, object of which is to prevent the dispersion of shots over a long distance thus increasing the effectiveness of weapons.

Calibre of shotgun: It is the size of a spherical lead ball which will exactly fit into the barrel and by the number of such balls that can be made out of 464 gm (one pound) of lead. Therefore, the calibre is less if the number of lead balls is more.

Cannelure: The bullet is held in the cartridge case by a groove called the cannelure.

Wad: In order to separate the shots from the gunpowder and to evenly distribute on the shots, the pressure generated by the explosion of gunpowder, shotgun cartridges are provided with a circular disc, in between the shots and gunpowder, made of compressed paper or felt termed as wad.

Turnover top wad: It is also a wad, situated over the lead shots, purpose of which is to keep the shots in place.

Abrasion collar/areola: During the bullet's attempt at perforating the skin while entering and because of its spin, the edges of the entrance wound may be abraded in the form of a collar, of some width around the entrance wound. This is termed as abrasion collar (outer zone).

Contusion collar: Contusion is associated with abrasion collar.

Grease collar/dirt collar/halo/cuff/areola: This results from spin of the bullet due to which it wipes its surface of lubricating oil, on the skin while entering (inner zone).

Tattooing/pepper pattern/stippled pattern: Refers to the grains of gunpowder being driven into the skin, each grain acting as an independent minute missile.

Blackening/metal ring: Refers to the superficial deposit of carbonaceous deposit (smoke) on the skin around entry wound in firearm discharge.

Lead ring/metal ring: Refers to the deposition in the form of a ring or collar around the entrance wound, of very small quantities of led or other metal, while the missile enters the skin.

Ricochet: Means the deflection in the direction of travel of missile as a result of striking against a hard object.

Tandem bullet/piggy-back bullet: Refers to an instance where a bullet tends to come out on firing but comes out along with second bullet on subsequent firing, both bullets entering the body through same entry wound.

Odd and even rule: When an even number (2, 4, 6...) of wounds are present, it generally means that missile has come out of the body, while if odd number (1, 3, 5...) of wounds are present, it generally means that missile is probably within the body.

Dermal nitrate test/paraffin test/paraffin glove test: Test performed to detect the presence of gunpowder residue on the hand of person who has fired the weapon, as some gunpowder residue generally escapes breech also and contaminates the hand holding the weapons.

Simple injury: One which is simple in nature does not fall in the domain of grieveous hurt, which is not extensive and heals rapidly without leaving any permanent disfiguration/disability.

Grievous hurt: An injury which results in any of the following is a grievous injury:

- Emasculation (deprivation of properties of male, to castrate or to remove the testicles, in females it refers to cutting off the pudenda).
- Permanent deprivation of sight of either eye.
- Permanent deprivation of hearing of either ear.
- Permanent impairment of powers of any member (part, organ or limbs of body) or joint.
- Permanent disfigurations of head or face (disfiguration means to mar the beauty of person by means of an injury).
- Fracture/dislocation of a bone/tooth (fracture of nasal/ear cartilages is grievous only when permanent disfiguration results therefrom).
- Any injury which directly endangers life, or causes the victim to be in severely body pain making him unable to follow his ordinary pursuits for at least a period of 20 days.

Dangerous injury: It is one in which life is in imminent danger, generally extensive or involving an important organ or structure.

Dangerous weapon: Defined as any instrument used for shooting, stabbing or cutting or any instrument which when used as a weapon of offence is likely to cause death.

Negative and positive vital reactions: In an antemortem wound, two district zones of enzyme activity are seen. There is a zone of diminished enzyme activity on either side of the edge of the wound known as negative vital reaction and still internally a zone of increased enzyme activity known as positive vital reaction.

Embolism: Defined as occlusion of blood vessel by an embolus.

Pulmonary fat embolism: A condition where many pulmonary capillaries get obstructed by droplets of fat, death resulting from asphyxia because gaseous exchange in lungs is imparied.

Systemic/arterial fat embolism: Conditions where fat droplets (emboli) pass from the pulmonary capillaries to the left side of heart and hence to the systemic circulation, reaching every organ of the body.

Election/preferential sites: A person thinks about the preferential sites for suicide attempt.

Self-inflicted wounds: Refer to wounds that are inflicted by the person on one's own body, motive being to falsely charge or accuse other person of having caused them, out of revenge, jealously or malice.

Primary and secondary impact injuries: Refer to those injuries on the victim, resulting from the first impact of vehicle on him. As a result of this impact, because of momentum of vehicle, the victim gets thrown down to the road and sustains some more injuries as a result of striking against the road surface. These latter injuries are called secondary injuries.

Coup injury: One which is situated immediately subjacent to the area of impact.

Contrecoup injury: An injury situated on the contralateral side of area of impact.

Cerebral compression: Condition resulting from pressure on the brain due to intracranial space occupying lesion.

Cerebral concussion/commotio cerebri: Condition of traumatic paralysis of brain, resulting in immediate suspended animation and unconsciousness.

Lucid interval: The interim period of consciousness between two bouts of unconsciousness is termed as lucid interval.

Amnesia: Loss of memory.

Retrograde amnesia: When a victim of concussion recovers from unconsciousness, he may be unable to recollect the exact manner in which he was injured. This is termed as retrograde amnesia.

Homicide (Homo—man; cide—to kill): Means killing of a human being by another human being.

Infanticide: Killing of an infant (below one year age).

Fratricide: Killing of a brother or sister.

Excusable homicide: Refers to death of a person caused unintentionally, by an act doen in good faith or for benefit of the person.

Justifiable homicide: Death resulting from administration of justice (above two are not punishable in law).

Culpable homicide not amounting to murder/man slaughter: An unlawful killing of a human being brought out by grave and sudden provocation, there being no wilful, delibrate or malicious intention to kill.

Murder: Unlawful killing of a human being when there is wilful, deliberate and malicious criminal intent to kill.

Accident: Unexpected mishap.

Suicide: Taking away one's own life.

Malingering: Defined as deliberate attempt on part of the patient to decieve the doctor.

Asphyxia/anoxia/anoxaemia/hypoxia suboxia: Refers to a condition where oxygen supply to blood and tissues is reduced because of interference with respiration.

Cyanosis (cyanos—blue): Refers to bluish discolouration resulting from deficient oxygen in blood and reduced haemoglobin to more than 5 gm%.

Tardieu's spots: In asphyxia, small round and discrete spots of haemorrhage about the size of pinhead, each are seen in parts where the capillaries are least supported. These spots are called Tardieu's spots.

Postmortem petechial haemorrhages: If a dead body remains suspended for some time (e.g. hanging), petechial haemorrhages may be seen on the skin of the lower limbs because of gravitation of blood to lower limbs and consequent rupture of capillaries from overdistension. These haemorrhages are called postmortem petechial haemorrhages.

Hanging: That form of death caused by complete or partial suspension of the body by a ligature tied around neck, the constricting force on ligature being the weight of the body or the head.

Complete hanging: When feet or any part of the body do not touch the ground, it is termed complete hanging.

Partial/incomplete hanging: When any part of the body is found touching the ground, it is termed partial hanging.

Lynching: When number of persons jointly overpower and hang an individual, it is called lynching.

Judicial hanging: In the legal execution of death sentence by hanging by the judge.

Strangulation: It is a form of death produced by constriction or pressure on the neck by any means other than the weight of victims body.

Throttling: When strangulation is effected by hands, it is called throttling.

Mugging: When the assailant compresses the victim's neck, within the angle of elbow, it is called mugging.

Bansdola: Conditions where the victim is asphyxiated to death by squeezing his neck in between two sticks, one placed in front and the other at back of his neck, one end tied and other end being brought together by means of rope.

Garroting: When a ligature is suddenly tied around the neck from behind and tightened by twisting it with lever in manner of tourniquet. It is called garroting.

Drowning: Form of death resulting from entry of water or any other liquid into the respiratory passages, when a person is submerged in that liquid.

Washerwoman's hands/dishwasher hands: These refer to the water sodden, bleached, puckered and wrinkled skin of hands and feet resulting from imbibition of water from prolonged immersion in water.

Oedema aquosum/emphysema aquosum: Term given to the appearance of lungs in case of drowning. The lungs are ballooned voluminous, weigh more, have a doughy and sodden feel, pit on pressure, are water-logged and show rib indentations when taken out.

Diatoms: These are small, microscopic, unicellular algae or plants contained in most samples of water.

Gettler's test: Estimation of electrolyte content of blood in case of drowning is termed Gettler's test.

Suffocation: This term embraces all those asphyxial deaths resulting from exclusion of air from lungs by means other than compression of neck (includes smothering, choking, traumatic asphyxia).

Smothering: Form of death caused by closure of the external respiratory orifices, namely nose and mouth.

Burking: A combination of smothering and traumatic asphyxia where the victim is thrown down and one assailant while sitting on his chest smothers the victim and the other assailant holds the victim down by pulling his legs.

Choking: Form of asphyxial death pro-duced by occlusion or impaction of air passages by a solid object.

Gagging: Type of choking caused by obstruction of mouth and throat by plugging them with a gag such as cloth or any other soft material.

Traumatic asphyxia: Type of asphyxial death resulting from pressure on and fixation of the chest.

Buckled sternum: In case of steering wheel impact, there may be transverse fracture of sternum at the junction of manubrium and body referred to as buckled sternum.

Rape: Defined as unlawful coitus by a man with a woman:
- Against her will.
- Without her consent.
- With her consent, when taken by putting her in fear of death or hurt of her dear ones.
- With or without consent by any girl under 16 years of age.
- With or without consent, if she is his wife under 15 years of age.
- With her consent when she knows that he is not her husband and that she consents believing that he is the man to whom she is lawfully wedded.
- With her consent when it is obtained under intoxication or by a girl of unsound mind.

Locard's principle of exchange: Professor Edmund Locard of Lyons, enunciated in 1928, a principle, stating that when any two objects come into contact with each other, there is always some transfer of material from one to the other. This is called Locard's principle of exchange.

Sexual perversion/deviation/paraphilia: Both law and custom permit only sexual intercourse between man and wife, with the sex organs intended for the purpose and generally related for reproduction. Anything which departs from this is abnormal and is termed sexual perversion or sexual deviation or paraphilia.

Pervert/deviate: A person who indulges in a sexual perversion is called a pervert or deviate.

Sodomy/buggery: A man is said to commit sodomy, if he has anal intercourse with another man or woman.

Catamite: The victim in a case of sodomy is referred to as catamite.

Paederasty/paedophilia: Type of sodomy where passive agent is a boy.

Bestiality: Means sexual intercourse by a human being with a lower animal.

Exhibitionism/indecent exposure: A sexual offence wherein sexual pleasure is obtained by indecently exposing the genitals to members of opposite sex in public.

Tribadism/lesbian love/lesbianism/female homosexuality/female sexual inversion: A sexual perversion wherein two women derive sexual pleasure by mutual friction of the external genitals.

Nymphomania: Exaggerated sexual desire in women.

Transvestism/eonism/cross-dressing: Asexual perversion wherein sexual pleasure is obtained by wearing the clothes of the opposite sex (transvestite—person exhibiting transvestism).

Sadism: Type of sexual perversion in which sexual pleasure is derived by beating, whipping, biting or otherwise torturing the sexual partner (such a pervert is called sadist) (rarely, a sadist may even murder the partner, which is termed as lust murder).

Masochism: Type of sexual perversion wherein sexual pleasure is ontained by being tortured by one's sexual partner, namely by submission to pain or cruelty.

Incest: Refers to coitus between persons who are within forbidden degrees of marital relationship.

Buccal coitus/coitus peros/sin of gomorrah: Refers to sexual intercourse through the mouth.

Fetichism/fetishism: Refers to that sexual perversion wherein sexual pleasure is obtained by contact with, or the site of an object belonging to opposite sex (persons who derives sexual pleasure in this manner is called fetichist).

Necrophila: Rare conditions wherein sexual pleasure is derived by indulging in coitus with a cadaver (necro—corpse: philia—to defile or foul).

Impotence: Defined as incapacity or inability to perform the act of coitus.

First night impotence: Refers to the impotence suffered by the bridegroom on the first bridal night.

Quod hanc: Refers to a condition where there is a psychological, but permanent impotence with reference to a particular female.

Sterility/infertility: Incapacity or inability to procreate.

Sterilization: Procedure deliberately practised in order to render a person sterile, namely incapable of reproduction.

Artificial insemination: Means introduction of semen (insemination) into the female genital tract by means of instrument to bring about conception, when natural methods fail.

AI-homologous: When semen derived for AI is from the woman's husband himself, it is termed as AI-homologous.

AI-heterologous/AI-donor: When the semen is obtained, not from the husband, but from a third person, namely a donor for AI, it is termed AI-donor. (Woman who receives the semen is called recipient or donee.)

Virginity: Refers to the state of female who has not experienced coitus.

Virgin/virgo intacta: Female who has not experienced coitus.

Defloration: Refers to loss of virginity, namely to an experience of coitus.

Hymen: It is a circular fold of connective tissue about 1 mm thick with a central aperture admitting tip of the little finger at vaginal opening.

Carunculae hymenalis/myrtiformis: After the birth of a child, the hymen is almost completely torn up, leaving only small remnant of it known as carunculae hymenalis or myrtiformis.

Pseudocyesis: Means false pregnancy.

Jacquemier's sign/Chadwick's sign: Refers to the bluish discolouration of vaginal mucosa, resulting from stasis of blood.

Therefore, pressure of gravid uterus impedes proper venous return, in case of pregnancy.

Hegar's sign: Refers to softening and compressibility of lower uterine segment at about 2 months of pregnancy.

Goodell's sign: Refers to softening of the cervix occurring from third month of pregnancy resulting from increased vascularity.

Quickening: Refers to the appreciation, by the mother, of movements of foetus within her womb, appearing from fourth month of pregnancy.

Braxton-Hick's sign: Refers to the appreciation, of intermittent contractions of uterus, detected by palpation of abdomen.

Ballottement: Refers to the method of eliciting the presence of foetus floating in liquor amnion. Two types: 1. Internal and 2. external.

Uterine souffle: It is a bruit or a soft blowing murmur synchronous with maternal pulse, which can be heard with a stethoscope applied just above the middle of inguinal ligament.

Delivery: Refers to the birth of a child or the products of conception.

Fullterm delivery: When delivery occurs after full period of gestation, i.e. 280 days it is termed fullterm delivery.

Pre-mature: If it occurs earlier than 280 days, it is clled premature delivery.

Post-mature: If it occurs beyond the full period of gestation, it is said to be postmature delivery.

Affiliation case: In law, father of an illegitimate child must support the child, such case is also called affiliation case.

Lochia: For about 2 weeks after delivery, there is a discharge from the uterus, which has a characteristic unpleasant odour and alkaline in reaction called lochia. For 1–3 days, it is bloody—lochia rubra. Next 3 days, it is pale and serous—lochia serosa (still later till it vanishes it is yellowish white of lochia alba).

Paternity: Literally, it means fatherhood.

Disputed paternity: When there is any dispute or doubt regarding the parentage of a child, it is termed disputed paternity.

Non-paternity: When one is sure that the alleged parents have not be gotten a particular child, case is of non-paternity.

Atavism: Resemblance of a child, not to one of the parents, but to one of the grand-parents or ancestors.

Superfecundation: Refers to the fertilisation of two ova of same ovulatory period, by different acts of coitus.

Superfoetation: Refers to fertilisation of two ova of different ovulatory periods by different acts of coitus.

Legitimacy: It is the status of a child born in lawful wedlock.

Illegitimate child/bastard: One who is born to parents not lawfully wedden to each other.

Abortion: Defined as premature expulsion of the products of conception from the womb at anytime before its period of gestation is complete.

Justifiable abortion/therapeutic abortion: Defined as one which is induced in:
- Good faith
- To save life or health of pregnant woman
- When there is a substantial risk that if the child was born, he may suffer from such physical and mental abnormalities as to be seriously handicapped

Health (as per WHO): A state of complete physical, mental and social well-being and not merely the absence of disease or infirmity.

Criminal abortion: Defined as abortion which is induced with criminal intent.

Ecbolics: These are the substances that act directly on the uterus and promote strong uterine contractions (e.g. ergot, quinine, pituitary extract).

Emmenagogues: There are drugs which promote or increase menstrual flow (e.g. borax, oil of savin, oestrogen).

Abortion stick: Any thin and long (12–18 cm) stick wrapped at one end with cotton wool and soaked in irritants like madar juice, marking nut juice, arsenic paste, used to procure abortion by introducing it in uterus. (A twig of calotropis or nerium odorum itself is sometimes used to procure abortion.)

Infanticide: Defined as delibrate and unlawful killing of an infant by an act of commission or omission.

Act of omission: Means wilful omission (failure) to do that which is necessary to preserve or maintain the life of an infant.

Act of commission: Means an act deliberately or positively done, as a result of which the infant dies.

Viability: Defined as capacity of an infant, after birth, to lead a separate existance apart from its mother, i.e. its ability to survive.

Ovum: Term applied to the products of conception during first two weeks of pregnancy.

Embryo: Term given to the product of conception from 3 to 5 weeks of pregnancy.

Foetus: Term given to product of conception from 5 weeks onward of pregnancy.

Lanugo: Refers to the fine, soft, downy, non-pigmented hair present on foetal body.

Meconium: Refers to the green viscid substance made up of inspissated bile and mucous present in foetal intestine.

Vernix caseosa: Refers to dirty, whitish, sticky, cheesy substance made up of sebaceous secretion and epithelial cells present on the skin of foetus.

Rule of Hasse: According to this rule, in earlier months of pregnancy, namely before 5 months, the square root of the length of foetus, measured from the crown to heel in centimeters gives the age of foetus in months. While in later months of pregnancy, namely after 5 month, one-fifth of the crown heel length measured in centimeters gives the age of foetus in months.

Alveolar duct membrane: A membrane made of fat, lines the alveolar duct, which when demonstrated by fat stains in foetal lung tissue, indicates live birth.

Stillborn infant: An infant is said to be stillborn if, after its birth, it did not breathe at all or show any other sign of life like kicking, crying, breathing, etc.

Dead born infant: A dead born infant is one which has died in uterus.

Maceration: It is a process of aseptic autolysis seen in dead born child.

Caput succedaneum: When precess of delivery is prolonged, tissues over the presenting part, usually the head (caput), gets engorged and edematous. This is called caput succedaneum. (When haemorrhages occur in this situation and there is great extravasation of blood, it is called cephalohaematoma.)

Immaturity: Refers to an infant under 2000 gm in weight.

Prematurity: Means birth prior to full gestation period (280 days).

Precipitate labour: Means labour which is quick and occurs without the knowledge of mother, in which three stages of labour are telescoped into one.

Burn: A lesion, resulting from application of dry heat to the body, such as flame or a hot object.

Scald: Lesion caused by application of moist heat like steam or hot liquids is called a scald.

Pugilistic attitude/boxing attitude/combat attitude/defence attitude/fencing attitude: Refers to an attitude of flexion, resulting from contraction of the muscles due to coagulation of muscle proteins on exposure to excessive heat.

Humidity: Refers to the degree of saturation of atmosphere with moisture.

Heat cramps/fireman's miner's or stoker's cramps: Refer to painful cramps of voluntary muscles occurring in persons working in hot, humid summer months.

Heat exhaustion/heat collapse/heat syncope/heat prostration: A condition characterized by headache, profuse perspiration, vomiting, subnormal temperature, muscular weakness, circulatory collapse and fainting seen in persons physically exerting themselves for a long period in hot and humid atmosphere.

Joule burns: Also called endogenous burns, are white, dry, insensitive crater-like burns centre being depressed and the margins raised.

Legal electrocution/judicial electrocution: It is the execution of death sentence by electrocution (practised in some states of America).

Lightning: It is an electrical discharge from the cloud to an object on the earth.

Arborescent markings/arborescent prints/ filigree burns/Lichtenberg's flowers/ lightning prints: In a case of lightning, sometimes one sees characteristic streaky burns on the skin, which resemble branches of a tree. These burns are called arborescent markings.

Frostbite: Refers to the local necrosis of tissues resulting from vascular thrombosis due to exposure to freezing temperature.

Insanity (unsoundness of mind): When a person suffers from a disease of mind, as a result of which his mental faculties, functions and emotions are manifested abnormal, he is said to be suffering from insanity (the person is called insane).

Hallucination: It is a false sense of perception which occurs without any external object or stimulus to produce it.

Illusion: It is a false interpretation by the senses, of an external object or stimulus which really exists.

Delusion: Means a false belief contrary to the fact.

Obsession: It is a constant idea occurring to a person with irresistable force.

Impulse: It is a sudden and irresistible desire compelling a person to do something without motive or forethought.

Lucid interval: Refers to the interval or period of time between two bouts of unsoundness of mind, during which the mind of the person is lucid or clear.

Feigned insanity: Means pretended insanity. In other words, the person is not really of unsound mind, but pretends to be so.

Idiocy (IQ—0–20): It is a condition where the behaviour of a person is below that of an animal, mental age being below that of a child of 2 years.

Imbecility (IQ—21–40): Minor form of idiocy where person's mental age is that of a child of 2–7 years.

Feeble mindedness (IQ—41–70) (moron): Condition where the intellect and the behaviour of a person is higher than an idiot but below that of a normal individual, mental age corresponding to a child of 7–12 years (such a person is also called moron).

Mania: State of excitement of both emotions and intellect, manifesting itself as a hyperactivity of mind and body.

Melancholia: A condition where there is an intense feeling of depression and misery.

Schizophrenia/split personality: A condition characterized by withdrawal from reality, person living in a dream world of his own and is apathetic to his surroundings.

Somnambulism (somnus—sleep: ambulare— walk): Also called sleepwalking. It is an abnormal mental state where in the person walks during sleep.

Somnolentia/semi-somnolence: It is a minor degree of somnambulism where the degree of awareness and wakefulness is a little more than in somnambulism.

Delirium: Condition characterized by restlessness, disorientation, incoordination and insomnia.

Hypnotism/mesmerism: Defined as a process which induces sleep or trance in which the susceptibility of mind of victim to suggestion, command or direction is used and in which he is generally insensible to pain.

Wandering lunatic: One who wanders aimlessly.

Dangerous lunatic: One, who because of his violent behaviour is dangerous to himself or to others or to the property.

Criminal lunatic: One who has committed a crime or a person who has become insane while undergoing a sentence in jail for same offence committed.

Testamentary capacity: Refers to a person's capacity to make a valid will.

Testament: It is a document executed by a person bequeathing his property to others.

Actus non-facit reum nisi mens sit rea: There cannot be a guilty act unless there is a guilty mind.

Durham's rule: A person is not criminally responsible, if the unlawful act was the result of mental disease or defect.

Toxicology: Subject that deals with study of poisons, their toxicity, lethal dose, treatment, their detection by chemical analysis or any other means and autopsy findings.

Poison: Substance which by its action is injurious to the health of the person or causes his death.
- Any substance which causes, undesirable effects in a poison.
- Only difference between a medicine and poison is the dose and intent with which it is given.

Addicts: Those persons who are habituated to a certain substance, can take even large quantities of the substance without suffering from toxic manifestations are called addicts.

Cumulative poisons: These are the poisons that accumulate in the body (e.g. ethyl/ methyl alcohol, barbiturates).

Antagonism: When two substances on mixing counteract each other or annual each other, it is termed antagonism.

Tolerance: Means refractoriness to a substance.

Emesis: Means vomiting.

Emetics: Substance which promotes vomiting.

Antidotes: They are the substances which neutralize the effects of poisons and render them innocuous.

Physical/mechanical antidotes: Those that neutralize poisons by sheer physical or mechanical action, there being no chemical interaction between the poison and antidote. *Example*:
- Animal charcoal
- Bulky food
- Demulscents

Demulscents: These are substances which form a protective coating on the gastric mucous membrane and thus do not permit the poison to cause any damage. *Example*:
- Egg white
- Fats
- Milk

Chemical antidotes: Substances which neutralize poisons by chemical interaction with the poison to form an inert or harmless substance.

Universal antidotes: An antidote that can be employed to neutralize a variety of poisons; used when exact nature of poison is obscure. Combination of both physical and chemical antidotes consists of:
- One part of MgO
- One part of tannic acid
- Two parts of animal charcoal.

Physiological/pharmacological antidotes: These substances counteract the physiological action of poisons.

Corrosive: It is a substance which causes corrosion and destruction of tissues with which it comes into contact.

Xanthoproteic reaction: Being a powerful oxidising agent, nitric acid reacts with organic matter to form picric acid, staining the tissues and teeth yellow. This is called xanthoproteic reaction.

Carbonisation: If sulphuric acid is ingested, mucous membrane of stomach is discoloured black and appears as charred, resulting from extraction of water and conversion of haemoglobin into haematin. This is termed carbonisation.

Vitriol throwing/vitriolage: Refers to throwing or application of a strong corrosive or any other destructive substance, generally on the face of another individual out of jealousy or revenge with a view to destroy vision, burn, maim, disable or disfigure the victim.

Oxaluria: Refers to the presence of calcium oxalate crystals in the urine.

Phosphorescence: Yellow phosphorus is luminous in dark and glows with pale yellow colour. This is termed phosphorescence.

Phossy jaw: It is an osteomyelitis and necrosis of jaw with formation of multiple sinuses, discharging foul smelling pus, seen in chronic phosphorus poisoning.

Aphrodisiac: An aphrodisiac is a substance which arouses sexual desire.

Hatter's shakes/glass blowers shakes: They refer to the tremors occurring in muscles of face, tongue and arms exaggerated by voluntary effort due to chronic mercurial poisoning in members engaged in hat and glass blowing industries.

Erethism: Refers to a peculiar change in personality of an individual characterized by nervousness, irritability, anxiety, timidity, sudden bouts of anger, amnesia and insomnia due to chronic mercury poisoning.

Mercuria lentis: Refers to discolouration of capsule of the lens of the eye due to deposition of mercury salts, characteristic feature of chronic mercury poisoning.

Chelating agent/sequestering agent: One which takes away the poison from blood and tissues, by preferentially combining with metallic ions, to form an inactive water-soluble complex which is readily excreted in urine.

Burtonian line/lead line: Refers to the blue-coloured line occurring at the junction of tooth and gums, only over carious tooth due to lead sulphide formation seen in chronic lead poisoning.

- Blue vitriol (copper sulphate).
- Verdigris (copper sub-acetate).

Toxalbumin/phytotoxin: A toxic protein which causes agglutination and lysis of red cells even in great dilution.

Strangury: Means painful micturition.

Priapism: It is persistent and painful erection of penis without sexual desire.

Alkaloid: It is a complex chemical substance found in variety of plants which behaves chemically like an alkali and combines with acids to form salts.

Stramonium cigarettes: Cigarettes made from the leaves of *dhatura* plant used to be smoked in former days for relief of bronchial asthma.

Truth serum/lie detector (hyosine): Lie detection is done by narcoanalysis. The underlying principle is that, when under the influence of a narcotis, person becomes semi-conscious and generally speaks the truth, hence called truth serum or lie detector.

Bhang: Mildest preparation of cannabis (15% concentration of active principle) made from dried leaves and fruit shoots of the plant.

Ganja/marihuana: Made from flowering and fruiting tip of the plant *Cannabis indica* containing 25% of active principles.

Reefers/weed: Refer to the doped cigarettes containing marihuana.

Hashish/charas: Resinous exudate obtained from the leaves of *Connabis indica* containing 25–40% of active principle.

Run amok: Name given to condition of person in chronic cannabis poisoning where the person indiscriminately kills the people coming in his way, finally committing suicide.

Magnan's symptom/cocaine bugs: Refers to the tactile hallucination experienced by the victim, who feels as though grains of sand are lying under his skin or that bugs are creeping under his skin, in chronic cocaine poisoning.

Narcotic: Substances which produce analgesia, unconsciousness and sleep.

Carbogen (gas containing 5% CO_2 + 95% O_2): It contains a mixture of 5% CO_2 and 95% O_2.

Addiction: Defined as a state of periodic or chronic intoxication, harmful to the individual and to the society resulting from repeated consumption of a drug.

Habituate/habitue: Refers to any person habituated to a drug.

Various postures seen in strychnine poisoning:

- *Opisthotonus*: Posture of extension where head is thrown backwards, back arched forwards and limbs extended.
- *Emprosthotonus*: Posture opposite to opisthotonus.
- *Pleurosthotonus*: Posture of lateral flexion, body being arched laterally either to left or to right.

Forensic medicine: Forensic medicine is the knowledge of all branches of medical sciences required in a court of law for purpose of administration of justice.

Medical jurisprudence: Means knowledge of law required by a registered medical practitioner to carry out proper medical practice.

Risus sardonicus/sardoning/sneering grin: Refers to grinning expression of the victim in strychnine poisoning from contraction of facial muscle and jaw.

Inebriant poison: A substance that causes depression of nervous system resulting in mental instability.

Gudamba (gud—jaggery): An alcoholic liquor formed by fermentation of jaggery with potassium bromide and chloral hydrate added as knock out agents. It is a local brew in Hyderabad area.

- **Absolute alcohol:** 99.95% ethyl alcohol
- **Rectified spirit:** 90% ethyl alcohol
- **Denatured spirit:** 95% ethyl alcohol + 5% methyl clcohol.

Analgesic: Drug which relieves pain without loss of consciousness.

Automatism: Refers to performance of non-reflex acts without conscious violation. The person takes the drug without realizing that he is repeating the dose (barbiturate poisoning).

Plant penicillin: Name given to endrin, a very toxic and popular insecticide used against a variety of plant pests.

Penal erasure: When a registered medical practitioner commits an offence and is convicted by law or is guilty of infamous conduct in professional respect, his name is erases/removed from state medcial register and named as penal erasure.

Professional death sentence: When the name of a registered medical practitioner is permanently removed, it is called professional death sentence.

Touting: When a medical practitioner uses non-medical people to send patients to him, it is called touting.

Dichotomy: When a registered medical practitioner shares his fees with other person (a medical man).

Waiver of professional secrecy: When a patient gives his express permission to the doctor to disclose professional secrets, it is termed waiver of professional secrecy.

Privileged communication: A statement made by a doctor in good faith to a concerned authority by virtue of his duty to protect the interest of community in general or of the state.

Statutory disclosure: Disclosure made because of statutory directives. A doctor has to divulge the professional secrets when asked as he owes a statutory duty to do so. This is termed as statutory disclosure, i.e. information regarding death, birth, infectious disease.

Professional misconduct: Any conduct on the part of medical practitioner, during his practice, which is considered disgraceful and dishonourable by professional brethren of good repute and competence is called professional misconduct.

Malpraxis (malpractice): Defined as want or absence of reasonable care and still and wilful negligence on the part of medical practitioner in treatment resulting in bodily injury or death of his patient.

Negligence: Defined as omission to do something which a reasonable prudent man will do or to do something which a reasonable prudent man will not do.

Civil negligence/civil malpraxis: Form of malpractice in which patient or his relatives bring a civil suit against a medical practitioner claiming compensation against the damage or injury suffered by him due to lack of reasonable care and skill or wilful negligence.

Criminal malpractice: Form of malpractice where a medical practitioner is prosecuted in a criminal court on charges of having caused death of his patient by a rash and negligent act not amounting to murder or when a patient dies because of gross carelessness in the treatment.

Res ipsa loquitur (the thing speaks for itself): When the act of negligence is such that it is self-explanatory like presence of gauze or small mosquito forceps inside abdomen after surgery it is called res ipsa loquitur.

Post hoc ergo propter hoc: The successive events being related causally.

Vicarious responsibility/vicarious liability: Means liability of an employer for negligence of his employee.

Respondent superior (let the master answer): The superior or the master is responsible for the act of his junior.

Qui facit per alum facit per se: He who acts through another, acts himself.

Contributory negligence: Refers to the negligent acts of the patient himself as a result of which he himself suffers injuries. This is the contribution on the part of the patient towards the damage caused to him by failing to follow the instructions of the doctor or following things not instructed by the doctor.

Curren's rule: An accused is not responsible for his unlawful act, if at the time of committing the act, he did not have the capacity to regulate his conduct as per requirement of the law due to mental disease or defect.

Doctrine of diminished responsibility: If it is proved that a person who committed a crime, suffers from aberration or weakness of mind, though not amounting to insanity (mental illness), then his responsibility for the act diminished from full to partial responsibility.

Agglutinins: Agglutinins are the naturally occurring antibodies present in the blood/serum, e.g. A and B.

Agglutinogens: Agglutinogens are the naturally occurring antigens present over RBC surface, e.g. A and B.

Bullet: It is the projectile that is fired from rifled firearms.

Cartridge/round: Basic unit of ammunition made up of case, primer, powder and pellets.

Catatonia (kata—down, tons—tone): Consists of excitable overactivity or bizarre posturing with abnormal muscle tone. It is seen in schizophrenia.

Chamber: It is receptacle for the projectile from where it is fired down the barrel.

Cheiloscopy/forensic stomatology: It is the study of lip prints.

Congnizable offence/cognizable case: Cognizable offence is an offence wherein the investigating officer can arrest an accused without a warrant.

Colliquative putrefaction: Progressive catalysis of a cell structure converting soft tissue of the body into thick, semi-liquid black pulpaceous mass.

Coma: State of deep unconsciousness from which a person cannot be aroused even with painful stimuli.

Consent: Consent is a willingness for an act to be done on oneself.

• Whenever two persons agree upon same thing, at the same time, in the same sense, they are said to consent over it (Indian Contract Act).

• A consent is no consent when consented to, by the consentor without knowing for which he is consenting to when consented.

Corpus delicti: Corpus delicti is the body of evidence or chain of evidence which is required to be proved beyond reasonable doubt to establish homicide.

Cross-examination: Cross-examination is the examination carried by the opposing counsel following examination in-chief.

Examination in-chief: It is an examination of the witness by counsel for the party that has cited him as witness.

Crural index: An index calculated by dividing length of tibia by length of femur multiplied by 100 for determination of race from skeleton.

Cryptorchid: Cryptorchid is a person with undescended testis (scrotum is like a pit without testis).

Cylinder: It is the rotating part of the revolver which contains several chambers for the projectiles.

Dementia: A condition in which mind has reached a certain stage of development and afterwards shows signs of deterioration.
• Dementia is a state of mind that fails to develop after a particular stage or does not develop at all.

Double action: It is a handgun mechanism in which single pull on the trigger cocks and releases the hammer, firing the round in the chamber.

Ejection port: A slot inside of semi-automatic pistol through which the empty casing of a fired round is ejected (in most pistols casing will eject to the right).

Embalming: A process by which a body may be mummified artificially for a purpose of preservation.

Firing action/fully automatic: Fires a succession of cartridges so long as the trigger is depressed or until the ammunition supply is exhausted.

Semi-automatic: Auto-loading action that will fire only a single shot for each pull of the trigger.

Firing pin: A firing pin is the pin which when stricken on the back of the cartridge ignites the primer.

Fugue: A state in which actions are performed without being aware of them.

Grain (firearm): It is a measure used to designate the weight of a bullet or the amount of gunpowder in cartridge (700 grains = 1 pound).

Holograph will: A will which is written by the testator in his own handwriting.

Heat haematoma: A soft, friable chocolate brown-coloured clot/haematoma seen in extradural space due to rupture of vessels with subsequent blood coagulation caused by exposure of head to intense heat.

Hammer (firearm): It is a firearm device trapped by movement of trigger, which impact the firing pin.

Hebephrenia: A type of schizophrenia where a person's thinking gets disorganized by hallucinations, illusions and delusions that he becomes impulsive and may commit any crime.

Hypospadias (hypo—below, spadias—penis): It is a birth defect where the urethral meatus opens on the under surface of the penis.

Indecent assault: An act committed with the intent or knowledge to outrage the modesty of a female is termed indecent assault (Section 354 of IPC).

Injury: As per Section 44 of IPC, any harm whatsoever illegally caused to a person in body, mind, reputation or property is called injury. In medical terminology, injury refers to physical trauma in contrast to the legal term injury, which includes harm to body, mind, reputation or property.

Kidnapping: It means carrying away a person from lawful guardianship by illegal means.

Magazine/clip: It is a device that holds cartridge in a repeating firearm, fitting into butt of a pistol.

Mutilomania: Irresistible desire to mutilate objects including body parts.

Muzzle: It is that end of the gun barrel from where the bullet emerges when gun is fired.

Oral evidence: Evidence carried in a court of law on oath, given orally.

Pistol: Any handgun which does not hold its ammunition in the revolving cylinder.

Pregnancy: A condition of having a developing embryo in the female, when ovum is fertilised by a spermatozoa.

Preternatural combustibility: A rare unnatural explosion due to hydrogen, methane, hydrogen sulphide accumulated in the intestine catching fire on exposure to galvanocautery or diathermy or to any flame near mouth or anus.

Primer: A volatile, highly inflammable compound that detonates when impacted by the firing pin, causing ignition of the gunpowder, e.g. mercury fulminate, lead azide.

Surrogate birth: Birth of a child from a woman who by contract agrees for preganancy to bear a child for someone else.

Syncope: Fainting attack or unconsciousness produced as a result of deficient blood supply to brain.

Trigger: Device that fires the gun when pulled by the index finger.

Vagitus uterinus and vagitus vaginus: Due to premature rupture of membranes with air entering into the sac, a foetus may cry with head still in vagina (vagitus vaginalis) or in uterus (vagitus uterinus). In vagitus uterinus, the foetus is dead in uterus.

In vagitus vaginalis the foetus is dead in vagina.

Wad cutter: A cylindrical-shaped bullet designed to cut clean holes in a paper target.

Prolonged labour: When the labour is inordinately delayed (more than 24 hours) since onset of labour it is called prolonged labour.

Reexamination: Examination of witness following cross-examination done by the counsel who conducted examination in-chief.

Rifling: Refers to twisting grooves cut in the barrel of a gun which puts a spin on the bullet, making its flight more stable.

Rugoscopy: Study of ridges and grooves in the palate.

Sexual offence: Defined as sexual intercourse performed in a way which is against the provision of the law of the land or sexual offence is an offence in which there is sexual violation upon a person contrary to law.

Starvation: Starvation is the state of a person who is deprived of his food and nutrition either suddenly or over a period of time leading to pillness or death, if not corrected.

MULTIPLE CHOICE QUESTIONS

FORENSIC MEDICINE

1. Forensic medicine deals with:

 a. Knowledge of law required for physicians
 b. Knowledge of medicine required for lawyers
 c. Knowledge of all medical sciences used in a court of law for administration of justice
 d. Knowledge of law and medicine required for lawyers

2. Medical jurisprudence deals with:

 a. Knowledge of medicine required for lawyers
 b. Knowledge of law required for docators for proper medical practice

 c. Knowledge of medicine required by doctors for practice
 d. Knowledge of law required for legal practice

3. Forensic toxicology means:

 a. Knowledge of poisons required for a forensic scientist
 b. Knowledge of poisons required for a medical man
 c. Knowledge of poisons utilized in administration of justice
 d. Knowledge of all aspects of substances causing desease, deformity of death, utilized in a court of law for administration of justice

4. The best form of inquest is:

a. Police

b. Coronor's

c. Magistrate's

d. Medical examiner system

5. Powers of first class magistrate are:

a. Three years imprisonment; Rs. 3,000 fine

b. Three years imprisonment; Rs.5,000 fine

c. One year imprisonment; Rs.1,000 fine

d. Five years imprisonment; Rs. 5,000 fine

6. Powers of second class magistrate are:

a. Six months imprisonment; Rs. 600 fine

b. One year imprisonment; Rs. 1,000 fine

c. One month imprisonment; Rs.100 fine

d. One year imprisonment; Rs. 3,000 fine

7. Powers of executive magistrate are:

a. One month imprisonment; Rs. 100 fine

b. One year imprisonment; Rs. 1,000 fine

c. Three years imprisonment; Rs. 3,000 fine

d. None of the above

8. Sessions judge cannot give this punishment:

a. Life imprisonment

b. Fine

c. Death sentence

d. None of the above

9. Maximum punishment an assistant session judge can award is:

a. Three years imprisonment

b. Five years imprisonment

c. Seven years imprisonment

d. Ten years imprisonment

10. An assistant session judge cannot award:

a. Fine

b. Rigorous imprisonment

c. Imprisonment up to 10 years

d. Death sentence

11. Exhumation is ordered by:

a. Civil surgeon

b. Superintendent of police

c. Circle inspector

d. District magistrate

12. Exceptions to oral evidence:

a. Death certificate

b. Postmortem report

c. Evidence recorded in lower court

d. None of the above

13. Following is not an exception to oral evidence:

a. Postmortem report

b. Expert opinion expressed in treatise

c. FSL report

d. Evidence recorded in lower court (medical)

14. Following punishment is removed in India:

a. Death sentence

b. Simple/rigorous imprisonment

c. Life imprisonment

d. Whipping

15. Subpoena means:

a. Document compelling witness to do his work

b. Document compelling witness to attend court of law

c. Document compelling attendence of a witness in a court of law under penalty

d. Document compelling the witness to handover a report in court

16. Purpose of taking oath is:

a. To speak truth

b. To speak truth and nothing but truth

c. To speak truth, whole truth and nothing but truth

d. To compel the witness to speak truth, the whole truth and nothing but truth

17. Purpose of cross-examination is:

    a. To test accuracy of statements of witness

    b. To help the accused

    c. To introduce the case to the judge

    d. To get replies for the questions of judge

18. Examination in-chief is:

    a. To roundup the whole case

    b. It is the first and main examination

    c. To discredit the witness

    d. To test the accuracy of statements made by witness

19. Re-examination is carried out by:

    a. Lawyer conducting main examination

    b. Lawyer conducting cross-examination

    c. Presiding officer of court

    d. None of the above

20. 'Evidence' means:

    a. Material produced before the court

    b. All documents produced for court's inspection

    c. Presence of accused

    d. Presence of victim

21. Leading question is one:

    a. Put by defence lawyer

    b. Put by prosecuting lawyer

    c. Which suggests its own answer

    d. None of the above

22. Documentary evidence includes:

    a. Dying declaration

    b. FIR

    c. Inquest report

    d. All of the above

23. Medicolegal report is:

    a. Report prepared by doctor and submitted in court

    b. Report prepared by doctor in obedience to demand by law enforcing authorities

    c. Medical certificate of death

    d. Medical certificate of sickness

24. Conduct money is tendered in:

    a. Summons from civil court

    b. Summons from criminal court

    c. Summons from the coronor

    d. Money paid by the appointing authority

25. In the following, who can record a dying declaration:

    a. Doctor attending the deceased in emergency

    b. Judicial magistrate

    c. Jail superintendent

    d. Commissioner of police

26. Dying deposition is recorded in the presence of:

    a. Doctor attending the deceased

    b. Magistrate

    c. Defence counsel

    d. All of the above

27. Volunteering of a statement is allowed for:

    a. Common witness

    b. Medical witness

    c. Police witness

    d. All of the above

28. Professional secrets can be divulged in court:

    a. If doctor feels so

    b. Cannot be divulged

    c. Can be divulged, if asked by court

    d. Can be divulged, if pressed by the court and under protest

29. Hostile witness is one who:

    a. Hosts the witness

    b. Does not answer leading questions

    c. Who delibrately utters falsehood

    d. All of the above

30. Perjury means:

    a. Breaking the oath

    b. Speaking the truth

    c. Submitting a document

    d. Not attending personally in court

31. Person who breaks the oath is said to have committed:

    a. No crime

    b. Perjury

    c. Obscene act

    d. Assault

32. Best type of evidence is:
   a. Oral evidence
   b. Documentary evidence
   c. Expert evidence
   d. Oral evidence proved in court

33. In 'hearsay evidence', the witness:
   a. Hears and says
   b. Sees and says
   c. Says what he writes
   d. Speaks and says what he is told by lawyer

34. On dying deposition:
   a. Leading questions are not permitted
   b. Cross-examination is allowed
   c. Doctor is not present
   d. Police is not allowed

35. Ballistics expert is specialized in:
   a. Ball pen writing
   b. Firearms and explosives
   c. Explosives
   d. Firearms

PERSONAL IDENTITY

36. Best method for identification is:
   a. DNA testing   b. Fingerprinting
   c. Photograph   d. Superimposition

37. Corpus delicti means:
   a. Postmortem certificate
   b. Body of evidence
   c. Viscera report
   d. None of the above

38. Cephalic index means:

   a. $\dfrac{\text{Max. breadth of skull}}{\text{Max. length of skull}} \times 100$

   b. $\dfrac{\text{Max. length of skull}}{\text{Max. breadth of skull}} \times 100$

   c. $\dfrac{\text{Max. length of skull}}{\text{Max. breadth of skull}} \times 100$

   d. $\dfrac{\text{Max. breadth of skull}}{\text{Max. length of skull}} \times 100$

39. Pure Aryans have cephalic index of:
   a. 80–84.9   b. 70–74.9
   c. 75–79.9   d. None of the above

40. Chinese are:
   a. Dolichocephalic
   b. Mesaticephalic
   c. Brachycephalic
   d. Mixed

41. Cephalic index of Europeans is:
   a. 70–74.9   b. 75–79.9
   c. 80–84.9   d. None of the above

42. 'Prenatal Diagnostic Techniques Act, 1994' helps in prevention and control of:
   a. Infanticide
   b. Suicide
   c. Selective abortion of female foetus
   d. None of the above

43. Polymorphonuclear luecocytes show:
   a. Barr body
   b. Davidson body
   c. No body
   d. Any body

44. Barr bodies are seen in the buccal mucosal cells of:
   a. Females
   b. Males
   c. Female pseudohermaphrodites
   d. None of the above

45. The chromosomes in human beings are normally:
   a. 22 pairs   b. 44 pairs
   c. 23 pairs   d. 46 pairs

46. The male determinant chromosome is:
   a. Y   b. X
   c. O   d. H

47. Klinefelter's syndrome is:
   a. 47, XXY   b. 46, XY
   c. 45, XO   d. 46, XX

48. In Klinefelter's syndrome:
   a. Testosterone level is decreased
   b. FSH level decreased

c. LH level is decreased

d. None of the above

49. The chromosomal pattern of Turner's syndrome is:

a. 46, XY   b. 45, XO

c. 46, XX   d. 45, YO

50. The nuclear sex in male hermaphrodite is:

a. 46, XY   b. 45, XO

c. 46, XX   d. 45, XY

51. In female pseudohermaphrodite, nuclear sex is:

a. 46, XX   b. 46, XY

c. 46, XO   d. 45, XY

52. First permanent molar errupts around:

a. 5–6 years   b. 6–7 years

c. 7–8 years   d. 9–11 years

53. Permanent canines erupt around:

a. 7–9 years   b. 9–11 years

c. 11–13 years   d. None of the above

54. Temporary set of teeth contains:

a. 18 teeth   b. 20 teeth

c. 22 teeth   d. 28 teeth

55. Premolars are absent in:

a. Temporary set

b. Permanent set

c. During mixed dentition

d. None of the above

56. In comparison of males, cranial capacity of females is:

a. 10% more   b. 10% less

c. 5% more   d. 5% less

57. The most reliable and best marked sex distinguishing characters are seen in:

a. Skull   b. Thorax

c. Pelvis   d. Femora

58. The male sacrum is:

a. Long and wide

b. Short and wide

c. Short and narrow

d. Long and narrow

59. The preauricular sulcus is well marked in:

a. Multiparous female

b. Elderly female

c. Nulliparous female

d. None of the above

60. In comparison to males, the acetabula in females are:

a. Wider   b. Narrower

c. Equal   d. Deeper

61. The ischial tuberosities in males are:

a. Inverted   b. Everted

c. Straight   d. Rounded

62. The neck of the femur in females forms an angle with the shaft of the nature of:

a. Obtuse angle

b. Nearly right angle

c. Very acute angle

d. Very obtuse angle

63. Greater sciatic notch in males in comparison of females is:

a. Larger   b. Wider

c. Deeper   d. Shallower

64. Body of the pubis in females is:

a. Triangular   b. Square

c. Round   d. Irregular

65. Subpubic angle in males is:

a. Inverted V-shaped

b. Inverted U-shaped

c. Inverted C-shaped

d. None of the above

66. Pelvic cavity in males is:

a. Broad and round

b. Conical and funnel shaped

c. Narrow and round

d. None of the above

67. Pelvic inlet in females is:

a. Heart shaped   b. Elliptical

c. Conical   d. Irregular

68. Chin in males is:

a. Rounded   b. Square

c. Pointed   d. None of the above

69. Ramus of mandible in males is:
   a. Inverted   b. Everted
   c. Straight   d. None of the above

70. Male skull capacity is:
   a. 1350–1400 cc   b. 1400–1450 cc
   c. 1450–1500 cc   d. 1500–1550 cc

71. Orbits in the female are:
   a. Rounded   b. Square
   c. Irregular   d. Triangular

72. In males, the body of the sternum in relation to the length of the manubrium is:
   a. More than twice
   b. Less than twice
   c. One-and-a-half times more
   d. One-and-a-half times less

73. Femoral bicondylar width in females is:
   a. 67–76 mm   b. 74–89 mm
   c. 49–66 mm   d. 89–102 mm

74. General pelvic shape in females is like:
   a. Flat bowl
   b. Deep funnel
   c. Long and curved
   d. Short and curved

75. The degree of accuracy of sexing adult skeleton with only pelvis is:
   a. 80%   b. 90%
   c. 95%   d. 100%

76. The degree of accuracy of sexing adult skeleton with only skull is:
   a. 100%   b. 95%
   c. 90%   d. 98%

77. The degree of accuracy of sexing adult skeleton with the pelvis and skull is:
   a. 80%   b. 95%
   c. 98%   d. 100%

78. The rudiments of all the temporary teeth are present:
   a. At birth   b. In three months
   c. In six months   d. By one year

79. Teeth calcification occurs:
   a. From crown to neck to roots
   b. From roots to neck to crown
   c. From neck to roots and crown
   d. From neck to crown and root

80. Deciduous teeth mean:
   a. Permanent teeth
   b. Temporary teeth
   c. Premolars
   d. Wisdom teeth

81. Temporary lateral incisors erupt:
   a. Earlier in upper jaw
   b. Earlier in lower jaw
   c. Before eruption of central incisors
   d. After eruption of canines

82. Temporary canines erupt at around:
   a. 7–9 months
   b. 17–18 months
   c. 6–8 months
   d. 12–14 months

83. Temporary first molar erupts at around
   a. 6–8 months   b. 12–14 months
   c. 7–9 months   d. 20–30 months

84. First premolar erupts at:
   a. 6–7 years   b. 7–9 years
   c. 9–11 years   d. 12–14 years

85. Permanent canine erupts before:
   a. First premolar   b. First molar
   c. Lateral incisor   d. Second molar

86. The most reliable of Gustafson's criteria is:
   a. Attrition
   b. Secondary dentine deposition
   c. Transparency of root
   d. Cementum opposition

87. When enamel is lost, the following is exposed:
   a. Dentine
   b. Dental pulp
   c. Root
   d. Periodontal membrane

88. Generally the first temporary tooth to appear is:
   a. Upper central incisor
   b. Lower central incisor

c. Upper lateral incisor

d. Lower lateral incisor

89. Canine teeth are used for:

a. Cutting the food

b. Tearing the food

c. Grinding the food

d. Biting

90. Molar teeth are used for:

a. Cutting the food

b. Tearing the food

c. Grinding the food

d. Biting

91. Centre for coracoid process of scapula unites at about:

a. 14 years   b. 15 years

c. 16 years   d. 18 years

92. Centre for acromion process of scapula appears around:

a. 14 years   b. 15 years

c. 16 years   d. 18 years

93. Triradiate cartilage of acetabulum is obliterated by:

a. 14 years   b. 15 years

c. 16 years   d. 18 years

94. Appearance of centre of ossification for ischial tuberosity is about:

a. 14 years   b. 15 years

c. 16 years   d. 18 years

95. Appearance of centre of ossification for inner end of collar bone is:

a. 15–16 years   b. 7–18 years

c. 18–19 years   d. 20–21 years

96. Pisciform bone appears at:

a. 10–11 years   b. 11–12 years

c. 12–13 years   d. 14–15 years

97. Appearance of olecranon is about:

a. 9 years   b. 12 years

c. 11 years   d. 14 years

98. Medicolegal autopsy cannot be carried out without the written order of:

a. Professor of forensic medicine

b. Subinspector of police

c. Medical superintendent

d. District collector

99. The main objective of medicolegal autopsy is:

a. To help investigating officer

b. To establish cause of death

c. To demonstrate to medical students

d. To trained doctors

100. Murder is:

a. Accidental death

b. Natural death

c. Homicide with intention to kill

d. Unexpected death

101. In a decomposed body:

a. Partial postmortem is done

b. Viscera need not be preserved

c. Complete and thorough autopsy should be done

d. Any of the above

102. Postmortem should not be done in night because:

a. Colour changes become deceptive

b. It is not a legal emergency

c. It is not a medical emergency

d. All of the above

103. The best way to conduct autopsy is by opining and examining first:

a. Head and cranial cavity

b. Thoracic cavity

c. Abdominal cavity

d. Any of the above

104. The stomach should be opened:

a. Along the greater curvature

b. Along the lesser curvature

c. On the front wall between the two curvatures

d. None of the above

105. The best way to examine testis is:

a. Without opening

b. By making incision on scrotum

c. By carefully bringing them up through inguinal canal

d. None of the above

106. For the histopathology examination, the tissues collected are preserved in:
   a. Common salt   b. Glycerine
   c. 10% formalin   d. None of the above

107. The commonest site of coronary artery block is:
   a. Left descending branch of anterior coronary artery
   b. Anterior descending branch of left coronary artery
   c. Circumflex artery
   d. Posterior descending branch of right coronary artery

108. In case of firearm injuries, before autopsy is started:
   a. Body should be washed
   b. X-ray examination should be done
   c. Clothes should be removed
   d. None of the above

109. The date and hour of postmortem examination should be noted to establish:
   a. Identity of person
   b. Scene of crime
   c. Body of evidence
   d. Time of death

110. All natural orifices should be examined at the time of autopsy for:
   a. Foreign bodies
   b. Bleeding
   c. Trauma
   d. All of the above

111. The injury report is incomplete:
   a. If antemortem/postmortem is not written
   b. If age of the injury is not written
   c. If nature of weapon causing it is not written
   d. All of the above

112. Partial postmortem is:
   a. Sometimes permitted
   b. Always allowed
   c. Never permitted
   d. None of the above

113. Postmortem examination should not be carried out until:
   a. Inquest report is given
   b. Medical report of treating doctor is given
   c. Forwarding letter of authorized person is not given
   d. All of the above

114. Cause of death should not be kept pending:
   a. When cause of death is obvious
   b. When viscera are sent for chemical analysis
   c. When histopathology examination is required.
   d. None of the above

115. Presence of detection of ingested poison in urine suggests that:
   a. Poison has passed through kidney
   b. Poison has passed through stomach
   c. Poison has passed through stomach, liver and kidney
   d. None of the above

116. Viscera for chemical analysis should generally be preserved in:
   a. Saturated solution of common salt
   b. Normal saline
   c. Sodium chloride solution
   d. None of the above

117. In all cases of advanced decomposition:
   a. Viscera should be kept for chemical analysis
   b. Viscera need not be kept for chemical analysis
   c. Chemical analysis is not necessary
   d. Cause of death should be given

118. The earliest site to show decomposition is:
   a. Right iliac fossa
   b. Left iliac fossa
   c. Hypochondrium
   d. Hypogastrium

119. The earliest site of decomposition in internal organs is:
   a. Ascending aorta
   b. Left ventricle

c. Portal vein

d. Inferior vena cava

120. **The last organ to get decomposed is:**

   a. Oesophagus

   b. Virgin uterus

   c. Multiparous uterus

   d. Ureter

121. **Rectified spirit should not be used as preservative in cases of:**

   a. Alcohol

   b. Carbolic acid

   c. Phosphorus (yellow)

   d. Any of the above

122. **After autopsy, postmortem room should be cleaned with solution of:**

   a. Formalin

   b. Saturated solution of saline

   c. Alcohol

   d. 10% solution of sodium hypochlorite

123. **Heart should be opened at autopsy from:**

   a. Right atrium, right ventricle, left atrium, left ventricle

   b. Left ventricle, left atrium, right ventricle, right atrium

   c. Left atrium, left ventricle, right atrium, right ventricle

   d. Right ventricle, right atrium, left ventricle, left atrium

124. **Autopsy, the kidneys are dissected from:**

   a. Outside to inside

   b. Inside to outside

   c. Above downwards

   d. Before backwards

125. **Liver should be dissected along the:**

   a. Long (transverse) axis, outside-to-inside

   b. Long (transverse) axis, inside-to-outside

   c. Vertical axis, outside-to-inside

   d. Vertical axis, inside-to-outside

126. **Spleen should be dissected:**

   a. Hilum-to-outside in long axis

   b. Outside-to-hilum in long axis (horizontal)

   c. Hilum-to-outside in vertical axis

   d. Outside-to-hilum in vertical axis

127. **The third lobe of left lung is:**

   a. Absent

   b. Present

   c. Represented by lingula

   d. None of the above

128. **On lifting the vault of cranium, one should look for:**

   a. Air embolism   b. Fat embolism

   c. Thrombi   d. None of the above

129. **Fat embolism can be demonstrated by fresh frozen section of suspected organ to:**

   a. Osmium tetroxide

   b. Haemotoxylin and eosin

   c. Leishman's stain

   d. Gram's stain

130. **Commonest site of thromboembolism at autopsy is:**

   a. Pulmonary trunk

   b. Aorta

   c. Left coronary artery

   d. Renal artery

131. **Hemopericardium can cause sudden death due to:**

   a. Cardiac tamponade

   b. Myocardial infarction

   c. Infective pericarditis

   d. Ventricular fibrilation

132. **Rigor mortis at autopsy is not found in some joints after 12 hours because of:**

   a. Cold weather

   b. Hot weather

   c. Rough handling

   d. None of the above

133. **Adipocere suggests that:**

   a. Dead body was in marshy place

   b. Dead body was in air conditioned room

   c. Dead body was covered with blankets

   d. None of the above

134. Presence of maggots on the body suggests after death a lapse of:
    a. Below 2 days   b. Below 3 days
    c. Below 4 days   d. Below 5 days

135. Presence of eggs suggests after death a lapse of:
    a. More than one day
    b. More than two days
    c. More than three days
    d. More than four days

136. The commonest eggs seen on the dead bodies are of:
    a. Mosquitoes   b. Spiders
    c. Houseflies   d. Butterflies

137. Presence of lathery froth at nostrils and mouth suggests:
    a. Insecticide poisoning
    b. Drowning
    c. Anaesthetic death
    d. Heart failure

138. Rupture of berry aneurysm of artery can cause death in age group of:
    a. First two decades
    b. Second two decades
    c. Third two decades
    d. Forth two decades

139. Decomposition takes longer time in the:
    a. Air
    b. Water
    c. Earth
    d. In a closed room

140. Consent from relatives is required in cases of:
    a. Medicolegal autopsy
    b. Non-medicolegal autopsy
    c. Partial autopsy
    d. All of the above

141. Panel postmortem is legaly allowed only in cases of:
    a. Dowry deaths
    b. Accident deaths
    c. Murder cases
    d. Poisoning cases

142. In police custody deaths, the postmortem examination requires to be:
    a. Radiographed
    b. Photographed
    c. Videographed
    d. None of the above

143. Multiple injuries of different age groups suggest:
    a. Repeated battering
    b. Motive to kill
    c. Accident proneness
    d. None of the above

144. Bumper fractures are seen in the cases of:
    a. Fall from height
    b. Vehicular accident
    c. Domestic accident
    d. None of the above

145. Pond fracture is seen in cases of:
    a. Children below 5 years
    b. Teenagers
    c. Adults
    d. Elderly people

146. Organisms of decomposition include:
    a. Gonococci
    b. *Treponema pallidum*
    c. HIV
    d. *Clostridium welchii*

147. Gases of decomposition do not include:
    a. Methane
    b. Hydrogen sulphide
    c. Oxygen
    d. Nitric oxide

148. A black contusion, after death:
    a. Remains black
    b. Becomes yellow
    c. Gets infected
    d. None of the above

149. Postmortem wounds do not show changes of:
    a. Vital reactions
    b. Infection
    c. Gaping
    d. Any of the above

150. Ant bites are mistaken for:

a. Lacerations
b. Abrasions
c. Contusions
d. None of the above

151. Injuries on the clothes:

a. Always correspond to injuries on the body
b. Generally correspond to injuries on the body
c. Never correspond to injuries on the body
d. Sometimes do not correspond with injuries on the body

152. Postmortem lividity suggests:

a. Time since death
b. Sudden death
c. Poisoning
d. None of the above

153. Cadaveric spasm is:

a. Antemortem process
b. Postmortem process
c. Type of rigor mortis
d. None of the above

154. In India, exhumation can be carried out after death within a period of:

a. 2 years   b. 5 Years
c. 30 years   d. Any time

155. Artefacts at autopsy may lead to diagnosis of:

a. Wrong cause of death
b. Wrong manner of death
c. Wrong time interpretation
d. Any of the above

156. A deep grove over the neck may be:

a. An artefact
b. A ligature mark
c. Axe wound
d. Any of the above

157. Diastatic fracture is:

a. Postmortem fracture
b. Suture separation
c. Separation of diaphysis
d. Rupture of diaphragm

158. In any medicolegal case brought for examination, the first duty is:

a. Informing the police
b. Instituting immediate treatment
c. Informing the consultant
d. Recording dying declarations

159. Postmortem burns do not show:

a. Red border
b. Fluid filled blisters
c. Infection
d. All of the above

DEATH AND MEDICOLEGAL ASPECTS

160. Death is declared when:

a. The heart sounds are not heard
b. The pain reflex is not elicited
c. All brainstem reflexes are absent
d. When the person does not respond to shouting his name

161. Organ transplantation team should not include:

a. Anaesthetist
b. General surgeon
c. Doctor certifying death
d. Any of the above

162. For transplantation, removal of organs should be authorized by:

a. Deceased person
b. The relatives
c. The deceased and the relatives
d. The doctor

163. The following is not a mode of death:

a. Coma   b. Syncope
c. Asphyxia   d. Shock

164. PVS means:

a. Persistant vegetative state
b. Persistant ventricular systole
c. Periodic ventricular systole
d. None of the above

165. The death rattle is due to:

a. Mucus in the oesophagus
b. Mucus in respiratory passages
c. Irregular breathing
d. Any of the above

166. In brainstem death:
    a. There is no corneal reflex
    b. The oculocephalic reflex is absent
    c. Vestibulo-ocular reflex is absent
    d. All of the above

167. After death:
    a. The elasticity of skin is lost
    b. The body temperature falls
    c. The pupils remain dilated and fixed
    d. Any of the above

168. The rate of fall of temperature in first six hours after death in a temperate climate is approximately:
    a. 1.5°F/hour   b. 1.5°C/hour
    c. 1.5°R/hour   d. 2.5°C/hour

169. Postmortem caloricity is due to:
    a. Yellow fever
    b. Sun stroke
    c. Cerebrospinal meningitis
    d. All of the above

170. The following is a test for circulation:
    a. Wredin's test
    b. Magnan's symptom
    c. Magnus test
    d. None of the above

171. The rate of cooling of the body is influenced by:
    a. Fat
    b. Body surface area
    c. Desease status
    d. All of the above

172. Cadaveric changes in muscles are due to:
    a. Fall of concentration of ATP
    b. Raise of concentration of ATP
    c. Fall of cholinesterase levels
    d. Absence of glycogenolysis

173. Autolysis in macerated foetus:
    a. Occurs in sterile conditions
    b. Occurs in presence of saprophytic organisms
    c. Occurs in presence of *Clostridium welchii*
    d. None of the above

174. After death, muscles respond to electrical stimuli, up to a maximum of:
    a. 4 hours   b. 8 hours
    c. 10 hours   d. 12 hours

175. Following putrefies soon:
    a. Lungs   b. Bladder
    c. Gravid uterus   d. Prostate

176. The following putrefies late:
    a. Adult brain   b. Stomach
    c. Liver   d. Prostate

177. Putrefaction is delayed in:
    a. Summer
    b. Damp climate
    c. Dry weather
    d. None of the above

178. Mummification occurs more commonly in:
    a. Rajasthan   b. Cherrapunji
    c. Himalayas   d. All of the above

179. Rate of growth of nails:
    a. 1 mm/month   b. 2 mm/month
    c. 3 mm/month   d. None of the above

180. The rate of growth of hair.
    a. 1–3 cm/week
    b. 1–3 mm/week
    c. 5–10 mm/week
    d. None of the above

181. Death is presumed, if a person lived for 30 years is not heard of, for a period of:
    a. 3 years   b. 5 years
    c. 7 years   d. 10 years

182. The question of presumption of survivorship can occur:
    a. In earthquake b. In air crash
    c. In air raids   d. Any of the above

183. The following is not a type of asphyxial death:
    a. Strangulation   b. Starvation
    c. Hanging   d. Lynching

184. Lynching is a type of:
    a. Homicidal hanging
    b. Accidental hanging

c. Suicidal hanging

d. None of the above

185. In hanging, the constricting force is:

a. Ligature

b. Weight of the body

c. Height of the body

d. Any of the above

186. Salivary stains around the angle of mouth suggest:

a. Antemortem hanging

b. Antemortem burns

c. Antemortem drowning

d. None of the above

187. In strangulation, asphyxia is due to:

a. Pressure around neck

b. Lump in the throat

c. Stricture of oesophagus

d. Any of the above

188. In bansdola:

a. Pressure is on front and back of the neck

b. Pressure is all around the neck

c. Pressure is inside respiratory passages

d. None of the above

189. The following is not a type of strangulation:

a. Garroting   b. Throttling

c. Choking   d. Mugging

190. Causes of suffocation do not include:

a. Choking

b. Inhalation of irrespirable gases

c. Traumatic asphyxia

d. Hanging

191. Cafe coronary is due to:

a. Reflex cardiac arrest

b. Burns

c. Electrocution

d. Hanging

192. Froth at nostrils is seen in:

a. Dry drowning

b. Secondary drowning

c. Immersion syndrome

d. Wet drowning

193. In salt water drowning, there is:

a. Pulmonary oedema

b. Cerebral oedema

c. Ascites

d. Any of the above

194. In starvation death, the body weight loss is up to:

a. 10% and above

b. 20% and above

c. 30% and above

d. 40% and above

195. The last tissue to be affected in starvation is:

a. Brain   b. Kidney

c. Intestines   d. Liver

196. Hypothermia causes death due to:

a. Lack of oxygen

b. Lack of nutrition

c. Lack of protection

d. Meningitis

197. Cold is endured longer by:

a. Women   b. Men

c. Children   d. Old people

198. Heat cramps are caused by loss of:

a. Potassium chloride

b. Sodium chloride

c. Magnesium chloride

d. Calcium chloride

199. In heat hyperpyrexia:

a. Heat regulation is impaired

b. Heart regulation is impaired

c. Hearing regulation is impaired

d. Any of the above

200. In heat cramps, main treatment consists of giving:

a. Sodium chloride

b. Artificial respiration

c. Glucose saline

d. Pethidine

201. Moist heat causes:

a. Burns

b. Scalds

c. Brush burn

d. None of the above

202. Pain in burns is due to:
- a. Nerve endings
- b. Coagulation of muscle proteins
- c. Loss of fluid
- d. None of the above

203. Non-exclusive first degree burns cause:
- a. Simple hurt
- b. Grieveous hurt
- c. Dangerous hurt
- d. Any of the above

204. In burns, death can occur due to carbon monoxide, if concentration of CoHb is:
- a. >10%
- b. <10%
- c. <5%
- d. None of the above

205. Postmortem burns do not show:
- a. Line of redness
- b. Singeing of hair
- c. Blisters
- d. Carbon monoxide in blood

206. Arboroscent marks of lightning show:
- a. Copper
- b. Nickel
- c. Iron
- d. None of the above

207. Highest resistance to electricity is offered by:
- a. Skin
- b. Muscles
- c. Blood
- d. Nerve tissue

208. Honeycomb vacuolisation is seen in cases of:
- a. Flame burns
- b. Scalds
- c. Joule's burns
- d. Arborescent marks

209. In electrocution, the following is seen:
- a. Gangrene
- b. Avascular necrosis
- c. Heat cracks
- d. None of the above

210. Palisading is seen in cases of:
- a. Lightning
- b. Burns
- c. Electrocution
- d. None of the above

211. The following metallic particles are seen in cases of Joule's burns:
- a. Copper
- b. Aluminium
- c. Zinc
- d. All of the above

212. The overlying skin is intact in cases of:
- a. Bruise
- b. Abrasion
- c. Ligature marks
- d. None of the above

213. Tailing of the wound suggests:
- a. Beginning of the wound
- b. Middle of the wound
- c. End of the wound
- d. Any of the above

214. Heaping up of epithelium suggests:
- a. Beginning of abrasion
- b. Middle of abrasion
- c. End of the abrasions
- d. No abrasion.

215. Scratch is a type of:
- a. Contusion
- b. Laceration
- c. Abrasion
- d. Incised wound

216. Colour changes in bruise are due to changes in:
- a. Haemoglobin
- b. Albumin
- c. Globulin
- d. Plasma

217. Deep bruises can be demonstrated by:
- a. Dissection
- b. X-ray examination
- c. Aspiration
- d. Any of the above

218. False bruises are caused by:
- a. Juice of marking nut
- b. Root of *chitra*
- c. *Lal chitra*
- d. All of the above

219. Crushed margins are seen in:
- a. Bruise
- b. Laceration
- c. Incised wound
- d. Stab wound

220. Infections are more common in:
- a. Abrasions
- b. Lacerations
- c. Incised wounds
- d. Any of the above

221. The following is a smooth-bored firearm:

a. Pistol   b. Muzzle loader

c. Revolver   d. Rifle

222. Rifling is seen:

a. On the bullet

b. On the barrel

c. Inside the barrel

d. Inside the bullet

223. Primer consists of:

a. Nitrocellulose

b. Potassium nitrate

c. Mercury fulminate

d. Nitroglycerine

224. Slug consists of:

a. Lead balls   b. Zinc pieces

c. Steel pieces   d. None of the above

225. Perforating wound shows:

a. Wound of entry

b. Wound of entry, wound of exit

c. Abraded collar

d. Tattooing

226. Any firearm consists of:

a. Barrel   b. Butt

c. Cartridge   b. All of the above

227. Choking is seen in:

a. Shotgun   b. Rifle

c. Pistol   d. Revolver

228. Wad is seen in the cartridge of:

a. Revolver

b. Rifle

c. Smooth-bored weapon

d. Any of the above

229. Cannelure is a part of:

a. Bullet

b. Pellet

c. Percussion cap

d. None of the above

230. X-ray examination in firearm injuries is carried:

a. To locate the bullets/pellets

b. To locate small metallic fragments left inside the body

c. To know the track

d. All of the above

231. Ammunition of rifled firearm consists of:

a. Nitroglycerine

b. Nitric acid

c. Carbon dioxide

d. Hydrogen sulphide

232. Flame effect of burning in rifled firearm occurs:

a. Up to 20 cm   b. Up to 40 cm

c. Up to 60 cm   d. None of the above

233. Involuntary tottooing occurs in shotguns:

a. Up to 75 cm

b. Up to 3 metres

c. Up to 6 metres

d. Up to 10 metres

234. Point blank range means:

a. Distant range   b. Contact range

c. Near contact   d. None of the above

235. Yaw means:

a. Ricochet phenomena

b. Balling of shot

c. Tumbling bullet

d. None of the above

236. When one bullet is behind the other like a piggy back, it is called:

a. Souvenir bullet

b. Tandem bullet

c. Dumdum bullet

d. Yawning bullet

237. Duplex cartridge contains:

a. One bullet   b. Two bullets

c. No bullet   d. Any of the above

238. Primary markings on bullet are due to:

a. Barrel

b. Firing pin

c. Gunpowder

d. Barrel irregularities

239. Individualisation of a firearm is possible by:

a. Primary markings on bullet

b. Secondary markings on bullet

c. a and b both

d. None of the above

240. Odd and even rule is helpful in:

a. Knowing the number of bullets

b. Knowing about the presence of bullets inside the body

c. Knowing the direction of fire

d. None of the above

241. Explosion due to bomb produces:

a. Burns   b. Fumes

c. Air blast   d. All of the above

242. Black gunpowder consists of:

a. Charcoal (75%), potassium nitrate (10%), sulphur (15%)

b. Charcoal (15%), potassium nitrate (75%), sulphur (10%)

c. Charcoal (10%), potassium nitrate (15%), sulphur (15%)

d. None of the above

243. Rifle is a:

a. Hand weapon

b. Shoulder weapon

c. Mounted weapon

d. Rocket launcher

244. Incendiary bullet contains:

a. Sulphur   b. Phosphorus

c. Wax   d. All of the above

245. Harrison and Gilroy test helps to detect:

a. Drowning

b. Pregnancy

c. Discharge of firearm

d. Infanticide

246. Scalp consists of:

a. Pericranium

b. Loose areolar tissue

c. Skin

d. All of the above

247. Ectopic contusion normally occurs around the:

a. Nose

b. Orbit

c. Ear

d. Any of the above

248. Comminuted fracture consists of:

a. Several fragments of bone

b. Communicates into a cavity

c. Depressed fracture

d. Compound fracture

249. Compound fracture shows:

a. Closed injury

b. Open injury

c. Comminuted fracture

d. None of the above

250. Lucid interval is seen in:

a. Extradural haemorrhage

b. Subdural haemorrhage

c. Subarachnoid haemorrhage

d. Intracerebral haemorrhage

251. Steering wheel impact causes:

a. Ruptured aorta

b. Buckled sternum

c. Myocardial trauma

d. Any of the above

252. Corneal ulcer is:

a. Simple injury

b. Grievous injury

c. Dangerous injury

d. Any of the above

253. Love bites are more common on:

a. Breast   b. Hands

c. Legs   d. Ears

254. Haemorrhage in anterior chamber of eye:

a. Leucoma   b. Glaucoma

c. Trachoma   d. Hyphema

255. Bleeding from Little's area is seen as:

a. Nasal bleeding

b. Bleeding from ear

c. Bleeding from mouth

d. None of the above

256. Whiplash injury is due to:

a. Hyperflexion

b. Hyperextension

c. a and b

d. None of the above

257. Commonest cause of impotence is:
- a. Psychological
- b. Physical in capacity
- c. Endocervical problem
- d. Infertility

258. In India, the lower age limit for presumption of impotence is:
- a. 18 years
- b. 16 years
- c. 14 years
- d. No such limit

259. Reduced fertility can occur due to:
- a. Diethyl stibestrol
- b. Polychlorinated biphenyls
- c. Organophosphorus pesticidis
- d. Any of the above

260. Impotence in woman is called:
- a. Frigidity
- b. Rigidity
- c. Geredity
- d. Any of the above

261. AID is recommended in cases of:
- a. Rh incompatibility
- b. Azoospermia
- c. Genetic abnormalities
- d. All of the above

262. Surrogate mother is a:
- a. Biological mother
- b. Hired mother
- c. Neither
- d. Either

263. Signs of defloration include:
- a. Elastic hymen
- b. Hymenal tears
- c. Lax vagina
- d. Any of the above

264. The question of virginity arises in cases of:
- a. Rape
- b. Fall from height
- c. Pregnancy
- d. Adultery

265. Any injury to hymen should be carefully examined for presence of:
- a. Blood
- b. Threadworms
- c. Foreign body
- d. All of the above

266. The surest sign of virginity is:
- a. Absence of hymen
- b. Presence of hymen
- c. Intact, inelastic hymen
- d. Imperforate hymen

267. Quickening is due to:
- a. Foetal movements
- b. Intestinal movements
- c. Flatulence
- d. Any of the above

268. Montgomery's tubercles are seen:
- a. On the breast
- b. In the axilla
- c. On the abdomen
- d. On the cheeks

269. Normal colour of vaginal mucosal membrane is:
- a. Pink
- b. Violet
- c. Blue
- d. Black

270. Positive sign of pregnancy is:
- a. Foetal heart sounds
- b. Skin pigmentation
- c. Ballottement
- d. Any of the above

271. Lochia is:
- a. Nasal discharge
- b. Discharge from ear
- c. Discharge from vagina
- d. None of the above

272. Lochia alba is seen during the:
- a. First three days after delivery
- b. First week after delivery
- c. Second week after delivery
- d. Fourth week after delivery

273. Spalding sign suggests:
- a. Foetal distress
- b. Foetal death
- c. Foetal abnormality
- d. Live foetus

274. Foetal death can be confirmed by:
- a. Palpation
- b. Auscultation
- c. Ballottement
- d. Sonography

275. Sonography in pregnancy is positive at the earliest by:
- a. 6 weeks
- b. 10 weeks
- c. 12 weeks
- d. 14 weeks

276. Foetal heart sounds are heard by:
- a. 6–8 weeks
- b. 10–14 weeks
- c. 8–16 weeks
- d. 18–20 weeks

277. Corpus luteum of pregnancy attains its largest size by:
- a. 8 weeks
- b. 10 weeks
- c. 14 weeks
- d. 16 weeks

278. Commonest cause of maternal death in pregnancy is:
- a. Haemorrhage
- b. Toxaemia
- c. Anaemia
- d. Jaundice

279. Feigning of pregnancy by a woman may be to get a benefit of:
- a. Blackmail
- b. Property right
- c. Mental illness
- d. Escape from punishment

280. Following is a sign of recent delivery:
- a. Big uterus
- b. Lochia
- c. Corpus luteum
- d. All of the above

281. Abnormal sexual offences include:
- a. Masturbation
- b. Sodomy
- c. Rape
- d. Incest

282. The sin of gonorrhoea means:
- a. Female homosexuality
- b. Male homosexuality
- c. Bestiality
- d. Buccal coitus

283. Rape is defined under Section:
- a. 376 of IPC
- b. 375 of IPC
- c. 377 of IPC
- d. 354 of IPC

284. Marital rape is:
- a. Man and his wife are under decree of separation
- b. When the husband helps another man to commirape on his wife
- c. When man has sexual intercourse with other's wife
- d. Any of the above

285. Section 376 C deals with:
- a. Sexual intercourse
- b. Sexual intercourse amounting to rape
- c. Sexual intercourse not amounting to rape
- d. Forcible sexual intercourse

286. Section 376 B deals with:
- a. Public servant
- b. Manager of jail
- c. Member of hospital management
- d. Man with decree of separation

287. The punishment for gang rape is not less than:
- a. One year
- b. Three years
- c. Five years
- d. Ten years

288. When the rape victim is below 12 years the punishment is not less than:
- a. Ten years
- b. Five years
- c. Three years
- d. One year

289. When a man has sexual intercourse with his wife during separation, punishment is:
- a. Up to six months
- b. Up to one year
- c. Up to two years
- d. None of the above

290. When a man commits rape on a known pregnant woman, the punishment is not less than:
- a. Ten years
- b. Twenty years
- c. Five years
- d. None of the above

291. Punishment for unnatural sexual offences extends up to:
- a. Two years
- b. Three years
- c. Five years
- d. Ten years

292. Catamite means:
- a. Rapist
- b. Active agent in sodomy
- c. Passive agent in sodomy
- d. Lesbian

293. Female homosexuality is called:
- a. Transvestism
- b. Transsexualism
- c. Tribadism
- d. Satyriasis

294. Satyriasis is opposite of:

a. Mutilomania
b. Dypsomania
c. Nymphomania
d. None of the above

295. Masochism causes sexual gratification:

a. By torturing   b. By being tortured
c. By both   d. By none

296. Wearing clothes of opposite sex to derive pleasure is called:

a. Transsexualism
b. Transvestism
c. Exhibitionism
d. Fetichism

297. Fetichism is seen in:

a. Males   b. Females
c. Both   d. None of the above

298. The following is not a sexual deviation:

a. Sadism   b. Masochism
c. Rape   d. Transvestism

299. Paederasty means:

a. Sexual intercourse with a girl
b. Sexual intercourse with woman
c. Anal sexual intercourse with a small boy
d. Sexual intercourse with animal

300. Death during sexual intercourse can be due to:

a. Bleeding
b. Vagal inhibition
c. Pressure on the neck
d. Any of the above

301. Presence of semen in the vaginal canal is a proof of:

a. Rape
b. Sexual intercourse
c. Indecent assault
d. Attempted rape

302. Shaving of the perianal hair is suggestive of:

a. Habitual passive agent
b. Habitual active agent
c. Rapist
d. None of the above

303. Presence of smegma:

a. Suggests sexual intercourse
b. Rules out sexual intercourse
c. Suggests rape
d. None of the above

304. Sexual intercourse by misinterpretation of facts is:

a. Rape
b. Not rape
c. Attempt to rape
d. Lawful sexual intercourse

305. Intact hymen suggests:

a. Virgin
b. False virgin
c. Attempted rape
d. Any of the above

306. The age limit for rape accused is:

a. 12 years   b. 16 years
c. 18 years   d. None of the above

307. A bastard child means:

a. Legitimate child
b. Illegitimate child
c. Child after pregnancy following rape
d. Within wedlock

308. Affliation cases require fixation of:

a. Paternity   b. Maternity
c. Both   d. None

309. A suppositions child is:

a. Legitimate child
b. Ilegitimate child
c. Posthumous child
d. Fictitious child

310. Posthumous child means:

a. Child born out of wedlock
b. Child born within wedlock
c. Child born without marriage
d. Child born after the death of father

311. The average duration of pregnancy is:

a. 40 weeks
b. 30 weeks
c. 35 weeks
d. 45 weeks

312. The minimum period of pregnancy with a viable child:

a. 7 months   b. 8 months

c. 9 months   d. 10 months

313. When the father is 'A' group and the mother is 'B group, the child can be:

a. 'A' group   b. 'B' group

c. 'O' group   d. Any of the above

314. When the father is 'A' group and the mother is 'O' group the child can be:

a. 'B' group

b. 'AB' group

c. 'A' group

d. None of the above

315. Adultery means:

a. Sexual intercourse between two adults

b. Sexual intercourse between two married persons

c. Sexual intercourse between a married person with another person who is not the wife of the person

b. None of the above

316. Infant is a child below the age of:

a. One month   b. Six month

c. One year   d. Two years

317. Acts of ommission include:

a. Not washing the baby

b. Washing the baby

c. Pressing the mouth of the baby

d. Pressing the baby tightly to the breast

318. Acts of commission do not include:

a. Feeding the baby

b. Applying opium and feeding the baby

c. Applying pressure on the chest of the baby

d. Drowning the baby in maternal fluids

319. Precipitate labour occurs when:

a. The baby is small

b. The vagina is roomy

c. Uterine contractions are powerful

d. All of the above

320. The commonest form of infanticide is:

a. Suffocation   b. Strangulation

c. Drowning   d. Poisoning

321. In concealment of birth the child might have died:

a. Before birth   b. During birth

c. After birth   d. Any of the above

322. Sudden infant death syndrome is due to:

a. Respiratory viral infection

b. Prolonged sleep apnoea

c. Hypersensitivity reaction

d. Any of the above

323. In battered baby syndrome:

a. Child is below one year

b. There are multiple fractures of different ages.

c. History does not suggest trauma

d. All of the above

324. Abortion means expulsion of products of conception up to:

a. 10 weeks   b. 20 weeks

c. 28 weeks   d. Full term

325. The commonest type of abortion is:

a. Natural abortion

b. Criminal abortion

c. Therapeutic abortion

d. None of the above

326. The conceptus is called embryo up to:

a. One week   b. Two weeks

c. Four weeks   d. Eight weeks

327. Medical termination of pregnancy by a single doctor is allowed up to:

a. 6 weeks   b. 12 weeks

c. 24 weeks   d. 28 weeks

328. There is no time limit for abortion in case of:

a. Risk to life of mother

b. When girl is below 18 years of age

c. When foetus is viable

d. Any of the above

329. Foetal abnormalities are caused due to:

a. Thalassaemia major

b. Rubella infection

c. Oral androgens and oestrogens

d. All of the above

330. Delayed complications of MTP are:

a. Incomplete abortion

b. Haemorrhage

c. Endometritis

d. Sterility

331. After MTP Act, abortions are:

a. Legalised

b. Liberalised

c. Criminalised

d. All of the above

332. Diachylon paste is used for:

a. Procuring abortion

b. Induction of labour

c. Lubrication

d. None of the above

333. Commonest cause of death in induced abortion is:

a. Septicaemia

b. Tetanus

c. Pulmonary embolism

d. Renal failure

334. Hasse's rule helps in determination of:

a. Duration of pregnancy

b. Age of foetus

c. Nature of placenta

d. Ectopic pregnancy

335. Viable foetus:

a. Is seven months old

b. Has pupillary membrane

c. Eyebrows are absent

d. Nails are not formed

336. Full term foetus:

a. 50 cm

b. 2 kg

c. Scalp hair rudimentary

d. Lanugo present everywhere

337. Vasectomy causes:

a. Impotence

b. Infertility

c. Impotence and infertility

d. None of the above

338. The tubes ligated in tubectomy are:

a. Uterus

b. Vas deferens

c. Fallopian tubes

d. None of the above

339. Commonest cause of death in laparo-scopic sterilisation is:

a. Vagal inhibition

b. Air embolism

c. Injury to aorta

d. Intestinal trauma

FORENSIC PSYCHIATRY

340. Unsoundness of mind is dealt with under Section:

a. 86 of IPC   b. 84 of IPC

c. 375 of IPC   d. 420 of IPC

341. Amnesia means:

a. Loss of speech

b. Loss of memory

c. Loss of emotions

d. Loss of sensations

342. The following are IQ tests:

a. Geltler's test   b. Binet-Simon test

c. Fodere's test   d. Wredin's test

343. Hallucination means:

a. Sensory perception with a sensory stimulus

b. Sensory perception without sensory stimulus

c. Altered sensory perception

d. Absence of sensory perception

344. Delusion is a:

a. True belief

b. False belief

c. False belief inspite of evidence to contrary

d. Altered sensory perception

345. Illusion is:

a. False belief

b. False sensory perception

c. False sensory perception due to distortion of sensory stimulus

d. None of the above

346. Insight means:
  a. The patient does not know that he is ill
  b. Patient knows that he is ill
  c. Patient does not know that he is not ill
  d. None of the above

347. Dipsomania means:
  a. Irresistible desire to drink alcohol
  b. Irresistible desire to set fire
  c. Irresistible desire to steal things
  d. Irresistible desire to break things

348. Lucid interval suggests:
  a. Abnormal mental state
  b. Normal mental state
  c. Altered mental state
  d. Confused state

349. Claustrophobia means:
  a. Fear of closed place
  b. Fear of open space
  c. Fear of water
  d. Fear of darkness

350. Anxiety disorder is:
  a. A neurotic state
  b. A psychotic state
  c. An impulse
  d. An obsession

351. In psychosis, the following are present:
  a. Empathy   b. Insight
  c. Cognition   d. Delusions

352. In anxiety neurosis:
  a. There is split personality
  b. No empathy
  c. No insight
  d. Normal contact with reality

353. Idiots have an IQ below:
  a. 5   b. 10
  c. 20   d. None of the above

354. Inbeciles show IQ:
  a. Below 20
  b. Above 20
  c. Above 50
  d. Above 60

355. In dementia, there is impairment of:
  a. Higher cerebral functions
  b. Cerebellar functions
  c. Brainstem functions
  d. Spinal activity

356. Alzheimer's disease occurs in:
  a. Infants   b. Children
  c. Adults   d. Old people

357. Korsakoff's psychosis occurs in:
  a. Chronic cocainism
  b. Chronic alcoholism
  c. Running amok
  d. None of the above

358. Admission to a psychiatric hospital can be:
  a. Voluntary
  b. On police demand only
  c. On magistrate order only
  d. Any of the above

359. Immediate restraint of mentally ill person can be done by:
  a. Anybody   b. By police
  c. By doctor   d. By magistrate

360. The human rights of mentally ill persons are protected in Mental Health Act under:
  a. Section 81   b. Section 83
  c. Section 39   d. Section 41

361. The civil responsibility not available for mentally unsound person:
  a. Testamentary capacity
  b. Contract of marriage
  c. Divorce
  d. Any of the above

362. McNaughten's rules are based on:
  a. Delusions
  b. Hallucination
  c. Illusion
  d. Obsession

363. Regulation of conduct is the basis of:
  a. Durham's rule
  b. Curren's rule
  c. ALI test
  d. IPC 84

364. **Postpartum psychosis is characterized by:**

   a. Delusions   b. Hallucinations
   c. Depressions   d. All of the above

365. **In catatonia, the patient may attempt:**

   a. Suicide   b. Homicide
   c. Both   d. Neither

366. **Fugue includes:**

   a. State of altered awareness
   b. Wandering state
   c. Individual forgets part/whole of his life
   d. All of the above

367. **Fugue occurs in:**

   a. Hysteria (somatisation disorder)
   b. Depression (bipolar disorder)
   c. Schizophrenia (split personality)
   d. All of the above

368. **Agoraphobia means:**

   a. Fear of open spaces
   b. Fear of heights
   c. Fear of closed spaces
   d. Fear of cockroaches

369. **Intelligence quotient is derived by:**

   a. Mental age × 100
   b. Biological age × 100
   c. Mental age/biological age × 100
   d. Mental age/biological age

370. **Jamais vu means:**

   a. New situation appears familiar
   b. An experienced situation appears unfamiliar
   c. A new situation remains new
   d. An unfamiliar situation remains unfamiliar

371. **Deja vu means:**

   a. New situation appears to be familiar
   b. Old situation appears to be new
   c. Fear of new places
   d. Fear of familiar places

372. **Nihilistic delusion means:**

   a. Person believes that the self or world is non-existing or going to end
   b. Person feels that he has done something wrong and sinful
   c. Person has unusual but fantastic belief
   d. Person feels that other people are planning to harm him

373. **In delirium:**

   a. Visual hallucinations are seen
   b. Insight and judgement lost
   c. Level of consciousness is variable
   d. All of the above

374. **In deciding competency to stand trial, the medical officer should see:**

   a. Whether the patient is of unsound mind
   b. Whether the patient is unable to understand court proceedings
   c. Whether he is unable to instruct his lawyers
   d. All of the above

375. **Section dealing with suicide in IPC is:**

   a. Section 309   b. Section 84
   c. Section 86   d. Section 320

376. **The Medical Council of India**

   a. Regulates medical education in India
   b. Punishes the erring registered medical practitioners
   c. Carries inspection for national board of examinations
   d. None of the above

377. **The term of office of Medical Council of India members is:**

   a. Two years   b. Three years
   c. Four years   d. Five years

378. **The state medical council looks after the:**

   a. Disciplinary control
   b. Regulation of medical education
   c. Recognition of degrees from other states
   d. All of the above

379. **Infamous conduct includes:**

   a. Association with quacks
   b. Advertisement
   c. Dichotomy
   d. Any of the above

380. A medical practitioner is liable for penal action for giving:

a. Medicolegal report
b. False medical certificates
c. Infectious disease certificates
d. Passport certificate

381. Professional secret includes:

a. Family matters
b. Matters connected with disease
c. Daughter's marriage
d. Son's education

382. Medical negligence includes:

a. Derilection of duty
b. Damage to the patient
c. Doctor–patient relationship
d. All of the above

383. Consumer Protection Act:

a. Covers registered medical practitioners
b. Excludes registered medical practitioners
c. Covers only the laboratory staff
d. Covers only the management

384. A doctor can be punished for prenatal sex determination:

a. Imprisonment up to 3 years, Rs. 10,000 fine
b. Imprisonment up to 5 years, Rs. 50,000 fine
c. Imprisonment up to 1 year, Rs. 1,000 fine
d. Imprisonment up to 10 years, Rs. 1,00,000 fine

385. Prenatal diagnostic tests are permitted for purpose of detection of:

a. Sex of foetus
b. Sex-linked genetic diseases
c. When women is below 35 years
d. When the woman did not have any abortion

386. Death certificate should be issued:

a. Without any delay
b. Without charging any fees
c. Mentioning exact cause of death
d. All of the above

387. Medicolegal documents:

a. Should be prepared in duplicate
b. Correction should be initiated
c. Signature and name of doctor must be mentioned
d. All of the above

388. The rights of patient include:

a. Due medical care
b. Human treatment
c. Full information about his conditions.
d. Any of the above

389. Duties of patient include:

a. To follow instructions of doctor
b. To pay the fees of the doctor
c. Not to leave the doctor without informing him.
d. All of the above

390. Professional death sentence means:

a. Permanent penal erasure of name of medical practitioner from medical register
b. Temporary removal of the name from the medical register
c. Boycott by all professional colleagues
d. Any of the above

391. Example of res ipsa loquitur:

a. Operation of hydrocele
b. Operation on young patient
c. Operation on wrong side
d. None of the above

392. Vicarious responsibility means:

a. Responsibility of various persons for negligence
b. Responsibility of laboratory technicians
c. Responsibility of senior for acts of juniors
d. None of the above

393. Professional indemnity insurance helps:

a. Doctor　　b. Patient
c. Lawyer　　d. None of the above

394. Medical examination without consent can be carried out on:

a. Accused
b. Victim

c. Person below 12 years

d. Prisoners

395. **Consent of both partners is required in cases of:**

a. Any operation

b. For artificial insemination

c. In medicolegal cases

d. Euthanasia

396. **Grievous hurt does not include:**

a. Emasculation

b. Fracture of tooth

c. Permanent loss of hearing

d. Scar

397. **Medical negligence in criminal law is tried under Section:**

a. 319 of IPC   b. 302 of IPC

c. 309 of IPC   d. 304A of IPC

398. **Physical torture includes:**

a. Twisting the nails

b. Humiliation

c. Disinformation

d. Any of the above

TOXICOLOGY

399. **Poisonous substances have:**

a. High therapeutic index

b. Low therapeutic index

c. No therapeutic index

d. None of the above

400. **Drugs can act as poisons:**

a. In higher doses

b. In lower doses

c. In routine doses

d. None of the above

401. **Idiosyncracy means:**

a. Toxic effect caused by any substance

b. Toxic effect caused by a very small dose of otherwise safe substance

c. Toxic effect caused by poisonous substance

d. None of the above

402. **Intentional overdosing of a substance is:**

a. Therapeutic misadventure

b. Medical negligence

c. Routine medical practice

d. None of the above

403. **MIC means:**

a. Medical Council of India

b. Methyl isocyanate

c. Methyl cyanide

d. Methyl carbide

404. **Teratogenicity means:**

a. Foetal abnormalities due to exposure of mother to thalidomide

b. Damage to the mother due to exposure to thalidomide

c. Damage to both mother and foetus due to exposure to thalidomide

d. None of the above

405. **The father of modern toxicology is:**

a. Discordes   b. Hippocrates

c. Orfila   d. Papyrus

406. **Baby powder contains:**

a. Boric acid

b. Barium sulphide

c. Potassium bromide

d. Sodium bicarbonate

407. **Depilatories include:**

a. Thallium   b. Aluminium

c. Zinc   d. Tartaric acid

408. **Rat poisons include:**

a. Aluminium phosphide

b. Sodium fluoride

c. Nitrobenzene

d. Methyl salicylate

409. **Moth balls means:**

a. Aniline   b. Iodine

c. Naphthalene   d. Gammaxene

410. **Fungicides include:**

a. Lead arsenate

b. Potassium chlorate

c. Sodium fluoride

d. Carbon tetrachloride

411. **Baking soda means:**

a. Sodium chloride

b. Sodium hydroxide

c. Sodium hypochlorate

d. Sodium bicarbonate

412. Matches contain:

a. Potassium chlorate

b. Potassium hydroxide

c. Potassium carbonate

d. None of the above

413. Hair bleach contains:

a. Hydrogen peroxide

b. Hydrogen sulphide

c. Hydrogen chloride

d. None of the above

414. Weed killers include:

a. Paraquat b. Permanganate

c. Perborates d. None of the above

415. Sleeping tablets contain:

a. Codeine b. Iodine

c. Barbiturate b. Dexidrine'

416. Nail polish remover contains:

a. Formaldehyde b. Acetaldehyde

c. Acetone d. Acetic acid

417. Schedule H contains a list of:

a. Poisons

b. Antibiotics

c. Antihistamines

d. None of the above

418. Commonly used homicidal poison is:

a. Arsenic b. Aspirin

c. Alcohol d. None of the above

419. Paediatric poison is:

a. Opium

b. Oleander

c. Organophosphorus compound

d. None of the above

420. Pakur murder was carried out using:

a. *Vibrio cholerae*

b. Plague bacilli

c. *Dhatura*

d. None of the above

421. Cattle poison includes:

a. *Abrus precatorius*

b. *Dhatura*

c. Carbolic acid

d. None of the above

422. Inebriant poison includes:

a. Cannabis b. Alcohol

c. Opium d. Strychnine

423. Somniferous poison includes:

a. Opium b. Barbiturates

c. Morphine d. All of the above

424. Cardiac poison includes:

a. Curare b. Cannabis

c. Chloroform d. Aconite

425. Peripheral nerves are affected by:

a. Curare b. Digitalis

c. *Dhatura* d. Barbiturates

426. Non-metallic inorganic irritant poison includes:

a. Aloes b. Cantharides

c. Copper d. Phosphorus

427. Mechanical irritant poisoning is caused by:

a. Croton oil b. Alcohol

c. Tobacco d. Powdered glass

428. Irrespirable gases do not include:

a. Carbon dioxide

b. Carbon monoxide

c. Coal gas

d. Ozone

429. On swallowing, poisoning occurs with:

a. *Abrus precatorius* seeds

b. *Nux vomica* seeds

c. *Dhatura* seeds

d. Castor seeds

430. Death occurs on swallowing.

a. Snake venom

b. *Nux vomica* seeds

c. *Abrus precatorius* seeds

d. None of the above

431. Priapism occurs in:

a. Snakebite

b. *Abrus precatorius* poisoning

c. Cantharidine poisoning

d. None of the above

432. Ricin occurs in:

  a. Rice   b. Croton

  c. Castor   d. Capsicum

433. Spectacle mark is seen on:

  a. Krait   b. King cobra

  c. Cobra   d. Russell's viper

434. Three rows of black spots are seen on the back of:

  a. Banded krait   b. King cobra

  c. Russell's viper   d. None of the above

435. The tail of the sea snake is:

  a. Round   b. Flat

  c. Triangular   d. None of the above

436. Round pupils are not seen in:

  a. Krait   b. Cobra

  c. Viper   d. Any of the above

437. Dry gangrene of the limbs can occur in:

  a. Viper bite

  b. Ergot poisoning

  c. Croton poisoning

  d. None of the above

438. Intravascular haemolysis gives rise to:

  a. Haemoglobinuria

  b. Glycosuria

  c. Carboluria

  d. Haematuria

439. Castor seeds contain:

  a. Crotin   b. Ricin

  c. Carlotropin   d. Cantharidin

440. *Dhatura* seeds have:

  a. Convex border with single edge

  b. Convex border with double edge

  c. Convex border with no edge

  d. Concave border with double edge

441. Arrow poison includes:

  a. Marking nut

  b. Calotropis

  c. *Abrus precatorius*

  d. *Croton tiglium*

442. Chilli seeds have:

  a. Concave border with single edge

  b. Convex border with single edge

  c. Concave border with double edge

  d. Convex border with double edge

443. Cyanosis occurs because of metha-emoglobinaemia in:

  a. Sodium nitrite

  b. Sodium chloride

  c. Sodium hydroxide

  d. None of the above

444. Cyanmethaemoglobin is:

  a. Highly toxic   b. Moderately toxic

  c. Non-toxic   d. Slowly toxic

445. Stupefying agent includes:

  a. Madar juice   b. Oleander

  c. *Dhatura*   d. Aloes

446. Spinal cord is affected by:

  a. Gelsemium

  b. Opium

  c. Nicotine

  d. Carbon monoxide

447. Hardening of the stomach mucosa is caused by:

  a. Hydrochloric acid

  b. Sulphuric acid

  c. Carbolic acid

  d. None of the above

448. Perforation of the stomach can occur in:

  a. Sulphuric acid poisoning

  b. Carbolic acid poisoning

  c. Copper sulphate poisoning

  d. All of the above

449. When a poison is detected in the stomach and not in viscera, the poison is:

  a. Not absorbed

  b. Introduced after death

  c. Ineffective

  d. Any of the above

450. When the poison is not detected from the viscera:

  a. Death is not due to poisoning

  b. The poison has disappeared from the body

  c. Death can be due to poisoning

  d. Any of the above

451. The medical officer should not give the cause of death as poisoning:
    a. If the poison is not detected in the viscera
    b. If the poison is detected in the viscera
    c. If the poison is detected only in the stomach
    d. None of the above

452. A private medical practitioner is bound to communicate to the nearest police officer or a magistrate in a case of:
    a. Homicidal poisoning
    b. Suicidal poisoning
    c. Accidental poisoning
    d. None of the above

453. In a case of attempt to commit suicide, the medical practitioner:
    a. Need not inform the police
    b. Must inform the police
    c. Must consult another doctor
    d. None of the above

454. A medical officer in government hospital should report to the police:
    a. All cases of suspected poisoning
    b. Only suicidal poisoning
    c. Only homicidal poisoning
    d. Only when the diagnosis of poisoning is certain

455. The treatment of poisoning should occur for:
    a. Removal of unabsorbed poison
    b. Elimination of poison
    c. Symptomatic relief
    d. All of the above

456. Diuresis may be forced by using:
    a. Frusemide   b. Barbiturates
    c. Insulin   d. Atropine

457. Pain is best relieved by:
    a. Morphine   b. Nicotine
    c. Aspirin   d. Paracetamol

458. Atropine is useful in:
    a. Dehydration   b. Abdominal colic
    c. Oliguria   d. None of the above

459. Stomach wash is not contraindicated in:
    a. Sulphuric acid poisoning
    b. Nitric acid poisoning
    c. Carbolic acid poisoning
    d. Corrosive sublimate poisoning

460. End of the stomach tube is kept rounded:
    a. To help inserting through mouth gag
    b. To prevent lying in oesophagus
    c. To prevent trauma to the stomach
    d. All of the above

461. In the case of infants, the length of the tube to reach the stomach should be about:
    a. 15 cm   b. 30 cm
    c. 45 cm   d. 55 cm

462. Stomach wash is repeated till:
    a. The fluid is yellow in colour
    b. The fluid is clear and odourless
    c. No more fluid comes
    d. None of the above

463. The first washing in stomach wash is useful for:
    a. Chemical analysis
    b. Determining the chloride level
    c. Determining glucose level
    d. All of the above

464. Gastric lavage is contraindicated in:
    a. Children
    b. Adults
    c. Women
    d. None of the above

465. Stomach tube can be used only in the following corrosive poison:
    a. Concentrated nitric acid
    b. Concentrated sulphuric acid
    c. Carbolic acid
    d. None of the above

466. While passing the stomach tube, absence of cough reflex suggests entry into:
    a. Any passage
    b. Right passage
    c. Wrong passage
    d. Any of the above

467. If the patient is conscious and responds to minimal stimuli, his level of consciousness is:

a. Grade IV   b. Grade III
c. Grade I   d. Grade II

468. Mechanical antidotes include:

a. Activated charcoal
b. Egg albumin
c. Potassium permanganate
d. Lime

469. Vinegar is used to counter the effects of:

a. Caustic soda
b. Carbolic acid
c. Hydrochloric acid
d. None of the above

470. Potassium permanganate is a very important antidote because of its:

a. Oxidising property
b. Reducing property
c. Alkaline property
d. Acidic property

471. Tannic acid precipitates:

a. Alkaloids
b. Glycosides
c. Many of the metals
d. All of the above

472. Hydrated ferric oxide is used as an antidote in the acute poisoning of:

a. Potassium cyanide
b. Potassium hydroxide
c. Arsenic
d. Zinc

473. Metallic mercury as a poison affects the:

a. Heart
b. Liver
c. Kidney
d. None of the above

474. Chelating agents include:

a. Calcium disodium versenate
b. Dimercaprol
c. Cuprimine
d. All of the above

475. Ventricular fibrillation can be treated by:

a. Lignocaine drip
b. Nitroglycerine
c. Amyl nitrite
d. None of the above

476. To control strychnine convulsions, the following is used:

a. Barbiturates
b. Morphine
c. Mephenteramine
d. None of the above

477. To give good sleep in children paraldehyde is injected:

a. Intravenously
b. Subcutaneously
c. Intramuscularly
d. Intraperitoneally

478. Universal antidote does not contain:

a. Activated charcoal
b. Tannic acid
c. Magnesium oxide
d. None of the above

479. Parasuicide means:

a. Completed suicide
b. Attempted suicide
c. Suicide by the parent
d. Pact suicide

480. Autolytic changes in the stomach are commonly found:

a. At the pyloric end
b. At the cardiac end
c. At the front wall
d. None of the above

481. If the medical practitioner gives false information to the police, he is liable to be charged under Section:

a. 193 of IPC   b. 176 of IPC
c. 201 of IPC   d. 202 of IPC

482. If he conceals information from the police, a registered medical practitioner is liable to be prosecuted under Section:

a. 175 of CrPC   b. 202 of IPC
c. 201 of IPC   d. 39 of CrPC

483. Homicidal poisoning should be informed to the police/magistrate by the RMP under Section:
   a. 201 of IPC   b. 39 of CrPC
   c. 176 of IPC   d. 193 of IPC

484. Copper oxychloride used as a fungicide is:
   a. Mildly toxic to the human body
   b. Comparatively harmless
   c. Highly toxic
   d. Virtually harmless

485. Paris green used as weed killer:
   a. Generally harmless to the human body
   b. Comparatively harmless
   c. Mildly toxic
   d. Highly toxic

486. Nicotine used as horticultural insecticide is:
   a. Highly toxic to the human body
   b. Mildly toxic
   c. Comparatively harmless
   d. Generally harmless.

487. The following is an insecticide vegetable origin:
   a. Malathion (Bugsoline)
   b. Diazinon (Tic-20)
   c. Endrine
   d. Pyrethrin

488. The following is not an organophosphorus poison:
   a. DDT   b. HETP
   c. OMPA   d. Methyl parathion

489. Organophosphorus compounds are:
   a. Acetylcholinesterase inhibitors
   b. Acetlycholinesterase stimulators
   c. No action on acetylcholinesterase
   d. None of the above

490. Chromodacryorrhoea is seen due to accumulation of:
   a. Atropine
   b. Acetylcholine
   c. Porphyrin
   d. All of the above

491. Pinpoint pupils are seen in poisoning with:
   a. Tic 20   b. DDT
   c. Gammaxane   d. None of the above

492. Atropinisation is done till the pupils become:
   a. Normal   b. Dilated
   c. Contracted   d. irregular

493. Protopan (pralidoxime chloride) is used in the treatment of poisoning with:
   a. Phosphorus
   b. Organophosphorus
   c. Chlorinated hydrocarbons
   d. All of the above

494. Plant penicillin is:
   a. Carbamate   b. Endrin
   c. Acetylcholine   d. DDT

495. Kerosene like smell of endrin is due to:
   a. Kerosene   b. Petrol
   c. Aromax   d. None of the above

496. Organochlorine compounds act on:
   a. Spinal cord
   b. Myoneural junction
   c. CNS
   d. None of the above

497. Metal fume fever is caused by:
   a. Aluminium   b. Zinc
   c. Mercury   d. Magnesium

498. In aluminium phosphide poisoning, the poisoning effect is due to:
   a. Phosphorus   b. Phosphine
   c. Phosgene   d. Phosphorylation

499. Treatment of aluminium phosphide poisoning consists of:
   a. Magnesium sulphate IV infusion
   b. Acidosis correction with IV sodium carbonate
   c. Adequate hydration with IV infusion
   d. All of the above

500. Baygon belongs to:
   a. Organochlorines
   b. Alkyl phosphates
   c. Aryl phosphates
   d. Carbamates

501. Specific antidote for carbamate poisoning is:

    a. Atropine
    b. Morphine
    c. Calcium gluconate
    d. Methylene blue

502. Rat poisons include:

    a. Aluminium phosphide
    b. DDT
    c. Gammaxane
    d. Endrin

503. Phosphorus causes preferential inhibition of:

    a. Sulphide group
    b. Cytochrome oxidase
    c. Cholinesterase
    d. None of the above

504. Cholinesterase inhibitors can be detected from the following:

    a. Fat   b. Tears
    c. Urine   d. None of the above

505. Muscarine-like action potentiates:

    a. Post-ganglionic parasympathetic activity
    b. Preganglionic activity
    c. Depression of CNS
    d. None of the above

506. Nicotine-like stimulation causes:

    a. Twitching of the eyelids and facial muscles
    b. Increased sweating
    c. Cardiac sinus node block
    d. Insomnia

507. In endrin poisoning, the treatment includes administration of:

    a. Calcium gluconate
    b. P2 AM
    c. Atropine
    d. None of the above

508. Aryl phosphates include:

    a. OMPA
    b. TEPP
    c. Diazinon
    d. Dimefox

509. Death due to phosphine poisoning may occur with:

    a. Zinc phosphide
    b. Aluminium phosphide
    c. Calcium phosphide
    d. All of the above

CORROSIVES

510. Corrosive acids produce:

    a. Coagulation
    b. Necrosis
    c. Coagulation necrosis
    d. None of the above

511. Vitriolage is caused by:

    a. Marking nut juice
    b. Sulphuric acid
    c. Madar juice
    d. Any of the above

512. Vitriolage is generally:

    a. Accidental   b. Suicidal
    c. Grievous hurt d. None of the above

513. In sulphuric acid poisoning, teeth become:

    a. Chalky white b. Black
    c. Yellow   d. None of the above

514. Perforation of stomach is more common in:

    a. Hydrochloric acid
    b. Carbolic acid
    c. Sulphuric acid
    d. All of the above

515. Xanthoproteic reaction is due to the production of:

    a. Citric acid   b. Picric acid
    c. Tartaric acid d. None of the above

516. In nitric acid poisoning, teeth turn:

    a. Black   b. Brown
    c. White   d. Yellow

517. Respiratory symptoms are more common in:

    a. Sulphuric acid poisoning
    b. Hydrochloric acid poisoning
    c. Oxalic acid poisoning
    d. None of the above

518. Fumes are emitted by:
  a. Sulphuric acid
  b. Oxalic acid
  c. Hydrochloric acid
  d. None of the above

519. Immediate death on exposure to nitric acid occurs due to:
  a. Suffocation
  b. Pulmonary oedema
  c. Bronchopneumonia
  d. None of the above

520. Corneal ulcer is common in chronic poisoning with:
  a. Hydrochloric acid
  b. Nitric acid
  c. Sulphuric acid
  d. Carbolic acid

521. Inflammation of gums is caused in chronic poisoning of:
  a. Hydrochloric acid
  b. H_2SO_4
  c. HNO_3
  d. Any of the above

522. Fatal dose of H_2SO_4 is:
  a. 1–2 ml   b. 5–10 ml
  c. 10–15 ml   d. 15–20 ml

523. Oxalic acid crystals resemble in appearance:
  a. Magnesium sulphate
  b. Calcium sulphate
  c. Sodium sulphate
  d. None of the above

524. Hypocalcaemia is seen in poisoning of:
  a. HCl   b. Acetic acid
  c. Oxalic acid   d. None of the above

525. Fatal period in oxalic acid poisoning is:
  a. 1–2 min   b. 1–2 hours
  c. 1–2 days   d. 10–12 hours

526. Fatal dose of oxalic acid is:
  a. 15–20 ml
  b. 15–20 g
  c. 5–10 g
  d. 5–10 ml

527. Treatment of oxalic acid poisoning includes:
  a. Calcium gluconate
  b. Calcium chloride
  c. Parathyroid extract
  d. All of the above

528. Ochronosis implies:
  a. Pigmentation caused by hydro-quinone and pyrocatechol in the cornea
  b. Poisoning by cobra bite
  c. Onchocerciasis
  d. Dracunculiasis

529. Carbolurea means:
  a. Carbolic acid in urine
  b. Hydroquinone and pyrocatechol in urine
  c. Haemoglobin in urine
  d. Nonof the above

530. In carbolic acid poisoning, stomach wash is:
  a. Indicated
  b. Not indicated
  c. Sometimes indicated
  d. Any of the above

531. Phenol's action on the nervous system:
  a. Depressant   b. Stimulant
  c. No action   d. Both a and b

532. Phenolic odour is seen in cases of:
  a. Carbonic acid
  b. Carbolic acid
  c. Carbon monoxide
  d. Carbonic anhydrate.

533. Pinpoint contracted pupils are seen in:
  a. Oxalic acid poisoning
  b. Carbolic acid
  c. H_2SO_4
  d. HNO_3

534. Treatment of carbolic acid poisoning includes:
  a. Magnesium sulphate
  b. Liquid paraffin
  c. Olive oil
  d. All of the above

535. Carbolic acid causes:
- a. Brownish scar on the skin
- b. Hardening of gastric mucosa
- c. Carboluria
- d. All of the above

536. If effervescence occurs with sodium carbonate, it is:
- a. Zinc sulphate
- b. Oxalic acid
- c. Magnesium sulphate
- d. None of the above

537. Aspirin is:
- a. Acetylsalicylic acid
- b. Acetanilide
- c. Acetic anhydride
- d. None of the above

538. Idiosyncracy to aspirin can cause death due to:
- a. Oedema of glottis
- b. Renal failure
- c. Hyperpyrexia
- d. None of the above

539. Death in aspirin poisoning is due to:
- a. Acidosis
- b. Uremia
- c. Shock
- d. Any of the above

540. Fatal blood aspirin level is:
- a. 25 mg%
- b. 50 mg%
- c. 75 mg%
- d. 100 mg%

541. Alkalies cause:
- a. Coagulative necrosis
- b. Liquefactive necrosis
- c. Necrosis
- d. None of the above

542. In alkali poisoning, the major long-term complication is:
- a. Oesophageal stricture formation
- b. Perforation of stomach
- c. Diarrhea
- d. Vomiting

543. Fatal dose of sodium hydroxide is:
- a. 1–2 gm
- b. 2–3 gm
- c. 4–6 gm
- d. 2–4 gm

544. Immediate death in ammonia vapour poisoning can be due to:
- a. Vagal inhibition
- b. Bronchopneumonia
- c. Perforation
- d. None of the above

545. Alkalies produce more severe injuries than acids because:
- a. They dissolve protein and saponify fat
- b. They produce liquefactive necrosis
- c. They cause deeper invasion or tissue
- d. All of the above

546. Black or brown scab is formed in the burns of:
- a. HCl
- b. Phenol
- c. Nitric acid
- d. Sulphuric acid

INORGANIC IRRITANTS (NONMETALLIC)

547. White phosphorus on exposure to air gets oxidised, so it is preserved in:
- a. Water
- b. Kerosene
- c. Liquid paraffin
- d. Any of the above

548. Red phosphorus is:
- a. Poisonous
- b. Non-poisonous
- c. Poisonous in commercial preparation only
- d. Poisonous in large quantities

549. The side of a match box contains:
- a. Red phosphorus
- b. Yellow phosphorus
- c. Antimony sulphide
- d. Potassium chlorate

550. Consumption of large dose of phosphorus causes death due to:
- a. Coma
- b. Haematemesis
- c. Renal failure
- d. Hepatitis

551. In fulminating phosphorus, poisoning patients usually die:
- a. Within one hour
- b. Within 12 hours
- c. Within 24 hours
- d. Instantaneously

552. Ordinary fatal dose of white phosphorus is:

    a. 10–15 mg   b. 15–30 mg
    c. 60–120 mg   d. 120–180 mg

553. Phosphorus content of a lucifer match head is about:

    a. 1 mg   b. 2 mg
    c. 3 mg   d. 0 mg

554. In phosphorescence:

    a. There is glow in darkness
    b. There is glow when we put a light
    c. There is no glow
    d. None of the above

555. In phosphorus poisoning, the patient feels a taste of:

    a. Garlic   b. Bitter
    c. Sour   d. None of the above

556. Antidote for acute phosphorus poisoning is:

    a. 0.1% $CuSO_4$ solution
    b. 0.2% $CuSO_4$ solution
    c. 2% H_2O_2 solution
    d. Egg

557. Chronic phosphorus poisoning can lead to:

    a. Phosphorism
    b. Phosphorescence
    c. Phossy jaw
    d. Any of the above

558. 'Phossy jaw' presents the following:

    a. Multiple sinuses
    b. Foul smelling pus
    c. Bone sequestration
    d. Any of the above

559. Phosphorus is not a homicidal poison because of:

    a. Death is not certain
    b. Typical taste
    c. Symptoms do not resemble any disease
    d. None of the above

560. Phosphorus is used in arsine because of its:

    a. Reduction property
    b. Oxidation property

    c. Hydrolysis
    d. None of the above

561. In acute phosphorus poisoning, necro-biosis is seen in:

    a. Heart   b. Kidneys
    c. Liver   d. Any of the above

562. In acute yellow atrophy, liver is:

    a. Greasy and leathery
    b. Big and yellow
    c. Big and greasy
    d. None of the above

563. Voluntary chlorine inhalation is a form of:

    a. Suicide   b. Self-abuse
    c. Homicide   d. None of the above

564. Potassium bromide is used as:

    a. Sedative   b. Convulsant
    c. Antipyretic   d. None of the above

565. Fatal dose of tincture iodine:

    a. 5–10 ml   b. 10–20 ml
    c. 20–30 ml   d. 30–60 ml

566. Postmortem appearances in chlorine poisoning are mainly of:

    a. Asphyxia   b. Syncope
    c. Coma   d. None of the above

567. Bromism includes:

    a. Papules and pustules on the body
    b. No skin changes
    c. Only macules
    d. Lichen planus

568. Bromoderma occurs:

    a. At the hair roots
    b. On the face
    c. Upper part of chest
    d. Any of the above

569. Radioactive iodine (I^{131}) causes:

    a. Hyperthyroidism
    b. Hypothyroidism
    c. Diabetes
    d. Euthyroidism

570. Iododerma consists of:

    a. Macules and papules
    b. Tubercles

c. Fungatus and granulomatous ulceration
d. Any of the above

571. Formalin is:

a. 10% formaldehyde in water
b. 20% formaldehyde in water
c. 40% formaldehyde in water
d. 100% formaldehyde in water

572. Stomach becomes hard and leathery in:

a. Carbolic acid poisoning
b. Formaldehyde poisoning
c. Bromine poisoning
d. All of the above

573. Brown discolouration at angles of mouth is seen in:

a. Sulphuric acid poisoning
b. Iodine poisoning
c. Carbolic acid poisoning
d. All of the above

574. In which of the following pure metallic state is not poisonous:

a. Metallic arsenic
b. Metallic mercury
c. Metallic copper
d. All of the above

575. White arsenic means:

a. Arsenious oxide
b. Potassium arsenite
c. Arsenic acid
d. Arsenic sulphide

576. Arsenic is popular as homicidal poison because:

a. Death occurs instantaneously
b. Sweet in taste
c. Resembles natural illness
d. All of the above

577. Fatal dose of arsenic is about:

a. 18 mg   b. 1.8 mg
c. 180 mg   d. None of the above

578. Arsenic is found in stomach as:

a. Big lump
b. Gritty, sandy, white particles
c. Crystalline substance
d. Irregular, small lumps

579. 'Mees lines' are seen on the:

a. Teeth
b. Gums
c. Nails
d. None of the above

580. Antidote in acute arsenic poisoning is:

a. Copper sulphate
b. Freshly prepared permanganate solution
c. Freshly prepared hydrated ferric oxide solution
b. Aluminium hydroxide

581. Death in fulminant type of arsenic poisoning is due to:

a. Shock
b. Coma
c. Perforation of stomach
d. Liver atrophy

582. Arsenic sinks to the bottom of milk because it has:

a. Low specific gravity
b. High specific gravity
c. Big crystals
d. Insoluble

583. Average fatal period in acute arsenic poisoning is:

a. <1 day   b. >1 day
c. >2 days   d. About a week

584. Inordinate delay in arsenic poisoning is due to:

a. Empty stomach
b. Full stomach
c. Unconsciousness
d. Small doses

585. Arsenic is deposited in maximum concentration in:

a. Hair   b. Brain
c. Spleen   d. Intestine

586. Disadvantage of arsenic as homicide poison is:

a. Delay in onset of symptoms
b. Death is certain
c. Can be given in milk
d. Resists decomposition

587. Arsenic is eliminated through urine for a period of:
   a. 2–3 days   b. 2–3 weeks
   c. 2–3 months   d. 2–3 years

588. Arsenophagists are those:
   a. Who eat arsenic
   b. Who commit suicide by eating arsenic
   c. Who commit murder by giving arsenic
   d. Who sell arsenic

589. Symptoms and signs resemble cholera in following poisoning:
   a. Phosphorus
   b. Sodium hydroxide
   c. Arsenic carbonate
   d. Bismuth

590. Arsenic interferes with cellular respiration by combining with sulphhydryl groups of:
   a. Pyruvate oxidase
   b. Cholinesterase
   c. Pyruvic acid
   d. Cytochrome oxidase

591. Arsenic inhibits the cell enzyme activity by binding to – SH groups:
   a. Succinic dehydrogenase
   b. ADP
   c. Cholinesterase
   d. Cytochrome oxidase

592. 'Mees lines' on the nails are:
   a. Longitudinal   b. Transverse
   c. Irregular   d. Diagonal

593. BAL is given in a dose of:
   a. 1–2 mg/kg/day
   b. 2–3 mg/kg/day
   c. 3–5 mg/kg/day
   d. 5–7 mg/kg/day

594. BAL is administered:
   a. Orally   b. Intramuscular
   c. Intravenous   d. Intraperitoneal

595. Arsenophagists can tolerate arsenic daily up to:
   a. 50 mg   b. 100 mg
   c. 200 mg   d. 300 mg

596. In fatal cases of arsenic poisoning, petechial haemorrhages are found in:
   a. Lungs
   b. Muscles of left ventricle
   c. Kidneys
   d. Liver

597. In chronic arsenic poisoning during the first stage, the following are seen:
   a. Cutaneous eruptions and laryngeal oedema
   b. Tingling and numbness of the extremities
   c. Peripheral neuritis and muscular atrophy
   d. Abdominal colic and loss of weight

598. White arsenic is mistaken for:
   a. Baking powder
   b. Sugar
   c. Flour
   d. All of the above

599. WHO's permissible limit of arsenic in water is below:
   a. 5 mg/100 ml
   b. 5 mg/1000 ml
   c. 50 mg/100 ml
   d. None of the above

600. Metallic mercury is:
   a. Solid   b. Liquid
   c. Gas   d. Mixture

601. Mercuric salts are:
   a. Intensely poisonous
   b. Poisonous
   c. Sometimes poisonous
   d. Non-poisonous

602. On swallowing, metallic Hg causes:
   a. Vomiting
   b. Diarrhoea
   c. Abdominal colic
   d. None of the above

603. Corrosive sublimate:
   a. Mercuric oxide
   b. Mercuric cyanide
   c. Mercuric chloride
   d. Mercurous chloride

604. Mercury is re-excreted into:

a. Stomach
b. Small intestine
c. Large intestine
d. Duodenum

605. Hatter's shakes means:

a. Mercurial tremors
b. Convulsions
c. Tongue tremors
d. None of the above

606. In mercuria lentis, the deposit on anterior lens capsule is:

a. Whitish   b. Brownish
c. Bluish   d. Greenish

607. Mercurial erethism means:

a. GIT symptoms
b. Urinary tract symptoms
c. Psychiatric symptoms
d. Skin symptoms

608. Blue line on gums is not seen in:

a. Chronic lead poisoning
b. Chronic copper poisoning
c. Chronic mercury poisoning
d. None of the above

609. Sodium formaldehyde sulfoxylate is given in Hg poisoning by:

a. Oral   b. Intramuscular
c. Intravenous   d. Subcutaneous

610. The following substance is not useful in mercury poisoning:

a. BAL
b. Penicillamine
c. Calcium disodium versenate
d. Magnesium sulphate

611. Pink disease is caused by:

a. Mercuric chloride
b. Mercurous chloride
c. Mercuric iodide
d. Mercuric sulphide

612. The fatal dose of mercuric chloride for an adult is:

a. 1–4 gm   b. 4–8 gm
c. 8–10 gm   d. 5–7 gm

613. The following metal is poisonous in metallic state:

a. Mercury   b. Copper
c. Iron   d. Lead

614. Sugar of lead means:

a. Lead carbonate
b. Lead monoxide
c. Lead tetroxide
d. Lead acetate

615. In acute lead poisoning, death may occur in:

a. 1–2 days   b. 3–4 days
c. 4–5 days   d. 5–6 days

616. Valuable screening test for lead poisoning is detection in urine of:

a. Coproporphyrin III
b. Coproporphyrin I
c. Coproporphyrin II
d. None of the above

617. In lead palsy, the following is not seen:

a. Wrist drop
b. Foot drop
c. Claw-shaped hand
d. Stiff hand

618. The typical anaemia in chronic lead poisoning is:

a. Hyperchromic
b. Hypochromic
c. Macrocytic
d. Nomochromic

619. Lead line of the gums is due to:

a. Lead oxide
b. Lead sulphide
c. Lead carbonate
d. Lead monoxide

620. Tetraethyl lead is used with:

a. Petrol   b. Turpentine
c. Alcohol   d. None of the above

621. Anti-knocking agent is:

a. Lead sulphide
b. Lead tetraethyl
c. Lead tetroxide
d. Lead chromate

622. In chronic lead poisoning, sterility is seen in:
a. Men
b. Women
c. Both
d. None of the above

623. Lead radio-opaque bands are seen in fuel poisoning in the long bones at:
a. Metaphysis
b. Epiphysis
c. Diaphysis
d. None of the above

624. Lead encephalopathy shows:
a. Ataxia
b. Anaemia
c. Anoxia
d. None of the above

625. Dry-belly ache is seen in:
a. Chronic lead poisoning
b. Chronic phosphorus poisoning
c. Chronic mercury poisoning
d. None of the above

626. Punctate basophilia is seen in:
a. Chronic arsenic poisoning
b. Chronic mercury poisoning
c. Chronic antimony poisoning
d. Chronic lead poisoning

627. For de-leading, the following gives better results:
a. IV calcium disodium versenate 80 mg/kg
b. BAL intramuscular 50–30 mg/kg/day
c. Oral penicillamine 0.3–1 g daily for 5 days
d. A combination of calcium disodium versenate and BAL

628. In chronic poisoning, lead is deposited in:
a. Brain
b. Bones
c. Bladder
d. All of the above

629. Saturnism means:
a. Mercurialism
b. Plumbism
c. Iodism
d. Silicon poisoning

630. Painters colic occurs in:
a. Chronic mercury poisoning
b. Chronic arsenic poisoning
c. Chronic lead poisoning
d. None of the above

631. In chronic lead poisoning, normally abortion occurs between:
a. 2–3 months
b. 3–6 months
c. 6–7 months
d. None of the above

632. Under UV lamp, coproporphyrism III looks like a fluorescence of:
a. Red colour
b. Yellow colour
c. Blue colour
d. Green colour

633. Lead workers should take diet-rich in:
a. Calcium
b. Sodium
c. Otassium
d. Magnesium

634. Potassium iodide administration in chlorine lead poisoning helps in elimination of lead through:
a. Skin
b. Lungs
c. Kidneys
d. None of the above

635. At the cellular level, lead interacts with:
a. –SH groups
b. Acetylcholine
c. Muscarine
d. Serotonin

636. Diachylon paste contains:
a. Lead tetraethyl
b. Lead tetroxide
c. Lead acetate
d. Lead monoxide

637. Diachylon paste is used as:
a. Astringent
b. Antiknocking agent
c. Abortifacient
d. None of the above

638. Blue vitriol means:
a. Dilute sulphuric acid
b. Rectified spirit
c. Copper sulphate
d. Copper subacetate

639. In copper sulphate poisoning, symptoms appear in:
a. 5–10 min
b. 15–30 min
c. 30–60 min
d. 60–120 min

640. Fatal dose of $CuSO_4$ is generally about:
a. 5 g
b. 15 g
c. 50 g
d. 25 g

641. Death occurs in CuSO$_4$ poisoning in:

  a. 1–24 hours   b. 24–72 hours
  c. 72–96 hours   d. 96–125 hours

642. Green line of gums is seen in:

  a. Paris green poisoning
  b. Blue vitriol poisoning
  c. Scheele's green poisoning
  d. None of the above

643. Greenish blue froth is found at mouth and nostrils in:

  a. Barbiturate poisoning
  b. Carbolic acid poisoning
  c. Copper sulphate poisoning
  d. Mercuric chloride poisoning

644. Rain drop type of pigmentation is seen in:

  a. Chronic mercury poisoning
  b. Chronic arsenic poisoning
  c. Chronic lead poisoning
  d. None of the above

645. Flaky/chocolate-coloured hypostasis is seen in:

  a. Sodium nitrate poisoning
  b. Sodium hydroxide poisoning
  c. Salicylic acid poisoning
  d. None of the above

646. Advantage of arsenic as homicidal poison:

  a. Delayed putrefaction
  b. Detected in decomposed bodies
  c. Detected in hair and nails
  d. Symptoms stimulate those of cholera

647. Oils and fats should not be given in the treatment of:

  a. Phosphorus poisoning
  b. Arsenic poisoning
  c. Copper sulphate poisoning
  d. Mercury poisoning

648. Ricin is a:

  a. Glycoprotein
  b. Alkaloid
  c. Amine
  d. Coumarin

649. Ricin is not present in:

  a. Pressed cake   b. Castor oil
  c. Broken seeds   d. Leaves

650. Ricin causes agglutination of:

  a. Red cells   b. White cells
  c. Platelets   d. All of the above

651. Fatal dose of ricin:

  a. 1–2 mg   b. 2–3 mg
  c. 4–5 mg   d. 6 mg

652. Croton oil is sometimes used as:

  a. Arrow poison
  b. Cooking oil
  c. For lighting lamps
  d. None of the above

653. Abrin resembles:

  a. Cobra venom   b. Scorpion venom
  c. Viper venom   d. None of the above

654. *Abrus precatorius* does not contain:

  a. Abrin   b. Abrine
  c. Abraline   d. Atropine

655. Abrus seeds are:

  a. Tasty   b. Sweet
  c. Tasteless   d. Bitter

656. Pieces of sui do not contain:

  a. Abrin   b. Atropine
  c. Morphine   d. Adrenaline

657. *Abrus precatorius* is commonly used as:

  a. Cattle poison
  b. Human poison
  c. Chicken poison
  d. None of the above

658. Abrus seeds are as:

  a. Abortifacient   b. Corrosive
  c. Suicide agent   d. Vitriolic

659. Adrenaline is:

  a. Alkaloid   b. Glycoside
  c. Amino acid   d. None of the above

660. In ergot poisoning, pupils are:

  a. Dilated
  b. Contracted

c. Alternately dilated and contracted
d. Non-affected

661. Ergotism includes:

a. No gangrene   b. Wet gangrene
c. Dry gangrene   d. Hyperaesthesia

662. Fatal dose of ergot:

a. 1–2 g   b. 2–3 g
c. 3–4 g   d. 0–1 g

663. Capsicum powder is thrown to:

a. Facilitate robbery
b. To commit homicide
c. To commit suicide
d. As a stupefying agent

664. Marking nut juice causes:

a. Abrasion   b. Laceration
c. Contusion   d. Artificial bruise

665. Madar juice is used for:

a. Abortion   b. Suicide
c. Homicide   d. None of the above

666. Active principles of calotropis do not include:

a. Calotropin   b. Uscharin
c. Procerin   d. Semicarpol

667. The active principle of spanish fly is:

a. Cantharidin   b. Calotropin
c. Cocaine   d. Capsicin

668. Marking nut does not contain:

a. Semicarpol   b. Bhilawinol
c. Anacardin   d. Tannic acid

669. Seeds of croton do not contain:

a. Crotonoside   b. Cronolic acid
c. Crotin   d. Tyramine

670. Ergot does not contain:

a. Ergotoxine   b. Ergometrine
c. Ergotamine   d. Purpurine

POISONOUS CREATURES

671. Ophitoxaemia means:

a. Manifestations of snake bite
b. Manifestations of scorpion sting
c. Manifestations of wasp sting
d. None of the above

672. Daboia elegans is:

a. Cobra
b. Krait
c. Russell's viper
d. None of the above

673. *Echis carinata* is:

a. Russell's viper
b. Pit viper
c. Saw-scaled viper
d. Krait

674. Pit viper bite is:

a. Highly fatal
b. Seldom fatal
c. Non-fatal
d. Moderately fatal

675. The most common poisonous snake is:

a. Common cobra
b. Common krait
c. Banded krait
d. Russell's viper

676. The banded krait has these alternate stripes on its back:

a. Jet black and deep yellow
b. Blue and orange
c. Steel blue and whiter
d. Black and white

677. The common krait has on its back:

a. Single or double white bands
b. Single or double yellow bands
c. Single or double orange bands
d. None of the above

678. The king cobra has:

a. Hood with no mark
b. Hood with binocular mark
c. Hood with monocellate mark
d. None of the above

679. The colour of common krait is:

a. Steel blue   b. Bluish black
c. Buff coloured   d. None of the above

680. Sea snakes have:

a. Round tails   b. Oval tails
c. Flat tails   d. All of the above

681. The poison glands of snake are modified:

    a. Salivary glands
    b. Sweat glands
    c. Sebaceous glands
    d. None of the above

682. All poisonous snakes have fangs:

    a. One   b. Two
    c. Three   d. Four

683. Snake venom when swallowed is:

    a. Non-poisonous
    b. Highly poisonous
    c. Sometimes poisonous
    d. Moderately poisonous

684. High proteolytic activity is seen in the venom of:

    a. Crotalidae   b. Clapidae
    c. Hydrophide   d. Viperidae

685. Neurotoxins are more predominant in:

    a. Cobra   b. Viper
    c. Scorpion   d. Sea snake

686. Haemolysins are more in:

    a. Russell's viper b. Krait
    c. Sea snake   d. King cobra

687. Venom of the following snake is myotoxic:

    a. Water snake   b. Rattle snake
    c. Rat snake   d. Sea snake

688. Semicircular set of teeth marks are found in the bite of:

    a. Cobra   b. Krait
    c. Viper   d. None of the above

689. If the third supralabial touches the eye and the nasal shield, the snake is:

    a. Non-poisonous
    b. Krait
    c. Viper
    d. Cobra

690. If the fourth infralabial is the largest among the existing four infralabials, then the snake is:

    a. Cobra   b. Water snake
    c. Krait   d. Viper

691. 'Lypholysed' means:

    a. Freeze dried   b. Sum dried
    c. Autoclaved   d. Microoven heated

692. Envenomation is treated with:

    a. Higher antibiotics
    b. Antivenin
    c. Chemotherapy
    d. None of the above

693. Antivenom is given in the dose of:

    a. 5 ml/min IV
    b. 5 ml/min IV repeated as required
    c. 5 ml/min IM
    d. 5 ml/min at the site of the wound

694. A white mark resembling a bird footprint or an arrow is seen on the upper surface of the head of:

    a. Saw-scaled viper
    b. Russell's viper
    c. Krait
    d. Cobra

695. Scorpion sting is:

    a. Neurotoxin
    b. Haemolysin
    c. Neurotoxin or haemolysin
    d. Neurotoxin and haemolysin

696. Site of scorpion sting shows:

    a. One hole
    b. Two marks
    c. One hole with red surrounding area
    d. Two holes into surrounding red area

697. The deadly danger of wasp or bee sting is:

    a. Laryngeal oedema
    b. Gastrointestinal disturbance
    c. Unconsciousness
    d. Sting site inflammation

FOOD POISONING

698. In the infection type of food poisoning, the symptoms occur:

    a. Soon after ingestion of food
    b. Six to twelve hours later
    c. Twenty-four hours later
    d. Three to six hours

699. Botulism is:
   a. Infection   b. Intoxication
   c. Infestation   d. Toxaemia

700. Botulism causes:
   a. Neurological symptoms
   b. Urinary manifestations
   c. Haematological symptoms
   d. Cardiac symptoms

701. Ptomaines are:
   a. Leucomaines
   b. Cadaveric alkaloids
   c. Vegetable alkaloids
   d. None of the above

702. 'Kesari dal' is:
   a. *Lathyrus sativus*
   b. *Amanita muscaria*
   c. *Argemone mexicana*
   d. *Claviceps purpurea*

703. Lathyrism causes:
   a. Paralysis   b. Arthritis
   c. Carditis   d. Bronchitis

704. The poison in the mushroom is:
   a. Muscarine
   b. Adrenaline
   c. Acetylcholine
   d. Serotonin

705. *Argemone mexicana* causes:
   a. Epididymitis   b. Epidemic dropsy
   c. Epistaxis   d. Diplopia

706. The alkaloid in argemone oil is:
   a. Sanguinarine   b. Berberin
   c. Protopin   d. None of the above

707. Ground nuts are contaminated with:
   a. Aflatoxins   b. Claviceps
   c. Lathyrus   d. None of the above

MECHANICAL IRRITANTS

708. Treatment of powdered glass intake is:
   a. Water
   b. Bulky food
   c. No treatment required
   d. Milk

COMMON POISONS

709. Opium is derived from:
   a. Unripe poppy capsules
   b. Cocoa plant
   c. Argemone plant
   d. Ophidia

710. Opium does not contain:
   a. Morphine
   b. Pethidine
   c. Papaverine
   d. Codeine

711. Benzyl isoquinoline group of alkaloid in opium is:
   a. Pethidine   b. Metopan
   c. Narcotine   d. Morphine

712. Phenanthrene group of alkaloid in opium does not include:
   a. Papaverine   b. Codeine
   c. Thebaine   d. Morphine

713. Poppy seeds are:
   a. Poisonous
   b. Non-poisonous
   c. Highly poisonous
   d. Poisonous only when crushed

714. Opium is:
   a. Solid   b. Liquid
   c. Smoke   d. Jelly

715. The following opium alkaloid has no narcotic effect:
   a. Narcotine   b. Codeine
   c. Morphine   d. Papaverine

716. Morphine causes:
   a. Hippus
   b. Pinpoint pupils
   c. Dilated pupils
   d. Irregular pupils

717. Hallucinations are seen in opium poisoning during the stage of:
   a. Narcosis
   b. Stupor
   c. Excitement
   d. Not seen at any stage

718. Opium normally causes:

a. Diarrhoea   b. Constipation

c. Convulsions   d. Hypertension

719: Fatal dose of opium is:

a. 0.2 g   b. 0.5 g

c. 1 g   d. 2 g

720. The following is the feature of opium coma:

a. Hyperpyrexia

b. Epileptiform convulsions

c. Dilated pupils

d. Low respiration rate

721. The following is not a feature of opium coma:

a. Pinpoint pupils

b. Slow pulse

c. Cheyne-Stokes breathing

d. Hyperpyrexia

722. Morphine content of standard opium is:

a. 10 g%   b. 5 g%

c. 15 g%   d. None of the above

723. Morphinism means:

a. Chronic morphine poisoning

b. Acute morphine poisoning

c. Opium withdrawal syndrome

d. None of the above

724. Morphine:

a. Stimulates the cortex

b. Stimulates the chemoreceptor trigger zones

c. Stimulates vomiting centre

d. Depresses the vagus

725. Opium was used as an infanticide:

a. By injection

b. By application to nipple

c. By mixing in the food

d. None of the above

726. The drug of choice in Rx of opium poisoning is:

a. Atropine

b. Nabrophine

c. Potassium dichromate

d. Naloxone

727. Ordinarily, the term 'Alcogol' is used for:

a. Methyl alcohol

b. Isopropyl alcohol

c. Ethyl alcohol

d. Ethylene glycol

728. The alcohol content of absolute alcohol is:

a. 100%   b. 90%

c. 95%   d. 99.95%

729. Methylated spirit contains:

a. 95% wood naphtha, 5% alcohol

b. 95% alcohol and 5% wood naphtha

c. 90% alcohol

d. 99.95% alcohol and 0.5% wood naphtha

730. Alcohol content of rum is:

a. 40–50%   b. 51–59%

c. 30–40%   d. 18–22%

731. Alcohol content of wine is:

a. 4–8%   b. 8–12%

c. 10–15%   d. 1–3%

732. Alcohol content of fenny is:

a. 1–2%   b. 2–4%

c. 4–8%   d. 8–12%

733. Proof spirit contains the following percentage by weight of absolute alcohol:

a. 29.24%   b. 24.49%

c. 49.24%   d. 24.29%

734. The alcohol content of rectified spirit is:

a. 95%   b. 90%

c. 85%   d. 80%

735. The rate of metabolism of absolute alcohol per hour is:

a. 10 ml   b. 15 ml

c. 20 ml   d. 25 ml

736. The lowering of blood alcohol level after consumption and metabolism is:

a. 5–10 mg/hr   b. 12–15 mg/hr

c. 15–18 mg/hr   d. None of the above

737. The metabolism of alcohol is carried out in:

a. Kidney   b. Duodenum

c. Liver   d. Pancreas

738. Alcohol is found in blood after it is drunk up to:
   a. 2 hours   b. 5 hours
   c. 10 hours   d. 20 hours

739. The energy liberated from alcohol on oxidation is about:
   a. 3 cal/g   b. 5 cal/g
   c. 7 cal/g   d. 9 cal/g

740. Vital centres are depressed, respiration and heart stop at an alcohol level of:
   a. 200 mg%   b. 400 mg%
   c. 500 mg%   d. >600 mg%

741. Alcohol absorbed by blood is deposited in tissues as liquids up to a percentage of:
   a. 5   b. 10
   c. 15   d. 20

742. The ratio useful for calculating the blood alcohol concentration from that of urine is:
   a. 1.55:   b. 1:1.33
   c. 1.33:1   d. None of the above

743. The alcohol concentration up to which a person is regarded as fit to drive a motor vehicle is:
   a. 0.05%   b. 0.15%
   c. 1.05%   d. None of the above

744. The following potentiate the action of alcohol:
   a. Barbiturate   b. Atropine
   c. Opium   d. None of the above

745. Widmark's formula is used for the estimation of the follwoing in the blood:
   a. Sugar
   b. Cholinesterase
   c. Ethyl alcohol
   d. Methyl alcohol

746. Section 84 of Bombay Prohibition Act deals with:
   a. Unsoundness of mind
   b. Workman's compensation
   c. Punishment for drinking
   d. None of the above

747. The following is used in varnish:
   a. Ether
   b. Chloroform
   c. Methyl alcohol
   d. None of the above

748. Death in methyl alcohol poisoning is due to:
   a. Acidosis
   b. Coma
   c. Respiratory failure
   d. All of the above

749. Blindness in methyl alcohol poisoning is due to:
   a. Retrobulbar neuritis
   b. Medullary haemorrhage
   c. Pontine haemorrhage
   d. CNS depression

750. Treatment of methyl alcohol poisoning consists of:
   a. Repeated administration of ethyl alcohol
   b. Repeated administration of denatured spirit
   c. Repeated administration of aluminium hydroxide gel
   d. Repeated administration of ethyl chloride

751. Fatal dose of methyl alcohol is:
   a. 10–20 ml   b. 20–40 ml
   c. 60–240 ml   d. 250–300 ml

752. 'Sukha sharab' means:
   a. Aconite
   b. Chloroform
   c. Chloral hydrate
   d. Ether

753. Death in chloral hydrate poisoning is due to:
   a. Paralysis of the respiratory centre
   b. Perforation of the stomach
   c. CNS depression
   d. None of the above

754. Long-acting barbiturates include:
   a. Gardinal   b. Amital
   c. Seconal   d. None of the above

755. Ultrashort-acting barbiturate includes:
a. Secobarbitol   b. Nembutol
c. Veronal   d. Pentothal

756. Forced diuresis means using of:
a. 500 ml of NS (normal saline)
b. 500 ml of 5% glucose solution
c. a and b
d. a and b and repeated

757. Tranquilizers are given to relieve:
a. Anxiety
b. Mental stress
c. Muscular tension
d. All of the above

758. Unintended death may occur in cases of:
a. Barbiturate automatism
b. Somnambulism
c. Somnolentia
d. None of the above

759. Fatal dose of nitroglycerine is:
a. 1–2 g   b. 0.1–0.2 g
c. 0.5–1 g   d. None of the above

DELIRIANT POISONS

760. Thorn apple is:
a. *Datura stramonium*
b. Calotropis
c. *Semicarpus anacardium*
d. *Nerium odorum*

761. The following does not belong to *dhatura* alkaloids:
a. Atropine
b. Hyoscyamine
c. Acetylcholine
d. Hyoscine

762. The hallucinations seen in *dhatura* poisoning are:
a. Visual   b. Tactile
c. Gustatory   d. None of the above

763. The following does not include a putrefaction resisting poison:
a. *Dhatura*   b. Strychnine
c. Endrine   d. Morphine

764. Mydriatic test does not help in case of:
a. Atropine   b. Hyoscine
c. Hyoscyamine   d. *Digitaline*

765. Cannabinol is:
a. Alkaloid   b. Glycoside
c. Phytotoxin   d. None of the above

766. Reefers are made from:
a. Tobacco   b. *Dhatura*
c. Cannabis   d. Calotropis

767. Majun is a sweet prepared from:
a. Bhang   b. Charas
c. Poppy seeds   d. Nutmeg

768. Charas is:
a. Smoked in a hukha
b. Taken as a gola
c. Taken as a sweet
d. None of the above

769. Hashish is:
a. Ganja   b. Bhang
c. Majun   d. Charas

770. Gynaecomastia is reported in chronic poisoning of:
a. Cocaine
b. Cannabis
c. Carbon monoxide
d. None of the above

771. Delta and THC is derived from:
a. Hydrocarbons
b. Ergot
c. HCN
d. Cannabis

772. Cocaine is:
a. Glycoside   b. Resin
c. Alkaloid   d. None of the above

773. Impotence is not caused by:
a. Opium   b. Cocaine
c. Arsenic   d. Alcohol

774. Dilated pupils are seen in:
a. Cocaine poisoning
b. Alcoholic intoxication
c. Pethidine poisoning
d. Any of the above

775. The following is not used in Pan:

    a. Cocaine   b. Calotropis

    c. Aconite   d. Catechu

776. The following is not a mushroom:

    a. *Amanita muscaria*

    b. *Amanita phalloides*

    c. Curarine

    d. None of the above

777. Meperidine is:

    a. Amphetamine b. Gardinal

    c. Diazepam   d. Pethidine

778. The following is not an arrow poison:

    a. Curare

    b. Aconite

    c. Alcohol

    d. *Abrus precatorius*

779. The following is not toxalbumin:

    a. Ricin   b. Crotin

    c. Abrine   d. Meperidine

780. Somniferous poisons include:

    a. Morphine   b. Pethidine

    c. Heroin   d. Pyridine

781. Kesari dal means:

    a. *Lathyrus sativus*

    b. *Paspalum scrobiculatum*

    c. *Argemona mexicana*

    d. None of the above

782. Nerine is:

    a. Cardiac poison

    b. Hepatic poison

    c. Nephrotoxin

    d. None of the above

783. Aconite is:

    a. Accidental poison

    b. Suicidal poison

    c. Homicidal poison

    d. Any of the above

784. Hydrocyanic acid does not act on:

    a. Respiratory system

    b. Heart muscle

    c. Central nervous system

    d. Kidneys

785. In atmospheric air, carbon dioxide exists up to:

    a. 1.0%   b. 0.4%

    c. 4.0%   d. 0.1%

786. Dry-ice contains:

    a. Carbon monoxide

    b. Carbon disulphide

    c. Carbon dioxide

    d. None of the above

787. The following is not a war gas:

    a. Mustard gas

    b. Phosgene

    c. Chloropicrine

    d. Sulphur dioxide (SO_2)

788. Aflatoxin contamination is seen in:

    a. Ground nuts b. Poppy seeds

    c. Kesari dal   d. Wheat

789. In case of insulin poisoning, insulin can be isolated after death up to:

    a. One day   b. One month

    c. One year   d. Six years

790. In botulism (a type of food poisoning), death is due to:

    a. Paralysis of respiratory muscles

    b. Dehydration and shock

    c. Convulsions

    d. None of the above

791. In kerosene poisoning, the following is not seen:

    a. Pulmonary oedema

    b. Bronchopneumonia

    c. Convulsions

    d. Contracted pupils

792. In carbamate poisoning, the following is indicated:

    a. Calcium chloride

    b. Atropine

    c. PAM

    d. All of the above

793. Aromax is used as a solvent for:

    a. DDT   b. Gammaxene

    c. Endrine   d. Malathion

794. Chlorpromazine is:

a. Neurotoxic
b. Nephrotoxic
c. Hepatotoxic
d. Non-toxic

795. Paraldehyde is administered:

a. Intravenously
b. Orally
c. Intramuscularly
d. Any of the above

796. Aspirin is:

a. Acetoacetic acid
b. Acetylsalicylic acid
c. Oxaloacetic acid
d. None of the above

797. Laughing gas is:

a. Nitric oxide
b. Nitrogen peroxide
c. Nitrous oxide
d. Ethane

798. Halothane anaesthesia can cause:

a. Massive hepatic necrosis
b. Acute left ventricular failure
c. Cerebral palsy
d. None of the above

MULTIPLE CHOICE QUESTIONS
(NEWLY ADDED)

1. DNA profile can be identical:

a. If samples are from same person
b. Samples different but error in collection or lab
c. If they are identical twins
d. Any of the above

2. SIDS is more common in:

a. Males
b. A few days to a few months
c. Premature infants
d. All of the above

3. Epithelial regeneration is clearly noted in a healing abrasion:

a. In 18 hours
b. In 1 day
c. In 2 days
d. In 3 days

4. A kick on the scrotum can cause immediate death due to:

a. Vagal stimulation
b. Haematocele formation
c. Urethral rupture
d. None of the above

5. Pulmonary fat embolism can occur:

a. In fractures
b. In burns
c. In criminal abortion
d. None of the above

6. Absence of bridging tissue in the depth of the wound indicates:

a. Stab wound
b. Lacerated wound
c. Firearm injury
d. Bomb blast injury

7. Hesitation cuts are seen in:

a. Suicidal cases
b. Homicidal cases
c. Accidental cases
d. Any of the above

8. Diameter of the bore measured from land to land in rifled firearm is equal to entry wound:

a. Caliber
b. Entry wound
c. Exit wound
d. Depth of the wound

9. Peppering or tattooing of firearm entry wounds:

a. Cannot be wiped
b. Are not burns
c. Are due to impregnation of carbon particles
d. All of the above

10. Recochet bullets cause:
 a. Typical entrance wounds
 b. Atypical entrance wounds
 c. Tattooing seen
 d. Grease collar is clearly seen

11. Pinprint pupils are seen in:
 a. Sulphuric acid poisoning
 b. Atropine poisoning
 c. Morphine poisoning
 d. Phosphorus poisoning

12. Hippus is seen in cases of:
 a. Carbolic acid poisoning
 b. Aconite poisoning
 c. Barbiturate poisoning
 d. Nicotine poisoning

13. Podogram deals with:
 a. Poroscopy   b. Fingerprints
 c. DNA   d. Footprints

14. Locard's method of identification uses:
 a. Study of pores which are the ducts of sweat glands
 b. Study of web transillumination
 c. Study of latent fingerprints
 d. Study of DNA chains

15. The number of specific loci to be studied in DNA profiling required for identification purpose:
 a. 13   b. 21
 c. 15   d. 2

16. For identification of hair, the following is significant:
 a. Long hair
 b. Cross-section
 c. Cuticular scale pattern
 d. None of the above

17. Lanugo hair is:
 a. Long
 b. Thin
 c. Grey
 d. All of the above

18. Abrasion heals by:
 a. 3 days   b. 5 days
 c. 10 days   d. 2 weeks

19. Shape of the palate in Negroes:
 a. Wedge   b. Horseshoe
 c. Rectangular   d. None of the above

20. Mixed dentition is seen in child of:
 a. 6 years   b. 4 years
 c. 21 years   d. None of the above

21. Prominent cheek bones are seen in:
 a. Negros   b. Caucasians
 c. Mongoloids   d. None of the above

22. Triangular orbits are seen in:
 a. Negros   b. Caucasians
 c. Mongoloid   d. All of the above

23. A person is presumed dead, if he is not heard for:
 a. 10 years   b. 5 years
 c. 7 years   d. 15 years

24. Histotoxic anoxia is seen in:
 a. Drowning
 b. Uraemia
 c. Heat smoke
 d. Carbon monoxide poisoning

25. Rigor mortis can be seen after:
 a. Cold stiffening
 b. Heat stiffening
 c. Gas stiffening
 d. None of the above

26. Green postmortem staining is seen in:
 a. HS poisoning
 b. CO poisoning
 c. Potassium nitrate poisoning
 d. Cyanide poisoning

27. Maggots are seen after:
 a. <24 hours   b. >2 days
 c. <5 days   d. After one week

28. Whole body rigor is seen by:
 a. 3 hours   b. 6 hours
 c. 12 hours   d. 1 hour

29. Gases of decomposition include:
 a. Methane
 b. Hydrogen
 c. Cyanogen
 d. None of the above

30. Blisters of decomposition contain:
   a. Albumen   b. High chloride
   c. Gases   d. Inflammation

31. After a week contusion is:
   a. Blue   b. Yellow
   c. Green   d. Black

32. Ectopic bruise is seen on:
   a. Nose   b. Leg
   c. Elbow   d. Eyelids

33. Avulsion is a type of:
   a. Abrasion   b. Stab
   c. Bruise   d. Laceration

34. Defence wounds are seen on:
   a. Palms   b. Back
   c. Buttocks   d. None of the above

35. Ring fracture of skull is seen on:
   a. Scalp   b. Temple
   c. Base   d. Vertex

36. Pond fracture is seen in:
   a. Old people   b. Adults
   c. Sick people d. Infants

37. Bumper fracture is seen in:
   a. Femur   b. Radius
   c. Tibia   d. Fibula

38. Spider fracture is seen when hit with:
   a. Pointed object b. Blunt object
   c. Pistol   d. None of the above

39. Balling of the shot is a feature of firing from:
   a. Revolver   b. Pistol
   c. Rifle   d. Shotgun

40. Scorching is due to:
   a. Carbon particles
   b. Flame
   c. Wood
   d. None of the above

41. AK-47 is:
   a. Shotgun
   b. Revolver
   c. Assault rifle
   d. Carbine

42. Saloon pistol is:
   a. Toy pistol   b. Carbine
   c. Stud gun   d. None of the above

43. Stud gun is:
   a. War weapon
   b. Suicide bomber
   c. Industrial gun
   d. Land weapon

44. Type of haemorrhage caused by rupture of bridging veins:
   a. Extradural   b. Subdural
   c. Subarachnoid   d. Pontine

45. Whiplash injury seen in:
   a. Front seat passengers
   b. Near back seat passengers
   c. Pedestrian
   d. Any of the above

46. Railway spine shows:
   a. Concussion
   b. Transections
   c. Laceration
   d. None of the above

47. Commoti cardis causes:
   a. Ventricular fibrilation
   b. Asystole
   c. Myocardial ischaemia
   d. Any of the above

48. Abduction fracture of hyoid bone is seen in:
   a. Throttling   b. Choking
   c. Hanging   d. Mugging

49. A dead body floats in water after:
   a. 6 hours   b. 12 hours
   c. 24 hours   d. 36 hours

50. A child is *doli incapax* before:
   a. 6 years   b. 10 years
   c. 7 years   d. 12 years

51. Widening of gyri and flattening of sulci is a characteristic feature of:
   a. Cephalhaematoma
   b. Extradural haematoma
   c. Cerebral oedema
   d. Papilloedema

52. To prevent AIDS, autopsy instruments should be washed with:
   a. 10% sodium hypochloride
   b. 10% formalin
   c. 10% carbolic acid
   d. 10% lysol

53. Postmortem rooms are disinfected by:
   a. 10% bleaching powder spray
   b. 10% gammaxene spray
   c. 10% saline
   d. Any of the above

54. Tissues for DNA are submitted as they are in case of:
   a. Hair   b. Blood
   c. Semen   d. Saliver

55. Common salt should not be used as preservative for chemical analysis of the viscera in:
   a. Alcohol
   b. Phosphorus
   c. Carbolic acid
   d. Aconite

56. Alcohol should not be used as preservative in cases of:
   a. Phosphorus
   b. Paraldehyde
   c. Kerosene
   d. All of the above

57. Ant bite marks resemble:
   a. Laceration
   b. Abrasion
   c. Contusion
   d. None of the above

58. Hyperpyrexia is caused by:
   a. Extradural haemorrhage
   b. Subdural haemorrhage
   c. Subarachnoid haemorrhage
   d. Pontine haemorrhage

59. In a fall from height, the following fracture is seen:
   a. Ring fracture of skull
   b. Fracture of humerus
   c. Fracture of sacrum
   d. None of the above

60. An oblique and above Adam's apple ligature mark indicates:
   a. Suicidal hanging
   b. Strangulation
   c. Partial hanging
   d. Homicidal hanging

61. Emphysaema aquosum suggests:
   a. Antemortem drowning
   b. Postmortem drowning
   c. Dry drowning
   d. Salt water drowning

62. In fresh water drowning, the chloride content on the left side of heart is:
   a. More than right side
   b. Less than right side
   c. Equal to right side
   d. None of the above

63. Dry drowning is due to:
   a. Laryngeal spasm
   b. Postmortem drowning
   c. Unconnected to drowning
   d. Secondary causes of drowning

64. Hydrocution in drowning means:
   a. Immesion syndrome
   b. Vagal inhibition
   c. Cold water stimulating tympanic membrame
   d. All of the above

65. When skin comes in contact with hot fluids at boiling point, the burns caused are:
   a. Contact burns b. Scalds
   c. Flame burns   d. Any of the above

66. Pugilistic attitude is:
   a. Boxer's attitude
   b. Putrefaction
   c. Mummification
   d. None of the above

67. Joule's burns are:
   a. Endogenous thermal burns
   b. Exogenous thermal burns
   c. Rediant burns
   d. Microwave burns

68. **High voltage electricity causes:**
    a. Exogenous thermal burns
    b. Endogenous thermal burns
    c. Fractures
    d. No effect

69. **Arborescent marks are greenish due to deposition of:**
    a. Copper
    b. Chrophyl
    c. Early decomposition
    d. None of the above

70. **Blighted ovum shows in sonography:**
    a. Loss of gestational ring
    b. Loss of fetal echos
    c. No progress of pregnancy
    d. All of the above

71. **Quickening is felt by mother in pregnancy by:**
    a. 4 weeks   b. 8 weeks
    c. 16 weeks   d. 20 weeks

72. **The product of conception is known as embryo up to:**
    a. 0–1 weeks   b. 1–2 weeks
    c. 2–3 weeks   d. 3–5 weeks

73. **Corpus luteum of pregnancy is seen in:**
    a. Cervix   b. Uterus
    c. Ovary   d. Broad ligament

74. **Munchausen syndrome by proxy is seen in:**
    a. Mother
    b. Child
    c. Father
    d. Any one

75. **Munchausen syndrome is:**
    a. Self-inflicted damage
    b. To get hospitalisation
    c. Without any extraneous stimulus
    d. All of the above

76. **Surrogate mother:**
    a. Womb on rent
    b. Not bilogical mother
    c. Has children already
    d. All of the above

77. **In undinism, a person derives sexual pleasure by watching:**
    a. Some one urinating
    b. Seeing wife having sex with another person
    c. Sexual organs of opposite sex
    d. By seeing clothes of opposite sex

78. **Zenanas have:**
    a. Intact sexual organs
    b. Penis cut off
    c. Wear dress of opposite sex
    d. None of the above

79. **In pederasty, child is:**
    a. Active agent
    b. Passive agent
    c. Not involved
    d. Involved in theft

80. **Bondage in a combination of:**
    a. Sadism and masochism
    b. Necrophilia and fetichism
    c. Trolism and frotteurism
    d. None of the above

81. **Lanugo is:**
    a. Fetal hair   b. Female hair
    c. Male hair   d. Bleached hair

82. **Antemortem artefacts are caused by:**
    a. Surgical interference
    b. Cardiac external massage
    c. Regurgitation of fluids
    d. Any of the above

83. **Bicuspids are seen as:**
    a. Milk teeth
    b. Premolars
    c. Molars
    d. Wisdom tooth

84. **SIDS occurs below:**
    a. 1 year   b. 2 years
    c. 3 years   d. 5 years

85. **Crib death is:**
    a. SIDS
    b. Caffey's syndrome
    c. Munchausen syndrome
    d. None of the above

86. Bridging tissue in the depth seen in:

a. Contusion

b. Laceration

c. Stab wound

d. Extradural haemorrhage

87. Death in stab wounds of neck is due to:

a. Exsanguination

b. Air embolism

c. Asphyxia

d. Any of the above

88. Chop wounds are caused by:

a. Axe   b. Hatchet

c. Matchet   d. Any of the above

89. In rifled firearm land-to-land measure denotes:

a. Caliber   b. Diameter

c. Speed   d. None of the above

90. Point blank range means:

a. Contact range b. Near contact

c. Intermediate   d. Distant

91. Abrasion ring is caused by:

a. Entry bullet   b. Flame

c. Greaze   d. Any of the above

92. Constriction of the gun bore at muzzle end is called:

a. Pellet   b. Choke

c. Rifling   d. Wad

93. Single round entrance in gunfire is seen:

a. Up to 5 ft   b. Up to 4 ft

c. Up to 3 ft   d. Up to 2 ft

94. Pinpoint pupils are seen in poisoning of:

a. Morphine   b. Methanol

c. Quinine   d. Any of the above

95. 3% sodium nitrite IV is given in poisoning of:

a. Nitric acid   b. Cyanide

c. Phosphorus   d. None of the above

96. Dimercaprol is used in the treatment of:

a. Arsenic

b. Lead

c. Mercury

d. Any of the above

97. Route of administration of pencillamine:

a. IV   b. IM

c. SC   d. Oral

98. BAL is administered:

a. Deep intramuscular

b. Intravenous

c. Intrathecal

d. Oral

99. The following poisons have odour, except:

a. Phenol

b. Cyanide

c. Hydrogen sulphide

d. Sulphuric acid

100. The following are stupefying agents, except:

a. *Dhatura*

b. Cannabis

c. Chloral hydrate

d. Aconite

101. Priapism is caused by:

a. Carbolic acid

b. Cantharides

c. Chloral hydrate

d. Cannabis

102. Chalky white teeth are seen in poising of:

a. Hydrochloric acid

b. Sulphuric acid

c. Arsenic

d. Aspirin

103. Brown pigmentation of skin is caused by:

a. Carbolic acid   b. Phosphorus

c. Nitrates   d. Mercuric salt

104. Pink disease is caused by:

a. Mercurous chloride

b. Mercuric chloride

c. Metallic mercury

d. Nitrates

105. Death cap is:

a. *Amanita muscaria*

b. *Amanita phalloides*

c. Allantiasis

d. None of the above

106. Botulism is a type of:
a. Neurological toxicity
b. Gastrointestinal lesion
c. Genitourinary irritant
d. None of the above

107. Pethidine causes:
a. Dilated pupils
b. Contracted pupils
c. Alternate contraction and dilatation
d. No pupillary changes

108. Marchiafava's syndrome in chronic alcoholics shows dementia of:
a. Substantia nigra
b. Pons
c. Corpus callosum
d. Red nucleus

109. McEwan's sign helps in detection of poisoning by:
a. Alcohol   b. Opium
c. Cannabis   d. Burbiturates

110. Example of ultrashort-acting barbiturate is:
a. Pentothal sodium
b. Seconal
c. Pentobarbitone
d. Gardinol

111. The following is known as dry liquor:
a. Oxalic acid   b. Cannabis
c. *Dhatura*   d. Chloral hydrate

112. Crack is a preparation of:
a. Cannabis   b. Cocaine
c. Alcohol   d. None of the above

113. Seven gases consist of:
a. Hydrogen sulphide
b. Carbon dioxide
c. Methane
d. All of the above

114. The following is vesicant:
a. Phosgene
b. Mustard gas
c. Chloropicrin
d. None of the above

115. Dry ice means:
a. Solid CO   b. CO
c. So   d. None of the above

116. Bag colour used for crushed synings:
a. Red   b. Yellow
c. Blue   d. Black

117. Beating to the soles of the feet is called:
a. Murcielago   b. Labandera
c. Jaok   d. Falanga

118. IPC 304-B deals with:
a. Medical negligence
b. Dwory death
c. Abetment of suicide
d. None of the above

MULTIPLE CHOICE QUESTION ANSWERS						
1. c	2. b	3. d	4. d	5. b	6. b	7. d
8. d	9. d	10. d	11. d	12. c	13. a	14. d
15. c	16. d	17. a	18. b	19. a	20. a	21. c
22. d	23. b	24. a	25. a	26. d	27. b	28. d
29. c	30. a	31. b	32. d	33. a	34. b	35. b
36. a	37. b	38. a	39. b	40. b	41. b	42. c
43. b	44. a	45. c	46. a	47. a	48. a	49. b
50. a	51. a	52. b	53. c	54. b	55. a	56. b
57. c	58. d	59. a	60. b	61. a	62. b	63. c
64. b	65. a	66. b	67. b	68. b	69. b	70. d
71. a	72. a	73. a	74. a	75. c	76. c	77. c
78. a	79. a	80. b	81. a	82. b	83. b	84. c

85. d	86. c	87. a	88. b	89. b	90. c	91. c
92. a	93. a	94. c	95. c	96. a	97. a	98. b
99. b	100. c	101. c	102. d	103. a	104. c.	105. c
106. c	107. b	108. b	109. d	110. d	111. d	112. c
113. d	114. a	115. c	116. a	117. a	118. a	119. a
120. b	121. d	122. d	123. a	124. a	125. a	126. a
127. c	128. a	129. a	130. a	131. a	132. c	133. a
134. c	135. a	136. c	137. b	138. a	139. c	140. b
141. a	142. c	143. a	144. b	145. a	146. d	147. c
148. a	149. d	150. b	151. d	152. a	153. a	154. d
155. d	156. d	157. b	158. b	159. d	160. c	161. c
162. c	163. d	164. a	165. b	166. d	167. d	168. a
169. d	170. c	171. d	172. a	173. a	174. a	175. c
176. d	177. c	178. a	179. c	180. b	181. c	182. d
183. b	184. a	185. b	186. a	187. a	188. a	189. c
190. d	191. a	192. d	193. a	194. d	195. a	196. a
197. a	198. b	199. a	200. a	201. b	202. a	203. a
204. a	205. a	206. a	207. a	208. c	209. b	210. c
211. d	212. a	213. c	214. c	215. c	216. a	217. a
218. d	219. b	220. b	221. b	222. c	223. c	224. d
225. b	226. d	227. a	228. c	229. a	230. d	231. a
232. a	233. a	234. c	235. d	236. b	237. b	238. a
239. b	240. b	241. d	242. b	243. b	244. b	245. c
246. d	247. b	248. a	249. b	250. a	251. d	252. d
253. a	254. d	255. a	256. c	257. a	258. d	259. d
260. a	261. d	262. b	263. d	264. a	265. d	266. c
267. a	268. a	269. a	270. a	271. c	272. c	273. b
274. d	275. a	276. d	277. d	278. a	279. d	280. d
281. b	282. d	283. b	284. a	285. c	286. a	287. d
288. a	289. c	290. a	291. d	292. c	293. c	294. c
295. b	296. b	297. a	298. c	299. c	300. d	301. b
302. a	303. b	304. a	305. d	306. d	307. b	308. a
309. d	310. d	311. a	312. a	313. d	314. c	315. c
316. c	317. a	318. a	319. d	320. a	321. d	322. d
323. d	324. d	325. a	326. d	327. b	328. a	329. d
330. d	331. b	332. a	333. a	334. b	335. a	336. a
337. b	338. c	339. b	340. b	341. b	342. b	343. b
344. c	345. c	346. b	347. a	348. b	349. a	350. a
351. d	352. d	353. c	354. b	355. a	356. d	357. b
358. c	359. a	360. a	361. d	362. a	363. b	364. d
365. c	366. d	367. d	368. a	369. c	370. a	371. a
372. a	373. d	374. d	375. a	376. a	377. d	378. a
379. d	380. b	381. b	382. d	383. a	384. a	385. b

386. d	387. d	388. d	389. d	390. a	391. c.	392. c
393. a	394. d	395. b	396. d	397. d	398. a	399. b
400. a	401. b	402. d	403. b	404. a	405. c	406. a
407. a	408. a	409. c	410. a	411. d	412. a	413. a
414. a	415. c	416. c	417. d	418. a	419. a	420. b
421. a	422. b	423. d	424. d	425. a	426. d	427. d
428. d	429. c	430. d	431. c	432. c	433. c	434. c
435. b	436. c	437. b	438. a	439. b	440. b	441. c
442. b	443. a	444. c	445. c	446. a	447. c	448. a
449. a	450. d	451. a	452. a	453. a	454. a	455. d
456. a	457. a	458. b	459. c	460. c	461. b	462. b
463. a	464. d	465. c	466. b	467. c	468. a	469. a
470. a	471. a	472. c	473. c	474. d	475. a	476. a
477. c	478. d	479. b	480. d	481. a	482. b	483. b
484. d	485. d	486. a	487. d	488. a	489. a	490. c
491. a	492. b	493. b	494. b	495. c	496. c	497. b
498. b	499. d	500. d	501. a	502. a	503. d	504. a
505. a	506. b	507. a	508. c	509. d	510. c	511. d
512. c	513. a	514. c	515. b	516. d	517. b	518. c
519. a	520. a	521. a	522. b	523. a	524. c	525. b
526. b	527. d	528. a	529. b	530. a	531. a	532. b
533. b	534. c	535. d	536. b	537. d	538. a	539. d
540. d	541. b	542. a	543. c	544. b	545. d	546. d
547. a	548. b	549. a	550. d	551. a	552. c	553. d
554. a	555. a	556. a	557. c	558. d	559. b	560. b
561. c	562. b	563. b	564. a	565. d	566. a	567. a
568. d	569. b	570. a	571. c	572. a	573. a	574. d
575. a	576. c	577. c	578. b	579. c	580. c	581. a
582. a	583. b	584. d	585. a	586. d	587. b	588. a
589. c	590. d	591. d	592. b	593. c	594. b	595. d
596. b	597. b	598. c	599. a	600. b	601. b	602. d
603. c	604. c	605. a	606. b	607. c	608. d	609. a
610. c	611. b	612. a	613. d	614. d	615. a	616. a
617. d	618. b	619. b	620. a	621. b	622. c	623. a
624. a	625. a	626. d	627. d	628. b	629. b	630. c
631. b	632. c	633. a	634. c	635. a	636. d	637. d
638. c	639. b	640. b	641. b	642. b	643. c	644. b
645. d	646. d	647. a	648. b	649. b	650. a	651. d
652. a	653. c	654. d	655. c	656. d	657. a	658. a
659. b	660. a	661. c	662. a	663. a	664. d	665. a
666. d	667. a	668. d	669. d	670. d	671. a	672. c
673. c	674. a	675. b	676. a	677. a	678. a	679. a
680. c	681. a	682. b	683. a	684. a	685. a	686. a

687. d	688. d	689. d	690. c	691. a	692. b	693. a
694. a	695. d	696. c	697. a	698. b	699. a	700. a
701. b	702. a	703. a	704. a	705. b	706. a	707. a
708. b	709. a	710. b	711. c	712. a	713. b	714. a
715. a	716. b	717. c	718. b	719. d	720. d	721. d
722. a	723. d	724. b	725. b	726. d	727. c	728. d
729. b	730. b	731. c	732. d	733. c	734. b	735. b
736. b	737. c	738. d	739. c	740. d	741. b	742. b
743. d	744. a	745. c	746. c	747. c	748. d	749. a
750. a	751. c	752. c	753. a	754. a	755. d	756. d
757. a	758. a	759. a	760. a	761. c	762. a	763. d
764. d	765. d	766. c	767. a	768. a	769. d	770. b
771. d	772. c	773. c	774. a	775. b	776. c	777. d
778. c	779. d	780. d	781. a	782. a	783. d	784. d
785. b	786. c	787. d	788. a	789. d	790. a	791. d
792. b	793. c	794. c	795. c	796. b	797. c	798. a

MULTIPLE CHOICE QUESTION ANSWERS (NEWLY ADDED)

1. d	2. d	3. d	4. a	5. a	6. a	7. a
8. a	9. d	10. b	11. c	12. b	13. d	14. c
15. a	16. b	17. d	18. b	19. c	20. a	21. c
22. b	23. c	24. b	25. d	26. a	27. b	28. c
29. a	30. c	31. b	32. d	33. d	34. a	35. c
36. d	37. c	38. a	39. d	40. b	41. c	42. a
43. c	44. a	45. a	46. a	47. d	48. c	49. d
50. c	51. c	52. a	53. a	54. a	55. d	56. d
57. b	58. d	59. a	60. a	61. b	62. a	63. a
64. a	65. b	66. a	67. a	68. d	69. a	70. a
71. c	72. a	73. c	74. a	75. b	76. a	77. a
78. a	79. b	80. a	81. a	82. d	83. b	84. a
85. a	86. b	87. b	88. a	89. a	90. a	91. a
92. b	93. a	94. a	95. c	96. d	97. d	98. a
99. d	100. d	101. b	102. b	103. d	104. b	105. b
106. a	107. a	108. c	109. a	110. a	111. d	112. a
113. d	114. d	115. a	116. c	117. d	118. b	

ADDITIONAL TOXICOLOGICAL ISSUES

Poison information and control centres provide:

- Immediate, round the clock toxicity assessment.
- Treatment recommendation over the telephone for all poisoning:
  - Affecting people of all ages
  - Ingestion of household products
  - Overdose of therapeutic medication
  - Use of illegal foreign and veterinary drugs
  - Chemical exposures during occupation
  - Hazardous material spills
  - Bites of snakes, spiders
  - Other venomous creatures
  - Plant and mushroom poisoning

On receiving a call, the poison information specialists take history:

- Assess the severity of the poisoning
- Provide treatment recommendations
- Refer the patient for further medical attention, if required.
- Follow-up with phone calls to assess progress
- Provide additional recommendations until poisoning is resolved.
- Pieces of information from the beginning of the call to the final outcome are noted case sheets, and quantifiable data is filled in by darkening respective bubbles on the sheet.

TOXIC SYNDROMES

Sedative Syndrome

- **Symptoms and signs:** Miosis, hypotension, bradycardia, hypothermia, CNS depression, hyporeflexia, coma, rarely convulsions.
- **Causative agents:** Barbiturates, benzodiazepines, ethanol, methaqualone, meprobamate, ethchlorvynol, glutethimide, clonidine.

Sympathomimetic Syndrome

- **Symptoms and signs:** Paranoia, delusions, tachycardia, hypertension, hyperpyrexia, sweating, mydriasis, seizures, arrhythmias.
- **Causative agents:** Cocaine, amphetamines, upper respiratory decongestants (phenylpropanolamine, ephedrine, and pseudoephedrine).

Cholinergic Syndrome

- **Symptoms and signs:** Confusion, CNS depression, salivation, lacrimation, urinary and faecal incontinence, vomiting, sweating, fasciculations, seizures, miosis, pulmonary oedema, tachy bradycardia.
- **Causative agents:** Organophosphates, carbamates, parasympathomimetic drugs, and some mushrooms.

Pupillary changes in drugs

Contracted	Dilated	Nystagmus
Barbiturates	Alcohol (constricted in coma)	Alcohol
Benzodiazepines	Amphetamines	Barbiturates
Caffeine	Antihistamines	Carbamazepine
Carbamates	Carbon monoxide	Phencyclidine
Carbolic acid (phenol)	Cocaine	Phenytoin
Clonidine	Cyanide	
Methyldopa	Datura (atropine)	
Nicotine	Ephedrine	
Opiates		
Organophosphates		
Parasympathomimetics		

Anticholinergic Syndrome

- **Symptoms and signs:** Delirium with mumbling speech, tachycardia, dry hot skin, mydriasis, myoclonus, urinary retention, decreased bowel sounds, convulsions and arrhythmias in severe cases.
- **Causative agents:** Antihistamines, antiparkinsonian drugs, atropine, scopolamine, amantadine, antipsychotic drugs, antidepressants, antispasmodics, skeletal muscle relaxants, many plants (especially Datura), and fungi (e.g. *Amanita muscaria*).

Skin changes in acute and chronic poisonings

Acute	
Substance	Manifestation
Datura, atropine	Dry, hot skin
Organophosphates, salicylates, arsenic,	Profuse sweating
LSD	Cherry pink colour
Carbon monoxide (CO)	Brick red colour
Cyanide	Blisters
Barbiturates, CO, imipramine, methadone, nitrazepam	Petechiae and purpuric spots
Warfarin	Flushing
Clonidine, ergot, niacin,	
Sympathomimetics, theophylline	

Chronic	
Substance	Manifestation
Heroin, barbiturates, morphine, phencyclidine	Needle marks
Bromides, iodides, coal tar products, phenytoin	Acne, brown colour
Arsenic	Rain drop pigmentation, hyperkeratosis, dermatitis, eczematous dermatitis, dark pigmentation
Chlorinated hydrocarbons, chloroquine, busulfan, clofazimine, phenothiazines, phenytoin, bromides, iodides, penicillin, salicylates, tetracycline	Erythema nodosum

Oral manifestations in poisoning

Feature	Substance
Glossitis	Piroxicam, erythromycin, amoxycillin, metronidazole, naproxen, diclofenac, trimethoprim-sulfamethoxazole
Stomatitis	Gentian violet dye, gold salts, penicillamine, cytotoxic drugs.
Sialadenitis	Iodine, nitrofurantoin, isoproterenol, phenylbutazone.
Parotitis	Thioridazine, phenyl and oxyphenbutazone, clonidine, methyldopa
Gingival hyperplasia	Verapamil, diltiazem, nifedipine, phenobarbitone, sodium valproate, phenytoin
Pigmentation	Antimalarials , oral contraceptives, cisplatin
Dental discolouration	Iron tonic syrups chlorhexidine, tetracycline, fluorides
Dental caries	Antibiotic suspensions, cough and vitamin syrups
Xerostomia	Centrally acting antihypertensives, diuretics, narcotics, anticonvulsants, anticholinergics, antihistamines, tricyclics, antipsychotics
Sialorrhoea	Iodides, parasympathomimetics

ELECTROLYTE DISTURBANCES—SODIUM, POTASSIUM, CALCIUM

1. Hyperkalaemia

Causes: Digitalis, beta-2 antagonists, potassium sparing diuretics, NSAIDs, fluoride, heparin, succinylcholine, and drugs producing acidosis.

Manifestations: Abdominal pain, diarrhoea, myalgia, and weakness. ECG changes are important—tall, peaked T waves, ST segment depression, prolonged PR interval, and QRS prolongation. In severe cases, there is ventricular fibrillation.

Treatment: Glucose, insulin infusion, sodium bicarbonate, and calcium gluconate. Haemodialysis and exchange resins may be required.

2. Hypokalaemia

Causes: Beta-2 agonists, theophylline, insulin, chloroquine, caffeine, dextrose, loop diuretics, thiazide diuretics, oral hypoglycaemics, salicylates, sympathomimetics, drug-induced gastroenteritis, and metabolic acidosis.

Manifestations: Muscle weakness, paralytic ileus, and ECG changes—flat or inverted T waves, prominent U waves, ST segment depression. In severe cases, there is AV block and ventricular fibrillation.

Treatment: Oral or IV potassium.

3. Hypernatraemia

Causes: Colchicine, lithium, propoxyphene, rifampicin, phenytoin, alcohol, mannitol, sorbitol, sodium salts, excessive water loss, IV saline solutions and salt emetics.

Treatment: Water restriction with or without loop diuretics.

4. Hyponatraemia

Causes: Carbamazepine, chlorpropamide NSAIDs, amitriptyline, biguanides, sulfonylureas, captopril and other ACE inhibitors, lithium, imipramine, oxytocin, and excessive water intake.

Treatment: Hypertonic saline.

5. Hypocalcaemia

Causes: Hydrogen fluoride, oxalates, aminoglycosides, ethanol, phenobarbitone, phenytoin, theophylline, and ethylene glycol.

Treatment: Calcium gluconate IV (10% solution, 10 ml at a time, slowly).

Forced Diuresis

Indications

- A substantial proportion of the drug is excreted unchanged.
- The drug is distributed mainly in the extracellular fluid
- The drug is minimally protein-bound.

Forced Alkaline Diuresis

- This is most useful in the case of phenobarbitone, lithium, and salicylates.
- Administer 1500 ml of fluid IV, in the first hour as follows:
  - 500 ml of 5% dextrose
  - 500 ml of 1.2 or 1.4% sodium bicarbonate
  - 500 ml of 5% dextrose.

Haemodialysis

Procedure: Three basic components blood delivery system, dialyser composition and method of delivery of the dialysate. For acute haemodialysis, catheters are usually placed in the femoral vein and passed into the inferior vena cava. Blood from one is pumped to the dialyser (usually by a roller pump) through lines that contain equipment to measure flow and pressure within the system. Blood returns through the second catheter. Dialysis begins at a blood flow rate of 50 to 100 ml/min, and is gradually increased to 250 to 300 ml/min, to give maximal clearance.

Activated charcoal adsorption			
Poorly adsorbed (+)	*Moderately adsorbed (++)*	*Well adsorbed (+++)*	
Alcohols	Antidiabetic drugs	Aflatoxins	Cimetidine
Carbamates	Kerosene	Amphetamines	Dapsone
Corrosives	Paracetamol	Antidepressants	Digitalis
Cyanide	Phenol	Antiepileptics	NSAIDs
Ethylene glycol	Salicylates	Antihistamines	Opiates
Heavy metals		Atropine	Phenothiazines
Hydrocarbons		Barbiturates	Quinine
Organophosphates		Benzodiazepines	Quinidine
		Beta blockers	Strychnine
		Chloroquine	Tetracycline
			Theophylline

Indications

Patients not responding to standard therapeutic measure as supportive care whether the toxicant is dialysable or not in the following situations:

- Stage 3 or 4 coma.
- Hyperactivity caused by a dialysable agent which cannot be treated by conservative means.
- Marked hyperosmolality which is not due to easily corrected fluid problems.
- Severe acid–base disturbance not responding to therapy.
- Severe electrolyte disturbance not responding to therapy.

Best indications

- Heavy metal chelation
- With renal failure
- Ethylene glycol
- Methanol ingestion

Very good indications

- Lithium
- Phenobarbitone
- Salicylates
- Theophylline

Fairly good indications

- Alcohol amphetamines
- Anilines
- Antibiotics
- Boric acid
- Barbiturates (short acting)
- Bromides
- Chlorates
- Chloral hydrate
- Iodides
- Isoniazid
- Meprobamate
- Paraldehyde
- Fluorides
- Quinidine
- Quinine
- Strychnine
- Thiocyanates

Poor indications

- Paracetamol
- Antidepressants
- Antihistamines
- Belladonna alkaloids
- Benzodiazepines
- Digitalis and related glycosides
- Glutethimide
- Opiates
- Methaqualone
- Phenothiazines
- Synthetic anticholinergics

Complications

- Infection (especially AIDS, hepatitis B)
- Thrombosis
- Hypotension
- Air embolism
- Bleeding (due to use of heparin as a systemic anticoagulant).

Haemoperfusion

A technique that is increasingly becoming popular since it is capable of removing many of the toxins that are not removed well by haemodialysis.

Haemoperfusion useful more efficiently than haemodialysis in toxicity of

Amanitin	Paracetamol
Barbiturates (all categories)	Paraquat
Carbon tetrachloride	Phenols
Chloral hydrate	Phenylbutazone
Chlorpromazine	Promethazine
Dapsone	Propoxyphene
Diazepam	Quinidine, quinine
Digoxin	Salicylates
Diphenhydramine	Theophylline
Organophosphates	Tricyclic antidepressants

Complications

- Bleeding (because of heparinisation)
- Air embolism
- Infection
- Thrombocytopenia
- Hypocalcaemia
- Hypotension

CHAPTER 34

Forms and Certificates

INJURY CERTIFICATE

From   To
Dr. ....   The Subinspector of Police
    ....
    ....
    ....
Sir,

Sub: Issuance of wound certificate registered.

Ref: Requisition no. .... Date ....

1. Name of individual ....

2. Sex ....

3. Age ....

4. Address ....

5. Identification marks:

    (a) ....

    (b) ....

6. Consent (signature or thumb impression) ....

7. Accompanying P.C. no., PS ....

8. Brief history ....

9. Date of examination ....

10. Time of examination:

    (a) Beginning ....

    (b) Conclusion ....

11. Place ....

12. Injuries:

Nature	Size	Site	Simple/ grievous	Nature of weapon	Dangerous weapon or not	Additional remarks

Signature of Medical Officer

Date ....

Name ....

Designation ....

Reg. no. ....

FORM FOR AGE DETERMINATION

1. Name of the subject ....

2. Address ....

3. Requisition from .... dated ....

4. Eperted by ....

5. History ....

6. Age .... as state by ....

7. Consent ....

8. Date and time of examination ....

9. Identification marks:

   (i) ....

   (ii) ....

10. Physical examination:

    Height .... Weight .... General build ....

    Voice .... Adam's apple ....

    Hair ....

         Moustache ....

         Pubic ....

         Axillary ....

    Breasts ....

    External genitalia ....

    Puberty/ejaculation ....

    Menstruation ....

    Other features ....

11. Dental examination:

    Total number of teeth .... Temporary...

                                                                 Permanent ....

    Details ....

12. Radiological examination .... On ....

Regions	Findings
1.	1.
2.	2.
3.	3.
4.	4.

Opinion:

Signature ....

Name of Dr. ....

Designation ....

Reg. no. ....

AGE CERTIFICATE

Date ....

1. Dr. ....

Certify as here under ....

A male/female person by name ....

Was sent by ....

With his requisition no. ....

dated .... for determination of age.

The subject was accompanied by ....

He/she was examined by me at .... on .... and the following findings

were observed:

Identification marks:

1. ....

2. ....

(a) Physical ....

(b) Dental ....

Total number of teeth .... Temporary ....

Permanent ....

(c) Radiological 9X-ray photographs taken on ....

no. ....

Opinion:

Based on the above physical, dental and radiological, I am of opinion that the person is
aged above .... and below .... years.

Signature...............................

Name ....

Designation ....

Forwarded to ....

Copy to ....

EXAMINATION OF POTENCY

Requisition received from the .... vide his letter no. .... dated .... through P.C./H.C. no. .... for examination of potency of .... Aged .... years involved in Cr. no. .... of .... Police Station.

1. Name and address of the subject ....

2. Age .... years (as stated by the subject)

3. Occupation ....

4. Accompanied by ....

5. Date, time and place of examination ....

6. Consent ....

7. Marks of identification:

   (i) ....

   (ii) ....

8. Clinical history: Diabetes/drug/addiction/trauma/exposure to venereal disease/ others if any ....

9. History of sexual development: Masturbation/night emissions/homosexual practice/ sexual intercourse ....

10. Physical examination:

   (a) General:

      (i) Height .... cm

      (ii) Weight .... kg

      (iii) Build: Good/moderate/poor

      (iv) Adam's apple ....

      (v) Hair: Pubic/axillary/facial/chest

   (b) Local:

      (i) Penis: Present/absent

         Length .... cm (flaccid state)

         Circumference .... cm (flaccid state)

         Disease (if any) ....

         Deformity (if any) ....

         Injury (if any) ....

         Sensations over glans penis ....

         Foreskin retractable/non-retractable ....

(ii) Scrotum: Pendulous/non-pendulous

Right testis: Present/absent

Left testis: Present/absent

Development of testes: Small/medium/adult size

Sensations ....

Disease, deformity, injury if any ....

Epididymis and cord ....

(c) Systemic examination

(i) CVS ....

(ii) GIS ....

(iii) CNS ....

(iv) RS ....

11. Special examinations (if relevant) ....

12. Opinion:

I. There is nothing to suggest that the above person is incapable of performing the sexual act.

II. The above subject is incapable of performing sexual act because of the following impediments:

Signature ....

Name ....

Designation ....

ALCOHOL CONSUMPTION CERTIFICATE
FORM "A"

Certificate by a registered medical practitioner showing whether a person examined by him hasn't consumed an intoxicant.

Serial no. ....

Name and location of the dispensary or hospital ....

Certified that Shri/Smt/Kumari .... of .... was brought

to this hospital/dispensary by .... (here state name and designation of the

officer) on .... 20 .... at .... AM/PM and was examined

by me on .... 20 .... at .... AM/PM

A clinical examination of the above named person disclosed the following:

    1. Age ....

    2. Weight ....

    3. Breath .... : Smelling/not smelling of alcohol/opium/charas/ganja/bhang

    4. Speech: Incoherent/normal ....

    5. Gait .... : Unsteady/steady

    6. Pupils.. : Dilated/normal

    7. Additional remarks, if any ....

    I find that the above named person has consumed alcohol/opium/charas/ganja/bhang has not consumed any intoxicant. I also find that he was/wasn't under the influence of alcohol.

    (N.B.: Blood from the body of the above named was/wasn't collected by me for chemical examination).

Date .... 20 ....   Signature..

Time .... AM/PM   Name ....

                                    Designation ....

                                    Reg. no. ....

Signature/thumb impression of
the person examined. (Marks of
identification of the person examined in case he refuses to give his
signature or thumb impression.)

ALCOHOL CONSUMPTION CERTIFICATE
FORM "B"

No. ....

From: (Name, designation and address of the registered Medical Practitioner).
To: (Name, designation and address of the Testing Officer).

From	To
Dr.	....
....	....
....	....
....	....

Sir,

I forward herewith, by post/with Shri (name, designation and address of the messenger with whom the phial containing the blood is forwarded for delivery to the Testing Officer) of .... a phial bearing serial no. .... containing .... ml of venous blood collected by me on .... at .... AM/PM from the body of Shri/Smt/Kumari .... of .... who was produced before me for medical examination and/or collection of blood from his/her body by (name and designation of the officer by whom the said person was produced for collection of blood) and request you to test the blood and issue a certificate (in duplicate) regarding the result of the test.

Yours faithfully

Facsimile of the seal or monogram
Used for sealing the phial containing
the blood.

Signature and designation of the
registered medical practitioner.

Reg. no. ....

ALCOHOL EXAMINATION CERTIFICATE
FORM "C"

No. ....

M.L. Case no. ....

From: The Director.

Forensic Science Laboratory

....

....

To

....

....

....

....

Your letter no. .... dated .... forwarding a phial containing blood of Shri/Smt/Kumari .... of .... bearing serial no. .... labelled .... received here on .... by post/with messenger Shri .... of .... sealed/unsealed, seals intact and as per copy sent/seals intact device. .... no copy sent.

Result of the Test of the Blood

The blood contained .... per cent W/V of ethyl alcohol

(W/V .... grams of ethyl alcohol in 100 ml of blood)

Date. ....

Signature and designation of
the Testing Officer.

DEATH CERTIFICATE

The following is the specimen of the certificate of cause of death (prescribed by the Bombay Municipal Corporation, Bombay).

To: The Municipal Commissioner, Bombay

....

I hereby certify that I attended the deceased (full name) ....

aged.................... residing at .... during his last illness and that to the best

of my belief the cause of death at (time) .... on (date) ....

was as stated as below.

Cause of Death

Approximate interval

between onset and death

1. Disease or condition   (a) ....   years   months

    directly leading to death   (due to or as consequence of) days   hours

    Antecedent cause morbid (b) .... years   months

    conditions, if any, giving   (due to or as consequence of) days   hours

    rise to the above cause,

    stating the underlying

    condition last

2. Other significant conditions

    contributing to the death   (c) .... years   months

    but not related to the disease .... days   hours

    or condition causing it. ....

                  ....

                  ....

Signature

Address or rubber stamp of   Designation

the institution   Degree

Registration number of

Medical Officer

MEDICAL CERTIFICATE

This is to certify that Mr .... aged about ....
bearing the following identification marks has been examined by me this day and I find
that he is suffering from ....

....

....

....

He is advised to take rest for a period of ....

Identification marks:

1. ....

2. ....

Place ....   **Signature and registration number**
                                                                        of the doctor

Date ....

PROFORMA FOR EXAMINATION OF SEXUAL OFFENCES
EXAMINATION OF THE VICTIM OF RAPE

Appearances found on the person of a female calling herself ....

aged stated .... years, an inhabitant of .... who was sent with

Letter/memo no. .... dated .... from .... and, injuries

or appearances said to have been caused on .... to be due to alleged rape.

Identification marks:

1. ....

2. ....

The person was seen by the undersigned..

on the .... and the examination was commenced

....................................on the .... when the following were found.

Instructions: (1) Obtain written consent for examination, and collection of specimens of blood, etc. and to supply copies of all medical reports to the police. (2) With a cotton swab, take vaginal material, and make four slides, and allow them to dry for two to three minutes. (3) Keep the same swab in test tube for acid phosphatase determination. (4) Insert a second swab in a test tube containing small amount of normal saline, and examine the fluid for motile spermatozoa. (5) Comb pubic hair and place loose hair in labelled envelope. (6) Cut sample of pubic hair (10 to 12 hairs) and place in labelled envelope. (7) Obtain blood samples (two) for comparison with grouping of the semen and for serological tests. (8) Obtain fingernail scrapings and place in labelled envelopes. (9) Collect any loose hair or fibres found on the person or clothes. (10) Collect dried blood stains and indicate the site from which collected. (11) Collect material from cervix for gonorrhoeal infection.

Preliminary particulars:

1. Name of the individual ....

2. Parent's or guardians's name ....

3. Address ....

4. Occupation ....

5. Caste ....

6. Age as alleged by the victim ....

7. Person accompanying or brought by ....

8. Consent of the individual for examination ....

9. Signature of the individual consenting his/her left thumb impression ....

10. In the case of minor, consent of the guardian and his/her signature or thumb impression

....

11. Name of female attendent/nurse present at the time of examination ....

History:

1. Age ....

2. Gravidity ....

3. Age of menarchy ....

4. Date of last menstrual period ....

5. Whether pregnant ....

6. Most rcent coitus prior to alleged assault ....

   Date .... Time .... Condom used or not ....

7. Patient's statement, whether she is a virgin ....

8. Is she suffering from any illness and taking any medicines? ....

9. History of any venereal disease (past or present) ....

10. History of emotional illness ....

11. Previous vaginal surgical procedure ....

12. Use of alcohol or drugs in 24 hours prior to alleged assault. If so amount and time of

    ingestion ....

13. About sexual offence/rape

    (a) Date and time when the rape was said to have been committed ....

    (b) Place where it was committed ....

    (c) Exact circumstances under which the rape was committed, i.e. whether the parties
        were standing or lying on the ground ....

    (d) Whether she was menstruating at the time ....

    (e) Whether she was sensible during the whole time the offence was committed or
        under the influence of alcohol or other intoxicants ....

    (f) Whether she uttered any cries or was she terrified ....

    (g) Did penis penetrate vulva? ....

    (h) Did assailant wear condom? ....

    (i) Since alleged assault has the victim ....

        1. Douched ....

        2. Bathed ....

        3. Defaecated ....

        4. Urinated ....

Physical examination:

1. (a) BP ....

    (b) Pulse ....

    (c) Temperature ....

    (d) Weight ....

    (e) Height ....

2. General appearance ....

3. Emotional status ....

4. Clothing ....

    (a) Blood stains ....

    (b) Seminal stains ....

    (c) Other discharge ....

    (d) Foreign material ....

    (e) Hair ....

    (f) Tears ....

5. Body surface (exact anatomical position)

    (a) Scratches ....

    (b) Bruises ....

    (c) Laceration ....

6. Mouth ....

7. Fingernails ....

8. Genitals: ....

    (a) Pubic hair, length, matted or not ....

    (b) Vulva ....

    (c) Hymen ....

    (d) Vagina ....

    (e) Fourchette ....

    (f) Perineum ....

    (g) Cervix ....

9. Is venereal disease present? ....

10. Smears taken from vagina, cervix, etc.:

    (a) Number ....

    (b) Gram's stain ....

    (c) Stain for spermatozoa ....

11. Any other findings ....

12. Material sent to the laboratory ....

13. Results of laboratory procedures:

    (a) Pregnancy test ....

    (b) Serology ....

    (c) Gonorrhoeal infection ....

    (d) Spermatozoa ....

    (e) Acid phosphatase ....

    (f) Grouping of blood and semen ....

    (g) Hair examination ....

Collection of evidence:

1. Blood in two tubes for serology and grouping ....

2. Fingernail scrapings ....

3. Loose pubic hair ....

4. Cut pubic hair ....

5. Hair, fibres and blood stains on body and clothing ....

6. Vaginal material for live spermatozoa ....

7. Four slides from vaginal material ....

8. Cervical material for gonorrhoea ....

9. Vaginal secretion on two cotton swabs:

    (a) Semen typing ....

    (b) Acid phosphatase ....

       Opinion ....

Station ....   Signature ....

Date ....   Name ....

                                                      Designation ....

                                                      Reg. no. ....

SEXUAL ASSAULT EXAMINATION OF MALE PATIENTS

Instructions: (1) Obtain written consent for examination and collection of specimens of blood, etc., and to supply copies of all medical reports to the police. (2) With a cotton swab, wipe the perianal area and put in a test tube for acid phosphatase determination. (3) Insert a cotton swab into the anal canal without touching the perianal area. Prepare two slides and dry for two to three minutes. (4) Place the same swab in a tube containing normal saline for acid phosphatase determination. (5) Collect blood for comparison with semen type. (6) In buccal coitus, swab the mouth of the patient, especially the gums and pharynx with a cotton swab, smear on a slide and dry. (7) Place the same cotton swab in a tube containing normal saline for acid phosphatase. (8) In the case of accused in a rape case, swab from coronal sulcus, prepuce, penile shaft for blood comparison with the victim's blood. (9) Urethral discharge for gonococcal infection. (10) Comb pubic hair and place loose hair in an envelope. (11) Obtain fingernail scrapings and place in labelled envelope.

Preliminary particulars: As in the case of the victim ....

Brief description of assault ....

Date of assault ....

Time ....

Physical examination:

Name .... Age ....

   1. (a) BP ....

      (b) Pulse ....

      (c) Temperature ....

      (d) Weight ....

      (e) Height ....

   2. General appearance and emotional status ....

   3. Clothing ....

      (a) Blood stains ....

      (b) Seminal stains ....

      (c) Foreign material ....

      (d) Hairs ....

      (e) Tears ....

   4. Injuries found on body ....

   5. Genitals:

      (a) Pubic hair: Length, matted or not ....

      (b) Penis:

         Length when flaccid .... when erect ....

         Smegma ....

Prepuce ....

Circumcised or not ....

Frenum ....

6. Anal examination ....

7. During alleged assault ....

   Did penis penetrate rectum? ....

   Did assailant had orgasm? ....

   Did assailant wear condom? ....

8. Since alleged assault:

   Bathed ....

   Urinated ....

   Defaecated ....

Collection of evidence:

1. Blood in two tubes for serology and grouping and for drug screening: ....
   ....

2. Perianal swab ....

3. Rectal swab ....

4. Oral swab ....

5. Loose pubic hair ....

6. Hair, fibres and blood stains on body and clothing ....

7. Urethral discharge for gonorrhoea ....

8. Fingernail scrapings ....

9. Suspected dried seminal stains on the skin or clothing ....

Opinion: ....

Station ....   Signature ....

Date ....   Name ....

                                                          Designation ....

                                                          Reg. no. ....

FORMAT OF ACCIDENT REGISTER

S. no. .... Date and Time ....

Name .... Sex .... Age ....

Occupation .... Address ....

....

Identification marks:

    1. ....

    2. ....

By whom brought ....

Police informed or not ....

Dying declaration required or not ....

If so, state action taken ....

History and alleged cause of injury ....

Nature of injury (simple or grievous) ....

Treatment ....

Investigation results, if any ....

X-ray no. .... Dated ....

Date of admission as inpatient and no. ....

Date of discharge ....

Condition on discharge ....

Opinion ....

Signature of Medical Officer

PROFORMAS AND CERTIFICATES
CONSENT TO SURGERY AND ANAESTHESIA

I authorise the performance upon myself or Shri/Smt .... the following operation .... to be performed by or under the direction of Dr. .... under administration of such anaesthetics as may be considered necessary or advisable by the physician responsible for this service with the exception of (general, "none", spinal anaesthesia, etc.) ....

I consent to the performance of operations and procedures in addition to or different from those now contemplated, whether or not arising from presently unforeseen conditions. Which the above named doctor or his assistants may consider necessary or advisable in the course of the operation.

For the purpose of advancing medical education, I consent to the admittance of observers to the operating room and allow for taking photographs and video-recording, provided my identity is not revealed.

The nature and purpose of the operation, possible alternative methods of treatment, the risks involved, and the possibility of complications have been fully explained to me in my own language. No guarantee or assurance has been given by anyone as to the results that may be obtained.

(Cross out any paragraphs above which do not apply)

Place ....   Date ....

Witness: 1. ....

2. ....

Signature (or left thumb impression)
(patient or person authorised to consent for patient)

N.B: It is advisable to write the above form in patient's mother tongue (if he does not know English).

PROFORMA FOR EXHUMATION

Requisition from .... Magistrate, of .... vide his

Letter no. .... dated ....

Letter no. .... dated .... from .... of police of PS ....

Time of departure ....

Time of arrival at the place of burial ....

Persons identifying the place of burial ....

Description of the burial place and grave ....

Location .... Length .... Breadth.............................

Height .... Covered with ....

Stone inscription, if any ....

Inquest conducted by ....

Grave identified by ....

Officers present at the time of exhumation ....

Condition of soil of buried site and surrounding area ....

Grave digging started at ....

Depth from ground level at which the body was seen ....

Position of the body in the grave ....

Description of coffin, if any ....

Body removed from the grave at ....

Description of clothes ....

Persons identifying the clothes ....

Body identified, by 1. .... 2. .... 3. ....

P.M. no. .... dated ....

P.M. commenced at .... P.M. concluded at ....

Instructions: (1) Describe clothing. (2) Determine sex, age and stature. (3) Describe identifying marks, if any. (4) Conduct autopsy in the usual manner and note all the findings. (5) Preserve viscera for chemical analysis. (6) Collect samples of earth (about half kg) from above, below, and from each side of the body. (7) Collect any fluid or debris in the coffin. (8) If the body is reduced to skeleton, collect all the bones and send them to the expert in sealed and labelled packets. (9) Handover the body to the concerned police after autopsy.

Approximate time of death ....

Opinion as to the cause of death ....

Place ....   Signature ....

Date ....   Designation ....

POSTMORTEM CERTIFICATE (SHORT OPINION)

P.M. no. .... Dated ....

Regarding the body of male/female named .... aged ....

About .... years, received on .... at .... hours

from the .... of police, ... P.S. with his

letter no. .... and incharge of P.C. no. ....

The dead body was first seen by the undersigned on .... at .... (hours)

and was identified by P.C. no. .... Postmortem commenced at

....

Opinion as to the cause of death: ....

Place ....

Signature ....

Date ....

Designation ....

REPORT OF A POSTMORTEM EXAMINATION

P.M./EX. OP. No ....

On the dead body of ....

Village/city ....

Taluka ....

District ....

By ....

I. GENERAL PARTICULARS

1. (a) By whom was the corpse sent ....

    (b) Name of place from which sent ....

    (c) Distance of place from which sent ....

2. By whom was the corpse brought ....

3. By whom identified ....

4. (a) The minute, hour and date of receipt ....

    (b) The minute, hour and date of beginning ....

       of postmortem examination.

    (c) The minute, hour and date of ending ....

       postmortem examination.

5. Substance of accompanying report from ....

   Police Officer or Magistrate, together with ....

   the date of death, if known, supposed cause ....
   of death or reason for examination.

6. If not examined at dispensary or hospital: ....

    (a) Name of place where examined. ....

    (b) Distance from dispensary or hospital...

    (c) Reason why the body was not sent to ....

       the dispensary or hospital. ....

II. EXTERNAL EXAMINATIONS

7. Sex, apparent age, race or caste description ....

   of clothes and ornaments on the body. ....

8. Condition of the clothes:

   Whether wet with water, stained with blood ....

   or soiled with vomit or faecal matter. ....

9. Special marks on the skin such as scars, ...
tattooing, etc. any malformation, peculiarities ....
or other marks of identification, state of teeth. ....
In newly born infants, the length and (if ....
possible) the weight of the body to be ....
recorded together with the state of hair, nails
and umbilical cord, its size and condition.

10. Condition of body: ....
Whether well-nourished, thin or emaciated, ...
Warm or cold'.

11. Rigor mortis: ....
Well-marked or slight or absent, whether ....
present in the whole body or part only. ....

12. Extent and signs of decomposition, presence
of postmortem lividity on buttocks, loin, ...
back and thighs or any other part, whether ....
bullae present, the nature of their contained ....
fluid, condition of the cuticle.

13. Features whether natural or swollen state
of eyes, position of tongue, nature of fluid ....
(if any) oozing from mouth, nostrils or ears. ....

14. Condition of skin-marks of blood, etc. in ....
suspected drowning the presence or absence ....
of cutis anserina to be noted.

15. Injuries to external genitals, indication of ....
purging.

16. Position of limbs, especially of arms and of ....
fingers in suspected drowning the presence ....
or absence of sand or earth within the nails ....
or on the skin or hands and feet.

17. Surface wounds and injuries:
(a) Their nature, position, dimensions, ...
directions and associated haemorrhage, ...
foreign body (if any to be accurately ....
stated their probable age and causes to be noted).

(b) If bruises be present, what is the ....

condition of the subcutaneous tissues? ....

N.B.: When injuries are numerous and cannot be mentioned within the space available they should be mentioned on a separate paper which should be signed.

18. Other injuries discovered by external ....

examination or palpation, as fractures, etc. ....

19. Can you say definitely that the injuries ....

shown against serial no.(17), (18), (20), ...

(21), (22), (23), and (24) are antemortem ....

injuries?

III. INTERNAL EXAMINATION

20. Cranial cavity ....

Head ....

(a) Injuries under the scalp, their nature. ....

(b) Skull vault and base—describe fractures

their sites, dimensions, directions, etc. ....

(c) Brain: The appearance of its coverings,

size, weight and general condition of ....

the organ itself and abnormality found ....

in its examination to be carefully noted. ....

21. Neck ....

22. Thoracic cavity ....

Thorax ....

(a) Walls, ribs, cartilages ....

(b) Pleura ....

(c) Larynx, trachea and bronchi ....

(d) Right lung ....

(e) Left lung ....

(f) Pericardium ....

(g) Heart with weight ....

(h) Additional remarks ....

23. Abdominal cavity:

(a) Abdomen ....

(b) Walls ....

(c) Peritoneum ....

(d) Buccal cavity ....

(e) Oesophagus ....

(f) Stomach and its contents ....

(g) Small intestine and its contents ....

(h) Large intestine and its contents ....

(i) Liver and gallbladder ....

(j) Pancreas ....

(k) Spleen ....

(l) Kidneys ....

(m) Suprarenals ....

(n) Bladder ....

(o) Organs of generation ....

(p) Additional remarks ....

VISCERA PRESERVED: YES OR NO

1. Stomach and one foot of small intestine and their contents ....

2. Pieces of liver and half of each kidney ....

3. Sample of blood ....

4. Sample of preservative ....

(The note should be made regarding the chemical analysis and examination of preserved viscera, if not required, it should be destroyed).

24. Spine and spinal cord:

....

....

....

....

....

....

....

....

....

....

Opinion as to cause or probable cause of death:

....

....

....

....

....

....

....

....

Dated ....   Signature ....

                                         Name ....

                                         Designation ....

                                         ....

CHAPTER 35

Sections of Law

RELEVANT SECTIONS OF INDIAN PENAL CODE

Section 40 of IPC—Offence: The word offence denotes a thing that is made punishable by this code.

Section 44 of IPC—Injury: It means any harm whatever illegally caused to a person in body, mind, reputation and property.

Section 51 of IPC—Oath: Any declaration required or authorized by law to be made before a public servant or to be used for the purpose of proof whether in court of justice or not.

Section 82 of IPC—Act of a child under seven years of age: Nothing is an offence which is done by a child under seven years of age.

Section 83 of IPC—Act of a child above seven and under twelve years of immature understanding: Nothing is an offence which is done by a child of above seven and below twelve years, who has not attained sufficient maturity to understand the nature and consequences of his conduct on that occasion.

Section 84 of IPC—Act of a person of an unsound mind: Nothing is an offence which is done by a person, who at the time of doing it, by reason of unsoundness of mind, is incapable of under standing the nature of the act or that he is doing what is either wrong or contrary to law.

Section 87 of IPC—Act not intended or not known to be likely to cause death or grievous hurt, done by consent: Nothing, which is not intended to cause death/ grievous hurt, is an offence by reason of any harm which it may cause to any person above 18 years of age, who has given consent, whether express or implied, to suffer that harm or by reason of any harm which it may be known by the doer to be likely to cause to any such person who has consented to take the risk to that harm.

Section 88 of IPC—Act not intended to cause death, done with consent in good faith for persons benefit: Nothing, which is not intended to cause death, is an offence by reason of any harm which it may cause to any person for whose benefit it is done in good faith, who has given consent whether express or implied, to suffer that harm or to take the risk of that harm.

Section 89 of IPC—Act done in good faith for benefit of a child or insane person by or by consent of guardian: Nothing which is done in good faith for the benefit of person under twelve years of age or unsound mind, by or by consent of the guardian or any other person in lawful incharge of that person, is an offence by reason of any harm which it may cause or be known by the doer to be likely to cause to that person.

Section 92 of IPC—Act done in good faith for benefit of a person, without his consent: Nothing is an offence by reason of any harm which it may cause to a person for whose benefit it is done in good faith, even without consent, if circumstances are such that it is impossible for person to give consent or it is not possible to obtain consent in time for the thing to be done with benefit.

Section 93 of IPC—Communication made in good faith: No communication made in good faith is an offence by reason of any harm to the person to whom it is made, if it is made for the benefit of that person.

Section 193 of IPC—Punishment for giving false evidence: Whoever, intentionally gives false evidence in any stage of judicial proceedings or fabricates false evidence for the purpose of using it in a judicial proceeding, shall be punished with imprisonment of either term up to seven years and shall also be liable to fine.

Section 197 of IPC—Issuing on signing false certificate: Whoever issues or signs any certificate required by law to be given or signed. Knowing or believing that such certificate is false in any natural point, shall be punished same as for giving false evidence (imprisonment up to seven years and fine).

Section 201 of IPC—Causing disappearance of evidence of offence or giving false evidence to screen the offender:

- *Firstly:* If offence is punishable with death, the punishment is imprisonment of either description for up to **seven years** and also fine.
- *Secondly:* If offence is punishable by life imprisonment, then punishment is imprisonment of either description **up to three years** and also fine.
- *Thirdly:* If offence is punishable with **less than ten years** imprisonment, then punishment is **one-fourth of the imprisonment** for that particular offence.

Section 202 of IPC—Intentional omission to give information of offence by person bound to inform: Shall be punished with imprisonment of either description for a term which may extend up to six months or fine or both.

Section 299 of IPC—Culpable homicide: Whoever causes death by doing an act with the intention of causing death or with the intention of causing such bodily injury as is **likely to cause death** or with the knowledge that he is likely by such act to cause death, commits the offence of culpable homicide.

Section 300 of IPC—Murder

- *Firstly:* A culpable homicide is murder, if the act by which the death is caused is done with the intention of causing death.
- *Secondly:* If it is done with intention by causing such bodily injury as the offender knows to be likely to cause death.
- *Thirdly:* If it is done with the intention of causing bodily injury **which is sufficient in the ordinary course of** nature to cause death.
- *Fourthly:* If the person committing the **act knows it is so immediately dangerous,** that it must **in all probability cause death** or such bodily injury as in likely to cause death and commits such act **without any excuse**.

Exceptions: Culpable homicide is not murder when, if the act by which death is caused is done:

- *Firstly:* Under grave and sudden provocation.
- *Secondly:* In good faith of right of private defence of person or property.
- *Thirdly:* For advancement of public justice.
- *Fourthly:* Without premeditation.
- *Fifthly:* When the person above the age of 18 years takes the risk of death with his own consent.

Section 301 of IPC—Culpable homicide by causing death of person other than person whose death was intended: The culpable homicide committed by the offender is of the description of which it would have been, if he had caused the death of person whose death he intended or knew himself to be likely to cause.

Section 302 of IPC—Punishment for murder: Whoever commits murder shall be punished with death or imprisonment for life and also shall be liable to fine.

Section 303 of IPC—Punishment for murder by a life convict: Whoever, being under sentence of imprisonment for life, commits murder shall be punished with death.

Section 304 of IPC—Punishment for culpable homicide not amounting to murder: Shall be punished with imprisonment for life or imprisonment of either description for a term which may extend up to ten years and shall also be liable to fine.

Section 304A of IPC—Causing death by negligence: Whoever causes the death of any person by doing any rash or negligent act not amounting to culpable homicide, shall be punished with imprisonment of either description for a term which may extend to two years or with fine or both.

Section 304B of IPC—Dowry death and its punishment: Where the death of a woman in caused by any burns/bodily injury or occurs otherwise than normal circumstances within **seven years of her marriage** and it is shown that before death she was subjected to cruelty or harassment by her husband or by any relative of her husband for or **inconnection with any demand or dowry.** Such death shall be deemed as dowry death and such husband or relative of that husband shall be deemed to have caused her death. Punishment— Whoever commits dowry death shall be punished with imprisonment for a term which **shall not be less than seven years** but which may extend to **imprisonment for life.**

Section 305 of IPC—Abetment of suicide of a child or insane person: If any person below eighteen years of age, insane delirious person, idiot or intoxicated person commits suicide, whoever abets the commission of such suicide, shall be punished with death or imprisonment for life or imprisonment for a term not exceeding ten years and shall also be liable for fine.

Section 306 of IPC—Abetment of suicide: If any person commits suicide, whoever abets the commission of such suicide shall be punished with imprisonment of either description for a term which may extend up to ten years and shall also be liable for fine.

Section 307 of IPC—Attempt to murder: If hurt is caused to any person by an act with such intention or knowledge and under such circumstances that, if he by that act caused death, the offender shall be liable either to imprisonment for up to ten years and shall also be liable for fine.

Section 308 of IPC—Attempt to murder by life convicts: When any person offending under this section if under sentence of imprisonment for life, he may, if hurt is caused, be punished with death.

Section 309 of IPC—Attempt to commit suicide: Whoever attempt to commit suicide and does any act towards the commission of such offence, shall be punished with simple imprisonment for a term which may extend to one year or with fine or both. It is not a crime now after recent amendment of mental health act.

Section 312 of IPC—Voluntarily causing miscarriage (even with consent):

- *Firstly*: Whoever voluntarily caused miscarriage is liable for imprisonment up to three years and/or fine.
- *Secondly*: If the woman was quick with child, the imprisonment may extend up to seven years (both are punishable).

Section 313 of IPC—Voluntarily causing miscarriage without woman's consent: Whether the woman was quick with child or not, the punishment is imprisonment for life or with imprisonment of either description for a term which may extend to ten years and shall also be liable to fine.

Section 314 of IPC: If a pregnant woman dies from an act intended to cause miscarriage, the offender is liable to be punished with imprisonment up to ten years and also fine.

Section 315 of IPC: Any person doing an act intended to prevent the child from being born alive or to cause to die after its birth is liable to be punished with imprisonment up to ten years or with fine or both.

Section 316 of IPC: Causing death of an unborn quick child by an act amounting to culpable homicide, shall be punished with imprisonment of either description for a term which may extend to ten years and shall also be liable to fine.

Section 317 of IPC: Exposure and abandonment of a child **under twelve year of age** by parents or person having care of it, shall be punished with imprisonment of either description for a term which may extend to seven years or fine or both.

Section 318 of IPC: Concealment of birth by secret disposal of dead body shall be punished with imprisonment of either description for a term which may extend to **two years or fine or both.**

Section 319 of IPC—Hurt: Whoever causes **bodily pain, disease** or **infirmity** to any person is said to have caused **hurt.**

Section 320 of IPC—Grievous hurt: The following constitutes grievous hurt.

- *Firstly*: Emasculation
  – Amputation of penis.
  – Cutting of testicles, crushing of testicles
  – Injury to lumbar spine.
- *Secondly*: Permanent privation of sight of either eys.
- *Thirdly*: Permanent privation of hearing of either ear.
- *Fourthly*: Privation of any member or joint.
- *Fifthly*: Destruction or permanent impairing of the powers of any members or joint.
- *Sixthly*: Permanent disfiguration of head or face.
- *Seventhly*: Fracture or dislocation of a bone or tooth.
- *Eighthly*: Any hurt which endangers life or which causes the sufferer during the span of 20 days in severe bodily pain or unable to follow his ordinary pursuits.

Section 323 of IPC: Punishment for voluntarily causing hurt shall be liable for imprisonment of either description for a term which may extend up to one year or with fine up to Rs. 1000 or both.

Section 324 of IPC: Any instrument used for shooting stabbing or cutting or any instrument which, used as a weapon of offence, is likely to cause death or by means of fire or any heated substance or by any means of any poison or any corrosive substance or by means of any explosive substance or by means of any substance which is deleterious to the animal is called dangerous weapon or means. Voluntarily causing hurt by dangerous weapons or means shall be punished with imprisonment of either description for a term which may extend to three years or fine or both.

Section 325 of IPC: Punishment for voluntarily causing grievous hurt shall be punished with imprisonment of either description for a term which may extend to seven years and also fine.

Section 326 of IPC: Whoever voluntarily causes grievous hurt by dangerous weapons or means shall be punished with imprisonment for life or with imprisonment of either description which may extend up to ten years and also fine.

Section 351 of IPC: Every attack or threat or attempt to apply force on the person of another in a hostile manner constitutes assault. 'Battery' means execution of an assault.

Section 359 of IPC—Kidnapping: Kidnapping is of two kinds:

1. From India.
2. From lawful guardianship.

Section 360 of IPC—Kidnapping from India: Whoever conveys any person beyond the limits of India, without his/her consent or of some person legally authorized to consent on behalf of that person, is said to kidnap that person from India.

Section 361 of IPC—Kidnapping from lawful guardianship: Whoever takes or entices any minor under 16 years of age, if male or under 18 years of age, if female or any person of unsound mind out of the keeping of the lawful guardian of such minor or person of unsound mind, without the consent of such guardian, is said to kidnap such minor or person from, lawful guardianship.

Section 362 of IPC—Abduction: Whoever by force compels or by any deceitful means induces, any person to go from any place, is said to abduct that person.

Section 363 of IPC: Punishment for kidnapping comprises imprisonment of either description for a term which may extend to seven years and shall also be liable to fine.

Section 377 of IPC—Unnatural offences: Whoever voluntarily has anal intercourse against the order of nature with any man, woman or animal shall be punished with imprisonment for life, imprisonment of either description up to ten years and also fine.

Section 497 of IPC—Defines and punishes adultery: Sexual intercourse with a woman known to be wife of another man, without consent or connivance of that man, shall amount to offence of adultery and not rape, shall be punished with imprisonment of either description up to five years or fine or both (the wife is not punishable as an abettor).

Section 498A of IPC: Whoever, being husband or relative of the husband of a woman subjects such woman to cruelty shall be punished with imprisonment for a term up to three years and also fine.

RELEVANT SECTIONS OF INDIAN EVIDENCE ACT

Section 107 of IEA—Burden of proving death of a person to have been alive within 30 years: When the question is whether a man is alive or dead and it is shown that he was alive within 30 years, the burden of proving that he is dead is on the person who affirms it.

Section 108 of IEA—Burden of proving that person is alive who has not been heard for seven years: Provided that when the question is whether a man is alive/dead and it diprived that he has not been heard of since last seven years by those who would have naturally heard him, if he had been alive, the burden of proving that he is alive is shifted to the person who affirms it.

Section 141 of IEA—Leading question: Any question suggesting the answer which the person putting it wishes or expects to receive is called a leading question.

RELEVANT SECTIONS OF CRIMINAL PROCEDURE CODE

Section 53 of CrPC—Examination of the accused by medical practitioners at the request of police officer: When a person is arrested on a charge of committing an offence of such a nature and alleged to have been committed under such circumstances that there are reasonable grounds for believing that examination of such a person will afford evidence as to the commission of an offence, it shall be lawful for a registered medical practitioner, acting at the request of a police officer not below the rank of a subinspector and for any person acting in good faith in his aid and under his direction, to make such an examination of the person arrested as is reasonably necessary in order to ascertain the facts which may afford such evidence and to use such force as is reasonably necessary for that purpose.

Section 174 of CrPC—Police to inquire and report: When any officer in-charge of a police station not below rank of PSI, receives information that a person has died in unnatural death, sudden death or in any manner raising suspicion of foul play, he shall immediately inform nearest executive magistrate empowered to hold inquest and shall proceed to the site where the dead body is and in the presence of two respectable inhabitants of neighbourhood, shall investigate and draw a report of apparent cause of death, which shall be signed by investigating officer and the other two persons and forwarded in sealed cover to the magistrate. If the investigating officer feels so, he can direct the body for postmortem examination by nearest civil surgeon or any other qualified man appointed for such postmortems.

Section 176 of CrPC—Inquiry by magistrate into cause of death: When any person dies in police custody, police firing, in jails and in cases of dowry deaths, the nearest magistrate empowered may hold an inquiry into cause of death or in any other case in addition to police inquest. Magistrate is also empowered for disinterment and examination of a dead body.

APPENDIX

AGE

From Ossification Activity of the Bones
Areas X-rayed to Determine Age

(Contributed by—Dr. I. Mohan Prasad, Asst. Professor, Department of Forensic Medicine, NMC, Nellore.)

- Wrist and hand—children
- Elbow, shoulder, pelvis and knee—adult
- Skull, vertebrae and sternum—old person

AT BIRTH

- Lower end of femur—½ cm in diameter
- Talus—7th month (IU)
- Calcaneum—5th month (IU)
- Cuboid—upper end of tibia and head of humerus

WRIST

- Number of carpal bone indicate age in years between 2 and 6 years
- Pisiform ossifies—10–12 years

Ossification of Carpal Bones

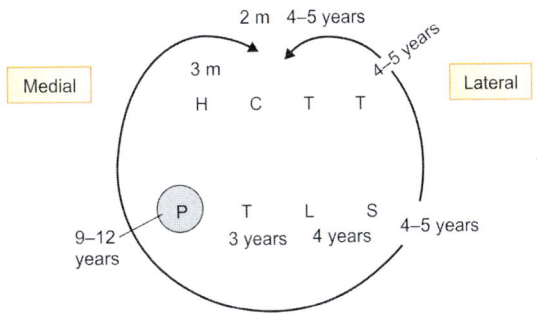

Hand X-ray—3 months age
One carpal bone is ossified.

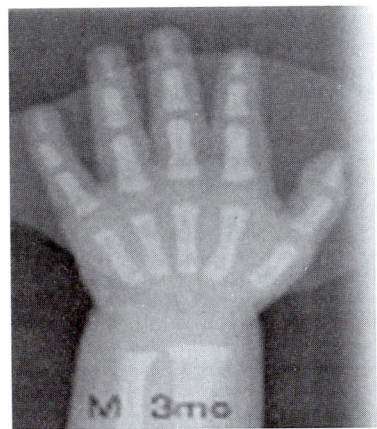

Hand X-ray—3 years
Three carpal bones are ossified.

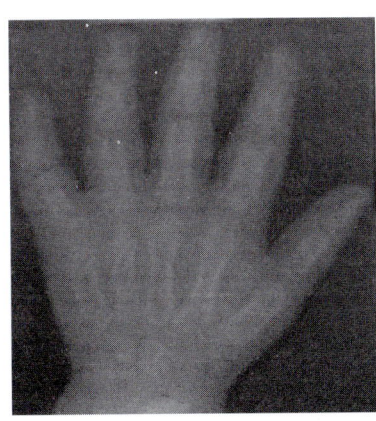

Hand X-ray—6 years
Six carpal bones are ossified.
Seven carpal bones are seen up to the age
of 9 years.

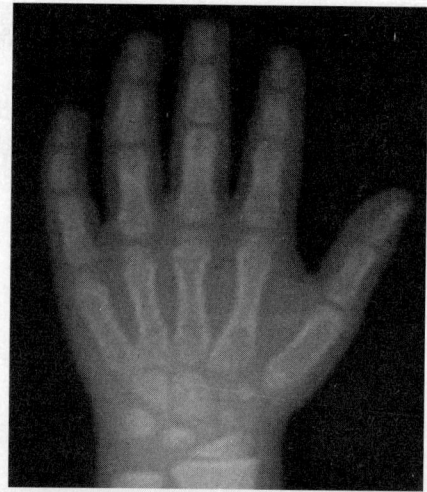

Hand X-ray—11 years
Appearance of pisiform is important.
A dense rim is fully developed around the
primary centre at the age of 11–12 years.

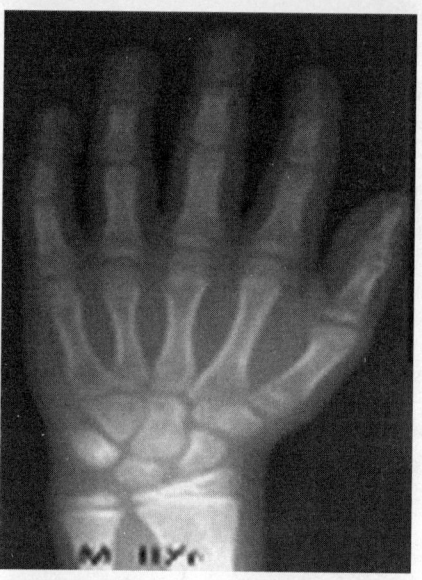

Elbow joint X-ray—1 year
Appear in medial epicondyle of humerus:
4 years (F); 6 years (M)

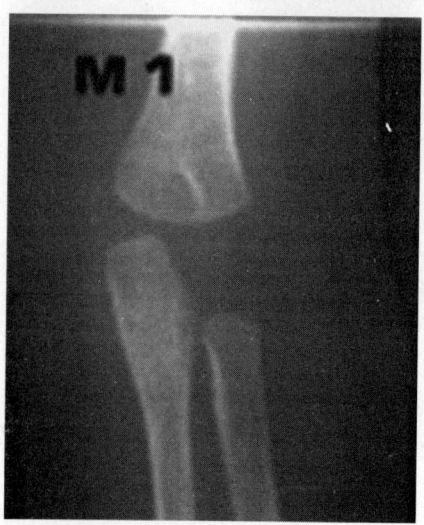

Appear in olecranon: **8–10 years**

Lateral epicondyle of humerus united with trochlea and capitulum: **13–14 years**

All epiphyses at elbow (except medial epicondyle) join respective shaft: **13–14 years** (F); **16–18 years** (M)

Elbow joint X-ray—9 years

Primary centre for lateral epicondyle appears at 9–12 years.

All the centres are open at the age of 11–12 years.

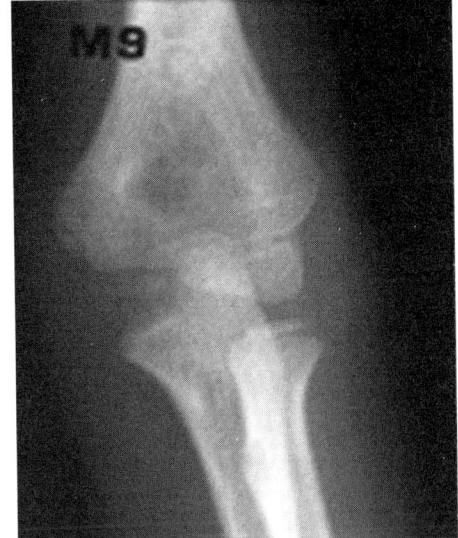

Elbow joint X-ray—14 years

Fusion occurs from 13 years

- **Starts from:**
  - Lateral epicondyle: 13 years
  - Radius: 14 years
  - Olecranon process: 14 years
  - Medial epicondyle: 15 years
  - Complete ossification occurs at the age of 16 years.

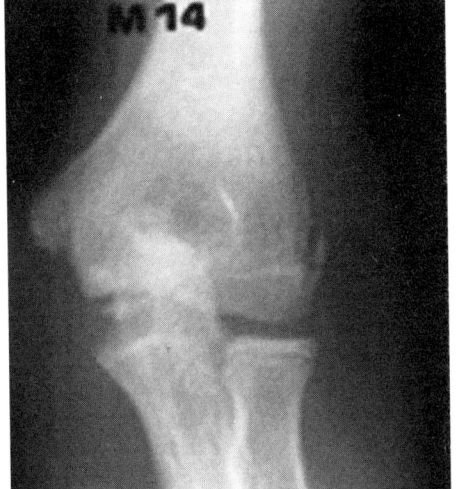

Wrist joint X-ray
Adult

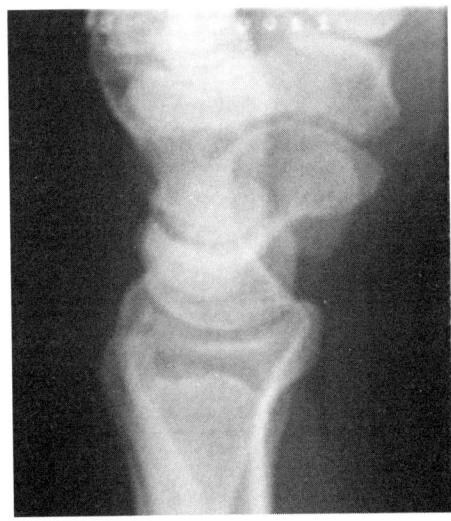

Wrist joint X-ray—15 years

Both distal ends of radius and ulna are open at the age of 15 years.

Fusion starts after 15 years.

Complete fusion occurs at 17 years.

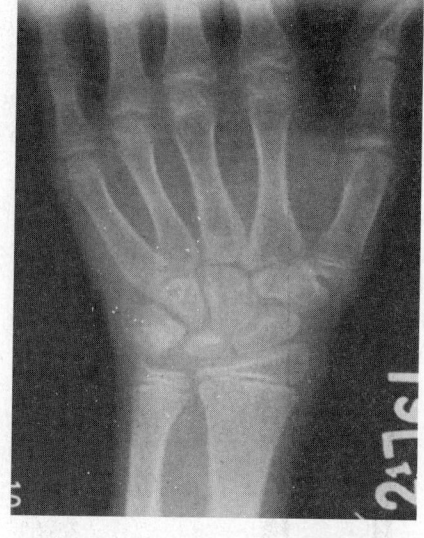

Wrist joint X-ray—fusion

Female	*Male*
Radius 16–16½	17
Ulna 17	17½–18

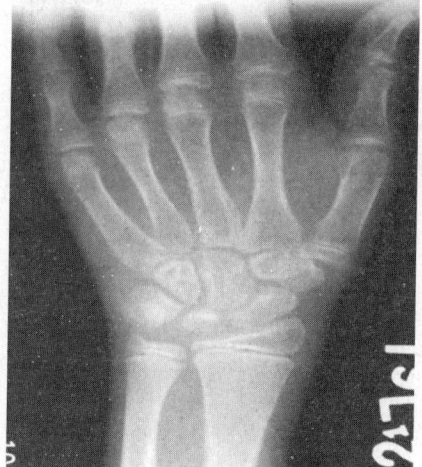

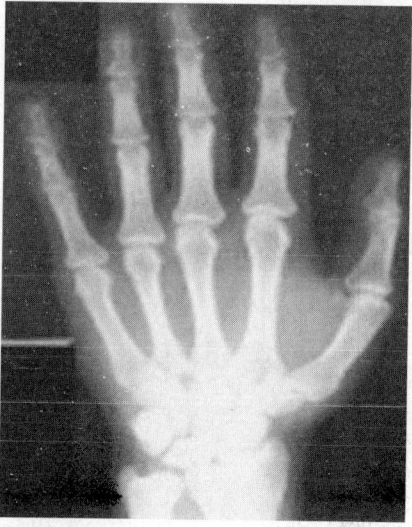

By 15–16 Years
- Epiphyses of calcaneum join the bone.
- Triradiate cartilage of acetabulum fused.
- Olecranon united to ulna, corocoid process to scapula.

By 16–18 Years
- All epiphyses at elbow (except medial epicondyle), head of femur and lower end of tibia—shaft.

By 18–20 Years
- All epiphyses at wrist, knee, crest of ilium, lateral end of clavicle—united.

By 22 Years
- The inner (secondary) epiphyses of clavicle fused.

X-ray Clavicle—Sternal End
Entire epiphysis is developed at 19 years
Complete fusion occurs:

Female	Male
20–21 years	22 years

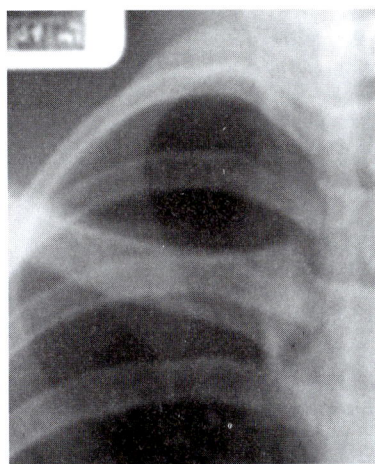

Age Determination in Adults Over 25 Years
After the age of 25 years, age estimation is uncertain.
- It is difficult after full, permanent eruption + fusion of all centres of ossification of long bones.
- The ossification of cartilage in the hyoid
- Fusion of greater horns of the hyoid to the body

- Manubrium + xyphisternum with body of the sternum
- Lipping of vertebrae

All occur between 40 and 60 years. May be suggestive of advancing age.

Symphyseal Surface in Estimation of Age
- **Below 20 years:** Symphyseal surfaces show even appearance
- **Between 20 and 30 years:** Looks markedly ridged
- **Between 25 and 35 years:** The billowing disappears
- **Between 35 and 45 years:** Articular surfaces smooth, oval
- **Between 45 and 50 years:** Narrow beaded rims
- **Above 50 years:** Shows erosion with breaking down of ventral margins.

Sternum

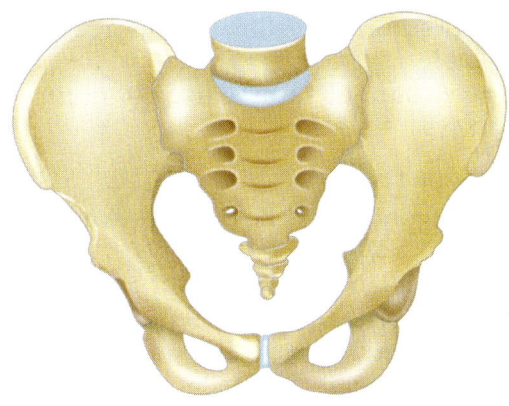

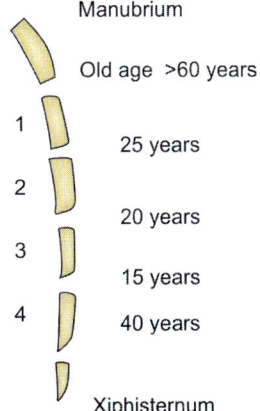

Manubrium
Old age >60 years
1
25 years
2
20 years
3
15 years
4
40 years
Xiphisternum

X-ray Sternum

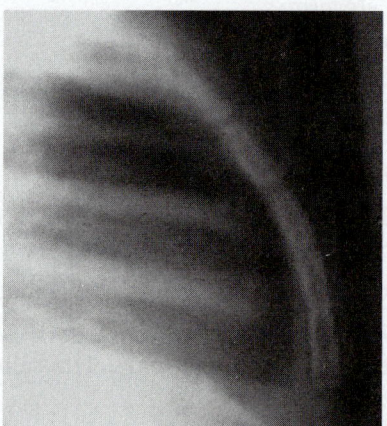

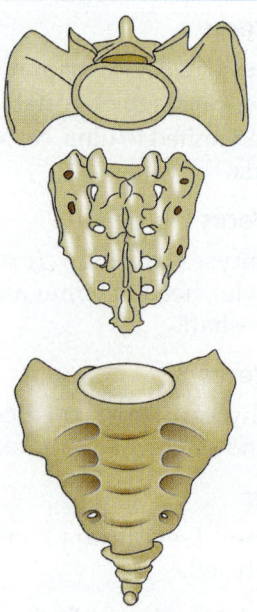

Sacrum

- Five sacral vertebrae remain separated by cartilage until puberty.
- **Onset of puberty:** Ossification of inter-vertebral disc starts from below upward
- **Fusion of sacral segment:** 20–25 years completed.

Skull suture in estimation of age is not reliable

The closure of sutures usually occurs as follows.

Fontanelle

- Posterior fontanelle closes between birth and 1.5 months
- Anterior fontanelle closes by the 2nd year.
- Posterolateral fontanelle closes within short period after birth.
- Anterolateral fontanelle closes within 6 months after birth.
- **Metopic suture:** 2–8 years between frontal bones
- **Basiocciput fuses with basisphenoid:**
  - 18–20 years (F)
  - 20–22 years (M)

Closure of Sutures

- Begins on the inner aspect by 5–10 years earlier than outer aspect.
- Early in males
- In order—sagittal, lambdoid, coronal.
  - a. Posterior one-third sagittal suture: 30–40 years
  - b. Anterior one-third sagittal + lower half of coronal: 40–50 years
  - c. Middle one-third sagittal + upper half of coronal: 50–60 years
  - d. Lambdoid suture: Start closure 25–30 years

Maximum closure—55 years

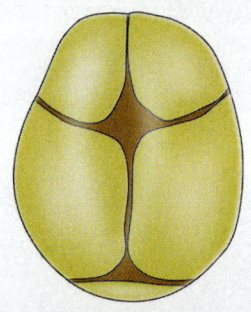

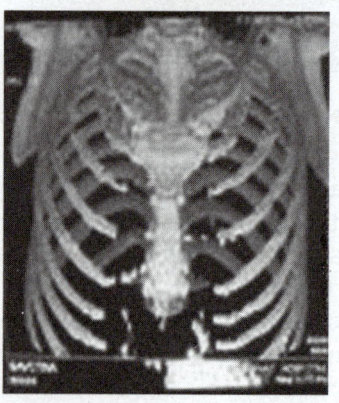

Fingerprints (Galton's Method—Dactylography)

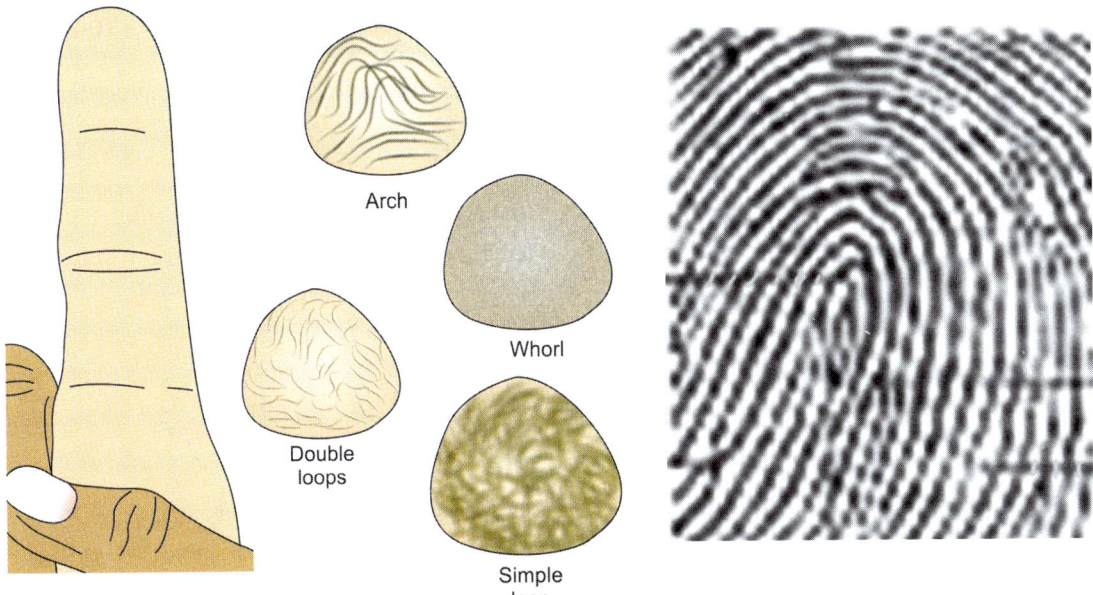

Arch

Whorl

Double loops

Simple loop

Principle

1. Skin of the balls of finger and thumb, part of palm and sole of feet are covered with ridges and grooves having characteristic patterns.
2. Each individual has its own constant pattern from birth till death.

Peculiarities of this Method (Advantages)

1. It is considered as the surest sign of identification because prints are present since birth and remain permanent till death until hands are totally destroyed.
2. Individualized character
3. No special instrument/trained person is required for taking prints.
4. Records can be kept easily for comparison at any time.
5. The print can be faxed from one place to another throughout the world.
6. The examiner needs simple training, simple (magnifying lens) for their recognition, classification and matching.
7. Computerization of the record is easy.

Classification

Main patterns

1. Arch	Less common
2. Loop	Most common open to ulnar side; open to radial side
3. Whorl	Less than loop
4. Composite	Less common

- Each ridge is further classified into:
  – Core
  – Island
  – Delta

There are two methods of taking finger impressions:

1. Plain
2. Rolled

PLAIN

It is obtained by lightly pressing the inked surface of finger or thumb upon plain paper without any turning movement.

Rolled impression: It is obtained by first inking the bulb surface of finger or thumb between the nail boundaries and then rolling the finger or thumb on the paper from one side to the other.

As rolled impression covers a larger area, it is preferred. While taking thumb impression, left thumb in males and 'right thumb in females are use.

Various Patterns Seen in Fingerprints

1. Arches
2. Loops
3. Whorls
4. Composite or compound

Arches: In arches, the ridges run from one side to the other without making back turn.

Loops or pocket formation: Here ridges either sway towards the thumb or little finger.

The loops which have a downward slop towards thumb from little fingers side are known as *radial loops*. The loops which have a downward slop towards little finger are known as *ulnar loops*.

Whorl: When the ridges run in a circular form around the central core. An ideal whorl consists of 3 things:

- A central core.
- Intersecting ridges.
- Two deltas which fall in the same straight plain.

A delta is formed when a single ridge bifurcates or by abrupt divergence of two ridges running side by side.

A recurrent whorl: It is one, which makes a circle in one direction and other in opposite direction.

Compound or composite: Means all the above three patterns, arches, loops and whorls are found mixed in the same impression.

Method of Taking Impression

1. Clean with sprit then dry
2. Take impression on an ordinary paper
3. Take impression of all the fingers (ten fingers)
4. Record personal data on back of paper

5. Fingerprints of person suffering from contagious disease like leprosy should not be recorded.
6. Obscure prints can be made prominent by using chemical ($AgNO_3$, iodide)
7. In dead (skin is hard, shriveled), first apply olive oil, then inject paraffin.
8. Use rolling method for recording.

Impression Instead of Plain Method

Medicolegal importance: Surest and easy method of identification especially for:

i. Habitual criminals
ii. Absconders
iii. Cases of impersonation
iv. People lost their memory
v. Decomposed bodies
vi. Mass disaster

Poroscopy

Devised by Mr Edmond Locard.

Principle: Sweat glands opening (pores) of the finger ridges varies in size, shape and position but are constant for a given individual. Number of pores varies 9–18 pores/mm.

Medicolegal importance: Method of identification, especially when fingerprints are not visible, fragmentary, blurred.

Portriat Parley System of Identification

In this system, the front and side views of photographs of faces of all international criminals are supplied to all international airports and sea ports so that a suspected criminal may not escape from suspected country.

Footprints

The impression of a foot or shoes left on ground at the site of crime may help in identifying a criminal. In other countries, at the time of birth, footprint of the newborn is taken so as to prevent exchange of children and is kept in record.

In most of the countries, footprints of air force personnel are taken because in case of crash as body is mutilated, foot is often preserved because of long and thick shoes.

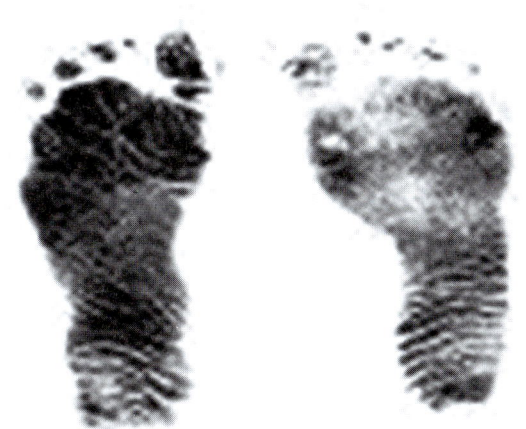

DNA Fingerprints

Useful

1. For identification in criminal investigations involving physical evidence such as blood, semen or hair.
2. In case of disputed paternity, developed by Dr. Alec Jeffreys, a British researcher value 100% accurate.

PRINCIPLE

In everyone's DNA chain, there are breaks (called stutters) which appear in a repetitive pattern throughout the DNA molecules. These portions of meolecules containing stutters can be isolated after a chemical treatment. Observations are compared with a suspected sample (control).

PROCEDURE

1. DNA is extracted and purified from the sample after a laboratory process.
2. DNA is cut apart with a restriction enzymes that fragments the DNA double strands at specific DNA sequences.
3. Fragmented portions are transferred to a nylon membrane where the probes are added.
4. The probes attach themselves to specific invisible bands of repetitive DNA.
5. The membrane is exposed to an X-ray film resulting in DNA fingerprinting.
6. On X-ray film, it looks like a bar code (bands).

7. The bands are analysed and compared to establish popsitive identity.

Advantages

Method is superior to other methods of identification because method is objective. Small amount of sample (tissue) is required. 1–2 drops of blood, 10 hair roots and trace of semen test can be performed on older samples. Less time-consuming comparison of fetal tissue and suspected father.

Disadvantage: Identical twins have identical patterns.

Cheiloscopy (Lip Prints)

Introduced by Japanese

Principle: Wrinkles, cracks, and crevices of lips are permanent and individualized characteristics.

Value: Accurate, useful in living and air-crash accident victims.

Disadvantage: Prints match in identical twins.

Speech Spectrogram (Identification from Voice)

Invented by: Mr. Lawerence G Kersta (New Jercy, 1963).

Principle: Method is to record and compare the speech pattern of chosen words and phrases uttered by a person on different occasions.

Method: The speech pitch and intensities at intervals of fraction of seconds are recorded and comparing the resultant spectrogram of same words when recorded from different sources (a telephone call or voice of suspect).

Superimposition Photography

Skull of deceased X-rayed in different views. Frontal and lateral photographs of the deceased when he was alive are enlarged to the size of radiographs. The positives of photographs and negatives of radiographs are technically superimposed to see if they tally in contour of the face and skull, if the radiographs and photographs belong to same person all surfaces, contours, orifices will match.

Frontal Sinus Pattern

Conisdered as surest method is an individualized character comparision of X-ray frontal sinuses taken during life and after death is done.

Neutron Activation Analysis

An extremely sensitive method to determine quantity of element present in a minute level in a given sample. The elements are detected from hairs, nails, blood and compared with previous values of a suspect.

Precipitin Test (Ring Test)

Use: To determine the source/species of some biological materials. Specimen bone commonly blood (fragmentary remains). Studied hairs skin, soft tissues and semen.

Technique

1. Take filtered isotonic saline extract of the material to be examined in a test tube.
2. Then put a drop of specific antisera in the tube.

3. A cloudy precipitate at the line of contact will be observed, if test is positive.

Trace Evidence

Definition: Any material (irrespective of its quantity) which helps in identification objectively, or give clues about crime or connect the criminal with crime.

Trace meaning

- To sketch, mark out
- Copy
- Follow the track or path of someone
- Track left by person
- Visible signs of what has existed or happened
- Small amount

Locard's Principle of Exchange

1. Every contact leaves a trace
2. The nature/character of trace must be confirmed by comparing it with a control, to give it an evidential value. Transfer of trace is may be and is often a two-way process.

CHAPTER 36

Tables at a Glance

Table 36.1: Weights and measurements of organs in adults

1. Brain: 1350 to 1400 g (males)	1250 to 1330 g (females)
2. Heart: 275 to 300 g (males)	225 to 250 g (females)
3. Thickness of walls of atria	1 to 2 mm
4. Thickness of wall of right ventricle	3 to 5 mm
5. Thickness of wall of left ventricle	10 to 15 mm
6. Circumference of aortic valve	6 to 7.5 cm
7. Circumference of pulmonary valve	7 to 9 cm
8. Circumference of mitral valve	9.5 to 10.5 cm
9. Circumference of tricuspid valve	10 to 12.5 cm
	360 to 570 g (mean 450 g)
	325 to 480 g (mean 400 g)
10. Right lung	1400 to 1500 g (males)
Left lung	1300 to 1400 g (females)
11. Liver	140 to 160 g (males)
12. Kidney	130 to 150 g (females)
13. Spleen	–

(This chapter is contributed by Dr. K. Rajesham, Asstistant Professor, Department of Forensic Medicine, Karimnagar, Telangana)

Table 36.2: Treatment of common acute poisoning

Name	Symptoms and signs	Management and treatment	Remarks
Acids and alkalies	1. Intense pain during the act of swallowing 2. Burns and ulcers on mucous membrane 3. Dysphagia 4. Shock due to pain 5. Oedematous glottis and difficulty in breathing	1. Acids can be neutralised by dilute alkaline substances, for example, magnesium oxide or aluminium hydroxide 2. Alkalies can be neutralised by weak acids like 10% vinegar or lemon juice 3. Demulcents 4. Supportive symptomatic treatment like intravenous fluids, analgesics	Acids are used for vitriolage
Acetaminophen (paracetamol)	Nausea and vomiting 1. 1–2 days: Abdominal pain, tender liver (liver function tests become abnormal, 12 to 36 hours after overdose) 2. ↑ Bilirubin, ↑ aspartate amino-transferase 3. ↑ Prothrombin time 4. 2–7 days: Liver failure (jaundice, hepatic encephalopathy), acute renal failure, cardiac arrhythmias, hypotension, tachycardia	1. Gastric lavage (useful if carried out within 4 hours of ingestion) 2. Antidote (best given within 10 hours after ingestion) 3. Methionine 2.5 g, orally, then 2.5 g, 4 hourly for further 3 doses **Total dose:** 10 g methionine over 12 hours 4. N-acetylcysteine 150 mg/kg intravenously, over 15 minutes in 200 ml of 5% dextrose, then 50 mg/kg in 500 ml of 5% dextrose intravenously, in the next 4 hours and 100 mg/kg in one litre of 5% dextrose intravenously, over the ensuing 16 hours Total dose: 300 mg/kg over 20 hours 5. Supportive measures 6. Vitamin K 10 mg intravenously, for 3 days (if prothrombin time is prolonged)	N-acetylcysteine and methionine are effective in the prevention of liver damage provided it is administered within 10 hours of ingestion of the overdose

(Contd.)

Table 36.2: Treatment of common acute poisoning (Contd.)

Name	Symptoms and signs	Management and treatment	Remarks
Aspirin (acetylsalicylic acid)	1. Nausea, vomiting, epigastric pain, hyperpyrexia, profuse sweating, irritability, tremors, roaring in the ears, deafness, blurring of vision, tachypnea, hyperapnoea, pulmonary-oedema 2. Dehydration due to vomiting, sweating and overbreathing 3. Respiratory alkalosis followed by metabolic acidosis (except in children) 4. Hyper-or hypoglycemia 5. Hypoprothrombinaemia (in an adult, moderate to severe toxicity will result from the ingestion of 50 or more standard 300 mg aspirin tablets, provided he has not vomited)	1. Heparinised blood should be withdrawn for immediate determination of the initial blood salicylate level (BSL) 2. Gastric aspiration and lavage, forced 'cocktail' diuresis. (Saline, 0.9%—0.5 L Dextrose 5%—1L Sodium bicarbonate 1.26%—0.5 L Potassium chloride 3 g) 3. As a mixture at 2 L/hour for 3 hours and thereafter 1 L/hour until BSL is 35 mg/ 100 ml when the drip may be stopped. The rate of infusion is most important. In the absence of accompanying sedative drug overdose, acidaemia should be suspected and corrected by prior infusion of ½ L of 5% sodium bicarbonate within 30 minutes prior to the start of forced cocktail diuresis 4. Haemoperfusion or haemodialysis if BSL >90 mg/100 ml 5. Copious fluid orally	1. BSL is the best guide to measure the severity of salicylate poisoning. They should be determined after 6 hours of ingestion of an overdose and repeated several hours later to make sure that the level is not rising. Generally, BSL ↓ 500 mg/L, 6 hours after ingestion of an overdose indicates *mild* toxicity; BSL between 500 and 750 mg/L is associated with *moderate* toxicity, BSL ↑ 750 mg/L at 6 hours may be associated with severe toxicity 2. Chart: (a) TPR ½ hourly (b) Fluid intake/output
Amphetamine	1. Restlessness, tremors, irritability, insomnia 2. Dryness of mouth, nausea, vomiting, diarrhoea, abdominal pain 3. Sweating hyperpyrexia, cardiac arrhythmias, tachycardia, hypertension or hypotension 4. Delirium, hallucinations, coma, convulsions	1. Gastric lavage. 2. Supportive treatment. 3. Chlorpromazine 50–100 mg intravenous and intramuscular/intravenous for sedation (repeated ½ to 1 hour intervals needed) 4. Forced acid diuresis may help those severely poisoned (as about 50% of drug is excreted in the urine)	1. Confusion, aggressiveness hallucinations, delirium, panic attacks; suicidal /homicidal tendencies may occur 2. Bizarre and inexplicable behaviour, often undistinguishable from paranoid schizophrenia, has been associated with amphetamine abuse

(Contd.)

Table 36.2: Treatment of common acute poisoning (*Contd.*)

Name	Symptoms and signs	Management and treatment	Remarks
Ammonia (gas is usually compressed into a liquid), ammonium hydroxide	1. Inhalation causes severe inflammation of respiratory tract—laryngitis, tracheobronchitis, pulmonary oedema, substernal pain, severe coughing, spasm of glottis, terminal pneumonia 2. Liquid ammonia causes dermatitis, necrosis, conjunctivitis, cataract, total loss of vision, etc.	1. Neutralise with vinegar 2. Demulcents 3. Antibiotics 4. Symptomatic treatment	1. Maximum permissible concentration of ammonia is 100 ppm 2. Strong odour on opening the body 3. The stomach contents are slippery 4. Accidental, suicidal, vitriolage
Bleaching solutions (3–6% solutions of sodium hypochlorite in water)	1. Severe irritation, corrosion mucous membrane, pain and vomiting 2. Pulmonary irritation with coughing, choking, oedema of pharynx, larynx, lungs 3. BP ↓ delirium, coma	1. Skin contact: Wash with running water until 'disappearance of soapiness' 2. Give milk, ice cream (melted) or beaten eggs . Give sodium thiosulphate orally 3. Do not use emesis, lavage or acid antidotes 4. Antacids, e.g. milk of magnesia or aluminium hydroxide are also useful	1. The strength of solution used for chlorinating swimming pools is 20% 2. Hypochlorous acid—released when bleaching solution comes in contact with acid gastric juice or acid solution is extremely irritating to the mucous membrane and skin
Barbiturate hypnotics (amylobarbitone, butobarbitone)	1. Drowsiness, ataxiz and dysarthria soon followed by coma, hypotension, respiratory depression and hypothermia, limbs hypotonic with loss of tendon reflexes 2. Plantar response, if present, flexor but in deep coma may be absent. Barbiturate blisters over presssure areas. Pupils—normal 3. Injection marks in addicts: (a) Hypostatic pneumonia and after apparent recovery, hepatocellular failure	1. Gastric aspiration and lavage 2. Supportive therapy. 3. Charcoal haemoperfusion in case of grade IV coma or if plasma concentration of following drug is above: 150 mg/L in phenobarbitone poisoning OR 50 mg/L in barbiturate hypnotic poisoning 4. Attend to 'burst' blisters 5. To a 5% glucose intravenous drip, add 15 mg of amiphenazol in	1. The treatment should be determined by the patient's clinical state rather than the plasma drug concentration 2. Plasma concentration frequently continue to rise in the first 48 hours after ingestion, when the patient may be improving clinically 3. Bladder catheterisation 4. Monitor fluid balance 5. Recovery within a week with supportive care and forced alkaline diuresis. Coma in severe poisoning lasts may several days

(Contd.)

Table 36.2: Treatment of common acute poisoning (*Contd.*)

Name	Symptoms and signs	Management and treatment	Remarks
	(b) Persons having pulmonary, hepatic and renal diseases succumb to the bad effects soon. Phenobarbitone As above, but coma, if present seldom deeper than grade 2 or 3, Gross coarse nystagmus on slightest movement of eyes. Disinhibited mental state (loquacious, argumentative)	slaline and 50 mg of bemigride in saline every 5 minutes, till pharyngeal and laryngeal reflexes return and a safe state is brought about OR Nikethamide (5–10 ml) intravenous, at 15–30 minutes interval can be used. 6. Gastric aspiration and lavage 7. Supportive therapy 8. Forced alkaline diuresis: 5% dextrose (0.5 L), 09% saline (0.5 L) and 1.26% sodium bicarbonate (0.5 L) in rotation at 0.5 L/hour 9. Frusemide 20 mg intravenously (if urinary output falls more than two litres behind fluid input). Antibiotics and good nursing	
Benzodiazepines (chlordiazepoxide)	Drowsiness, apathy, ataxia, dysarthria, partial ptosis and nystagmus	1. Gastric aspiration and lavage 2. Supportive therapy 3. Flumaxenil	1. Overdose of nitrazepam in man result in bullous skin lesions. Many benzodiazepines have active metabolites with long plasma half-lives, so that performance in skilled task, e.g. driving motor vehicles may be impaired for several days or weeks after apparent recovery from overdose. Persons poisoned with benzodiazepine recover considerably within 24 hours 2. Benzodiazepines are taken with other psychotropic drugs, and potentiate CNS depressant effects of alcohol barbiturate and tricyclic antidepressants

(*Contd.*)

Table 36.2: Treatment of common acute poisoning *(Contd.)*

Name	Symptoms and signs	Management and treatment	Remarks
Diazepam (flurazepam, lorazepam, etc.)	1. Coma (Grade-II usually) 2. Hypotension	As above	As above
Beta-adrenergic blocking drugs (atenolol, metoprolol, propranolol)	1. Pallor, cold, clammy cyanosed/limbs 2. Ataxia, coma, convulsions 3. Severe bradycardia (sinus in origin) 4. Marked QRS prolongation and ST and T wave changes in ECG 5. Bronchospasm	1. Gastric aspiration and lavage 2. Atropine 3 mg intravenously (or 0.04 mg/kg) for bradycardia and hypotension; followed if required, by isoprenaline 2 mg/ 500 ml normal saline or 5% glucose 20/40 drops/min, depending upon response 3. Glucagon 5–10 mg intravenously (a safe alternative to isoprenaline and is the treatment of choice) 4. Supportive therapy	Severe bronchospasm responds to salbutamol inhalations.
Cannabis (marihuana)	1. If smoked or ingested, mild anxiety, excitement followed by a feeling of calmness euphoria, uncontrollable laughter. Perception of colour and sound often enhanced. Purposeless muscular exercises, later drowsiness and sleep (intoxication may result from the rupture of ingested cannabis—filled balloons (condoms) in which the drug is being smuggled) 2. Chronic use—results in increased desire and decreased sexual power, leading to sexual perversions	1. Generally not required, if inhaled or ingested 2. Symptomatic treatment if necessary	Intravenous injection of canabistea results in nausea, vomiting, abdominal pain, watery diarrhoea, fever, rigor, BP ↓, shock, later renal impairment, cholestatic jaundice, lethargy, hypoglycaemia, ECG may show ischaemic changes. The alterations in perception and cerebral functions seen after cannabis has been ingested or smoked

(Contd.)

Table 36.2: Treatment of common acute poisoning (Contd.)

Name	Symptoms and signs	Management and treatment	Remarks
Chlorine (gas)	Lacrimation, conjunctivitis, cough followed by breathlessness, wheezing, hoarseness due to laryngeal oedema, tachypnoea, central cyanosis with bronchi and crepitations in lungs	1. Remove patient from the toxic atmosphere 2. Symptomatic therapy 3. O_2 inhalation 4. Bronchodilators 5. Prednisolone 60 mg/daily until symptoms disappear and on X-ray clear lungs, then withdraw over about 2 weeks	1. Observe for 12 hours, in case of those exposed minimally 2. Inhalation of chlorine results in oedema of lungs, patchy necrosis or respiratory mucosa (chlorine combines with moisture to form HCl)
Dhatura	1. Fixed dilated pupils 2. Diplopia 3. Dysphagia 4. Difficulty in speaking 5. Drunken gait 6. Delirium (muttering type) mental confusion, excitement, hallucinations 7. Rolling movements (may be because of pillo) movements or drawing imaginary threads 8. Hyperpyrexia 9. Tachycardia	1. Gastric aspiration lavage if needed 2. Carbachol 0.125 mg test dose, if no untoward effect gives 0.5 mg subcutaneously or neostigmine (0.25 mg) or physostigmine salicylate 1–4 mg subcutaneously, intramuscularly or intravenously slowly to be repeated 1–2 hours later if necessary 3. Ice bag 4. Diazepam intravenously for seizures 5. Catheterisation	1. It is used by road-side robbers to stupefy travellers to rob them of their belongings 2. Avoid promethazine, phenothiazine and morphine
Iodine	1. Nausea, vomiting (brown/blue), diarrhoea, Burning sensation in mouth, throat, epigastric pain, salivation 2. Albuminuria, oliguria	1. Gastric lavage with starch solution. Intravenous 10% sodium thiosulphate 10 ml / 4 hourly 2. Intravenous fluids and supportive therapy	Tincture iodine should not be used for cleaning skin before withdrawing blood for alcohol estimation

(Contd.)

Table 36.2: Treatment of common acute poisoning (Contd.)

Name	Symptoms and signs	Management and treatment	Remarks

Iron poisoning	1. Epigastric pain, nausea, vomiting, diarrhoea, haematemesis, malena, circulatory collapse
	2. Later complications: Acute encephalopathy (headache, confusion, coma, convulsions) cyanosis, pulmonary oedema, metabolic acidosis, acute renal failure circulatory collapse and death, hepatic failure, high gastrointestinal obstruction, black line at the junction of gum and teeth
		1. Gastric aspiration and lavage with
		  (a) 5% $NaHCO_3$ or
		  (b) Desferrioxamine solution
		    2 g in 1 L of warm water
		2. Following lavage, leave desferrioxamine solution (5 g in 50–200 ml of water) to chelate any free iron in gastrointestinal tract. In addition, intravenous slow drip of desferrioxamine not exceeding 15 mg/kg body weight (maximum 80 mg /kg body weight in 24 hours)
		3. Inject desferrioxamine (2 g in 10 ml water in adult and 1 g in 5 ml water in a child) intramuscularly every 12 hourly according to clinical state and plasma concentration level
		4. If oliguria/anuria develops peritoneal dialysis or haemodialysis	

Methyl alcohol (methanol)	Latent period of 12–24 hours or more, later headache, weakness, blurring of vision, breathlessness, nausea, vomiting, abdominal pain, rarely diarrhoea, pupils dilated, not responding to light. Hyperaemia of optic disc in acute stage, later peripapillary oedema (up to	1. Gastric aspiration and lavage. In minor intoxication: Absolute alcohol (0.5 ml / kg) orally followed by 0.25 ml/kg 2 hourly. In severe poisoning absolute alcohol (5–10 g/hour) until the plasma methanol concentration is less than about 200 ml/L	May cause optic atrophy, central scotoma, etc. Cerebral oedema, necrosis in the putamen and haemorrhagic pancreatitis may be found on postmortem

(Contd.)

Table 36.2: Treatment of common acute poisoning (*Contd.*)

Name	Symptoms and signs	Management and treatment	Remarks
	8 weeks). Sweating, excitement, drowsiness, coma, convulsion, atrophy of optic nerve and blindness	2. Haemodialysis to be considered if the plasma methanol concentration ↑ 500 g/L, if visual symptoms have developed and there is significant metabolic acidosis. Continue dialysis till plasma concentration falls below 250 mg/L 3. Intravenous sodium bicarbonate to correct metabolic acidosis	
Methaemoglobinaemia due to: *Direct oxidants:* Nitroglycerin, amyl nitrite, $AgNO_3$ (burns), quinones (choloroquine, primaquine), food-rich in nitrates, nitrous gases seen in arc welders, food adulterated with nitrites, well water (nitrates) *Indirect oxidants:* Aniline dye derivatives (for example, wax crayons, moth ball), phenacetin, benzocaine, nitrobenzenes, sulphonamides, lime, sulfanilamide, sulfapyridine, sulfamethizole, etc.)	1. ↑30–40% concentration of methaemoglobin: Headache, giddiness, weakness, dyspnoea, cyanosis 2. 40–60% concentration: Stupor, respiratory depression, chocolate-coloured blood 3. ↑60% concentration: Death	1. Gastric aspiration or lavage—wash skin throughly with soap and water 2. Give 100% O_2 by mask when Met-Hb concentration is ↑ 40% or in presence of symptoms give antidote 3. Methylene 1 or 2 mg/kg of 1% solution intravenously, over a 10 minutes period or vitamin C, 1 g slowly intravenous—supportive therapy 4. Exchange transfusion	1. Methaemoglobin is formed by oxidation of the ferrous ion of Hb to the ferric form by the action of a number of chemicals including nitrites, chlorates and amino and nitro-organic compounds 2. Caution: Intravenous administration of therapeutic doses of methylene blue may cause nausea, giddiness, rise in BP 3. Spectrophotometric analysis gives the Met-Hb concentration in blood
Narcotic analgesics—opium, morphine, heroin (dextropropoxyphene, pentazocine, pethidine, codeine)	1. Exhiliration and physical case followed by depression, coma, pinpoint pupils, marked reduction of the respiratory rate are the hallmarks	Naloxone 1.2 mg intravenously (0.4 mg for child) to be repeated every 15–30 minutes, till pupils begin to dilate (as much as 75 mg naloxone in 24 hours has	Poisoning or death may result from the rupture of ingested opium or heroin filled condoms in which the drug is being smuggled. Acute withdrawal syndrome may precipitate after

(*Contd.*)

Table 36.2: Treatment of common acute poisoning (Contd.)

Name	Symptoms and signs	Management and treatment	Remarks
Methadone, lomotil tablet (diphenoxylate and atropine)	2. BP ↓, temperature ↓, sweating 3. Presence of injection marks	been given without obvious adverse effects). Once the patient is resuscitated from the CNS depression, carry out gastric aspiration and lavage whether taken orally or parenterally	administration of naloxone to poisoned narcotic addict, however, it is short-lived and seldom severe
Naphthalene (moth repellent)	1. Nausea, vomiting, diarrhoea 2. Haemolysis in patient with G6PD deficiency in red cells 3. Oliguria, haematuria, anuria 4. In more serious poisoning excitement, coma convulsions	1. Gastric lavage 2. Alkalinisation of urine (give sodium bicarbonate, 5 g orally every 4 hour or as necessary) 3. Diuretics (give up to 15 ml/ kg/hr or fluids with furosemide 1 mg /kg for maximum diuresis and to reduce injury to the kidney from Hb products) 4. Dialysis if necessary	Avoid fats, milk and castor oil, etc.
Oxalic acid (binoxalate of potassium salts of sorrel or essential salts of lemon)	Local irritation and corrosion of mouth, oesophagus and stomach with pain and greenish-brown or black vomiting. Muscular tremors, convulsions and collapse. Later acute renal failure from blocking of renal tubules by calcium oxalate urine contains calcium oxalate crystals, RBC and albumin	1. Precipitate oxalates by saccharated solution of lime water orally 2. Inject calcium gluconate, 10% 10 ml slowly intravenously 3. Fluid orally 2–4 L/day to prevent precipitation of calcium oxalate in the ranal tubules	Present in stain removers so must be kept away from children
Organophosphorus compounds and carbamates (baygon)	1. Kerosene like odour 2. Early: Headache, nausea, giddiness, tightness of chest, dimness of vision, miosis, twitching of eye muscles, tremors of tongue profuse frothing 3. Late: Vomiting, sweating salivation oronasal froth, muscular	1. Remove soiled clothes. Throughly wash contaminated skin gastric aspiration and lavage 2. Atropine 2 mg intravenous every 10–30 minutes till signs of atropinisation (the total dose	1. Before starting treatment blood sample should be collected for estimation of cholinesterase activity. Measurement of plasma cholinesterase activity is useful for confirming the diagnosis of poisoning

(Contd.)

Table 36.2: Treatment of common acute poisoning (*Contd.*)

Name	Symptoms and signs	Management and treatment	Remarks
	fasciculations, bronchospasm, cyanosis pulmonary oedema, disorientation, drowsiness, coma, convulsions, incontinence (CNS manifestations less in carbamate poisoning)	required may be much as 30 mg or more in first 24 hours) 3. Pralidoxine (P$_2$AM, 2-PAM, PAM, P$_2$S), 1 gm slow intravenous (to be given witin 12–24 hours of exposure/ ingestion) (contraindicated in carbamate poisoning) 4. Intensive supportive therapy. Remove respiratory secretions. Artificial respiration and anticonvulsants, perrectum, O$_2$ inhalation paraldehyde	2. Miosis may appear late (mydriasis may be present in up to 10% of cases) 3. Before giving atropine, oxygenation should be adequate
(a) Oleander	Due to: 1. Gastrointestinal irritation, nausea, vomiting, epigastric pain, diarrhoea 2. Digitalis like action on heart, cardiac arrhythmias and heart block 3. General: Profuse frothy salivation, difficulty in swallowing/ talking, lock jaw, giddiness, muscular twitching, coma	1. Gastric aspiration and lavage. 2. Phenytoin 100–200 mg orally every 6 hours until arrhythmia is reverted 3. Propranolol 1–3 mg intravenous, slowly 4. Morphine sulphate 10–15 mg subcutaneously	1. All parts of the plant poisonous 2. Active principles (cardiac glycosides nerin, oleandrin)

(b) *Cerbera thevetia* (yellow oleander), Pilakaner	Burning pain in mouth with dryness of throat, tingling and numbness of the tongue, nausea, vomiting, diarrhoea, headache, giddiness, loss of muscular power, varying degrees of heart block, fainting, collapse, tetanoid convulsions	1. Gastric aspiration and lavage
		2. Molar sodium lactate intravenously
		3. SIntravenous injection by drip method of 5% glucose solution with 1.2 mg of atropine, 2 ml of adrenaline (1:1000) (and 2 mg of noradrenaline if blood pressure is low)
			1. All parts of plant poisonous
			2. Active principles glycosides:
			  (a) From plant:
			    • Thevetin
			    • Cerberin: Peruvoside and ruvoside, the other two glycosides are digitaloidin action

(*Contd.*)

Table 36.2: Treatment of common acute poisoning (Contd.)

Name	Symptoms and signs	Management and treatment	Remarks

(c) *Cerbera odallam* (Dabur)	1. Due to:
	  (a) Gastrointestinal irritation
	  (b) Like action on heart
	  (c) Vomiting, diarrhoea, respiration irregular, collapse, general paralysis
	2. ECG may show sinus bradycardia
	3. S-A block, combination of SA and AV block, other cardiac arrhythmias
		Treatment similar to that of *Nerium odorum*	(a) From kernel of seeds (glycosides):
			  • Thevetin
			  • Thevetoxin
			  • Nerifolin
			  • Cerberin
			
			Fruit resembles an unripe mango and kernel contains glycosides, cerboris, cerebroside

Petroleum distillates and turpentine benzine, diesel fuel, furniture polish, kerosene, naphtha, paraffin, petrol	1. Smell of hydrocarbon in breath. Nausea, vomiting, diarrhoea rarely 2. Excitation, more often drowsiness coma in severe poisoning, convulsions rarely 3. Cough, choking, cyanosis breathlessness are the pulmonary complications 4. X-ray: Hydrocarbon pneumonitis (usually involves 2 or more lobes and occassionally perihilar) 5. Fever, polymorph leukocytosis (diagnosis of hydrocarbon ingestion may be confirmed by finding a double fluid level in stomach taken in the erect posture	1. Gastric lavage after insertion of a cuffed endotracheal tube in a case (a) showing serious poisoning or (b) when a solution contains another poison, (c) if a 2- or 3-year old child has swallowed a mouthful (4–5 ml) 2. Supportive therapy 3. Antibiotics if necessary	1. Petroleum distillates are a group of fuel solvents, containing a variety of aliphatic and aromatic hydrocarbons in different proportions. While turpentine refers to a mixture of pinenes, camphenes and other terpenes 2. Turpentine substitute (white spirit) is a mixture of long chain hydrocarbons and is used as paint thinner
Snakebite (poisonous) (ophitoxaemia)	1. Bite marks. (a) *Local features:* Severe local pain, tingling, swelling spreading from bite, bleeding from the site, local ecchymosis, serum filled bullae, later	1. *First aid measures:* To transport the victim to the nearest hospital. Do not use tourniquet. Do not apply ice. Do not incise or apply suction to the punctured wounds, keep bitten limb immobilised at	1. Skin or conjunctival tests for sensitivity to antisnake venom serum is mandatory before its administration. Adrenaline should be available for immediate use, should allergic reactions occur, despite a negative sensitivity test (inject

(Contd.)

Table 36.2: Treatment of common acute poisoning (Contd.)

Name	Symptoms and signs	Management and treatment	Remarks
	extensive sloughing, ulceration. Necrosis with putrid smell • Cramps in abdominal muscles • Myalgia and myoglobinuria (b) *Systemic features:* Nausea, vomiting, headache, fever and allergic rash • CNS: Muscular paralysis (ascending), cannot talk, swallow or protrude the tongue. Paraesthesia, muscle spasm, convulsions, ptosis, squint, diplopia • CVS: Tachycardia, BP↓, cardiac arrhythmias, nonspecific ECG changes (c) *Haemopoietic system:* Haemorrhagic tendencies, bleeding from site, ecchymosis, bleeding from gums, haematemesis, haemoptysis, haematuria, intra-abdominal/retroperitoneal haemorrhage	the level of the heart. The victim should avoid exertion. Reassurance of the victim is important aspect of first aid 2. *Specific treatment:* Perform skin test for sensitivity to antisnake venom serum. If no reaction or urticaria, inject slowly intravenous 20 ml reconstituted, antisnake venom serum; repeat 2 hours later, further dose 6 hourly till symptoms disappear 3. In presence of sensitivity reactions to serum, desensitisation or the administration of serum under cortisone cover may be undertaken 4. Neostigmine 5 mg, intravenous (in elapid snakebite case). Repeat ½ hourly, after 5 such injections at an interval of 2–12 hours depending on response	promptly adrenaline 0.5 ml of 1:1000, which must be drawn into the syringe before giving antivenom) 2. Admit under observation for 24 hours. A patient with minimal or no local reaction and who is given first aid treatment only 3. Monitor vital signs 4. Record pulse and BP hourly for 48 hours 5. Record daily the girth of proximal and distal parts of the bitten limb (measured about the mid-point) 6. Blood grouping should be done at the earliest; since venom may interfere with blood grouping
Solvent abuse (acetone, butane, ether, florinated hydrocarbons, petrol, toluene, trichloroethylene, etc.). *Synonyms:* Solvent inhalation, glue sniffing	1. Skin irritation (excitation, followed by depression, hypoxia) 2. Dizziness, disorientation, hallucination, convulsions, coma 3. Later complications: Jaundice, renal damage (toluene, carbon tetrachloride) 4. Acute and chronic encephalopathy (petrol with its tetraethyl lead content). Cerebellar degeneration (toluene). Predominantly motor, mixed, polyneuropathy (hexane)	1. Stop solvent inhalation (considerable improvement by the time patient is brought to hospital) 2. Supportive therapy	1. Abstinence from further solvent abuse is vitally important 2. Halogenated hydrocarbons sensitise the heart to endogenous catecholamines leading to fatal cardiac dysarrhythmias

Table 36.3: Differences among rigor mortis, heat stiffening and cold stiffening

Traits	Rigor mortis	Heat stiffening	Cold stiffening
1. Time of onset	Usually in the tropics in Eastern India, it occurs approximately 2 hours after death.	Occurs just after death when dead body is exposed to temperature above 65°C temperature	May occur just after death, if body is exposed to temperature below 3.5°C temperature
2. Cause	Loss of ATP in muscle fibres along with rise of lactic acid level	Exposure of dead body to raise temperature above 65°C temperature	Exposure of dead body to freeze temperature below 3.5°C with solidification of body fat, fluids and muscles
3. Predisposing cause	It occurs in all types of death natural or unnatural	It occurs in all cases of deaths or dead bodies exposed to temperature above 65°C as in bodies recovered from burnt building, motor cars, aeroplanes or on exposure to high voltage current causing coagulation of muslce proteins	It occurs in all cases of death with bodies recovered from ice caves, arctic areas, etc. or when it is exposed to temperature below 3.5°C
4. Important characteristic features	Body is hard and stiff like log of wood but no shortening of muscle fibres. On thawing after cold stiffening, it appears. Rigor mortis does not appear after heat stiffening. No shortening of muscle fibres occurs	It can occur in muscles under influence of rigor mortis. Body may assume pugilistic attitude with great shortening of muscle fibres, unlike rigor mortis	If body is exposed to freeze temperature before onset of rigor, rigor mortis will be delayed in onset unless and until after thawing. No shortening of muscle fibres occurs
5. Mode of onset and progress	Onset is gradual. The course and progress are along a fixed and definite order, both in respect of appearance and disappearance	Onset is very rapid. No definite order in respect of progress, development and appearance, disappears on putrefaction	Onset is quick; course and progress are not in fixed or definite order, both in respect of its appearance and disappearance
6. Any particular attitude attained	Dead body will attain particular attitude aproximate to the position in which it is kept after death allowing RM to appears	Attainment of "Pugilistic attitude" is the characteristic feature in this state	The body will assume the attitude in which cold stiffening will affect and remain in body
7. How it can be broken down	By mechanical extension of limbs RM can be broken	It cannot be broken down by mechanical extension of limbs or joints	As long as cold freezing surroundings persist, it cannot be disturbed much by mechanical means

(Contd.)

Table 36.3: Differences among rigor mortis, heat stiffening and cold stiffening (Contd.)

Traits	Rigor mortis	Heat stiffening	Cold stiffening
8. Further progress	Rigor mortis terminates into state of putrefaction	The state will ultimately merge into stages of putrefaction in due course of time without RM in-between	Body remains in the state indefinitely, so long as freezing surroundings are present. On thawing, rigor mortis appears and disappears rapidly to be followed by putrefaction
9. Medicolegal importance	It gives idea about time past since death; may also suggest the position and attitude of the body at the time of death, about cause and nature of death in some cases	It suggests the circumstances, etc. leading to death; the evidence of burn injuries on the body point to nature, cause of death whether the burn and injuries were antemortem or postmortem. A dead body, if exposed to such high temperature or fire can undergo this change	It suggests the condition and surroundings, in which the body was present after death. As the dead body in this state remains fresh, it may help in identification, in fixing cause and nature of death

Table 36.4: Number of teeth at different ages

Name of teeth	Number of teeth	Temporary/permanent	Age
CI, LI, first molar	8/12 teeth	Temporary	12 months
CI, LI, first molar	8/12 teeth	do	15 months
CI, LI, first molar, canine	8/12 teeth	do	18 months
CI, LI, first molar, canine, second molar	8/12 teeth	do	24 months
All temporary teeth + first permanent molar	24 (temporary 20 + permanent 4)	Permanent	6 years
Permanent 1st molar and CI + rest temporary teeth	24 (temporary 16 + permanent 8)	Permanent	7 years
Permanent 1st molar and CI and LI + rest temporary teeth	24 (temporary 12 + permanent 12)	Permanent	8 years
Permanent IM, CI, LI, first premolar + rest temporary teeth	24 (temporary 8 + permanent 16)	Permanent	9 years
Permanent IM, CI, LI, first premolar, second premolar + no canine, no temporary	24 (temporary 4 + permanent 20)	Permanent	10 years
Permanent IM, CI, first and second premolar canine, no temporary	24 (temporary nil + permanent 24)	Permanent	11 years
Permanent IM, CI, first	28 (temporary nil + permanent 28)	All permanent	12–14 years
All except third molars erupted with space behind second molars present	28 (all permanent)	All permanent	14–17 years
All permanent teeth including third molars erupted	32 (all permanent)	All permanent	17–25 years

CI: Central incisor, LI: Lateral incisor, IM: 1st molar

Table 36.5: Age from toot calcification of teeth

Root calcification	Teeth	Appearance of calcification
Approx 9–10 years	Permanent first molar	At birth
Approx 9–10 years	Central incisor	About 4 months
Approx 10–11 years	Lateral incisor	About 12 months
Approx 13–15 years	Permanent canine	About 5 months
Approx 12–13 years	First premolar	About 18 months
Approx 14–15 years	Second premolar	About 24 months
Approx 14–16 years	Second molar	About 30–36 months
Approx 18–25 years	Third molar	About 9–10 months

Table 36.6: Differences between summons case and warrant case

Summons case	Warrant case
1. Instituted in respect of non-cognizable offence.	1. Instituted in respect of cognizable offence
2. Magistrate has discretion to convict the accused without going into evidence	2. Magistrate has no discretion to convict the accused without any hearing
3. No charge need be framed	3. A charge sheet need be framed against the accused
4. When instituted on complaint and the complainant, absent himself on date of hearing, the accused is entitled to be acquitted.	4. When instituted upon complaint, magistrate can discharge the accused when: • Charge has been framed • Charge is compoundable or non-recognizable
5. The case can be withdrawn at any time before the passing of final orders	5. The complainant can withdraw the case only when the accused has been convicted of some of the charges, when rest of the charges can be withdrawn

Table 36.7: Differences between dying deposition and dying eclaration

Dying deposition	Dying declaration
1. **Statement**: Always made to a magistrate	1. Need not be made to magistrate; in his absence, doctor can record it
2. **Oath**: Always taken	2. Not required to be taken
3. **Accused or his counsel:** Present to cross examine the declarant	3. Not present
4. **Role of doctor:** (a) To assess if the patient is compos mentis (b) The statement is recorded by the magistrate	4. (a) To assess if the patient is compos mentis (b) To record statement in absence of magistrate but in presence of witness
5. **Legal value:** Bedside court	5. Only if the person dies

Table 36.8: Differences between infamous conduct and professional negligence

Infamous conduct	Professional negligence
1. **Nature of offence:** Violation of code of medical ethics	1. Wilful negligence or utter disregard for case and attention
2. **Damages:** May be present	2. Always present
3. **Due care:** May be present	3. Expected, but violated
4. **Tried by**: By state medical council	4. By both civil and criminal courts
5. **Punishment**: Be assure of name from register or issue of warning notice by the council	5. Imprisonment or fine as per law
6. **Appeal**: To MCI and central government	6. To higher court of law

Table 36.9: Differences between criminal and civil negligence

Criminal negligence	Civil negligence
1. **Type of negligence:** Gross, wilful, wanton and culpable negligence	1. Absence or care, skill and proper performance
2. **Type of offence:** There is clear, specific and outright violation of particular criminal law in question	2. Not specific and clear. Outright violation of law need not be proved
3. **Doctor's conduct:** It is unbecoming and infamous conduct of the doctor in the professional sense	3. It is compared to generally accepted standard of professional conduct of doctor of same standing
4. **Consent of the patient:** Consent of the patient gives no protection. Doctor can be prosecuted for his wanton wilful negligence	4. Where patient gives consent, doctor has some protection
5. **Trial court:** Criminal court	5. Civil court
6. **Evidence:** Sufficient evidence is required to prove guilt beyond reasonable doubt	6. Evidence of that high standard not required
7. **Punishment:** Liable for imprisonment with or without fine	7. Liable to pay damages or compensation
8. **Double jeopardy:** Cannot be tried twice for the same crime	8. Can be tried twice for the crime

Table 36.10: General characters of mandible

Female	Male
1. **Size:** It is smaller, thinner and lighter	1. It is usually larger, thicker and heavier
2. **Symphysis menti:** It is smaller and shorter	2. The height of symphysis menti is greater and higher up
3. **Ramus:** It has rather smaller breadth	3. The ascending ramus has greater breadth
4. **Shape of chin:** Chin is pointed or rounded (V-shaped)	4. Chin is square/U-shaped
5. **Anatomical angle:** The anatomical angle is more obtuse, less prominent and inverted	5. The anatomical angle is the angle between the body and the ramus on outer aspect will be less obtuse, under 125, more prominent and everted
6. **Condyles:** Condyles will be smaller	6. These will be bigger and larger
7. **Impression:** These are less prominent	7. Impressions for the muscular attachments are prominent

Table 36.11: Chief homologous parts in female and male

Female	Male
1. Clitoris	Glans penis
2. Nymphae	Prepuce
3. Labia majora	Scrotum
4. Uterus	Sinus pocularis
5. Fallopian tube	vas deferens
6. Round ligament	Gubernaculum testis
7. Ovary	Testicles

Table 36.12: Distinguishing characters of female and male

Female	Male
1. (a) A person is considered as female, if she does possess at least one ovary and has periodic discharge of blood from near about the genitals (b) The uterus, fallopian tubes, vagina are appendages only (c) A subject is ascertained as female, if she has got an uterus or an opening or cul-de-sac behind the urethral canal and in front of rectum	1. A person will be considered a male, if he possess at least one testicle which secretes spermatozoan. The prostate, seminal vesicles, penis are mere appendages
2. External genitalia is being represented by vulva, vagina, etc.	2. External genetalia is characterised by penis, testicles, etc.
3. Usually thinly built, delicate and less muscular in constitution. Bones are rather slender lighter with relatively smaller shafts, wider medullary canals, subcutaneous fat more	3. General build is usually strong, stout and muscular subcutaneous fat less, bones bigger, stronger, heavier with less wide medullary canals
4. Hips broader than shoulder	4. Shoulders broader than hips
5. Pomum adami not well developed, voice low modulated. Face smaller than cranium, chin less projecting; lower jaw usually narrower	5. Pomum adami well developed and prominent; voice usually deep
6. Breasts are well developed after puberty; may get pendulous after childbirth	6. Breasts are rudimentary get developed only in case of 'Gynecomastia'
7. Hairness of the body parts is absent—a definite feminine feature. Scalp hair longer, thinner and finer	7. Hairness of face, chest with beard and moustache after puberty are characteristic. Scalp hair shorter, thicker and coarser
8. Pubic hair are of thin growth turned downwards, over mons veneris; never extend above the line joining anterior superior iliac spines	8. Pubic hair are thick, reach upwards conically up to the naval
9. Thoracic dimensions less, abdominal girth comparatively larger. Abdominal segment is larger	9. Dimension of thorax is more, the abdominal girth is smaller, unless very obese; abdominal segment is also smaller
10. The length of the larynx is usually 1.5" in size; is smaller than that of the males	10. Size of larynx and length of trachea are greater in males; length of larynx from upper border of thyroid cartilage to lower border of cricoid cartilage is approximately 2" in males
11. The waist is well defined in females, with gluteal regions well developed round and fully formed	11. The waist is ill-defined in males
12. Female thighs are conical for more deposition of fat, greater developed adductor muscles and shorter femurs. Circumference of upper part of female thighs usually are greater than males. Legs in females are more plumps and rounded. The wrists, ankles and nails are more delicate and slender. Limbs are shorter and slender, arms are cylindrical usually; on cross section, they are usually circular. Limbs in females compared to the body are shorter; as a result the centre of gravity is situated lower down, hence lordois is noticed in many cases	12. Male thighs are more cylindrical but legs are rounded; wrists, ankles and nails not delicate in males. Limbs are longer, arms are flatter usually, on cross section from side to side

Table 36.13 : General characteristic features of skull

Female	Male
1. **Size:** Lighter, smaller, contour smoother and less rugged	1. Bigger, heavier, contour is more rough and rugged
2. **Capacity:** Less capacious capacity 10% less than that of males	2. Cranial capacity is approximately 10% more than that of females (approximately 200 cc more)
3. **Glabella, etc.:** All these are more delicate, small, smooth and less prominent. Condylar facets are small, broad and short	3. Glabella, supraorbital ridges, zygomatic arches, mastoid processes, occipital condyles of adult male skulls are well marked and prominent. Condylar facets are long (length or height > width) slender
4. **Areas of muscular attachments:** These are less prominent, and marked in females occipital bony surface is relatively smooth. Digastric grooves are less deep	4. Muscular attachments and impression over occipital region of skull are well marked and prominent. Occipital surface is rough and protuberant more so in those who carry heavy weight on head, irrespective of sex. Digastric grooves are more deep
5. **Base of skull:** It is less rough and rugged; more smooth and plain. Foramen magnum small.	5. It is more rough and rugged. Foramen magnum is large
6. **Frontal sinuses:** Frontal sinuses are less developed. Frontal and parietal eminences are large comparatively. Frontal sinuses get unduly developed in hyperpituitarism in females	6. These are more well developed. Frontal and parietal eminences are small. Frontal sinuses may get atrophied in males in Kartagener's syndrome which is characterised by sinusitis, dextrocardia and bronchiectasis
7. **Orbital cavities:** These are bigger, nearly circular and placed higher up with sharp upper edges. Sizes being larger relative to the face as a whole	7. These are comparatively smaller square and placed low down with round upper edges.
8. **Forehead:** It is rounded and full with tendency of bugling	8. It is steeper and less round with no tendency to buldge
9. **Frontonasal junction:** It is smooth curve from forehead to upper part of bridge of nose	9. There is distinct angulation at the junction
10. **Facial bones:** These are less massive; rather smaller, delicate and more compressed sideways	10. These are massive, rough and heavier are more laterally arched
11. **Palate:** Usually smaller and narrower, is parabola shaped due to relative length of cheek-tooth-jaw	11. The breadth of palate is larger, wider and broader tends to be like "U" shape, due to relative length of cheek-tooth-jaw.
12. **Chin:** Chin is less prominent	12. It is more prominent and square in male.
13. **Cervical vertebrae:** The mean breadth is 72 mm (65–76 mm). Female atlas is never more than 76 mm	13. Mean breadth of 1st cervical vertebrae is 83 mm (74–90 mm). Male atlas is approx. 11 mm greater than female; male adult atlas is never less than 76 mm
14. **Teeth:** Teeth are smaller in size, molars are more often tricuspid	14. Teeth are larger in males than the females. Lower first molars are often five cusped.
15. **Nasal apertures:** Nasal apertures in females are low down and broader	15. These are usually placed high up and are narrower in breadth
16. **Larynx:** In females it is 3.8 cm. Anteroposterior diameter of female larynx is 2.6 cm	16. Average height of the larynx measured from upper border of thyroid to lower border of cricoid cartilage in midline is 4.8 cm. Anteroposterior diameter of male larynx is 3.6 cm

Table 36.14: Pelvis

Female	Male
1. **General framework :** Shallow, wide, smooth, less massive, more gracile	1. Deep rather narrow but is massive rough and rugged
2. **Build:** Lighter in construction, height is less. The transverse oblique and anteroposterior diameter is greater than in males, is bigger	2. Rather heavy in built in case of adult; height is bigger
3. **True pelvis:** It is wide and shallow; brim is nearly circular in outline	3. It is narrow deep and funnel shaped. The brim of true pelvis is typically heart shaped
4. **Ileum:** Ilia are less sloped and more expanded; walls more displayed posteriorly and borders more rounded	4. This is less expanded, more sloped; posterior borders less rounded but more rough. The curve of iliac crest is more prominent and reaches higher level than in females
5. **Anterior superior iliac spines:** These are widely separated	5. These are comparatively closer and not widely separated
6. **Symphysis pubis:** It is lower, smaller and shorter, wide and rounded. The pubic arch margins are not everted and are smooth. The dorsal border of pubic symphysis is irregular in case of adult female, in case of women who have born children, there will be scars of parturition in the form of depression or pits on dorsal surface/border of pubic symphysis due to childbearing	6. This is higher and bigger in depth and narrower in width; the margins of the pubic arch tends to be everted due to large size of the crura of penis getting attached to it. The dorsal border of pubic symphysis is not so irregular and does not show depression or pits, as in parous females
7. **Subpubic angle:** It is wide and obtuse, 90° and above. Distance between the ischia on two sides hence is more in females subpubic arch is more or less U-shaped	7. This is less than a right angle, i.e. is acute angled between 70 and 75 degrees; distance between ischium on two sides is less for the narrow pubic arch. Subpubic arch is V-shaped here
8. **Greater sciatic notches:** These are larger, wider, shallower, forming almost a right angle	8. These are smaller, narrow, angular less than right angle
• It varies between 5 and 6 in females	$$\frac{\text{Width of sciatic notch}}{\text{Depth of sciatic notch}} \times 100$$ • It varies between 4 and 5 in males
9. **Pre-auricular sulcus:** This is always broad and deep with sharp margins specially in parous women, for attachment of anterior sacro-iliac ligament and more mobile sacroiliac joints	9. It is not prominent; is usually narrow, shallow with margin prominent
10. **Obturator foramen:** It is triangular in shape with its apex directed forward	10. This is oval in shape with the base directed upwards
11. **Ischial tuberosities:** They are everted.	11. These are more or less inverted
12. **Pubis:** The body of pubis is broad and square. Its ramus is having a narrow appearance. Ischiopubic rami less everted	12. The body of pubis is narrow and triangular; its ramus being like continuation of the body. Ischiopubic rami more everted
13. **Acetabula:** It is smaller and narrower, the diameter average 46 mm	13. Are large wider deeper; the diameters average 52 mm

(Contd.)

Table 36.14: Pelvis *(Contd.)*

Female	Male
14. **Sacrum:** Female sacrum is short and wide with less prominent sacral promontory; body of 1st sacral vertebrae is small. The anterior curvature of sacrum is almost straight in the lower half, i.e. in its three segments but it is sharply curved in the lower half, i.e. from below the centre of 3rd sacral vertebrae. As a rule it has five segments	14. This is long and narrow with the sacral promontory well marked; body of 1st sacral vertebrae larger. The anterior curvature is distributed equally over its whole length. It may have more than five segments
15. **Sacroiliac articular surface:** Small and extend up to 2 to 2.5 sacral vertebral bodies	15. Large and extend up to 2.5 to 3 vertebral bodies
16. **Sacral index:** Sacral index in females is 116	16. $\dfrac{\text{Breadth of base}}{\text{Anterior length}} \times 100$
17. **Corporobasal index of sacrum:** It is approximately 40.5 females	17. Transverse diameter or breadth of: $\dfrac{\text{1st sacral vertebral body}}{\text{Transverse diameter or breadth of base of sacrum}} \times 100$
18. **Illiopectineal lines:** They are rounded and smooth	18. These are sharp and rough
19. **Ischiopubic index:** Ischiopubic index varies between 91 and 115 in females	19. $\dfrac{\text{Ischial length in mm}}{\text{Pubic length in mm}} \times 100$ It varies between 73 and 94 in males. The lengths of ischium and pubic are measured from the point at which they meet at the acetabulum
20. **Coccyx:** It is movable	20. It is less movable

Table 36.15: Sternum

Female	Male
1. **Body:** The body of the sternum is shorter, and is less than twice the length of the manubrium	1. The body of the sternum is bigger and is at least twice or more the length of the manubrium
2. **Level:** The upper border of the sternum is usually at the level of lower part of the body of the third thoracic vertebra	2. The upper border of the sternum is usually at the level of lower part of the body of the 2nd thoracic vertebra
3. **Ashely's rule:** As per Ashley's rule of 149, it is less than 149 mm	3. As per Ashley's rule of 149, the combined midline length of manubrium and mesosternum, equals or exceeds 149 mm. This rule applies to Europeans only
4. **Manubrium:** It is somewhat bigger	4. Manubrium is somewhat smaller
5. **Sternal index:** $54.3 = \dfrac{\text{Length of manubrium}}{\text{Length of mesosternum}} \times 100$	5. Sternal index is 46.2

Table 36.16: Thorax and ribs

Female	Male
1. Thorocic cage shorter and wider	1. Longer and narrower
2. Ribs are thinner and delicate in texture	2. Ribs are thicker and comparatively massive in texture
3. Ribs are disposed more obliquely	3. Ribs are disposed not so obliquely
4. Costal arches are longer	4. Costal arches are not larger
5. Ribs have greater curvatures	5. Ribs have lesser curvatures

Table 36.17: Femur

Female	Male
1. The neck of the femur forms almost a right angle with its shaft as because the female pelvis is wide	1. The neck of femur forms an obtuse angle of about 125 with its shaft, as the male pelvis is usually narrow
2. Acetabula narrower and shallower	2. Acetabula wider and deeper
3. The head of femur is smaller, forming less than 2/3 of a sphere	3. Head of the femur is larger forming almost about 2/3 of a sphere
4. The vertical diameter of the femoral head is less than 44 mm (43–45 mm)	4. The vertical diameter of the femoral head is usually greater than 48 mm (47–49 mm)
5. The bicondylar width varies between 67–76 mm and 72 mm approx	5. The bicondylar width usually varies between 74–89 mm and 78 mm approx

Table 36.18: Radius and ulna

Female	Male
1. Smaller, thinner and lighter	1. Generally larger, thicker and heavier
2. Radius is more curved	2. Radius is less curved

Table 36.19: Differences between abduction and kidnapping

Abduction	Kidnapping
1. It can be done in respect of any person of any age	1. It can be committed in respect of a minor or a person of unsound mind
2. Element of force or fraud is always present in abduction	2. Element of force or fraud is absent in kidnapping
3. Abduction can occur without removal from the protection of law or lawful guardianship	3. In kidnapping, there must be removal from the protection of law or lawful guardianship
4. Abduction will not be an offence unless there is presence of one of the evil intentions as detailed under Section 364 and Section 369 of IPC	4. Intention is not the essence of the offence

Table 36.20: Death and its medicolegal aspect

Inflammatory congestion	Internal hypostasis
1. **Position:** Congestion is present irrespective of position	1. Present only in the dependent part of an organ
2. **Distribution:** Redness will be uniform and all over the organ	2. Redness will be discrete and irregular
3. **Mucosa:** Mucous membrane may be angry looking	3. Mucous membrane will be dull and lustreless
4. **Inflammatory reaction:** Exudation, oedma, etc. are concomitant findings of inflammatory reaction	4. Absence of inflammatory exudation, oedema, etc.
5. **Hollow viscus put before light:** Uniform congestion	5. A stretch of intestinal coil, if held before light, will show alternating stained and unstained areas. According to the position of the coils

Table 36.21: Humerus

Female	Male
1. The average length of the bone is 30 cm	1. The average length of the bobe is 32.5 cm
2. The vertical diameter of the head is usually less than 41.5 mm, the transverse diameter is 38.9 mm	2. The vertical diameter of the head of humerus is 48.7 mm while its transverse diameter is 44.6 mm usually

Table 36.22: Differences between permanent tooth and temporary tooth

Permanent tooth	Temporary tooth
1. Longer and larger than temporary teeth except permanent bicuspids replacing temporary molars	1. Smaller in size usually, except in case of temporary molars which are larger than the permanent bicuspids replacing them
2. Strong broad and heavy; temporary molars are bigger and longer than premolars replacing them	2. They are lighter and more delicate than the permanent ones except molars
3. Permanent incisor teeth are more or less inclined forwards. Have small irregularities on its cutting edges, known as "developing mamelons"	3. The anteriorly placed milk teeth are vertical "No developing mamelons" on the cutting edges
4. Neck is less constricted	4. Neck is more constricted
5. Crowns are usually ivory white in colour	5. Crowns are China white in colour
6. No ridges	6. A ridge or thick edge is present, at the junction of the crown and fangs
7. Biscuspids replace temporary molars	7. Temporary molars have their cusps flat, roots smaller and more divergent
8. Presence of tooth germs beneath the tooth is not visible in X-ray in case of permanent tooth	8. Presence of tooth germs beneath the tooth if seen in X-ray will suggest that the tooth is temporary

Table 36.23: Changes in mandibles in infancy, adult and old age

Traits	Infancy	Adult	Old age
1. Medicolegal angle (i.e. angle formed by the ramus with body)	Right angle	Obtuse	Obtuse
2. Body	Shallow and small	Thick and elongated	Shallow and big

(Contd.)

Table 36.23: Changes in mandibles in infancy, adult and old age *(Contd.)*

Traits	Infancy	Adult	Old age
3. Ramus	Short and oblique	Short and acute angled	Long and oblique
4. Condyloid process	Lies at a lower level than the process	Projects above the level of coronoid process	Condyloid process lies with its neck bent backward
5. Mental foramen	Placed near the lower border of the ramus of mandible	Opens midway between the upper and lower borders	Placed near the alveolar margin

Table 36.24: Differences between bruise and hypostasis

Traits	Bruise	Hypostasis
1. Nature of distribution	It is always superficial being confined to epidermis as the area of skin discolouration. When hypostasis gets fixed, the discolouration of skin is due to staining of tissues from haemolysis.	It always lies under the epidermis in between layers of dermis, deep burises may further lie deep still
2. Situation	It may occur anywhere on the body depending on the area of its infliction, but is usually seen over prominent body parts	It occurs in the dependent part of the body, appearing first in patches later on coalescing together to spread over a wide area
3. Appearance	Bruised area is raised above its surroundings, due to extravasation and oedematous swelling of tissue under seat of violence. It usually takes the shape and pattern of the weapon used	Hypostatic area always flush with body surface, is never swollen, as the blood is still inside the vessels or has stained overlying skin tissue. It does not take any shape or pattern except that due to position from lying on a particular place or surface
4. Margins	Its edges and margins are never well defined, because of the tissue reaction as per age of the injury	Margins of hypostasis are always sharply defined specially over those adjacent to area of contact flattening
5. Nature	Bruising in the areas of contact flattening remains red and shows tissue reaction as to its age	Hypostasis is absent in the areas of contact flattening
6. Changes due to altered position	Change of position of body, has no part to play	Position of hypostasis may get altered with changed position of the body, before it is 'fixed' before 6 to 8 hours after death
7. Associated findings	Overlying abrasion resulting from the same trauma that cause bruise, may be present together	Not likely to have overlying abrasion accompanying, unless present from before
8. Colour	Colour change indicative of vital reaction present in and around the bruise due to the extravasated blood and its haemoglobin	The colour of hypostasis is uniform and depends upon its cause. Colour green on onset of putrefaction, on blood decomposing, its colouring matter permeates into surrounding tissue producing general discolouration. In advanced putrefaction, it is difficult to distinguish between bruise and hypostasis by histological examination of tissue it is possible

(Contd.)

Table 36.24: Differences between bruise and hypostasis *(Contd.)*

Traits	Bruise	Hypostasis
9. Effect of pressure	Pressure makes it lighter than the rest of the bruised area	Colour of hypostasis "blanches" on application of pressure and reappears on its release
10. On section	On incision shows extravasation and infiltration in and around the seat of bruising with fluid blood this cannot be washed by washing with a stream of water	On incision, liquid blood oozes out of the cut ends of capillaries and venules and this blood can be easily washed out with gentle stream of water. There is no evidence of extravasation and infiltration of tissue with fluid or clotted blood in and around

Table 36.25: Differences between postmortem blister and antemortem blister

Postmortem blister	Antemortem blister
1. Contents: It contains large amount of putrefying gases, a little or no liquid. If fluid is present, it is never inflammatory in nature; hence contains very little albumin; may look reddish tinged from decomposing blood	1. Contains inflammatory fluid which is rich in albumin; is little turbid in colour amount being large enough to keep the blisters turgescent
2. Inflammatory ring: There is no red ring of inflammation around the margins of postmortem blister	2. There is invariably a red ring of inflammatory zone around the margin of the blister
3. Base: The base of postmortem blister is usually white and glistening, except when the decomposition is advanced in nature	3. The base of antemortem blister is dull, congested and oedematous
4. Vital reaction: No such evidence is ever noted in case of postmortem blister	4. There will be evidence of inflammation and repair in and around the blister
5. Other evidences: No evidence of such is expected in postmortem blisters at all. Evidence of other putrefactive changes will be all apparent	5. Evidence of burning, singeing of hair, trickling down of fluid, smell of burning flesh and body tissues may all be evident in blisters of antemortem burns

Table 36.26: Differences between gangrene and putrefaction

Gangrene	Putrefaction
1. Usually pus formation is a feature	1. No pus is formed
2. Sign of inflammation and repair are present invariably	2. No evidence of inflammation and repair present as it is a postmortem phenomenon
3. There is always a line of demarcation between living and dead tissue	3. No line of demarcation between the living and dead tissue
4. Localised feature of gangrene with no evidence of generalised putrefaction	4. Features of putrefaction will be manifested all over the body

Table 36.27: Differences between postmortem abrasion and antemortem abrasion

Postmortem abrasion	Antemortem abrasion
1. Appears brown and parchment like	1. Looks brownish or reddish in colour
2. No scab formation	2. Scab formation noticed
3. No bleeding	3. May show bleeding surface, when fresh.
4. Nore pair	4. Healing changes evident
5. Seen over bony prominence	5. Seen on any part of body
6. Surface looks dry; there is no evidence of bleeding or exudation of serum and blood	6. Surface feels moist from exudation of serum and blood

Table 36.28: Differences between incised wound and lacerated wound

Incised wound	Lacerated wound
1. **Manner of production:** Caused by weapons with sharp cutting edges	1. Caused by blunt weapons
2. **Situation:** Any where on the body	2. Over bony prominences
3. **Shape, gaping of wound:** Usually linear or fusiform shaped, gaping is common	3. Usually irregular, varies as per causative agent, gaping uncommon
4. **Margins:** Regular, clean cut, smooth and everted	4. Ragged, irregular, uneven and often undermined, accompanied with bruising and abrasions
5. **Dimension:** Length is greater than the depth and breadth. Deeper tissues cleanly cut and evenly divided; may gap deeply, in cut throat injuries	5. Shallow or in deep with gaping and irregular margins
6. **Condition of tissues surrounding or underneath:** Soft tissue underneath clean cut hairs and hair bulbs clean cut. Bones cut with cut ends showing comminuted and fissured fractures depending upon force	6. Soft tissues underneath show tearing and spliting strands of tissue bridging between the margins. Exposed hair and hair bulbs crushed cut
7. **Bleeding:** Profuse, spurting of blood common	7. Not pronounced; spurting of blood uncommon
8. **Other features:** Tentative cuts and tailing of the wound are seen	8. Tentative cuts, tailing of the wound not noticed
9. **Multiplicity:** Multiple superficial incised wounds over accessible body parts, suggest suicidal infliction; multiple deep incised wounds over different body parts with defence wounds indicate homicidal nature	9. Multiple lacerated wounds with bruised and abrasions over different parts of the body indicate traffic accidents or fall from a height, assaults by several persons, extensive lacerated wounds with fracture of bones over vital body parts suggest homicide
10. **Complications:** Due to severe haemorrhage with shock; involvement of vital organs deaths	10. Sepsis haemorrhage vital organ damage
11. **Foreign matter:** Not common	11. Trace evidence left in the wounds, connects the crime with the offending object and place of occurrence
12. **Wearing:** Covering over the affected site, usually show corresponding cuts on clothings; when garment is loose or folded, there may be multiple cuts on the clothing	12. Coverings over the affected site

Table 36.29: Differences between chilly seeds and *dhatura* seeds

Chilly seeds	Dhatura seeds
1. Yellow in colour	1. Brown in colour
2. Round in shape	2. Kidney shaped
3. Pungent smell	3. No smell
4. Convex border is single edged	4. Convex border is double edged
5. Embryo of seed is turned inwards	5. Embryo turned outwards

Table 36.30: Differences between rigor mortis and cadaveric spasm

Rigor mortis	Cadaveric spasm
1. Onset: 3–6 hours after death	1. Instantaneous
2. Occurs all over the body	2. Occurs in small group of muscles
3. Involves both voluntary and involuntary muscles	3. Involves only voluntary muscles
4. Seen in all deaths	4. Not seen in all deaths
5. Underlying mechanism known	5. Mechanism not clear

Table 36.31: Differences between firearm entry wound and firearm exit wound

Entry wound (firearm)	Exit wound (firearm)
1. Small with regular **edges**	1. Large with irregular **edges**
2. Margins **inverted**	2. Margins **everted**
3. Margins abraded	3. No abrasions
4. **Grease collar** seen	4. No grease collar
5. **Burning, snigeing** and **tattooing** present	5. Absent
6. Bleeding is **slight**	6. Bleeding is **more**
7. **Radiography** reveals lead ring	7. No such lead/metal ring

Table 36.32: Differences between arsenic poisoning and cholera

Arsenic poisoning	Cholera
1. Vomiting followed by diarrhoea	1. Diarrhoea followed by vomiting
2. Eyes congested	2. No such congestion
3. Initially rice water stools followed by bloody diarrhoea	3. Rice water stools throughout
4. Tenesmus prominent	4. No tenesmus
5. Arsenic positive	5. *V. cholerae* positive

Table 36.33: Differences between hanging and strangulation

Hanging	Strangulation
1. Usually suicidal	1. Usually homicidal
2. Ligature mark oblique, above thyroid cartilage in front and deficient over site of knot	2. Ligature mark transverse, complete, at or below the level of thyroid cartilage
3. Neck usually stretched	3. Not stretched
4. Dissection of ligature mark reveals dry glistening tissue	4. Neck tissues ecchymosis
5. Saliva running out through either angle of mouth	5. No such dribbling of saliva

Table 36.34: Differences between strychnine poisoning and tetanus

Strychnine poisoning	Tetanus
1. No **history** of injury	1. History of injury
2. Onset **sudden**	2. Onset **gradual**
3. All **muscles of body** involved simultaneously	3. **Lock jaw** prominent
4. Convulsions **tonic-clonic**	4. Convulsions **tonic**
5. Rapidly fatal	5. Not so

Table 36.35: Differences between poisonous snakes and nonpoisonous snakes

Poisonous snakes	Nonpoisonous snakes
1. **Tail**: Compressed, flat	1. Rounded
2. **Fangs**: Long and hollow	2. Short and solid
3. **Bite marks**: Two clear puncture wounds with/without small teeth marks	3. A number of small teeth marks in a row
4. **Oedema** and discolouration at the site of bite	4. No **oedema**/discolouration

Table 36.36: Differences between antemortem wound and postmortem wound

Antemortem wound	Postmortem wound
1. Copious haemorrhage	1. A little or no haemorrhage
2. Stained edges, not removed by washing	2. Stained edges removed by washing
3. Gaping present	3. Gaping absent
4. Signs of repair present	4. No signs of repair
5. Enzyme histochemistry positive	5. Enzyme histochemistry negative

Table 36.37: Common domestic poisons

1. Depilatories	1. Barium sulphide, thallium
2. Nail polish removers	2. Acetone
3. Sun-tan lotion	3. Denatured alcohol, methyl salicylate
4. Baby powder	4. Boric acid
5. Baking powder	5. Tartaric acid (50%)
6. Baking soda	6. Sodium bicarbonate
7. Dish washers	7. Sodium polyphosphates, sodium carbonates
8. Fire extinguishing fluids	8. Carbon tetrachloride, methyl bromide
9. Matches	9. Antimony, phosphorus, potassium chlorate
10. Rat paste	10. Aluminium phosphide, zinc sulphide, arsenious oxide, zinc phosphide

Table 36.38: Differences between apoplexy haemorrhage and post-traumatic haemorrhage

Apoplexy haemorrhage	Post-traumatic haemorrhage
1. Caused by hypertension/atherosclerosis	1. Caused by head injury
2. Seen in elderly	2. May be seen at all ages
3. Usually occurs in ganglionic region	3. White matter or temporoparietal region
4. No contrecoup haemorrhage	4. Contrecoup haemorrhage may be present

Table 36.39: Differences between virginity and defloration

Virginity	Defloration
1. **Labia majora:** Developed, in apposition completely close vaginal orifice	1. Not in apposition, vaginal orifice may be seen
2. **Labia minora:** In contact and fully covered by labia majora	2. Not in contact; can be seen through labia majora
3. **Hymen:** Intact, inelastic and rigid, margins regular, Admits only tip of little finger	3. Intact loose and elastic; allows passage of two or more fingers
4. **Vagina:** Narrow, rugose, vault is more conical	4. Grows in length, smooth
5. **Fossa navicularis:** Intact	5. Disappears
6. **Fourchette:** Intact	6. Usually torn

Table 36.40: Differences between true bruise and artificial bruise

True bruise	Artificial bruise
1. Produced by trauma	1. Produced by juice of marking nut, calotropis, plumbago rosea
2. Seen anywhere	2. Commonly on exposed parts
3. Margins irregular and ill-defined	3. Margins regular, well defined, surrounded by tiny vesicles
4. No itching	4. Itching present
5. No vesicles on fingertips	5. Vesicles on fingertips present
6. Chemical tests negative	6. Chemical test positive

Table 36.41: Differences between suicidal wounds and homicidal wounds

Suicidal wounds	Homicidal wounds
1. Seen usually on accessible body areas	1. Seen anywhere
2. Usually superficial	2. Usually deep
3. Multiple hesitation cuts present over other parts of body	3. Cut absent
4. Tailing present in incised wounds	4. May be absent
5. Weapon present	5. Present or absent

Table 36.42: PNDT Act: Indications and contraindications

Indications	Contraindications
• Congenital anomalies	• Pregnant woman
• Chromosomal anomalies	– >35 years of age
• Genetic metabolic diseases	– Has undergone two or more spontaneous of abortions or fetal loss
• Sex-linked genetic diseases	– Has been exposed to teratogenic agent Q as drug radiation infection and chemical
• Haemoglobinopathies	– Has family history of mental retardation or physical deformity such as plasticity or any other genetic diseases
• Any other diseases may be specified by the Central Supervisory Board	

Table 36.43: Methods of torture

By	Beating
Falanga/Falaka/Baatinada	Beating on soles of feet with blunt object
El-Telefono	Simultaneous beating of both ears with palms of hands
El-Quirofano	Beating on abdomen while upper half of body lying unsupported on table
	Electricity
Piacana	Placing electric wires in vagina, anus, mouth or over nipples and testicles
Black slave	Heated metal skewer inserted into anus
	Near suffocation
Dry submarine	Tying a plastic bag covering head and face
Wet submarine, Labaneva, Latina, Pileta	Forced immersion of victim's head in water, often contaminated with urine, vomit or blood

Table 36.44: Methods of torture by suspension

La-Bandera	By wrist
Mercelago	By ankles
Forced postures	
El-Planton	Prolonged standing
El-Cabellete or Sawhorse	Forced straddling of a bar
Parrot's perch, Jack, Paude Grava	Head down, by a horizontal pole placed under knees, with the wrists bounds to the ankles
Chepuwa	Tight clamping of thighs or legs with bamboo, and the torturer may press two sides of clamps with his legs or may stand on two sides of clamps. Practiced on Bhutanese refugees in Nepal

Table 36.45: Odour of poison

Poison	Odour
H_2S (Hydrogen sulphide)	Rotten egg
Zinc phosphide	Fishy
Arsenic zinc phosphide, aluminium phosphide (celphos)	Garlic odour
Ethyl alcohol	Fruity
Cyanide	Bitter almonds
Organophosphates and kerosene	Kerosene-like
Carbolic acid	Phenolic
Cannabis	Burnt rope

Case Studies

EXAMINATION OF VICTIM OF SEXUAL OFFENCE

Ms A, a 19-year-old girl living in Housing Board quarters, is a vendor in the local market, selling bangles, chains, etc. Four days back, her mother found that she did not go to work but was with Mr B, 26-year-old man. That evening she did not come home and her parents gave the report "Girl missing" to the local police station. Today, she was apprehended by the police and the findings of the lady medical officer, who examined her are:

- Well nourished female.
- No injuries seen anywhere on the body.

Examination of Genitals

Vulva   : Normal
Vagina   : Normal

Hymen   : Old healed tears at 3.6 and 9'o clock position.

Perineum   : Intact

Fourchette : Normal

Note: Vaginal and cervical smears show motile spermatozoa.

Examine the Victim and Issue the Certificate

1. Can Ms A give a legally valid consent for sexual act? Yes/No
2. Can a male medical officer examine Ms A? Yes/No
3. What the healed tears hymen suggest? Sexual intercourse/rape?
4. What is the significance of motile spermatozoa? Recent sexual intercourse/delayed?

EXAMINATION OF VICTIM OF SEXUAL OFFENCE

Ms C, 15-year-old girl, daughter of Mr D was married to a 21-year-old man. He took her with him to a picnic place. At that place he was alleged to have sexually assaulted her and presented by the police patrol party for medical examination. The findings of the lady medical officer who examined her are:

1. Semilunar 2 mm sized contused abrasion red in colour on the aerola of both breast.
2. Scratches on the inner aspect of both thighs.

Examination of Genitals

Vulva   : Red and tender
Vagina   : Red and tender
Hymen   : Clotted blood, tears at 3.6 and 9'o clock positions
Perineum   : Intact
Fourchette : Normal

Examine the Victim and Issue the Certificate

1. Mrs C is wife of a 21-year-old man. Can the husband be charged for the rape? Yes/No
2. What do genital findings suggest? Assault/No crime

CASE STUDY 3

CASE STUDY 3

EXAMINATION OF VICTIM OF SEXUAL OFFENCE

Ms E, an 18-year-old girl was returning home from college. A resident of their locality known to her, came in an auto with three accomplices forcibly made the girl get into the auto, took her to a remote area outside the town. She was molested, and the following injuries were noted during examination, by the lady medical officer.

1. Contusion 4 × 4 cm on right cheek
2. Swelling of the upper lip
3. Abrasion 7 × 3 cm upper part of right side of back
4. Abrasion 4 × 2 cm on back of left elbow.
5. Multiple discoid contusions of 2 × 2 cm present around both wrists.

Examination of Genitals

Vulva   : Red and tenderness present
Vagina   : Red and tender
Hymen   : Blood clots present, tears at 3 and 6'o clock position
Perineum   : Intact
Fourchette   : Normal

Examine the Victim and Issue the Certificate

1. Injury number 5 is caused by? Cigarette butts/heated ladle
2. Is it statutory rape? Yes/No
3. What is the present rape called? Group rape/gang rape.

CASE STUDY 4

EXAMINATION OF INJURED PERSON

Mr K, 28-year-old is brought to the casualty by his wife along with P.C. no. 625 with the history of assault by two known persons, due to previous enmity with a log of wood and knife at his residence at 7.00 AM.

Identification Marks

1. A 0.2 cm diameter black-coloured mole without hair on the inner side of left forearm at about 2 cm from the wrist joint.
2. A 0.1 cm diameter black-coloured mole without hair on the right side of forehead above the right eyebrow at a distance of 2 cm.

The following Injuries were seen on the Victim

1. Contused laceration 2 × 1 × 0.5 cm on the inner aspect of right side of lower lip with partly broken canine tooth.

2. An incised wound 2.5 × 1 cm front of abdomen 5 cm to navel at 3° clock position.
3. An incised wound 6 × 2 × 1 cm, 6 cm below sternum in middle line of the abdomen, angled, towards the right and directed from above downwards.
4. Reddish contusion 8 × 4 cm with swelling on the lateral aspect of middle of right forearm. X-ray of right forearm: Fracture middle third of right radius.
5. A lacerated wound 5 × 2 cm bone deep on the left side of forehead, vertically placed, upper end at the hairline and lower end touching the inner end of the left eyebrow.

Examine the Victim and Issue the Certificate

Injury number 1: Simple/grievous injury. Number 3: Simple/grievous injury. Number 5 caused by logwood/knife.

CASE STUDY 5

EXAMINATION OF INJURED PERSON

A young adult named Mr L about 20 years was brought to the casualty by P.C. no. 354 with a history of assault during a quarrel with the neighbours. The injuries were said to be caused by a hockey stick and a vegetable knife. The following identification marks were seen on the victim.

- A 0.2 cm diameter black-coloured mole with hair on the medial aspect of left forearm at a distance of 4 cm from wrist.
- A old healed scar triangular in shape measuring 1.5 × 1.5 × 1 cm at the medial side of elbow joint.

The following Injuries were seen on the Victim

1. Multiple linear abrasions of 1.5 × 0.5 cm each red in colour, on the medial aspect of right forearm in its upper one third.
2. 4 × 3 cm reddish contusion on the front of the chest running from a point 3 cm below the angle of sternum going obliquely downwards to the right.
3. An incised wound 2.5 × 1.25 × 1.25 cm over the forehead just above the right eyebrow.
4. A linear abrasion which is red in colour, 2.25 × 0.25 cm over the left shoulder blade towards its lower part.
5. Reddish contusion 5 × 5 cm on the lateral aspect of left forearm, at a distance of 6 cm below the elbow joint with swelling and deformity present.

Examine the Victim and Issue the Wound Certificate

1. Which injuries are caused by vegetable knife? 1/2/3/4/5
2. Which injuries are caused by hockey stick? 1/2/3/4/5

CASE STUDY 6

EXAMINATION OF INJURED PERSON

Mr M, 27-year-old is brought to the casualty by P.C. no. 701, with the history of assault by blade while going to his workplace.

Identification Marks

- A scar 2.5 cm in length and 0.5 cm in breath, on the left side of forehead just above the eyebrow.
- A 0.2 cm diameter black-coloured mole with no hair on the back side of right little finger near the nail bed.

The following Injuries are seen on the Victim

1. Two vertical linear cuts each 1.5 × 0.5 cm and 0.5 cm apart on the left side of the chest above the left nipple.
2. Two vertical superficial incised wounds, measuring 2.5 × 0.5 cm and 1 cm apart along the inner border of upper part of the right thigh.
3. A reddish abrasion 3 × 2 cm on the right side of chest 4 cm from nipple at 11° clock position.
4. Reddish contusion of 5 × 3 cm on the right cheek.
5. Multiple contusions and abrasions of 0.5 to 1 × 0.5 to 1 cm each. On the right hand over the knuckles of 4th and 5th fingers and was unable to move his fingers.
6. Linear parallel incised wounds four in number measuring 1 to 2 × 0.25 to 5 × 0.25 cm, 0.5 cm apart on the left cheek bleeding present.

Examine the Victim and Issue the Certificate

1. Are they self-inflicted injuries? Right/ Wrong
2. Are all injuries possible by blade? Yes/No
3. Are injuries 4 and 5 caused by? Blow/ friction

CASE STUDY 7

CERTIFICATE FOR DRUNKENNESS

Mr X, a 27-year-old male working in the harbour was brought today at 11:00 AM to the casualty department of government hospital with the history that he was found smelling of alcohol while working as a mechanic in the Power Room. He was brought by P.C. no. 111 of harbour Police Station.

Identification Marks

1. A black mole on the back of wrist of left hand.
2. A scar of 1 × 1 cm on the front of right forearm.

On Examination

- Patient was abusive and shouting
- Breath smells of alcohol
- Face dirty
- Clothing shows dried vomitus
- Unable to tell name and address
- Eyelids swollen, conjunctiva congested
- Papillary reaction to light is sluggish
- He could not stand and was staggering.

Examine the Subject and Issue the Certificate

Finding suggests

a. Not under influence of alcohol. Right/ Wrong
b. Under influence of alcohol. Right/Wrong

CASE STUDY 8

CERTIFICATE FOR DRUNKENNESS

Inspector of police brought Mr Y, aged 31 years, a driver today at 2:00 PM with the history that while patrolling traffic and checking vehicles, he was found driving the car and he was alleged to have assaulted the police constable who stopped the car for checking.

Identification Marks

1. A black mole on the left side of forehead
2. A scar 2 cm below the right ear.

On Examination

- Patient conscious
- Breath smells of alcohol
- Eyes congested
- Uniform: Dressed properly
- Cooperative during examination
- Speech: Normal
- Able to walk properly
- Reflexes are normal
- Voluntarily submitted for an examination.

Examine the Subject and Issue the Certificate

1. Consumed alcohol, not under influence. Right/Wrong
2. Consumed alcohol, under influence. Right/Wrong

CASE STUDY 9

CERTIFICATE FOR DRUNKENNESS

Mrs Z aged 35 years, at around 10:30 AM this day, was brought to the casualty of government hospital, by W.P.C. 16 of Mahila P.S., with the history of possessing arrack packets.

Identification Marks

1. A black mole on the left side of chin.
2. A scar of 1 × 1 cm on the right side of forehead.

On Examination

- Patient is cooperative
- She stated her address
- She wrote down her name and signed
- Breath does not smell of alcohol
- Eyes: Normal
- Gait: Normal
- Speech: Normal
- Reflexes: Normal
- Muscular
- Coordination: Able to perform simple tests
- No signs or symptoms of any disease.

Examine the Subject and Issue the Certificate

1. Mrs Z not consumed alcohol, not under influence. True/False
2. Mrs Z consumed alcohol, not under influence. True/False

MCQs Revision Test

1. Forensic medicine means:
a. Knowledge of law required for physicians
b. Knowledge of medicine required for lawyers
c. Knowledge of all medical sciences used in a Court of Law for administration of justice
d. Knowledge of law and medicine required for lawyers

2. Medical jurisprudence means:
a. Knowledge of medicine required for lawyers
b. Knowledge of law required for doctors for proper medical practice
c. Knowledge of medicine required by doctors for practice
d. Knowledge of law required for legal practice

3. Forensic toxicology means:
a. Knowledge of poisons required for a forensic scientist
b. Knowledge of poisons required for a medical man
c. Knowledge of poisons utilized in administration of justice
d. Knowledge of all aspects of substances causing disease, deformity or death, utilized in a court of law for administration justice

4. Leading question is one:
a. Put by defense lawyer
b. Put by prosecuting lawyer
c. Which suggests its own answer
d. None of the above

5. Purpose of taking oath is:
a. To speak truth
b. To speak truth and nothing but truth
c. To speak truth, whole truth and nothing but truth
d. To compel the witness to speak truth, the whole truth and nothing but truth

6. Professional secrets can be divulged in court:
a. If doctor feels so
b. Cannot be divulged
c. Can be divulged, if asked by court
d. Can be divulged, if pressed by the court and under protest

7. The medical council of India
a. Regulates medical education in India
b. Punishes the erring registered medical practitioners
c. Carries inspection for National Board of Examinations
d. None of the above

8. Example of "Res Ipsa Loquitur":
a. Operation of hydrocele
b. Operation on young patient
c. Operation on wrong side
d. None of the above

9. Medical negligence in criminal law is tried under Section:
a. 319 of IPC
b. 302 of IPC
c. 309 of IPC
d. 304 A of IPC

10. Prenatal diagnostic tests are permitted for purpose of detection of:
a. Sex of foetus
b. Sex-linked genetic diseases
c. When woman is below 35 years
d. When the woman did not have any abortion

11. **Death is declared when:**
    a. The heart sounds are not heard
    b. The pain reflex is not elicited
    c. All brain stem reflexes are absent
    d. When the person does not respond to shouting his name

12. **The following is not a mode of death:**
    a. Coma   b. Syncope
    c. Asphyxia   d. Shock

13. **Physical torture includes:**
    a. Twisting the nails
    b. Humiliation
    c. Disinformation
    d. Any of the above

14. **Dry waste is disposed in:**
    a. Black bags   b. Yellow bags
    c. Red bags   d. Blue bags

15. **Ear torture is called:**
    a. Dry submarine
    b. Telephony
    c. Falanga
    d. la Bandera

16. **Beating the soles of the feet is called:**
    a. Bastinado
    b. Wet submarine
    c. Sawhorse
    d. la Picana

17. **MTP is carried out in case of:**
    a. Pregnancy followed by rape
    b. Any pregnancy
    c. Only in married woman
    d. Below 30 years only

18. **AIH is done:**
    a. If the husband is impotent
    b. If the husband is infertile
    c. If there is Rh incompatibility
    d. None of the above

19. **Surrogacy is advocated if:**
    a. Woman has repeated abortions
    b. If the woman has pelvic infection
    c. If the woman does not want to bear pregnancy
    d. If the woman is below 30 years

20. **Surgical reason for death on operation table:**
    a. Cutting large vessels
    b. Giving anaesthesia to wrong patient
    c. Wrong posture of the patient
    d. Choosing wrong anaesthetic agent

21. **Bumper fractures are seen in the cases of:**
    a. Fall from height
    b. Vehicular accident
    c. Domestic accident
    d. None of the above

22. **Pond fracture is seen in cases of:**
    a. Children below 5 years
    b. Teenagers
    c. Adults
    d. Elderly people

23. **Postmortem wounds do not show changes of:**
    a. Vital reactions
    b. Infection
    c. Gaping
    d. Any of the above

24. **Ant bites are mistaken for:**
    a. Lacerations
    b. Abrasions
    c. Incised wounds
    d. Contusions

25. **Injuries on the clothes:**
    a. Always correspond to injuries on the body
    b. Generally correspond to injuries on the body
    c. Never correspond to injuries on the body
    d. Sometimes do not correspond with injuries on the body

26. **Diastatic fracture is:**
    a. Postmortem fracture
    b. Suture separation
    c. Separation of diaphysis
    d. Rupture of diaphragm

27. **A black contusion, after death:**
    a. Remains black
    b. Becomes yellow

c. Gets infected

d. None of the above

28. Heaping up of epithelium suggests:

a. Beginning of abrasion

b. Middle of abrasion

c. End of the abrasions

d. No abrasion

29. Deep bruises can be demonstrated by:

a. Dissection

b. X-ray examination

c. Aspiration

d. Any of the above

30. Tailing of the wound suggests:

a. Beginning of the wound

b. Middle of the wound

c. End of the wound

d. Any of the above

31. Decomposition takes longer time in the:

a. Air   b. Water

c. Earth   d. In a closed room

32. Presence of maggots on the body suggests after death a lapse of:

a. Below 2 days

b. Below 3 days

c. Below 4 days

d. Below 5 days

33. Adipocere suggests that:

a. Dead body was in marshy place

b. Dead body was in air-conditioned room

c. Dead body was covered with blankets

d. None of the above

34. The earliest site of decomposition in internal organs is:

a. Ascending aorta

b. Left ventricle

c. Portal vein

d. Inferior vena cava

35. The death rattle is due to:

a. Mucus in the oesophagus

b. Mucus in respiratory passages

c. Irregular breathing

d. Any of the above

36. In brain stem death:

a. There is no corneal reflex

b. The oculo-cephalic reflex is absent

c. Vestibulo-ocular reflex is absent

d. All of the above

37. The rate of fall of temperature in first six hours after death in a temperate climate is approximately:

a. 1.5°F/hour

b. 1.5°C/hour

c. 1.5°R/hour

d. 2.5°C/hour

38. Postmortem caloricity is due to:

a. Yellow fever

b. Sun stroke

c. Cerebrospinal meningitis

d. All of the above

39. Pain in burns is due to:

a. Nerve endings

b. Coagulation of muscle proteins

c. Loss of fluid

d. None of the above

40. Antemortem burns can show:

a. Line of redness

b. Singeing of hair

c. Carbon monoxide in blood

d. All of the above

41. In hanging the constricting force is:

a. Ligature

b. Weight of the body

c. Height of the body

d. Any of the above

42. In strangulation asphyxia is due to:

a. Pressure around neck

b. Lump in the throat

c. Stricture of oesophagus

d. Any of the above

43. Salivary stains around the angle of mouth suggest:

a. Antemortem hanging

b. Antemortem burns

c. Antemortem drowning

d. None of the above

44. The following is not a type of asphyxial death:

a. Strangulation   b. Starvation

c. Hanging   d. Lynching

45. Whiplash injury is due to:

a. Hyperflexion

b. Hyperextension

c. a and b

d. None of the above

46. Steering wheel impact cases:

a. Ruptured aorta

b. Buckled sternum

c. Myocardial trauma

d. Any of the above

47. Lucid interval is seen in:

a. Extradural haemorrage

b. Subdural haemorrage

c. Subarachnoid haemorrage

d. Intracerebral haemorrage

48. Ectopic contusion normally occurs around the:

a. Nose   b. Orbit

c. Ear   d. Any of the above

49. Presence of semen in the vaginal canal is a proof of:

a. Rape

b. Sexual intercourse

c. Indecent assault

d. Attempted rape

50. Shaving of the perianal hair is suggestive of:

a. Habitual passive agent

b. Habitual active agent

c. Rapist

d. None of the above

51. Presence of smegma:

a. Suggests sexual intercourse

b. Rules out sexual intercourse

c. Suggests rape

d. None of the above

52. Paederasty means:

a. Sexual intercourse with a girl

b. Sexual intercourse with woman

c. Anal sexual intercourse with a small boy

d. Sexual intercourse with animal

53. Female homosexuality is called:

a. Transvestism

b. Transsexualism

c. Tribadism

d. Satyriasis

54. Highest resistance to electricity is offered by:

a. Skin

b. Muscles

c. Blood

d. Nerve tissue

55. Pain in burns is due to:

a. Nerve endings

b. Coagulation of muscle proteins

c. Loss of fluid

d. None of the above

56. The following is not a sexual deviation:

a. Sadism   b. Masochism

c. Rape   d. Transvestism

57. Death during sexual intercourse can be due to:

a. Bleeding

b. Vagal inhabitation

c. Pressure on the neck

d. Any of the above

58. Intact hymen suggests:

a. Virgin

b. False virgin

c. Attempted rape

d. Any of the above

59. Sudden infant death syndrome is due to:

a. Respiratory viral infection

b. Prolonged sleep apnoea

c. Hypersensitivity reaction

d. Any of the above

60. Quickening is due to:

a. Foetal movement

b. Intestinal movements

c. Flatulence

d. Any of the above

61. Spalding sign suggests:
   a. Foetal distress
   b. Foetal death
   c. Foetal abnormality
   d. Live foetus

62. Hasse's rule helps in determination of:
   a. Duration of pregnancy
   b. Age of foetus
   c. Nature of placenta
   d. Ectopic pregnancy

63. In battered baby syndrome:
   a. Child is below one year
   b. There are multiple fractures of different ages
   c. History does not suggest trauma
   d. All of the above

64. Positive sign of pregnancy is:
   a. Fetal heart sounds
   b. Skin pigmentation
   c. Ballottement
   d. Any of the above

65. Precipitate labour occurs when:
   a. Baby is small
   b. The vagina is roomy
   c. Uterine contractions are powerful
   d. All of the above

66. Viable foetus:
   a. Is 7-month-old
   b. Has papillary membrane
   c. Eyebrows are absent
   d. Nails are not formed

67. A bastard child means:
   a. Legitimate child
   b. Illegitimate child
   c. Child after pregnancy following rape
   d. Within wedlock

68. Infant is a child below the age of:
   a. 1 month   b. 6 months
   c. 1 year   d. 2 years

69. *Dhatura* seeds have:
   a. Convex border with single edge
   b. Convex border with double edge
   c. Convex border with no edge
   d. Concave border with double edge

70. Tannic acid precipitates:
   a. Alkaloids
   b. Glycosides
   c. Many of the metals
   d. All of the above

71. Antidote for acute phosphorus poisoning is:
   a. 0.1% $CuSO_4$ solution
   b. 0.2% $CuSO_4$ solution
   c. 2% H_2O_2 solution
   d. Egg

72. In acute phosphorus poisoning necrobiosis is seen in:
   a. Heart
   b. Kidneys
   c. Liver
   d. Any of the above

73. Metal fume fever is caused by:
   a. Aluminium   b. Zinc
   c. Mercury   d. Magnesium

74. Baygon belongs to:
   a. Organochlorines
   b. Alkyl phosphates
   c. Aryl phosphates
   d. Carbamates

75. Antidote in acute arsenic poisoning is:
   a. Copper sulphate
   b. Freshly prepared permanganate solution
   c. Freshly prepared hydrated ferric oxide solution
   d. Aluminium hydroxide

76. The alcohol content of absolute alcohol is:
   a. 100%   b. 90%
   c. 95%   d. 99.95%

77. Reefers are made from:
   a. Tobacco
   b. *Dhatura*
   c. Cannabis
   d. Calotropis

78. **Dilated pupils are seen in:**
    a. Cocaine poisoning
    b. Alcoholic intoxication
    c. Pethidine poisoning
    d. Any of the above

79. **Botulism is:**
    a. Infection   b. Intoxication
    c. Infestation   d. Toxaemia

80. **Lathyrism causes:**
    a. Paralysis   b. Arthritis
    c. Carditis   d. Bronchitis

81. **The alkaloid in argemone oil is:**
    a. Sanguinarine
    b. Berberin
    c. Protopin
    d. None of the above

82. **Marking nut juice causes:**
    a. Abrasion   b. Laceration
    c. Contusion   d. Artificial bruise

83. **The poison glands of snake are modified:**
    a. Salivary glands
    b. Sweat glands
    c. Sebaceous glands
    d. None of the above

84. **The king cobra has:**
    a. Hood with no mark
    b. Hood with binocular mark
    c. Hood with monocellate mark
    d. None of the above

85. **If the third supralabial touches the eye and the nasal shield, the snake is:**
    a. Non-poisonous
    b. Krait
    c. Viper
    d. Cobra

86. **The active principle of spanish fly is:**
    a. Cantharidin   b. Calotropin
    c. Cocaine   d. Capsaicin

87. **Abrin resembles:**
    a. Cobra venom
    b. Scorpion venom
    c. Viper venom
    d. None of the above

88. **The following is not a war gas:**
    a. Mustard gas
    b. Phosgene
    c. Chloropicrine
    d. Sulphur dioxide (SO_2)

89. **Exceptions to oral evidence:**
    a. Death certificate
    b. Postmortem report
    c. Evidence recorded in lower court
    d. None of the above

90. **Perjury means:**
    a. Breaking the oath
    b. Speaking the truth
    c. Submitting a document
    d. Not attending personally in court

91. **The best form of inquest is:**
    a. Police
    b. Coroner's
    c. Magistrate's
    d. Medical examiner system

92. **Conduct money is tendered in:**
    a. Summons from civil court
    b. Summons from criminal court
    c. Summons from the coroner
    d. Money paid by the appointing authority

93. **Hostile witness is one who:**
    a. Hosts the witness
    b. Does not answer leading questions
    c. Who deliberately utters falsehood
    d. All of the above

94. **Following punishment is removed in India:**
    a. Death sentence
    b. Simple/rigorous imprisonment
    c. Life imprisonment
    d. Whipping

95. **Cephalic index means:**
    a. Max. breadth of skull
    b. Max. length of skull × 100 × Max. length of skull × Max. breadth of skull
    c. Max. length of skull
    d. Max. breadth of skull × 100 × Max. breadth of skull × Max. length of skull

96. Cephalic index of Europeans is:
a. 70–74.9	b. 75–79.9
c. 80–84.9	d. None of the above

97. The chromosomes in human beings are normally:
a. 22 pairs	b. 44 pairs
c. 23 pairs	d. 46 pairs

98. In comparison of males, cranial capacity of females is:
a. 10% more	b. 10% less
c. 5% more	d. 5% less

99. Ramus of mandible in males is:
a. Inverted	b. Everted
c. Straight	d. None of the above

100. The chromosomal pattern of Turner's syndrome is:
a. 46, XY	b. 45, XO
c. 46, XX	d. 45, YO

101. Re-examination is carried out by:
a. Lawyer conducting main examination
b. Lawyer conducting cross examination
c. Presiding officer of court
d. None of the above

102. The overlying skin is intact in cases of:
a. Bruise
b. Abrasion
c. Ligature marks
d. None of the above

103. Colour changes in bruise are due to changes in:
a. Haemoglobin	b. Albumin
c. Globulin	d. Plasma

104. Infections are more common in:
a. Abrasions
b. Lacerations
c. Incised wounds
d. Any of the above

105. Scratch is a type of:
a. Contusion
b. Laceration
c. Abrasion
d. Incised wound

106. False bruises are caused by:
a. Juice of marking nut
b. Root of *chitra*
c. *Lal chitra*
d. All of the above

107. In police custody deaths, the postmortem examination requires to be:
a. Radiographed
b. Photographed
c. Videographed
d. None of the above

108. The main objective of medicolegal autopsy is:
a. To help investigating officer
b. To establish cause of death
c. To demonstrate to medical students
d. To train doctors

109. Rifling is seen:
a. On the bullet
b. On the barrel
c. Inside the barrel
d. Inside the bullet

110. Cannelure is a part of:
a. Bullet
b. Pellet
c. Percussion cap
d. None of the above

111. Flame effect of burning in rifled firearm occurs:
a. Up to 20 cm
b. Up to 40 cm
c. Up to 60 cm
d. None of the above

112. Involuntary tattooing occurs in shotguns:
a. Up to 75 cm
b. Up to 3 metres
c. Up to 6 metres
d. Up to 10 metres

113. Point-blank range means:
a. Distant range
b. Contact range
c. Near contact
d. None of the above

114. Yaw means:

  a. Ricochet phenomenon

  b. Balling of shot

  c. Tumbling bullet

  d. None of the above

115. Primary markings on bullet are due to:

  a. Barrel

  b. Firing pin

  c. Gunpowder

  d. Barrel irregularities

116. The stomach should be opened:

  a. Along the greater curvature

  b. Along the lesser curvature

  c. On the front wall between the two curvatures

  d. None of the above

117. Autolysis in macerated foetus:

  a. Occurs in sterile conditions

  b. Occurs in presence of saprophytic organisms

  c. Occurs in presence of *Clostridium welchii*

  d. None of the above

118. The following putrefies late:

  a. Adult brain   b. Stomach

  c. Liver   d. Prostate

119. The following is not a type of strangulation:

  a. Garroting   b. Throttling

  c. Choking   d. Mugging

120. Café coronary is due to:

  a. Reflex cardiac arrest

  b. Burns

  c. Electrocution

  d. Hanging

121. Lynching is a type of:

  a. Homicidal hanging

  b. Accidental hanging

  c. Suicidal hanging

  d. None of the above

122. Froth of nostrils is seen in:

  a. Dry drowning

  b. Secondary drowning

  c. Immersion syndrome

  d. Wet drowning

123. In salt water drowning there is:

  a. Pulmonary oedema

  b. Cerebral oedema

  c. Ascites

  d. Any of the above

124. In case of firearm injuries, before autopsy is started:

  a. Body, should be washed

  b. X-ray examination should be done

  c. Clothes should be removed

  d. None of the above

125. The commonest form of infanticide is:

  a. Suffocation   b. Strangulation

  c. Drowning   d. Poisoning

126. Scalp consists of:

  a. Pericranium

  b. Loose areolar tissue

  c. Skin

  d. All of the above

127. Sudden infant death syndrome is due to:

  a. Respiratory viral infection

  b. Prolonged sleep apnoea

  c. Hypersensitivity reaction

  d. Any of the above

128. In concealment of birth the child might have died:

  a. Before birth   b. During birth

  c. After birth   d. Any of the above

129. In delirium:

  a. Visual hallucinations are seen

  b. Insight and judgement lost

  c. Level of consciousness is variable

  d. All of the above

130. Nihilistic delusion means:

  a. Person believes that the self or world is non-existing or going to end

  b. Person feels that he has done something wrong and sinful

  c. Person has unusual but fantastic belief

  d. Person feels that other people are planning to harm him

131. Hallucination means:

a. Sensory perception with a sensory stimulus
b. Sensory perception without sensory stimulus
c. Altered sensory perception
d. Absence of sensory perception

132. Hypothermia causes death due to:

a. Lack of oxygen
b. Lack of nutrition
c. Lack of protection
d. Meningitis

133. In burns, death can occur due to carbon monoxide if concentration of CoHb is:

a. >10%   b. <10%
c. <5%   d. None of the above

134. Postmortem burns do not show:

a. Line of redness
b. Singeing of hair
c. Blisters
d. Carbon monoxide in blood

135. Cold is endured longer by:

a. Women   b. Men
c. Children   d. Old people

136. Corrosive acids produce:

a. Coagulation
b. Necrosis
c. Coagulation necrosis
d. None of the above

137. Illusion is:

a. False belief
b. False sensory perception
c. False sensory perception due to distortion of sensory stimulus
d. None of the above

138. Leading questions can be asked in:

a. Cross examination
b. Hostile hotness
c. Judge
d. All of the above

139. Bed side court is:

a. Dying declaration
b. Dying deposition

c. Juvenile court
d. Family court

140. Cephalic index helps to determine:

a. Race   b. Sex
c. Age   d. Stature

141. First permanent tooth to erupt is:

a. Central incisor
b. First premolar
c. First molar
d. Canine

142. Best criteria for identification in Gustafson's method is:

a. Attrition
b. Secondary—dentin
c. Transparency of root
d. Cementum apposition

143. Which rule is used for foetal age examination:

a. Haase   b. Boyde
c. Quetelets   d. Gustafson

144. Which is not a mode of death:

a. Asphyxia   b. Shock
c. Coma   d. Syncope

145. Warning notice is given by:

a. Executive magistrate
b. Indian medical association
c. State medical council
d. Judicial magistrate

146. Red Cross emblem can be used by:

a. Doctors and all paramedical staff
b. Doctors and nurses only
c. Doctors only
d. Army medical corps

147. Privileged communication is an exception to:

a. Professional secrecy
b. Infamous conduct
c. Consent
d. Negligence

148. Res ipsa loquitur means:

a. The thing itself speaks
b. Let the master answer

c. New thing comes in-between

d. Contributory negligence

149. Mercy killing is also known as:

a. Euthanasia   b. Assisted suicide

c. Aid-in-dying   d. All of the above

150. The earliest site to show decomposition is:

a. Right iliac fossa

b. Left iliac fossa

c. Hypochondrium

d. Hypogastrium

151. Presence of maggots on the body suggests after death a lapse of:

a. Below 2 days

b. Below 3 days

c. Below 4 days

d. Below 5 days

152. The following putrefies late:

a. Adult brain   b. Stomach

c. Liver   d. Prostate

153. Cadaveric spasm is:

a. Antemortem process

b. Postmortem process

c. Type of rigor mortis

d. None of the above

154. Dark colour of an organ during postmortem examination is due to:

a. Contusion   b. Congestion

c. Hypostasis   d. All of the above

155. Tissue bridges are seen in:

a. Abrasion   b. Contusion

c. Laceration   d. Incised wound

156. Blue colour of contusion is due to:

a. Bilirubin

b. Haemosiderin

c. Haematoidin

d. Deoxyhaemoglobin

157. Incised-like wound is due to:

a. Sharp object

b. Blunt object

c. Pointed object

d. Heavy cutting weapon

158. Rape is defined under Section:

a. 299 of IPC   b. 302 of IPC

c. 320 of IPC   d. 375 of IPC

159. Hesitation cuts are seen in case of:

a. Homicide

b. Suicide

c. Accident

d. Fabricated wounds

160. Duplex cartridge contains:

a. One bullet   b. Two bullets

c. No bullet   d. Two cartridges

161. Choking is seen in:

a. Shotgun   b. Rifle

c. Pistol   d. Revolver

162. Catamite means:

a. Rapist

b. Active agent in sodomy

c. Passive agent in sodomy

d. Lesbian

163. Female homosexuality is called:

a. Transvestism

b. Transsexualism

c. Tribadism

d. Satyriasis

164. Posthumous child means:

a. Child born out of wedlock

b. Child born within wedlock

c. Child born without marriage

d. Child born after the death of father

165. Who cannot ask a leading question:

a. Defense lawyer

b. Judge

c. Public prosecutor

d. All of the above

166. Duces tecum is:

a. Summon

b. Panchanama

c. Perjury

d. Judgement

167. Dying declaration cannot be taken by:

a. Magistrate

b. Doctor

    c. Police

    d. None of the above

168. Section 304-B of IPC deals with:

    a. Murder

    b. Culpable homicide

    c. Dowry death

    d. Inquest

169. Death sentence can be awarded by:

    a. Supreme court

    b. High court

    c. Sessions court

    d. All of the above

170. If the patient survives after giving dying declaration then DD stands as:

    a. No value

    b. Corroborating evidence

    c. Stands during 1st trial only

    d. All of the above

171. Quickening appears at about:

    a. 6 weeks

    b. 8–10 weeks

    c. 16–20 weeks

    d. 20–24 weeks

172. Bluish discolouration of the vagina seen in pregnancy is known as:

    a. Chadwick's sign

    b. Goodell's sign

    c. Hegar's sign

    d. Palmar's sign

173. Quod hanc means:

    a. Medically impotent

    b. Legally impotent

    c. Impotent towards all women

    d. Impotent towards a particular woman

174. Most common cause of first trimester abortion is:

    a. Chromosomal defect

    b. Endocrine disturbances

    c. Anatomic abnormality of uterus

    d. Infections

175. Lendrum's stain is done for:

    a. Air embolism

    b. Fat embolism

    c. Amniotic fluid embolism

    d. Pulmonary embolism

Bibliography

1. Agarwal P, Handa R, Wali JP. Common Poisonings in India. J. Forensic Medicine and Toxicology. 15:73–79, 1998.
2. Age Determination, AJPA, 15:9, 1957.
3. Alcohol and Road Traffic Proceedings of the Third International Conference, 113, 1962.
4. All India Major Criminal Acts. Central Law Agency, 1989.
5. Anderson L. A Microscopic Study of Dermal Gunshot Wounds, AJCP 38.393–402, 1961.
6. Archives of Pathology (1929), 7:63; Cited in BNJ.
7. B. Hughes and HS Banks. Levels of Potassium in Vitreous Humour after Death, Medicine, Science and Law, Vol V, 1965.
8. Ballantine B, Marrs T and Turner P. General and Applied Toxicology, Abridged, 1 (Edn), Macmillan, 1993.
9. Burgess AW and Holmstorn. American Journal of Psychiatry, 131. 981, 1974.
10. Cameron J and Suis BG. Forensic Dentistry, 1974.
11. Camps FE. Gradwohl's Legal Medicine, 1976.
12. Camps FE. Recent Advances in Forensic Pathology, 1969.
13. Camps FE and Cameron JM. Practical Forensic Medicine; 191, 192;1971.
14. Camps FE. Gradwohl's Legal Medicine, 3 (Edn), 1963.
15. Camps FE. Recent Advances in Forensic Pathology, 1969.
16. Chandran MR. Human Organ Transplantation, J Karnataka, Medicolegal Society, 18:3–5, 1999.
17. Chopras Indigenous Drugs of India, 2 (Edn), 657.
18. Coombs RRA and Dodd B. Possible Application of the Principle of Mixed Agglutination in the Identification of Blood Stains; Medicine, Science and Law, 1:359, 1961.
19. Crawford Adams J, Livingstone ES. Outline of Fractures, 5 (Edn), 1970.
20. Crompton R. Closed Head Injury. Its Pathology and Legal Medicine, Edward Arnold Ltd,; 1985.
21. Daftary SN and Chakravarty S. Holland and Brews, Mannual of Obstetrics, 15 (Edn) 1991.
22. Davidson. Medical Ethics; 1957.
23. Di Maio DJ, Di Maio VJM. Wounds due to Blunt Trauma, In. Forensic Pathology, Elsevier, New York; 87–107, 1989.
24. Dutta DC. Textbook of Obstetrics, 1992
25. Electrolysis for Removal of Tattoo Marks, Medical Council, Philadelphia, 13, 374, 1908; JAMA, 185, 1928.
26. Ellenhorn MJ. Medical Toxicology, Diagnosis and Treatment of Human Poisoning 2(Edn), Williams and Wilkins, Baltimore, USA, 1084, 1997.
27. Encyclopaedia Americana, 25, 1975.
28. Fingerprint and Identification. Magazine, Chicago, 1968.
29. Flanagan RJ, Braithwaite RA, Brown SS, Widdep B and De Wolf FA. Basic Analytical Toxicology, WHO, 26–30, 1995.
30. Freeman MDA. Cruelty at Home.
31. Friedman IJ. Virgin Wives, 1962.

32. Goldfrank's Toxicological Emergencies, 5 (Edn), Appleton and Frank, 1994.

33. Gonzales. Firearm and Firearm Injuries.

34. Gonzales TA and M Umberger GJ. Legal Medicine and Toxicology, 2 (Edn).

35. Gordon and Shapiro. Forensic Medicine, London, Churchill Livingstone, 40, 1975.

36. Gordon I, Turner R and Price TW. Medical Jurisprudence, 3 (Edn), 1953.

37. Gresham GA, Tumer AF. The Postmortem Examination in Forensic Medicine, 3 (Edn), Churchill Livingstone, London, 63–79, 1988.

38. Gurdijian ES. Impact Head Injury, 1978.

39. Gustafson G. Age Determination of Teeth, J. Amer Dental Association, 41–45–54, 1950.

40. Hardman JG and Limbird LE, Goodman and Gilman. The Pharmacological Basis of Therapeutics, 9 (Edn), McGraw-Hill, 1996.

41. Hicks DJ. Rape Sexual Assault, Obstetrics and Gynaecology, Annual, New York, 1978.

42. Hopkins P. Lancet, 145, 1945.

43. Houlbourn AHS. Mechanism of Brain Injury, Lancet, 2438, 1943.

44. Ismond R (Ed). Pathology and Treatment of Sexual Deviation, 1964.

45. JFMT, Vol. XI No 2–94, 1–12.

46. Jhala RM. Regional Injuries. In: Jhala and Raju's Medical Jurisprudence, 5 (Edn), Eastern Book Company, Lucknow, 323, 1990.

47. Journal of Criminal Law, Criminology, Police Science, 46, 468, 1957.

48. Journal of Forensic Science. The significance of diatoms in diagnosis of drowning, Vol. 9, 11, 1964.

49. Journal of Industrial Hygiene (JIH), Blyth, Poisons, their Effect and Detection, 5 (Edn), 233, 1925.

50. Kapse CS. Medical Investigation of Aircraft Fatalities. Dissertation submitted to the University of Bombay for MD (Forensic Medicine), 1958.

51. Keating Hast, Waltes V. Survival in cold water, Oxford and Edinburgh, 1969.

52. Knight B. The Pathology of Wounds in Forensic Pathology, 2 (Edn), 133–69 Arnold, London, 1996.

53. Knight B, Sahai VB. Injuries from Firearms; In. HWV Cox's Medical Jurisprudence and Toxicology, 6 (Edn), The Law Book Company (P) Ltd., Allahabad, 327–54, 1992.

54. KrogmanWM. The Human Skeleton in Legal Medicine, 1962.

55. Landsteiner K and Levine P. PSEB, 124. 1941, R. Sanger and RR Race, Lancet, 18, 1962.

56. Major Criminal Acts, Published by Central Law Agency, Allahabad, 1989.

57. Mant AK. Modern Trends in Forensic Medicine; Vol. III, 1973.

58. Mant AK. Taylor's Principle and Practice of Medical Jurisprudence.

59. Mason JK. Aviation Pathology—A study of fatalities; Butterworths, London, 1962.

60. Mason JK, McCall Smith RA. Medicolegal Encyclopaedia, Butterworth, London, UK. 276–77, 1987.

61. Masters WN and Johnson VE. Homosexuality in perspective, 1979.

62. Medical Aspects of Artificial Insemination, JAMA, 1958.

63. Mehta HS. Medical Law and Ethics in India, The Bombay Samachar Pvt. Ltd. 1963.

64. Meyerhof, JAMA, 1751, 1930.

65. Miles S. BMJ, 3, 597, 1968 and D.G. Rushton. Drowning—A Review, MJ, 29:90.

66. Mollison IPC. Blood Transfusion in Clinical Medicine, 15 (Edn), 1972.

67. Moritz AR. The Pathology of Trauma.

68. Mukherjee JB. Forensic Medicine and Toxicology, 1 Vol., 2 (Edn), 1994.

69. Mukherjee JB. Violent Asphyxial Deaths; In: Forensic Medicine and Toxicology, 2 (Edn), Amold Associates, India. 475–593,1994.

70. Nathan Lord. Medical Negligence, Butterworth, 1955.

71. Snakes of India. National Book Trust, New Delhi, 1965.

72. Nature. Oct. 1956 cited in JAMA; Dec. 1957, 1818.

73. Negroes, 10:463, 1952.
74. Nickolls LC and Pereira M. A Study of Modern Method of Grouping Dried Blood Stains; Medicine Science and Law, 2:172, 1962.
75. Peterson, Haines and Webster. Legal Medicine and Toxicology, 2 (Edn) Vol. 1; 294.
76. Pillay VV. Brain Stem Death. The Real Moment of Death. JIAFM, 13:9–11, 1991.
77. Pillay VV. Modern Medical Toxicology. 2 (Edn), Jaypee Brothers Medical Publishers, 1999.
78. Pillay VV. Krishnan's Handbook of Forensic Medicine, 13 (Edn), Paras, 2003.
79. Polson CJ and Marshall TK. The Disposal of Dead Bodies, 1975.
80. Polson CJ, Gee DJ, Bernard Knight. Essentials of Forensic Medicine, 1985.
81. Recognition of Intoxication, 2 (Edn), 1958.
82. Reddy MP. Euthanasia. The Emerging Scenario. The Lawyers, 13–16, 1991.
83. Rentoul E and Smith H. Glaisters Medical Jurisprudence and Toxicology, 1973.
84. Rhodes HTF. Forensic Chemistry, 1946.
85. Safertein R. Criminalistics. An Introduction to Forensic Science, 1981.
86. Sevitt S. Fat Embolism, Butterworths, London, 1962.
87. Shapiro HA, et al. The Significance of Fingernail Abrasion of the Skin, JFAM, 9, 17, 1962.
88. Simpson CK (Editor). Modern Trends in Forensic Medicine, Vol, II, 1967.
89. Simpson K. Forensic Medicine, 1957.
90. Simpson K. Cold and starvation. Modern Trends in Forensic Medicine, 1953.
91. Smith S and Friddes. Forensic Medicine, 10 (Edn), 1959.
92. Spencer H. Lightening Stroke and its Treatment London, T Balliers and Cox, 1932.
93. Stevens PJ, Williams and Wilkins. Fatal Civil Aircraft Accident, 1970.
94. Stewart TC. Distortion of Pubic Symphyseal Surface in Females and its Effect on Age Estimation, AJPA, 15:9, 1957.
95. Stuart HJ. Blood Stain Pattern Interpretation, Blood Evidence in Crime Scene Investigation, 10–76.
96. Subrahmanyam BV. Legal Procedure in Criminal Courts; Modi's Medical Jurisprudence and Toxicology, 22 (Edn), Butterworths, India, 1999.
97. Taylor. On Poisons, 3 (Edn), 119.
98. Taylor. Medical Jurisprudence, 11 (Edn), pp 19.
99. Tedischii CG, Gtedischii L. Forensic Medicine—A Study in Trauma and Environmental Hazards, Vol. III, 1997.
100. The Identification of Blood Stains; Medicine Science and Law, 1:395, 1961.
101. The Indian Journal of Criminology and Criminalistics (IJCC), 1, 167, 1981.
102. The Mental Health Act, 1987; Ministry of Law and Justice, Government of India.
103. Theives CH, Halley J. Clinical Toxicology, 5 (Edn), 1972.
104. Thomson WAR. Sex and its problems, 1968.
105. Thomas CC. The Human Skeleton in Forensic Medicine, 94, 1962.
106. Trotter M and Glesser GC. Estimation of Stature from Long Bones of American Whites and Negroes, 10:463, 1952.
107. Valdes-Dapena MA. A Review of Medical Literature, Paediatrics 66(4): 597–614, 1974.
108. Vincent T Devita, A Rosenberg. AIDS Aetiology, Diagnosis, Treatment and Prevention, 1988.
109. Walls HJ. Forensic Science, 2 (Edn), 1974.
110. Whitlock FA. Criminal Responsibility in Mental Illness, 1963.
111. Wigglesworth JS. Perinatal Pathology, 2 (Edn), WB Saunders; Philadelphia, USA, 1996.
112. Wintrobe MW. Clinical Haematology, 7 (Edn), 1975.

Index